INVERSE AND ILL-POSED PROBLEMS SERIES

# Poorly Visible Media in X-ray Tomography

## Also available in the Inverse and Ill-Posed Problems Series:

Dynamical Inverse Problems of Distributed Systems
*V.I. Maksimov*
Theory of Linear Ill-Posed Problems and its Applications
*V.K. Ivanov, V.V. Vasin and V.P. Tanana*
Ill-Posed Internal Boundary Value Problems for the Biharmonic Equation
*M.A. Atakhodzhaev*
Investigation Methods for Inverse Problems
*V.G. Romanov*
Operator Theory. Nonclassical Problems
*S.G. Pyatkov*
Inverse Problems for Partial Differential Equations
*Yu.Ya. Belov*
Method of Spectral Mappings in the Inverse Problem Theory
*V. Yurko*
Theory of Linear Optimization
*I.I. Eremin*
Integral Geometry and Inverse Problems for Kinetic Equations
*A.Kh. Amirov*
Computer Modelling in Tomography and Ill-Posed Problems
*M.M. Lavrent'ev, S.M. Zerkal and O.E. Trofimov*
An Introduction to Identification Problems via Functional Analysis
*A. Lorenzi*
Coefficient Inverse Problems for Parabolic Type Equations and Their Application
*P.G. Danilaev*
Inverse Problems for Kinetic and Other Evolution Equations
*Yu.E. Anikonov*
Inverse Problems of Wave Processes
*A.S. Blagoveshchenskii*
Uniqueness Problems for Degenerating Equations and Nonclassical Problems
*S.P. Shishatskii, A. Asanov and E.R. Atamanov*
Uniqueness Questions in Reconstruction of Multidimensional Tomography-Type Projection Data
*V.P. Golubyatnikov*
Monte Carlo Method for Solving Inverse Problems of Radiation Transfer
*V.S. Antyufeev*
Introduction to the Theory of Inverse Problems
*A.L. Bukhgeim*
Identification Problems of Wave Phenomena - Theory and Numerics
*S.I. Kabanikhin and A. Lorenzi*
Inverse Problems of Electromagnetic Geophysical Fields
*P.S. Martyshko*
Composite Type Equations and Inverse Problems
*A.I. Kozhanov*
Inverse Problems of Vibrational Spectroscopy
*A.G. Yagola, I.V. Kochikov, G.M. Kuramshina and Yu.A. Pentin*
Elements of the Theory of Inverse Problems
*A.M. Denisov*
Volterra Equations and Inverse Problems
*A.L. Bughgeim*
Small Parameter Method in Multidimensional Inverse Problems
*A.S. Barashkov*
Regularization, Uniqueness and Existence of Volterra Equations of the First Kind
*A. Asanov*
Methods for Solution of Nonlinear Operator Equations
*V.P. Tanana*
Inverse and Ill-Posed Sources Problems
*Yu.E. Anikonov, B.A. Bubnov and G.N. Erokhin*
Methods for Solving Operator Equations
*V.P. Tanana*
Nonclassical and Inverse Problems for Pseudoparabolic Equations
*A. Asanov and E.R. Atamanov*
Formulas in Inverse and Ill-Posed Problems
*Yu.E. Anikonov*
Inverse Logarithmic Potential Problem
*V.G. Cherednichenko*
Multidimensional Inverse and Ill-Posed Problems for Differential Equations
*Yu.E. Anikonov*
Ill-Posed Problems with A Priori Information
*V.V. Vasin and A.L. Ageev*
Integral Geometry of Tensor Fields
*V.A. Sharafutdinov*
Inverse Problems for Maxwell's Equations
*V.G. Romanov and S.I. Kabanikhin*

Inverse and Ill-Posed Problems Series

# Poorly Visible Media in X-ray Tomography

*D.S. Anikonov, V.G. Nazarov and I.V. Prokhorov*

///VSP///

Utrecht • Boston

2002

VSP
P.O. Box 346
3700 AH Zeist
The Netherlands

Tel: +31 30 692 5790
Fax: +31 30 693 2081
vsppub@compuserve.com
www.vsppub.com



First published in 2002

ISBN 90-6764-374-2



*Printed in The Netherlands by Ridderprint bv, Ridderkerk.*

# Preface

This book is devoted to explanation of certain difficulties in solving a problem of X-ray tomography. The problem consists in determining the internal structure of an unknown medium using the results of measurements of X-ray radiation passing through the medium.

The introduced notion "the measure of visibility" allows authors to define invisibility media as those which have measure of visibility equals to zero. However, these definitions seem to be too complex for their practical applications. Therefore, a more simple notion "a poorly visible medium" is added for a case when the measure of visibility is close to zero. A very simple version of such definition is represented in this book. Namely, a medium is called poorly visible under its radiography by X-ray, if the coefficient of absorption (the difference between the coefficient of total attenuation and the coefficient of scattering) is continuous on the interface between different materials in the unknown medium.

The book contains a certain theoretical foundation of the notions introduced and the tables of many pairs of different substances forming poorly visible media. The represented numerical experiments confirm the theoretical results. It is not improbable that some cases of unsuccessful reconstruction in X-ray tomography appear to be the cases described in this book, and the authors give certain advices devoted to how to improve the reconstructions.

# Contents

# Introduction

The tomography problem considered consists in finding an essential part of information about the internal structure of an unknown medium. More precisely, the contact boundaries between various materials in the medium are sought for. The known information is given by measurements of X-ray radiation passing through the medium. The investigation is implemented by studying an appropriate mathematical model which is represented as a transport equation (linear Boltzmann's equation) together with certain boundary conditions. We used both theoretical and numerical methods. The results consist in the proved theorems, computer testing of the corresponding algorithms and certain tables.

This book can be considered as the continuation and application of author's book "Transport Equation and Tomography" also published by VSP in 2002. Here we focus on the aspects connected with the problem of invisibility or poor visibility for media under their radiography by X-ray radiation.

The major role plays the notion of "the measure of visibility" introduced in D.Anikonov (1994) and advanced in many consequent papers (for example, see Anikonov, 1997; Anikonov, Nazarov and Prokhorov, 1997; Anikonov, 1998; Anikonov, 1999; Anikonov and Prokhorov, 1999; Anikonov, Kovtanyuk and Prokhorov, 1999; Anikonov and Prokhorov, 1999; Anikonov and Prokhorov, 2000; Anikonov and Nazarov, 2001; Anikonov and Prokhorov, 2002). In particular, many similar results are collected in the book mentioned above.

The medium is called invisible under its radio-diagnosis, if the measure of visibility for this medium equals to zero, at least, on the boundary of inclusion. The proved theorem guarantees that the internal structure of such medium can't be determined by tomography methods (of course, in the framework of the admitted mathematical model). Note, that the positiveness of the measure provides determination of the internal structure.

However, the definition of the invisible medium appears to be too complicate for practical application. Therefore, for this purpose, we prefer the notion of a poorly visible medium the measure of visibility of which is close to zero. Naturally, there exist many ways for introduction of the similar exact definitions. While, we choose a very simple version. Namely, the medium is called poorly visible if its coefficient of absorption (the difference between the coefficient of total attenuation and the coefficient of scattering) is continuous on the boundaries between various materials in the medium. This property provides the closeness of the measure of visibility to zero, in particular, in many, traditionally difficult cases for tomography. In other words the coefficient of absorption appears to be more important characteristic in X-ray tomography than the coefficient of scattering and the coefficient of total attenuation.

The most part of the book is devoted to tables of poorly visible pairs of different substances. For this purpose, we used the well-known paper Hubbell J. H. and Seltzer S. M. (1995). Below, in the beginning of Chapter 2 we explain how to interpret and apply this tables. Here we only note that the interfaces within the pointed pairs turn out to be difficult cases for their finding on the certain levels of photon energy. This means that the attempt of determining the contact boundaries for the pairs pointed in our tables can be unsuccessful in view of the reasons described in this book. Therefore we dare to give an advice to tomography specialists to look into these tables before application of similar tomography methods in practice. At the same time we represent a method which enables to improve the situation.

It is important to notice that we use the mathematical model including the monoenergetic transport equation which means neglecting the loss of photon energy in acts of interactions. Because of this simplification we restrict our consideration by the photon energy levels from 1 keV up to 60 keV, i. e. mainly by X-ray radiation. Moreover, we are obliged to use approximated data for creation of our tables. In the whole, this book can be considered as a preliminary investigation in the pointed scientific direction.

Now we give a short overview of the book. Considerably, Chapter 1 is devoted to generalization and modification of the results proved in Anikonov, Kovtanyuk and Prokhorov (2002). Section 1.1 contains investigation of the boundary value problem for the monoenergetic transport equation, i. e. the direct problem. Here the previous results are adapted for our new purpose and are represented completely for the convenience of the reader.

In Section 1.2, in the corresponding terms, we represent two settings of the tomography problem and compare them. Some restrictions are added and discussed as well.

Section 1.3 is devoted to proving several auxiliary statements.

Section 1.4 contains the investigation of the modified indicator of heterogeneity. The properties of this indicator allow us to prove the theorem of uniqueness for the tomography problem and to construct the corresponding algorithm.

Section 1.5 seems to be the most important from the theoretical point of view. Here we introduce and substantiate the notions of invisible and poorly visible media under their radiography. The theoretical results are confirmed by the numerical experiments. In the comments to the third numerical test we dare to advise how to improve the reconstruction of the medium. At the end of this section we try to explain the physical sense of the poorly visible medium and discuss the real conditions of measurement of radiation flux.

In the Section 1.6 we give the theoretical examples of the invisible media.

Section 1.7 concludes the first chapter of the book. It is devoted to discussion of the hypothesis connected with the extension of the obtained results onto other applications. Probably, this section is so important as Section 1.5.

The second chapter of the book contains the tables of the poorly visible pairs of different substances, as well as the directions devoted to using these tables. We take the necessary data from Hubbell J. H. and Seltzer S. M. (1995), for 92 chemical elements and 48 complex substances.

Note that each section has its own numeration of statements and formulae. Therefore, if we refer to another section, its number is indicated together with the number of the referred item.

A big volume of the tables of poorly visible pairs of substances appeared to be unexpected for the authors. Just by this reason we decide to publish this book without full and complete investigation of the corresponding problems. Perhaps, we will research such problems more carefully in future.

# Main notations

$\mathcal{E}^3$ — three-dimensional Euclidean space.
$e_1, e_2, e_3$ — the vectors of the main orthonormal basis in $\mathcal{E}^3$.
$r$ — a point in $\mathcal{E}^3$.
$\omega$ — a point in the unit sphere $\Omega$ in $\mathcal{E}^3$.
$r = (r_1, r_2, r_3)$, $\omega = (\omega_1, \omega_2, \omega_3)$ — the representations of the vectors $r$ and $\omega$ in the main basis.
$G$ — a convex bounded domain in $\mathcal{E}^3$ where a process of radiation is considered.
$G_0$ — the union of the domains (inclusions) $G_i, i = 1, \ldots, p$, such that $G_i \cap G_j = \varnothing$, $i \neq j$, $\overline{G} = \bigcup_{i=1}^{p} \overline{G}_i$.
$\partial G, \partial G_0, \partial G_i$ — the boundaries of the sets $G, G_0, G_i$ respectively.
$E$ — the scalar variable that stands as energy, $E \in [E_1, E_2]$.
$d(r, \omega)$ — the distance from the point $r \in \overline{G}$ to the boundary $\partial G$ in the direction $\omega$.
$\Gamma^-$ — the set of points $(\xi, \omega, E)$ such that $\xi \in \partial G$, $\omega \in \Omega$, $E \in [E_1, E_2]$ and the following representation holds: $\xi = r - d(r, -\omega)\omega$, $r \in G_0$.
$\Gamma^+$ — the set of points $(\eta, \omega, E)$ such that $\eta \in \partial G$, $\omega \in \Omega$, $E \in [E_1, E_2]$ and the following representation holds: $\eta = r + d(r, \omega)\omega$, $r \in G_0$.
$h(\xi, \omega, E)$ — the distribution of the input flux.
$H(\eta, \omega, E)$ — the distribution of the output flux.
$f(r, \omega, E)$ — the distribution of the particle flux at the point $r \in G$ having the direction $\omega$ and the level of energy $E$.
$\nabla_r f(r, \omega, E)$ — the gradient of the function $f$ with respect to $r_1, r_2, r_3$.
$\mu(r, E)$ — the coefficient of the total attenuation of the flux at the point $r$ and for the particles with energy $E$.
$\mu_s(r, E)$ — the coefficient of scattering at the point $r$ and for the particles with energy $E$.
$\mu_s^*(r, E)$ — the dual coefficient of scattering at the point $r$ and for the particles with energy $E$.

$\mu_a(r, E)$ — the coefficient of absorption at the point $r$ and for the particles with energy $E$.
$\mu_a^*(r, E)$ — the dual coefficient of absorption at the point $r$ and for the particles with energy $E$.
$\mu_{en}(r, E)$ — the energy-absorption coefficient at the point $r$ and for the particles with energy $E$.
$k(r, \omega \cdot \omega', E, E')$ — the indicatrix of scattering of the particles at the point $r$ changing their state from $(\omega', E')$ to $(\omega, E)$.
$J(r, \omega, E)$ — the distribution of the internal sources at the point $r$ in the direction $\omega$ and for the level of energy $E$.
$N(r, \omega, E)$ — the collision integral.
$[\![\mu(z, E)]\!]$, $[\![\mu_s(z, E)]\!]$, $[\![\mu_a(z, E)]\!]$, $[\![\mu_s^*(z, E)]\!]$, $[\![\mu_a^*(z, E)]\!]$, $[\![\mu_{en}(z, E)]\!]$, $[\![k(z, \omega \cdot \omega', E, E')]\!]$, $[\![J(z, \omega, E)]\!]$, $[\![f(z, \omega, E)]\!]$ and $[\![N(z, \omega, E)]\!]$ — the jumps of the corresponding functions at the contact point $z$ which is common for two boundaries $\partial G_l$ and $\partial G_j$, $1 \leq l < j \leq p$. These jumps are equal to the difference of the boundary values of the function depended on $r$, when the point $r$ is passing from $G_l$ to $G_j$ $(l < j)$.

Also, in this book the monoenergetic case is considered, dependence on energy loss being neglected. Accordingly, we use the following designations: $\Gamma^+, \Gamma^-$, $h(\xi, \omega)$, $H(\eta, \omega)$, $f(r, \omega)$, $\mu(r), \mu_s(r), \mu_a(r), \mu_{en}(r)$, $k(r, \omega \cdot \omega')$, $J(r, \omega)$ and $N(r, \omega)$, whose physical meaning is the same as in the general case, but the level of energy is assumed to be fixed.
$\tilde{h}(r, \omega)$ — the function given by the equality: $\tilde{h}(r, \omega) = h(r - d(r, -\omega)\omega, \omega)$, $(r, \omega) \in G_0 \times \Omega$.
$\mathrm{Ind}(r)$, $\mathrm{Ind}^*(r)$ — the integro-differential indicators of heterogeneity in the medium $G$ at the point $r \in G_0$.
$|mv(z, \omega)|$ — the measure of visibility of the medium $G$ at the point $z \in \partial G_l \cap \partial G_j$ $(l < j)$ in the direction $\omega$, $m_1(z, \omega)$ — the main multiplier in the measure of visibility $|mv(z, \omega)|$.

# Chapter 1.

# The theoretical aspects of invisibility in X-ray tomography

## 1.1. THE DIRECT PROBLEM TO THE MONOENERGETIC TRANSPORT EQUATION

Consider the stationary integro-differential transport equation

$$\omega \cdot \nabla_r f(r,\omega) + \mu(r) f(r,\omega) = \int_\Omega k(r, \omega \cdot \omega') f(r,\omega')\, d\omega' + J(r,\omega), \qquad (1)$$

where $r \in G$, $G$ is a convex bounded domain in the Euclidean space $\mathcal{E}^3$, $\omega \in \Omega = \{\omega \in \mathcal{E}^3 \mid |\omega| = 1\}$. The function $f(r,\omega)$ is interpreted as density (or intensity) of the particle flux at the point $r$ with direction $\omega$. The functions $\mu(r), k(r, \omega \cdot \omega'), J(r,\omega)$ describe the medium $G$ and are called to be the coefficients of total attenuation, indicatrix of scattering and the density (or intensity) of the internal sources of the radiation, respectively.

We mean that the intensity is equal to the density multiplied by the corresponding value of energy. Thus, if $f(r,\omega,E)$ means the density of the particle flux, then the intensity is $f(r,\omega,E)\cdot E$ (see Case and Zweifel, 1972). Further, for generality, we use the term "distribution of the particle flux" for the function $f(r,\omega,E)$. The difference in the choice becomes important starting from Section 1.7 and further, where we try to apply the theoretical results.

We introduce a subset $G_0$ of the domain $G$ to characterize the heterogeneity of the medium $G$, ($G_0 \subset G$, $\overline{G}_0 = \overline{G}$)

$$G_0 = \bigcup_{i=1}^{p} G_i, \qquad G_i \cap G_j = \varnothing, \quad i \neq j,$$

where $p$ is a positive integer number. Each domain $G_i$ can be interpreted as a certain material (substance) included in $G$. We also call domains $G_i$, $i = 1, \dots, p$ as zones, inclusions or heterogeneities.

This and a more general transport equation are represented in more details, for example, in Anikonov, Kovtanyuk and Prokhorov (2002) (see also Section 1.7 of this book).

Here we only point out our intention to use (1) as the main part of the mathematical model for the description of $X$-ray radiation passing through the medium $G$.

Let a ray with the initial point $r$ and the direction $\omega$ be denoted as $L_{r,\omega} = \{r + \omega t \mid t \geq 0\}$. We set

$$d(r, \omega) = \text{mes}_1(L_{r,\omega} \cap G),$$

where the symbol $\text{mes}_1$ means the Lebesgue measure on a straight line. The function $d(r, \omega)$ is a distance from the point $r \in \overline{G}$ to the boundary $\partial G = \overline{G} \setminus G$ of the domain $G$ in the direction $\omega$.

Consider the sets $\Gamma^{\pm}$ of the point $(\xi, \omega) \in \partial G \times \Omega$, $(\eta, \omega) \in \partial G \times \Omega$ such that the following representations hold

$$\Gamma^- = \{(\xi, \omega) \in \partial G \times \Omega \mid \xi = r - d(r, -\omega)\omega, \; r \in G_0\},$$
$$\Gamma^+ = \{(\eta, \omega) \in \partial G \times \Omega :\mid \eta = r + d(r, \omega)\omega, \; r \in G_0\}.$$

The set $\Gamma^+$ will be used bellow. Here we add the boundary condition to the equation (1):

$$f(\xi, \omega) = h(\xi, \omega), \qquad (\xi, \omega) \in \Gamma^-. \tag{2}$$

The function $h$ means the distribution of the input flux of the radiation on the boundary of $G$.

**Problem (1), (2).** *The boundary value problem of determination the function $f$ from* (1), (2), *with the given $\mu, k, J, h$, is called the direct problem to the equation* (1).

Hereinafter we use the following functional spaces. The symbol $C_b(G_0 \times \Omega)$ denotes the Banach space of continuous and bounded in $G_0 \times \Omega$ functions, with the norm:

$$\|\phi\| = \sup_{(r,\omega)\in G_0\times\Omega} |\phi(r,\omega)|. \tag{3}$$

The space $C_b(G_0)$ is defined in the similar way, i.e. it is the set of the functions from $C_b(G_0 \times \Omega)$ which are independent on $\omega$. The traditional designation $L_1(Y)$ stands for space of functions such that their absolute values are integrable in the sense of Lebesgue in $Y \subset \mathcal{E}^m$ (see Schwartz, 1981). The norm in the space is

$$\|\phi\|_{L_1} = \int_Y |\phi(y)|\, dy. \tag{4}$$

Now we formulate the main restrictions for the functions $\mu, k, J, h$. Assume that all of them are nonnegative and $\mu(r) \in C_b(G_0)$, $J(r,\omega) \in C_b(G_0 \times \Omega)$. The function $k(r, \omega \cdot \omega')$ can be represented as a finite sum

$$k(r,\omega\cdot\omega') = \sum_{i=1}^{M} \sigma_i(r) S_i(\omega\cdot\omega'), \tag{5}$$

where $\sigma_i(r) \in C_b(G_0)$ and $S_i(\omega \cdot \omega')$ is a composition of a function from $L_1[-1,1]$ and the scalar product $\omega{\cdot}\omega'$. Without loss of generality, we assume that

$$\int_\Omega S_i(\omega\cdot\omega')\, d\omega' = 2\pi \int_{-1}^{1} S_i(\nu)\, d\nu = 1. \tag{6}$$

In particular, these restrictions imply that there exists the value called the coefficient of scattering

$$\mu_s(r) = \int_\Omega k(r,\omega\cdot\omega')\, d\omega' = \sum_{i=1}^{M} \sigma_i(r). \tag{7}$$

It is easy to see that $\mu_s(r)$ belongs to $C_b(G_0)$.

The class $\mathrm{D}(G_0 \times \Omega)$ consists of functions $\phi$ that are bounded on $G_0 \times \Omega$ and continuous at each point $r \in G_0$ for almost all $\omega \in \Omega$; furthermore, a function $\phi(r,\omega)$ is measurable with respect to $\omega$ for all fixed $r \in G_0$. The linear set $\mathrm{D}(G_0 \times \Omega)$ with the norm (3) is closed in the Banach space of bounded functions with the same norm (3) (see Schwartz, 1981). Therefore, $\mathrm{D}(G_0 \times \Omega)$ itself is a Banach space. Note that the functions $\mu, k$ and $J$ are defined for all $r \in \overline{G}$ but their values on $\overline{G}\backslash G_0$ do not change the considerations.

As far as the function $h(\xi,\omega)$, $(\xi,\omega) \in \Gamma^-$ is concerned, it is nonnegative and such that $\tilde{h}(r,\omega) = h(r - d(r,-\omega)\omega, \omega) \in \mathrm{D}(G_0 \times \Omega)$.

The set $G_0$ satisfies the traditional condition of generalized convexity (see Vladimirov, 1961; Germogenova, 1986): each straight line having a common point with $G_0$ intersects $\partial G_0$ at a finite number of points. It is not hard to prove that, in such a case, the 3-d measure of $\partial G_0$ is equal to zero, i. e. $\mathrm{mes}_3(\partial G_0) = 0$ (see Anikonov, Kovtanyuk and Prokhorov, 2002).

Let $lf(r, \omega)$ denote the following differential expression:

$$lf(r, \omega) = \frac{df(r + t\omega, \omega)}{dt}\bigg|_{t=0} + \mu(r)f(r, \omega).$$

The integral in the right-hand side of (1) is called the collision integral:

$$N(r, \omega) = \int_\Omega k(r, \omega \cdot \omega')f(r, \omega')\, d\omega'.$$

**Definition 1.** The function $f(r, \omega) \in \mathrm{D}(G_0 \times \Omega)$ is a solution of the direct problem (1), (2), if for every point $(\xi, \omega) \in \Gamma^-$ the function $f(\xi + t\omega, \omega)$ satisfies the following conditions:

1) it is absolutely continuous with respect to $t$, $t \in [0, d(\xi, \omega)]$;

2) the condition (2) is valid for $t = 0$;

3) for almost all points from $\{\xi + t\omega \mid t \in [0, d(\xi, \omega)]\}$ the following equality holds:

$$lf(\xi + t\omega, \omega) = N(\xi + t\omega, \omega) + J(\xi + t\omega, \omega).$$

**Remark 1.** The definition implies that the case of a nonconvex domain $G$ can also be included into consideration as well as the case with planar parts of the surface $\partial G_0$ (see Anikonov, Kovtanyuk and Prokhorov, 2002).

**Lemma 1.** *The operator $\mathcal{S}$ defined by the equality*

$$(\mathcal{S}\phi)(r, \omega) = \int_\Omega k(r, \omega \cdot \omega')\phi(r, \omega')\, d\omega', \tag{8}$$

*maps the space* $\mathrm{D}(G_0 \times \Omega)$ *into* $C_b(G_0 \times \Omega)$.

**Proof.** Let a function $\phi(r, \omega)$ belong to $\mathrm{D}(G_0 \times \Omega)$. We take into account the representation (5) and consider the function

$$\psi(r, \omega) = (\mathcal{S}\phi)(r, \omega) = \int_\Omega k(r, \omega \cdot \omega')\phi(r, \omega')\, d\omega'$$

$$= \sum_{i=1}^{M} \sigma_i(r) \int_\Omega S_i(\omega \cdot \omega')\phi(r, \omega)\, d\omega'.$$

The functions $\sigma_i(r)$ belong to $C_b(G_0)$. Therefore the function $\psi(r,\omega)$ belongs to $C_b(G_0 \times \Omega)$ if the following functions:

$$\psi_i(r,\omega) = \int_\Omega S_i(\omega \cdot \omega')\phi(r,\omega')\,d\omega', \qquad i = 1,\dots,M$$

belongs to $C_b(G_0 \times \Omega)$. The boundedness of these functions follows from integrability of $S_i(\omega \cdot \omega')\phi(r,\omega')$ with respect to $\omega'$ uniformly for $(r,\omega) \in G_0 \times \Omega$. Let us prove the continuity of the considered functions.

As follows from Kolmogorov and Fomin (1999) the function $S_i(\nu) \in L_1[-1,1]$ can be approximated by continuous functions with respect to the metric of $L_1[-1,1]$. Let $S_i^n(\omega \cdot \omega')$ be such a sequence, i. e.

$$\int_{-1}^{1} |S_i^n(\nu) - S_i(\nu)|\,d\nu \to 0, \quad n \to \infty.$$

We define the sequence:

$$\psi_i^n(r,\omega) = \int_\Omega S_i^n(\omega \cdot \omega')\phi(r,\omega')\,d\omega'.$$

As the function $S_i^n(\omega \cdot \omega')\phi(r,\omega')$ is bounded in $G_0 \times \Omega$ and continuous in each point $r \in G_0$ for almost all $\omega' \in \Omega$, then $\psi_i^n(r,\omega) \in C_b(G_0 \times \Omega)$ (see Schwartz, 1981).

Since $G_0$ is open then for any point $r_0 \in G_0$ there exists a $\delta$-neighborhood of $r_0$: $V_\delta(r_0) = \{r' \in \mathcal{E}^3 \mid |r - r_0| < \delta\}$ such that $\overline{V}_\delta(r_0) \subset G_0$. Let us prove that the sequence $\psi_i^n(r,\omega)$ uniformly converges to $\psi_i(r,\omega)$ as $n \to \infty$ in the closed set $\overline{V}_\delta(r_0) \times \Omega \subset G_0 \times \Omega$. We estimate the difference:

$$|\psi_i^n(r,\omega) - \psi_i(r,\omega)| \le \int_\Omega |\, S_i^n(\omega \cdot \omega') - S_i(\omega \cdot \omega')|\,|\phi(r,\omega')|\,d\omega'$$
$$\le \text{const} \int_{-1}^{1} |S_i^n(\nu) - S_i(\nu)|\,d\nu.$$

Since $S_i^n(\nu) \to S_i(\nu)$ as $n \to \infty$ in the metric of $L_1[-1,1]$, then the sequence $\psi_i^n(r,\omega)$ uniformly converges to $\psi_i(r,\omega)$ in the compact set $\overline{V}_\delta(r_0) \times \Omega$ for any point $r_0 \in G_0$. Therefore the limit function $\psi_i(r,\omega) \in C_b(G_0 \times \Omega)$ and, hence, $\psi = \mathcal{S}\phi \in C_b(G_0 \times \Omega)$, that completes the proof. □

**Lemma 2.** *Let a function $\phi(r,\omega) \in C_b(G_0 \times \Omega)$, and a function $\psi(r,\omega,t')$ be continuous in a certain compact set $K = (\overline{V}_\delta(r_0,\omega_0) \cap (\overline{G} \times \Omega)) \times [0,t]$, where $V_\delta(r_0,\omega_0)$ is a $\delta$-neighborhood of the point $(r_0,\omega_0) \in \overline{G} \times \Omega$*

$$V_\delta(r_0,\omega_0) = \{(r,\omega) \in \mathcal{E}^3 \mid |r - r_0| < \delta,\ |\omega - \omega_0| < \delta\}.$$

*Then the equality*

$$mes_1(L_{r,\omega} \cap \partial G_0) = 0, \tag{9}$$

*which is valid for every* $(r, \omega) \in \overline{V}_\delta(r_0, \omega_0) \cap (\overline{G} \times \Omega)$ *implies that the function*

$$\Phi(r, \omega, t) = \int_0^t \psi(r, \omega, t')\phi(r - t'\omega, \omega)\, dt'$$

*is continuous at the point* $(r_0, \omega_0, t) \in \overline{G} \times \Omega \times [0, d(r_0, -\omega_0)]$.

**Proof.** We introduce the function which is equal to the distance from the point $r \in \mathcal{E}^3$ to the boundary $\partial G_0$ of the set $G_0$:

$$\rho(r) = \inf_{r' \in \partial G_0} |r - r'|.$$

In view of closeness of $\partial G_0 = \overline{G_0} \backslash G_0$ this function is continuous in $\mathcal{E}^3$ and it is equal to zero only for $r \in \partial G_0$ (see Schwartz, 1981, p.83). We define the sequence of functions:

$$\phi_n(r, \omega) = \phi(r, \omega)(1 - \exp(-n \cdot \rho(r)))$$

for $r \in G_0$ and $\phi_n(r, \omega) = 0$, for $r \in \partial G_0$. The function $\phi_n(r, \omega)$ is continuous in $\overline{G}_0 \times \Omega$. In fact, for any $r \in G_0$ the function $\phi_n(r, \omega)$ is continuous as the product of two continuous functions $\phi(r, \omega)$ and $1 - \exp(-n \cdot \rho(r))$. The function $\phi_n(r, \omega)$ tends to zero as $r \to z$, $z \in \partial G_0$. This follows from the boundedness of the function $\phi(r, \omega)$ and from the convergence to zero of the function $1 - \exp(-n \cdot \rho(r))$ as $r \to z \in \partial G_0$.

Consider the sequence

$$\Phi_n(r, \omega, t) = \int_0^t \psi(r, \omega, t')\phi_n(r - t'\omega, \omega)\, dt'.$$

Since $\phi_n \in C_b(\overline{G}_0 \times \Omega)$ and $\psi(r, \omega, t') \in C(K)$ , then $\Phi_n$ are continuous in $K \subset G_0 \times \Omega \times [0, t]$, where $K$ is a compact set.

Now we prove that $\Phi_n \to \Phi$ as $n \to \infty$ uniformly in $K$. For every $(r, \omega, t) \in K$ we estimate the value $|\Phi(r, \omega, t) - \Phi_n(r, \omega, t)|$ as follows

$$\begin{aligned} &|\Phi(r, \omega, t) - \Phi_n(r, \omega, t)| \\ &\qquad \le \int_0^t |\psi(r, \omega, t')|\, |\phi_n(r - t'\omega, \omega)| \exp(-n \cdot \rho(r - t'\omega))\, dt' \\ &\qquad\qquad \le C \int_0^t \exp(-n \cdot \rho(r - t'\omega))\, dt' = T_n(r, \omega, t), \quad C = \text{const}, \end{aligned}$$

and obtain that the sequence $\{\Phi(r,\omega,t) - \Phi_n(r,\omega,t)\}$ is majorized by the sequence $T_n(r,\omega,t)$. Thus, it is enough to prove that $T_n(r,\omega,t)$ uniformly converges to zero, as $n \to \infty$ for proving the uniform convergence to zero of the sequence $\Phi_n(r,\omega,t)$.

The nonnegative continuous functions $T_n(r,\omega,t)$ in the compact set $K$ can be considered as a non-increasing sequence. Therefore, by the Dyne theorem (see Shilov and Gurevich, 1964) we need only to prove that $T_n(r,\omega,t) \to 0$ as $n \to \infty$ for each point from $K$. Let $(r,\omega,t)$ be an arbitrary fixed point from $K$. Consider the limit

$$T_\infty = \lim_{n\to\infty} T_n(r,\omega,t) = \lim_{n\to\infty} C \int_0^t \exp\left(-n \cdot \rho(r - t'\omega)\right) dt'.$$

In view of (9) the function $\rho(r - t'\omega)$ can be equal to zero only in a set $\{t'\} \subset [0,t]$ with the zero measure ($\mathrm{mes}_1\{t'\} = 0$). Therefore $\exp\left(-n \cdot \rho(r - t'\omega)\right) \to 0$, as $n \to \infty$ almost everywhere in $[0,t]$. Using the theorem about limit convergence under the Lebesgue integral (see Kolmogorov and Fomin 1999), we obtain

$$T_\infty = C \int_0^t \lim_{n\to\infty} \exp\left(-n \cdot \rho(r - t'\omega)\right) dt' = 0.$$

Thus, $T_n(r,\omega,t) \to 0$ as $n \to \infty$ uniformly in $K$ and this implies convergence of $\Phi_n$ to $\Phi$. It follows that the limit function $\Phi(r,\omega,t)$ is continuous in $K$, in particular, at the point $(r_0,\omega,t) \in \overline{G} \times \Omega \times [0, d(r_0,-\omega)]$ (see Schwartz 1981, p. 155). The lemma is proved. □

**Corollary 1.** *Since* $\phi(r,\omega) \in C_b(G_0 \times \Omega)$, $\psi(r,\omega,t') \in C_b(G_0 \times \Omega \times [0,t])$, *then the function*

$$\Phi(r,\omega,t) = \int_0^t \psi(r,\omega,t')\phi(r - t'\omega,\omega)\, dt'$$

*belongs to the space* $C_b(G_0 \times \Omega \times [0, d(r,-\omega)])$.

**Proof.** As the set $G_0$ is open, then for each point $r_0 \in G_0$ there exists a neighborhood $V_\delta(r_0) = \{r \mid |r - r_0| < \delta\}$ such that $\overline{V}_\delta(r_0) \in G_0$. For all points $(r, \omega) \in \overline{V}_\delta(r_0) \times \Omega$ the condition of generalized convexity holds and the condition (9) takes place. Since $r_0$ is arbitrary, Lemma 2 yields that $\Phi(r, \omega, t)$ is continuous in $G_0 \times \Omega \times [0, d(r, -\omega)]$.

The boundedness of $\Phi$ follows from the boundedness of the integrand and of the interval $[0, t]$. The corollary is proved. □

**Corollary 2.** *The function $d(r, \omega)$ belongs to $C_b(G_0 \times \Omega)$.*

**Proof.** In view of convexity of $G$ the function $d(r, \omega)$ can be given as follows

$$d(r, \omega) = \text{mes}_1(L_{r,\omega} \cap G) = \int_0^d \chi(r + t\omega)\, dt,$$

where $\chi(r)$ is the characteristic function of $G$, $d$ is the diameter of $G$. As $\chi(r) \in C_b(G)$, then Corollary 1 implies that $d(r, \omega) \in C_b(G_0 \times \Omega)$, which completes the proof. □

Lemma 2, Corollary 1 and Corollary 2 yield the following statement.

**Corollary 3.** *Since $\phi(r, \omega) \in C_b(G_0 \times \Omega)$, and $\psi(r, \omega, t) \in C_b(G_0 \times \Omega \times [0, d(r, -\omega)])$, then the function*

$$\Phi(r, \omega) = \int_0^{d(r,-\omega)} \psi(r, \omega, t)\phi(r - t\omega, \omega)\, dt$$

*belongs to space $C_b(G_0 \times \Omega)$.*

Consider the functions

$$\tau(r, \omega, t) = \int_0^t \mu(r - t'\omega)\, dt', \qquad \tau(r, \omega) = \int_0^{d(r,-\omega)} \mu(r - t'\omega)\, dt'.$$

The function $\tau(r, \omega, t)$ is called the optical distance between the points $r$ and $r - t\omega$, and $\tau(r, \omega)$ is the optical distance between the point $r$ and the boundary point $r - d(r, -\omega)\omega$.

We define the linear operator $\mathcal{A}$ by the equality

$$(\mathcal{A}\phi)(r, \omega) = \int_0^{d(r,-\omega)} \exp\left(-\tau(r, \omega, t)\right)\phi(r - t\omega, \omega)\, dt, \tag{10}$$

considering $C_b(G_0 \times \Omega)$ as the domain of definition.

**Lemma 3.** *The operator $\mathcal{A}$ maps $C_b(G_0 \times \Omega)$ into $C_b(G_0 \times \Omega)$.*

**Proof.** Since $\mu(r) \in C_b(G_0)$, then Lemma 2 implies that $\tau(r,\omega,t) \in C_b(G_0 \times \Omega \times [0, d(r,-\omega)])$. Hence, Corollary 3 yields that $(\mathcal{A}\phi)(r,\omega) \in C_b(G_0 \times \Omega)$ for any $\phi(r,\omega) \in C_b(G_0 \times \Omega)$. The lemma is proved. □

Note that in the case of absence of planar parts in the surface $\partial G_0$, the condition (9) is valid everywhere in $\overline{G} \times \Omega$. In this case we can easy prove that $\tau(r,\omega,t) \in C_b(\overline{G} \times \Omega \times [0, d(r,-\omega)])$, $d(r,\omega), \tau(r,\omega) \in C_b(\overline{G} \times \Omega)$ and consequently, $(\mathcal{A}\phi) : C_b(G_0 \times \Omega) \to C_b(\overline{G} \times \Omega)$.

As follows from Lemmas 1 and 3 the operator $\mathcal{AS}$ maps $\mathrm{D}(G_0 \times \Omega)$ into $C_b(G_0 \times \Omega) \subset \mathrm{D}(G_0 \times \Omega)$. Therefore, the operator $\mathcal{AS} : \mathrm{D}(G_0 \times \Omega) \to \mathrm{D}(G_0 \times \Omega)$.

It is easy to see that by Lemma 1 the collision integral $N = \mathcal{S}f$ belongs $C_b(G_0 \times \Omega)$, where $f$ is a solution to the direct problem (1),(2). This means that $\mathcal{A}N = \mathcal{AS}f \in C_b(G_0 \times \Omega)$ and $\mathcal{A}N \in \mathrm{D}(G_0 \times \Omega)$.

Furthermore, we prove that the direct problem (1),(2) is equivalent to the following equation:

$$f(r,\omega) = f_0(r,\omega) + (\mathcal{AS}f)(r,\omega), \quad (r,\omega) \in G_0 \times \Omega, \tag{11}$$

where

$$f_0(r,\omega) = h(r - d(r,-\omega)\omega, \omega) \exp(-\tau(r,\omega)) + (\mathcal{A}J)(r,\omega).$$

For brevity we shall use the designation: $P(r,\omega) = N(r,\omega) + J(r,\omega)$. The following statement takes place.

**Lemma 4.** *A function $f(r,\omega)$ is a solution of the direct problem (1), (2) if and only if the function $f(r,\omega)$ satisfies the following equation for all $(r,\omega) \in G_0 \times \Omega$:*

$$f(r,\omega) = h(r - d(r,-\omega)\omega, \omega) \exp(-\tau(r,\omega)) + \int_0^{d(r,-\omega)} \exp(-\tau(r,\omega,t)) P(r - t\omega, \omega)\, dt, \tag{12}$$

*in the class $\mathrm{D}(G_0 \times \Omega)$.*

**Proof.** *The necessity.* Let a function $f(r,\omega)$ be a solution of the direct problem. Then $f(r,\omega) \in \mathrm{D}(G_0 \times \Omega)$ and for every point $(r,\omega) \in G_0 \times \Omega$ we have

$$lf(r - t\omega, \omega) = P(r - t\omega, \omega) \tag{13}$$

almost everywhere in the set $\{r - t\omega, t \in [0, d(r, -\omega)]\}$. As the function $f(r - t\omega, \omega)$ is absolutely continuous in the set $\{r - t\omega \mid t \in [0, d(r, -\omega)]\}$, the expression $lf(r - t\omega, \omega)$ is an integrable function with respect to $t$ for any fixed $(r, \omega) \in G_0 \times \Omega$. We multiply the equality (13) by the function $\exp(-\tau(r, \omega, t))$ and integrate the obtained result over $t \in [0, d(r, -\omega)]$. Thus, we have

$$\int_0^{d(r,-\omega)} \exp(-\tau(r, \omega, t)) lf(r - t\omega, \omega)\, dt = \int_0^{d(r,-\omega)} \exp(-\tau(r, \omega, t)) P(r - t\omega, \omega)\, dt. \quad (14)$$

Since the function $\tau(r, \omega, t)$ is absolutely continuous with respect to $t$, and the function $lf(r - t\omega, \omega)$ is integrable, we can apply the formula of integration by parts in the left-hand side of the equality (14) (see Kolmogorov and Fomin, 1999). As a result, we obtain

$$\begin{aligned}\int_0^{d(r,-\omega)} &\exp(-\tau(r, \omega, t)) lf(r - t\omega, \omega) dt \\ &= f(r, \omega) - f(r - d(r, -\omega)\omega, \omega) \exp(-\tau(r, \omega)) \\ &\quad - \int_0^{d(r,-\omega)} \exp(-\tau(r, \omega, t))(-\mu(r - t\omega) f(r - t\omega, \omega) \\ &\quad + \mu(r - t\omega) f(r - t\omega, \omega))\, dt. \quad (15)\end{aligned}$$

Taking into account the boundary condition (2) $f(r - d(r, -\omega)\omega, \omega) = h(r - d(r, -\omega)\omega, \omega)$, it is possible to derive the following equality from (15):

$$\int_0^{d(r,-\omega)} \exp(-\tau(r, \omega, t)) P(r - t\omega, \omega)\, dt = f(r, \omega) - h(r - d(r, -\omega)\omega, \omega) \exp(-\tau(r, \omega)).$$

This means that the function $f(r, \omega)$ satisfies the equation (12) for all $(r, \omega) \in G_0 \times \Omega$. The necessity is proved.

*The sufficiency.* Let a function $f(r, \omega)$ satisfy the equation (12). Then taking into account that $d(\xi + t\omega, -\omega) = t$, for every $(\xi, \omega) \in \Gamma^-$ the equation (12) implies the following equality

$$f(\xi + t\omega, \omega) = \exp(-\tau(\xi, -\omega, t))(h(\xi, \omega) + \int_0^t \exp(\tau(\xi, -\omega, t')) P(\xi + t'\omega, \omega)\, dt'). \quad (16)$$

Here the integral is an absolutely continuous function with respect to $t$ because the integrand is an integrable function. The sum and the product of absolutely continuous functions are also absolutely continuous functions (see Shilov and Gurevich, 1964; Kolmogorov and Fomin, 1999). Therefore, from (16) we see that the function $f(\xi + \omega t, \omega)$ is absolutely continuous in the set $\{\xi + t\omega \mid t \in [0, d(\xi, \omega)]\}$ for any fixed $(\xi, \omega) \in \Gamma^-$. It is easy to prove that the function $f(\xi + \omega t, \omega)$ satisfies the boundary condition (2) for $t = 0$.

It is known that for the product of two absolutely continuous functions $\varphi(t)$ and $\psi(t)$ the equality $(\varphi(t)\psi(t))' = \varphi'(t)\psi(t) + \psi'(t)\varphi(t)$ holds almost everywhere. Hence, for almost all $t \in [0, d(\xi, \omega)]$ we have

$$\begin{aligned} lf(\xi + t\omega, \omega) = & -\mu(\xi + t\omega) \exp(-\tau(\xi, -\omega, t))(h(\xi, \omega) \\ & + \int_0^t \exp(\tau(\xi, -\omega, t'))P(\xi + t'\omega, \omega)\, dt') + \\ & + \exp(-\tau(\xi, -\omega, t)) \exp(\tau(\xi, -\omega, t))P(\xi + t\omega, \omega) \\ & + \mu(\xi + \omega t) \exp(-\tau(\xi, -\omega, t))(h(\xi, \omega) \\ & + \int_0^t \exp(\tau(\xi, -\omega, t'))P(\xi + t'\omega, \omega)\, dt') = P(\xi + t\omega, \omega). \end{aligned}$$

Thus, the function $f(r, \omega)$ from $\mathrm{D}(G_0 \times \Omega)$ which is a solution of the equation (12) satisfies all requirements for a solution of the boundary value problem (1), (2). This completes the proof of the lemma. □

We set

$$\lambda(r) = \mu_s(r)/\mu(r),$$

if $\mu(r) \neq 0$ at a point $r$, and $\lambda(r) = 0$, if $\mu(r) = 0$ at a point $r$ . The function $\lambda(r)$ is often called the single scattering albedo. We require the existence of the following value:

$$\bar{\lambda} = \sup_{r \in G_0} \lambda(r) \neq \infty.$$

Put

$$\bar{\tau} = \sup_{(r,\omega) \in G_0 \times \Omega} \tau(r, \omega).$$

The value $\bar{\tau}$ is called the optical diameter of the domain $G$. Bellow we shall assume that if $\mu(r) = 0$ at a point $r$, then $\mu_s(r) = 0$ at the same point.

**Lemma 5.** *The following estimate is valid*

$$\|\mathcal{AS}\| \leq \bar{\lambda}(1 - e^{-\bar{\tau}}). \tag{17}$$

**Proof.** The definition of a norm of a linear operator implies that

$$\begin{aligned} \|\mathcal{AS}\| \leq & \sup_{(r,\omega)\in G_0\times\Omega} \int_0^{d(r,-\omega)} \exp(-\tau(r,\omega,t))\mu_s(r-t\omega)\,dt \\ = & \sup_{(r,\omega)\in G_0\times\Omega} \int_0^{d(r,-\omega)} \exp(-\tau(r,\omega,t))\lambda(r-t\omega)\mu(r-t\omega)\,dt \\ & \leq \bar{\lambda} \sup_{(r,\omega)\in G_0\times\Omega} \int_0^{d(r,-\omega)} \exp(-\tau(r,\omega,t))\mu(r-t\omega)\,dt. \end{aligned}$$

Using analytical calculation of the latter integral, we obtain

$$\|\mathcal{AS}\| \leq \bar{\lambda} \sup_{(r,\omega)\in G_0\times\Omega} (1-\exp(-\tau(r,\omega))) \leq \bar{\lambda}(1-\exp(-\bar{\tau})).$$

The lemma is proved. □

**Theorem 1.** *If the inequality*

$$\bar{\lambda}(1-e^{-\bar{\tau}}) < 1 \tag{18}$$

*is valid, then there exists a unique solution of the boundary value problem* (1), (2), *which can be represented as the following uniformly convergent series*

$$f(r,\omega) = \sum_{n=0}^{\infty}((\mathcal{AS})^n f_0)(r,\omega), \quad (r,\omega)\in G_0\times\Omega. \tag{19}$$

**Proof.** Lemma 4 implies that it suffices to consider the equation (11). We rewrite it in the form:

$$(\mathcal{I}-\mathcal{AS})f = f_0,$$

where $\mathcal{I}$ is the identity operator. From the estimate (17) and the condition (18) it follows that $\|\mathcal{AS}\| < 1$. Since $\mathrm{D}(G_0\times\Omega)$ is a Banach space, there exists the inverse operator $(\mathcal{I}-\mathcal{AS})^{-1}$ and $f = (\mathcal{I}-\mathcal{AS})^{-1}f_0$. Moreover, if $\|\mathcal{AS}\| < 1$, then

$$(\mathcal{I}-\mathcal{AS})^{-1} = \mathcal{I}+\mathcal{AS}+(\mathcal{AS})^2+\dots.$$

Therefore, the solution of the equation (11) can be represented as a sum of the corresponding Neumann series (19) (see Kolmogorov and Fomin, 1999). This series can be majorized by a convergent number series. It guarantees the uniform convergence of such Neumann series. This completes the proof of the theorem. □

## 1.2. SETTING THE TOMOGRAPHY PROBLEMS AND PRELIMINARY REMARKS

In this section we put the exact mathematical tomography problems which correspond to more general problem represented in the very beginning of the introduction.

In addition to (1.1.2) we consider the boundary condition

$$f(\eta,\omega) = H(\eta,\omega), \quad (\eta,\omega) \in \Gamma^+, \tag{1}$$

where the set $\Gamma^+$ was defined in Section 1.1. The function $H(\eta,\omega)$ means the distribution of the output particle flux on the boundary of $G$.

Now we can set the following tomography problem, which has been firstly considered in Anikonov (1994).

**Tomography problem 1.** Determine the surface $\partial G_0$ from the transport equation (1.1.1) and the boundary conditions (1.1.2), (1), where only the function $H(\eta,\omega)$, $(\eta,\omega) \in \Gamma^+$ is given.

The problem seems to be consistent with the physical point of view. Indeed, the surface $\partial G_0$ is treated as the contact boundaries between various materials inside the medium $G$ and the information about $\partial G_0$ is rather useful for tomography. At the same time the distribution of the output radiation $H(\eta,\omega)$ can be measured by real detectors.

Note, that from the mathematical point of view, the surface $\partial G_0$ is the discontinuity surface for the coefficients of the transport equation because of the restrictions formulated in Section 1.1 for these coefficients. It is easy to see that $\partial G_0$ coincides with the union of all surfaces $\partial G_i$, $i = 1,\dots,p$.

Thus far the introduced restrictions were quite insignificant. Further investigation requires additional assumptions for the coefficients of the equation (1.1.1) and the function $h(\xi,\eta)$, $(\xi,\omega) \in \Gamma^-$. However, we intend to preserve the importance of the tomography problems with regard to applications.

Firstly, we suppose that every surface of $\partial G_i$, $i = 1,\dots,p$, consists of a finite number of smooth surfaces of the class $C^2$, as defined, for example, in Ladyzhenskaya and Uralt'seva (1964); furthermore, every $\partial G_i$ is a Lipshitz surface (see Ladyzhenskaya, 1973).

Also we make more precise the definition of generalized convexity. Assume that every ray $L_{r,\omega}$, $r \in G_0, \omega \in \Omega$ intersects $\partial G_0$ at a finite number of the points $r + t_j(r,\omega)\omega$ (in addition to $r$), and, accordingly, the intersection of $L_{r,\omega}$ and $G_0$ consists of the intervals $\{r + t\omega \mid t \in$

$(t_{j-1}(r,\omega), t_j(r,\omega))\}$, $j = 1, \dots, l(r,\omega)$, so that each of them belongs to one of the domains $G_i$, $i = 1, \dots, p$. Suppose that

$$0 < t_1(r,\omega) < t_2(r,\omega) < \cdots < t_{l(r,\omega)}(r,\omega),$$
$$t_0(r,\omega) = 0, \qquad \sup_{(r,\omega)\in G_0\times\Omega} l(r,\omega) < \infty.$$

The conditions to be imposed on the coefficients of the equation (1.1.1) are as follows. Let a nonnegative function $\mu(r)$, $r \in \mathcal{E}^3$ vanish outside $\overline{G}$. It can be zero at some points in $G$, but there exists at least one domain $G_i$ where $\mu(r) > 0$ for all $r \in G_i$. The function $\mu(r)$ is assumed to be uniformly continuous along with the first and the second partial derivatives in every $G_i$. The function $k(r, \omega\cdot\omega')$ is nonnegative, vanishing outside $\overline{G}$, and the functions $\sigma_i$ are as smooth as $\mu(r)$, and the functions $S_i(\nu) \in C^2[-1,1]$.

Suppose that nonnegative function $J(r,\omega)$ $(J(r,\omega) = 0,\ r \notin \overline{G})$ and $h(\xi,\omega)$ has all partial derivatives up to the second order which are uniformly continuous for $(r,\omega) \in G_i \times \Omega$, $i = 1, \dots, p$, and $(\xi,\omega) \in \Gamma^-$, respectively. The precise definition of the differentiation of functions defined on a surface was given, for example, in Anikonov, Kovtanyuk, Prokhorov (2002, p. 87).

Evidently these conditions imposed on the coefficients $\mu, k, J$ do not rule out the existence of discontinuities of the first kind for $z \in \partial G_0$. Introduce the following notation for the corresponding jumps. Assume $z \in \partial G_0$ and $z$ is a common point of the boundaries of two domains $G_l$ and $G_j$ only $(1 \le l < j \le p)$. Then

$$[\![k(z,\omega\cdot\omega')]\!] = \lim_{r'\to z} k(r',\omega\cdot\omega') - \lim_{r''\to z} k(r'',\omega\cdot\omega'),\ r' \in G_l,\ r'' \in G_j.$$

The jumps $[\![\mu(z)]\!]$ and $[\![J(z,\omega)]\!]$ are defined analogously.

Tomography Problem 1 was firstly investigated in D.Anikonov (1994) and more thoroughly in Anikonov (1999) and Anikonov, Kovtanyuk and Prokhorov (2002), under additional restrictions which were appropriate for practical applications.

For this, the following function

$$\mathrm{Ind}(r) = \left|\nabla_r \int_\Omega f(r + d(r,\omega)\omega, \omega)\, d\omega\right|, \tag{2}$$

was defined for $r \in G_0$. This function was called the indicator of heterogeneity. Due to some condition of visibility $\mathrm{Ind}(r)$ tends to infinity if and only if the distance $\rho(r, \partial G_0)$ between the point $r \in G_0$ and the boundary $\partial G_0$ tends to zero. The condition of visibility will be explained in detail in Section 1.5.

However, in 3-D space, $H(\eta, \omega)$, $(\eta, \omega) \in \Gamma^+$ depends on four independent scalar variables and simultaneous measuring of such big amount of information seems to be too difficult for practical application. It is also difficult to use $\mathrm{Ind}(r)$ in simulated numerical experiments in view of the needed long computer time. Consequently, there is a problem of reduction the volume of necessary information or use of such information by parts. In what follows we represent a version of solving this problem.

In addition, introduce the following designations and assumptions. Let $\mathcal{P}$ be a plane in $\mathcal{E}^3$ such that $\mathcal{D} = G \cap \mathcal{P} \neq \varnothing$. Since the domain $G$ is bounded and convex, and an arbitrary interval $(a, b)$ from $\mathcal{E}^1$ is connected, then the set $\mathcal{D}$ appears to be a convex and bounded domain in $\mathcal{P}$. Assume that each nonempty set $G_i \cap \mathcal{P}$ is a union of a planar domains the number of which is finite. The set of such domains (in $\mathcal{P}$) is denoted as $\mathcal{D}_1, \mathcal{D}_2, \ldots, \mathcal{D}_q$.

We suppose that $q \geq 2$ and the following conditions hold:

$$\overline{\mathcal{D}} = \bigcup_{i=1}^{q} \overline{\mathcal{D}}_i, \quad \mathcal{D}_i \cap \mathcal{D}_j = \varnothing, \text{ for } i \neq j, \quad i, j = 1, \ldots, q.$$

Note, that these conditions are similar to the conditions for the domains $G_i$. We denote $\mathcal{D}_0$ as a union for all $\mathcal{D}_i$, $i = 1, \ldots, q$. Let $\mathcal{P}^*$ be a plane parallel to $\mathcal{P}$ and the origin of the coordinates belongs to $\mathcal{P}^*$; $\Omega_1 = \Omega \cap \mathcal{P}^*$.

**Tomography problem 2.** Determine the boundary $\partial\mathcal{D}_0$ from the transport equation (1.1.1) and the boundary conditions (1.1.2), (1), where only the function $H(r + d(r, \omega)\omega, \omega) = f(r + d(r, \omega)\omega, \omega)$ is given for $(r, \omega) \in \mathcal{D}_0 \times \Omega_1$.

The trace of $f(r, \omega)$ on the set $\mathcal{D}_0 \times \Omega_1$ is designated by $f^*(r, \omega)$. Hence, in the formulated problem, the known function $H^*(\eta, \omega) = f^*(r + d(r, \omega)\omega, \omega)$ depends only on two independent variables instead of $H(\eta, \omega)$ which depends on four variables. At the same time, only a part $\partial\mathcal{D}_0$ of the set $\partial G_0$ is sought for in the problem.

To simplify the formulation of the problem, we assume that the whole set $\partial\mathcal{D}_0$ is to be determined. Since its part $\partial\mathcal{D}$ is known, we need to determine only the part of $\partial\mathcal{D}_0$ which is internal for the domain $\mathcal{D}$.

From the physical point of view, it is clear that the distribution of output radiation $H^*(\eta, \omega)$ can be measured and even partial information about the coefficients provides certain important data about the internal structure of the medium.

Note that the distribution of the input radiation is not given. However, it is not arbitrary. We remind that $h(\xi, \omega)$ is nonnegative and $h(\xi, \omega) \in C^2(\overline{\Gamma}^-)$.

In addition, suppose that $\partial\mathcal{D}_0 \in C^2$ and each $\partial\mathcal{D}_i$, $i = 1, \ldots, p$ consists of a finite number of smooth curves belonging to the class $C^2$. Without loss of generality we can assume that the plane $\mathcal{P}$ is defined by the equality $r_3 = 0$ and therefore the plane $\mathcal{P}$ is designated by $\mathcal{E}^2$.

For brevity suppose that $J^2(r,\omega) + \tilde{h}^2(r,\omega) > 0$ for $(r,\omega) \in D_0 \times \Omega_1$. This provides positiveness of $f(r,\omega)$ for $(r,\omega) \in \overline{\mathcal{D}} \times \Omega_1$ in which the formula (1.1.12) holds.

Let $\beta(r,\omega)$ be an arbitrary differentiable function. Its partial derivatives with respect to $r_k$ are denoted by $D_k\beta(r,\omega)$ and its partial derivatives with respect to $\omega_k$, are denoted by $D_{k+2}\beta(r,\omega)$, $k = 1,2$, $r = (r_1, r_2)$, $\omega = (\omega_1, \omega_2)$.

Introduce a class of functions $W$. A function $v(r,\omega)$, $(r,\omega) \in \mathcal{E}^2 \times \Omega_1$, belongs to $W$, if

a) $v(r,\omega) = 0$ for $r \notin \overline{\mathcal{D}}$, $\omega \in \Omega_1$;

b) $v(r,\omega)$ satisfies the Holder condition for some $\alpha$, $0 < \alpha < 1$. More precisely,

$$|w(r',\omega') - w(r'',\omega'')| \leq \text{const} \cdot \{|r' - r''|^\alpha + |\omega' - \omega''|^\alpha\},$$
$$r', r'' \in \mathcal{D}_i, \quad i = 1, \ldots, q, \quad \omega', \omega'' \in \Omega_1. \tag{3}$$

Here and in what follows the symbol "const" stands for a positive number independent of all variables of the relation in which it is used;

c) $v(r,\omega)$ has all first order partial derivatives which are continuous in $\mathcal{D}_0 \times \Omega_1$, so that $|D_{k+2}\, v(r,\omega)| \leq \text{const}$, and

$$|D_k v(r,\omega)| \leq \text{const} \cdot \{|\ln \rho(r, \partial\mathcal{D}_0)| + 1\}, \quad (r,\omega) \in \mathcal{D}_0 \times \Omega_1, \quad k = 1,2, \tag{4}$$

where $\rho(r, \partial\mathcal{D}_0)$ denotes the distance between the point $r$ and the set $\partial\mathcal{D}_0$.

Let $\beta(r)$, $r \in \mathcal{E}^3$ be an arbitrary function continuous uniformly in each $G_i$, $i = 1, \ldots, p$ and equal to zero outside of $\overline{G}$. The following lemma has been proved in Prokhorov (1996) (see also Section 1.1).

**Lemma 1.** *The function*

$$\int_{t_1}^{t_2} \beta(r + t\omega)\, dt$$

*is continuous for* $(r, \omega, t_1, t_2) \in G_0 \times \Omega \times [-d, d] \times [-d, d]$, *where the number* $d$ *is a diameter of the domain* $G$.

It is clear that $\mu(r)$ can be taken equal to $\beta(r)$. Lemma 1.1 allows us to use the proper results from Germogenova (1986) and to consider the trace of the collision integral $N(r,\omega)$ on $\mathcal{E}^2 \times \Omega_1$ as a function from $W$.

Introduce the following designations. Let $\Pi_i^{(\varepsilon)} = \{r \in \mathcal{D}_i \mid \rho(r, \partial\mathcal{D}_i) < \varepsilon\}$, $\mathcal{D}_i^{(\varepsilon)} = \mathcal{D}_i \backslash \overline{\Pi}_i^{(\varepsilon)}$, $i = 1, \ldots, q$, $0 < \varepsilon \leq \varepsilon_0$. Later on $V$ denotes an arbitrary open set in $\mathcal{E}^2$ such that $\overline{V} \subset \mathcal{D}_0$. Obviously $\rho(\overline{V}, \partial\mathcal{D}_0)$ is positive. Assume that there exists sufficiently small $\varepsilon_0 > 0$ such that all $\mathcal{D}_i^{(\varepsilon)}$ and $\Pi_i^{(\varepsilon)}$ are domains in $\mathcal{E}^2$ with their piecewise smooth boundaries of the class $C^2$ and the following condition holds:

$$\Psi(\overline{V}, \varepsilon) = \sup_{(r,\omega)\in\overline{V}\times\Omega_1} \operatorname{mes}_1\Big(L_{r,\omega} \cap \Big(\bigcup_{i=1}^{q} \Pi_i^{(\varepsilon)}\Big)\Big) \to 0, \qquad \text{for} \quad \varepsilon \to 0. \tag{5}$$

Symbol $\operatorname{mes}_k(T)$ means a measure in $\mathcal{E}^k$ of a set $T$, $T \subset \mathcal{E}^k$, $k = 1, 2$. In particular, $\operatorname{mes}_1(T)$ is a measure of the set $T$ on the straight line.

Analogously to Anikonov (1999) we introduce the following functions $g_i^{(\varepsilon)}(r)$: $\mathcal{E}^2 \to [0, 1]$, $i = 1, \ldots, q$, such that $g_i^{(\varepsilon)}(r) = 1$ for $r \in \mathcal{D}_i^{(\varepsilon)}$, $g_i^{(\varepsilon)}(r) = 0$ for $r \notin \mathcal{D}_i$ and $g_i^{(\varepsilon)}(r) \in C^\infty(\mathcal{E}^2)$. These functions are often used for smoothing discontinuous functions. The following estimate holds (see Anikonov, Kovtanyuk and Prokhorov, 2002)

$$|D_k g_i^{(\varepsilon)}(r)| \leq \text{const} \cdot \varepsilon^{-1}, \quad r \in \mathcal{E}^2, \quad k = 1, 2. \tag{6}$$

Let a function $\chi(r, \omega)$ be uniformly continuous in $\mathcal{D}_i \times \Omega_1$, $i = 1, \ldots, q$. We define $\chi_i(r, \omega)$, $i = 1, \ldots, q$, as follows. Each function $\chi_i(r, \omega)$ coincides with $\chi(r, \omega)$ for $(r, \omega) \in \mathcal{D}_i \times \Omega_1$. For $r \in \partial\mathcal{D}_i$, it is equal to the limit of $\chi(r, \omega)$ as $r \to \partial\mathcal{D}_i$, $r \in \mathcal{D}_i$. For $r \notin \overline{\mathcal{D}}_i$, $\chi_i(r, \omega) = 0$ for all $\omega \in \Omega_1$. It is clear that the equality $\chi(r, \omega) = \chi_1(r, \omega) + \ldots + \chi_q(r, \omega)$ can fail only for $(r, \omega) \in \partial\mathcal{D}_0 \times \Omega_1$, if $\chi(r, \omega)$ is defined for these arguments.

We set $\chi_\varepsilon(r, \omega) = \chi_1(r, \omega) g_1^{(\varepsilon)}(r) + \ldots + \chi_q(r, \omega) g_q^{(\varepsilon)}(r)$. It is well-known (see Anikonov, 1999) that if $\chi(r, \omega)$ belongs to the class $W$, then $D_k \chi_\varepsilon(r, \omega)$ are continuous for $(r, \omega) \in \mathcal{E}^2 \times \Omega_1$, $k = 1, 2$, $0 < \varepsilon \leq \varepsilon_0$. In this case the functions $\chi_\varepsilon(r, \omega)$ and $D_k \chi_\varepsilon(r, \omega)$, $k = 1, 2$ are equal to zero if $(r, \omega) \in \partial\mathcal{D}_0 \times \Omega_1$. The introduced definitions easily imply the inequality $|\chi_\varepsilon(r, \omega)| \leq |\chi(r, \omega)|$, $(r, \omega) \in \mathcal{D}_0 \times \Omega_1$.

The functions $\mu(r)$, $N(r, \omega)$ and $J(r, \omega)$ hold the condition imposed for $\chi(r, \omega)$, therefore assuming $\chi(r, \omega) = \mu(r)$, $\chi(r, \omega) = N(r, \omega)$, $\chi(r, \omega) = J(r, \omega)$ we introduce $\mu_i(r)$, $N_i(r, \omega)$, $J_i(r, \omega)$, $i = 1, \ldots, q$ and $\mu_\varepsilon(r)$, $N_\varepsilon(r, \omega)$, $J_\varepsilon(r, \omega)$, respectively. Remind that for brevity we define the function $P(r, \omega) = N(r, \omega) + J(r, \omega)$.

## 1.3. THE PRELIMINARY STATEMENTS

In this section we prove or represent some lemmas to be used in the following sections. Proofs of the first two lemmas do not differ from the proofs of similar lemmas for 3-dimensional case in Anikonov (1999), Anikonov, Kovtanyuk and Prokhorov (2002). At the same time there is some difference in the designations. Therefore we represent the formulations of these lemmas completely.

**Lemma 1.** *The function $d(r,\omega)$ is continuous in $G \times \Omega$ as well as its derivatives $D_k\, d(r,\omega)$, $k = 1,2,3$.*

The proof of this lemma is contained in Anikonov (1996).

**Lemma 2.** *Let the function $\chi(r,\omega)$: $\mathcal{E}^2 \times \Omega_1 \to \mathcal{E}^1$, $(r,\omega) \in \mathcal{E}^2 \times \Omega_1$, be equal to zero for $r \notin \overline{\mathcal{D}}$, and be uniformly continuous in each set $\mathcal{D}_i \times \Omega_1$, $i = 1,\dots,q$, then for any neighborhood $V, \overline{V} \subset \mathcal{D}_0$ we have*

$$\lim_{\varepsilon\to 0} \int_{t_1}^{t_2} \chi_\varepsilon(r+t\omega,\omega')\,dt = \int_{t_1}^{t_2} \chi(r+t\omega,\omega')\,dt, \tag{1}$$

*The convergence is uniform with respect to $r \in \overline{V}$, $\omega,\omega' \in \Omega_1$, $t_1,t_2 \in [0,d]$.*

**Proof.** The functions $\chi_\varepsilon(r,\omega)$ and $\chi(r,\omega)$ may have different values only for $(r,\omega) \in \overline{\Pi}_i^{(\varepsilon)} \times \Omega_1$, $i = 1,\dots,q$; therefore two integrands in (1) may differ only for the values $t \in [0,d]$, such that $r + t\omega \in L_{r,\omega} \cap (\bigcup_{i=1}^q \overline{\Pi}_i^{(\varepsilon)})$. Since $|\chi_\varepsilon(r,\omega)| \le |\chi(r,\omega)| \le \text{const}$, then

$$\left| \int_{t_1}^{t_2} \chi_\varepsilon(r+t\omega,\omega')\,\mathrm{dt} - \int_{t_1}^{t_2} \chi(r+t\omega,\omega')\,dt \right| \le \text{const} \cdot \Psi(\overline{V},\varepsilon) \to 0$$

for $\varepsilon \to 0$. Due to the condition (1.2.5) the convergence appears to be uniform on the set $\overline{V} \times \Omega_1 \times \Omega_1 \times [0,d] \times [0,d]$. The lemma is proved. □

Lemma 2 easily implies the following remark.

**Remark 1.** In the particular case $t_1 = 0$, $t_2 = d(r,\omega)$ the following convergence

$$\lim_{\varepsilon\to 0} \int_0^{d(r,\omega)} \chi_\varepsilon(r+t\omega,\omega')\,dt = \int_0^{d(r,\omega)} \chi(r+t\omega,\omega')\,dt, \tag{2}$$

is uniform with respect to $r \in \overline{V}$; $\omega,\omega' \in \Omega_1$, and the right-hand sides in (1) and (2) are continuous for $r \in \mathcal{D}_0$; $\omega,\omega' \in \Omega_1$, $t_1,t_2 \in [0,d]$.

Introduce the functions $f^{(\varepsilon)}(r,\omega)\colon \overline{\mathcal{D}} \times \Omega_1 \to \mathcal{E}^1$

$$f^{(\varepsilon)}(r,\omega) = \tilde{h}(r,\omega) \exp\Big( - \int_0^{d(r,-\omega)} \mu_\varepsilon(r - t\omega)\, dt\Big)$$
$$+ \int_0^{d(r,-\omega)} \exp\Big( - \int_0^t \mu_\varepsilon(r - t'\omega)\, dt'\Big) \big\{N_\varepsilon(r - t\omega,\omega) + J_\varepsilon(r - t\omega,\omega)\big\}\, dt, \tag{3}$$

where $\tilde{h}(r,\omega) = h(r - d(r,-\omega)\omega,\omega)$.

The function $f^{(\varepsilon)}(r,\omega)$ will approximate the function $f(r,\omega)$.

**Lemma 3.** *For any $\varepsilon$, $0 < \varepsilon \le \varepsilon_0$, the function $f^{(\varepsilon)}(r,\omega)$ belongs to $C(\mathcal{D} \times \Omega_1)$. For any neighborhood $V$, $(\overline{V} \subset \mathcal{D}_0)$ the sequence $f^{(\varepsilon)}(r,\omega)$ converges to $f(r,\omega)$ as $\varepsilon \to 0$ uniformly with respect to $r \in \overline{V}$, $\omega \in \Omega_1$. The function $f(r,\omega)$ belongs to the class $C(\mathcal{D}_0 \times \Omega_1)$.*

**Proof.** All integrands in (3) belong to $C(\overline{\mathcal{D}} \times \Omega_1)$. For any domain $\mathcal{D}'$ such that $\overline{\mathcal{D}}' \subset \mathcal{D}$, the functions $d(r,-\omega)$ and $\tilde{h}(r,\omega)$ belong to $C(\overline{\mathcal{D}}' \times \Omega_1)$. Therefore $f^{(\varepsilon)}(r,\omega) \in C(\overline{\mathcal{D}}' \times \Omega_1)$. Since $\mathcal{D}'$ is arbitrary, $f^{(\varepsilon)}(r,\omega) \in C(\mathcal{D} \times \Omega_1)$.

Now we prove that $f^{(\varepsilon)}(r,\omega)$ converges to $f(r,\omega)$ $(r,\omega) \in \overline{V} \times \Omega_1$ uniformly as $\varepsilon \to 0$.

We denote the first and the second terms in the right-hand side of (1.1.12) by $A_1(r,\omega)$ and $A_2(r,\omega)$, respectively. The first and the second term in the right-hand side of (3) are denoted by $A_1^{(\varepsilon)}(r,\omega)$ and $A_2^{(\varepsilon)}(r,\omega)$, respectively. Then these formulas can be rewritten as follows

$$f(r,\omega) = A_1(r,\omega) + A_2(r,\omega), \qquad f^{(\varepsilon)}(r,\omega) = A_1^{(\varepsilon)}(r,\omega) + A_2^{(\varepsilon)}(r,\omega).$$

By virtue of the evident inequality $|\exp(-t_1) - \exp(-t_2)| \le |t_1 - t_2|$, $t_1, t_2 \ge 0$, we obtain

$$|A_1(r,\omega) - A_1^{(\varepsilon)}(r,\omega)| \le \text{const} \cdot \Big| \int_0^{d(r,-\omega)} \mu(r - t\omega)\, dt - \int_0^{d(r,-\omega)} \mu_\varepsilon(r - t\omega)\, dt \Big|.$$

This inequality and Remark 1 with $\chi(r,\omega) = \mu(r)$ imply that $A_1^{(\varepsilon)}(r,\omega) \to A_1(r,\omega)$ as $\varepsilon \to 0$ uniformly with respect to $(r,\omega) \in \overline{V} \times \Omega_1$.

Taking into account boundedness of $P = N + J$ and $P_\varepsilon = N_\varepsilon + J_\varepsilon$ we see that

$$|A_2(r,\omega) - A_2^{(\varepsilon)}(r,\omega)| \le \text{const} \cdot \Big\{ \int_0^{d(r,-\omega)} \int_0^t |\mu(r - t'\omega) - \mu_\varepsilon(r - t'\omega)|\, dt'\, dt + \int_0^{d(r,-\omega)} |P(r - t\omega, \omega) - P_\varepsilon(r - t\omega, \omega)|\, dt \Big\}.$$

Lemma 2 and Remark 1 imply that $A_2^{(\varepsilon)}(r,\omega) \to A_2(r,\omega)$ as $\varepsilon \to 0$ uniformly with respect to $\overline{V} \times \Omega_1$.

Thus, we have proved that the continuous function $f^{(\varepsilon)}(r,\omega)$ converges to $f(r,\omega)$ as $\varepsilon \to 0$ uniformly with respect to $(r,\omega) \in \overline{V} \times \Omega_1$. Hence, $f(r,\omega) \in C(\overline{V} \times \Omega_1)$. Since $V$ is arbitrary, $f(r,\omega) \in C(\mathcal{D}_0 \times \Omega_1)$. The lemma is proved. □

Suppose that a continuous bounded function $Q^{(\varepsilon)}(r,y)$, $r \in \mathcal{D}_0$, $y \in \overline{\mathcal{D}}$, $r \ne y$ is defined for all $\varepsilon$ such that $0 < \varepsilon \le \varepsilon_0$. Let $Q(r,y)$ be also continuous and bounded function defined for $r \in \mathcal{D}_0$, $y \in \overline{\mathcal{D}}$, $r \ne y$. For every neighborhood $V$, $\overline{V} \subset \mathcal{D}_0$, the functions $Q^{(\varepsilon)}(r,\omega)$ converge to $Q(r,\omega)$ as $\varepsilon \to 0$ uniformly with respect to $r \in \overline{V}$, $y \in \overline{\mathcal{D}}$, $r \ne y$. All first order partial derivatives of the functions $Q^{(\varepsilon)}(r,y)$ are assumed to be continuous in their domains of definition. Finally, we assume that for $k = 1,2$ and $0 < \varepsilon \le \varepsilon_1$, where $\varepsilon_1$ is sufficiently small number, $\varepsilon_1 \le \varepsilon_0$, the following inequality holds:

$$\Big| \frac{\partial}{\partial y_k} Q^{(\varepsilon)}(r,y) \Big| \le \text{const} \cdot \{1 + \varepsilon^{-1} \cdot \Psi(\overline{V}, \varepsilon)\}, \quad r \in \overline{V}, \quad y \in \bigcup_{i=1}^{q} \Pi_i^{(\varepsilon)}. \tag{4}$$

Under these assumptions, we formulate the following statement.

**Lemma 4.** *If $\chi(r,\omega)$ belongs to the class $W$, then the integrals*

$$X^{(\varepsilon)}(r) = \int_{\mathcal{D}} \frac{D_k\, \chi_\varepsilon(y, (y-r)/|y-r|)}{|r-y|}\, Q^{(\varepsilon)}(r,y)\, dy \qquad (k = 1,2),$$

*converge to $X(r)$, as $\varepsilon \to 0$ uniformly with respect to $r \in \overline{V}$. Here*

$$X(r) = \sum_{i=1}^{q} \int_{\mathcal{D}_i} \frac{D_k\, \chi_i(y, (y-r)/|y-r|)}{|r-y|}\, Q(r,y)\, dy + \sum_{i=1}^{q} \int_{\partial \mathcal{D}_i} \frac{(n_i(y) \cdot e_k) \chi_i(y, (y-r)/|y-r|)}{|r-y|}\, Q(r,y)\, d\sigma_y,$$

*where $n_i(y) \cdot e_k$ is the inner product. The vector $n_i(y)$ is the unit vector of the inward normal to $\partial\mathcal{D}_i$ at $y$; $e_k$ is the unit vector of the $k$-th coordinate axis. The integrals in the second sum are understood as the line integrals of the first kind (integration is implemented with respect to a length of the curve).*

**Proof.** Differentiating the equality

$$\chi_\varepsilon(y,\omega) = \chi_1(y,\omega)g_1^{(\varepsilon)}(y) + \ldots + \ldots + \chi_q(y,\omega)g_q^{(\varepsilon)}(y)$$

with respect to $y_k$, we obtain

$$D_k\chi_\varepsilon(y,\omega) = \sum_{i=1}^{q}\{\chi_i(y,\omega)D_k g_i^{(\varepsilon)}(y) + g_i^{(\varepsilon)}(y)D_k\,\chi_i(y,\omega)\},$$

$$y \in \mathcal{D}_0, \qquad \omega \in \Omega_1.$$

We recall that $D_k g_i^{(\varepsilon)}(y) = 0$ for $y \notin \Pi_i^{(\varepsilon)}$ and $\chi_i(y,\omega) = 0$ for $y \notin \overline{\mathcal{D}}_i$, $i = 1,\ldots,q$. Therefore

$$X^{(\varepsilon)}(r) = \sum_{i=1}^{q}\int_{\mathcal{D}_i}\frac{D_k\chi_\varepsilon(y,(y-r)/|y-r|)}{|r-y|}Q^{(\varepsilon)}(r,y)\,dy$$
$$= \sum_{i=1}^{q}\int_{\mathcal{D}_i}\frac{g_i^{(\varepsilon)}(y)\cdot D_k\chi_i(y,(y-r)/|y-r|)}{|r-y|}Q^{(\varepsilon)}(r,y)\,dy$$
$$+\sum_{i=1}^{q}\int_{\Pi_i^{(\varepsilon)}}\frac{\chi_i(y,(y-r)/|y-r|)D_k g_i^{(\varepsilon)}(y)}{|r-y|}Q^{(\varepsilon)}(r,y)\,dy = X_{1,\varepsilon}(r)+X_{2,\varepsilon}(r),$$

where $X_{1,\varepsilon}(r)$ and $X_{2,\varepsilon}(r)$ are the first and the second sums in the left-hand side of the last equality, respectively. First, we analyze $X_{1,\varepsilon}(r)$. For this purpose, we write

$$X_{1,\varepsilon}(r) = \sum_{i=1}^{q}\Big\{\int_{\mathcal{D}_i}\frac{D_k\chi_i(y,(y-r)/|y-r|)}{|r-y|}Q^{(\varepsilon)}(r,y)\,dy$$
$$+\int_{\mathcal{D}_i}\frac{(g_i^{(\varepsilon)}(y)-1)D_k\chi_i(y,(y-r)/|y-r|)}{|r-y|}Q^{(\varepsilon)}(r,y)\,dy\Big\}.$$

Since $\mathcal{D}_i = \overline{\mathcal{D}}_i^{(\varepsilon)} \cup \Pi_i^{(\varepsilon)}$ and $g_i^{(\varepsilon)}(y) = 1$ for $y \in \mathcal{D}_i^{(\varepsilon)}$, we have

$$X_{1,\varepsilon}(r) = \sum_{i=1}^{q} \Big\{ \int_{\mathcal{D}_i} \frac{D_k\chi_i(y,(y-r)/|y-r|)}{|r-y|} Q^{(\varepsilon)}(r,y)\,dy + \int_{\Pi_i^{(\varepsilon)}} \frac{(g_i^{(\varepsilon)}(y)-1)D_k\chi_i(y,(y-r)/|y-r|)}{|r-y|} Q^{(\varepsilon)}(r,y)\,dy \Big\}. \quad (5)$$

Because $Q^{(\varepsilon)}(r,y)$ uniformly converge to $Q(r,y)$ as $\varepsilon \to 0$, we establish

$$\lim_{\varepsilon\to 0} \int_{\mathcal{D}_i} \frac{D_k\chi_i(y,(y-r)/|y-r|)}{|r-y|} Q^{(\varepsilon)}(r,y)\,dy = \int_{\mathcal{D}_i} \frac{D_k\chi_i(y,(y-r)/|y-r|)}{|r-y|} Q(r,y)\,dy,$$

and this convergence is uniform with respect to $r \in \overline{V}$.

Starting from this point, we will assume that $\varepsilon \le \varepsilon_1$ and $\varepsilon_1$ is sufficiently small, so that $|r-y| \ge \text{const} > 0$ for $r \in \overline{V}$, $y \in \Pi_i^{(\varepsilon)}$, $i = 1,\dots,q$. Then in (5), the absolute values of the integrands are not greater than $\text{const}\cdot|\ln\rho(y,\partial\mathcal{D}_0)|$. Since the function $|\ln\rho(y,\partial\mathcal{D}_0)|$ is integrable in $\mathcal{D}_i$ and

$$\text{mes}_2(\Pi_i^{(\varepsilon)}) \le \text{const}\cdot\varepsilon, \qquad i = 1,\dots,q,$$

it follows that the integrals over $\Pi_i^{(\varepsilon)}$ in (5) converge to zero as $\varepsilon \to 0$ uniformly with respect to $r \in \overline{V}$. Thus, we have established the uniform convergence of the functions $X_{1,\varepsilon}(r)$, $(r \in \overline{V})$ to $X_1(r)$ as $\varepsilon \to 0$, where

$$X_1(r) = \sum_{i=1}^{q} \int_{\mathcal{D}_i} \frac{D_k\chi_i(y,(y-r)/|y-r|)}{|r-y|} Q(r,y)\,dy. \quad (6)$$

We now turn to $X_{2,\varepsilon}(r)$. Integrating by parts (see Tikhonov and Samarskii, 1990; Vladimirov, 1967), we obtain

$$X_{2,\varepsilon}(r) = \sum_{i=1}^{q} \Big\{ -\int_{\Pi_i^{(\varepsilon)}} g_i^{(\varepsilon)}(y) \frac{\partial}{\partial y_k}\Big(\frac{\chi_i(y,(y-r)/|y-r|)}{|r-y|} Q^{(\varepsilon)}(r,y)\Big)\,dy + \int_{\partial\Pi_i^{(\varepsilon)}} \frac{(n_i^{(\varepsilon)}(y)\cdot e_k)\chi_i(y,(y-r)/|y-r|)}{|r-y|} g_i^{(\varepsilon)}(y) Q^{(\varepsilon)}(r,y)\,d\sigma_y \Big\},$$

where $n_i^{(\varepsilon)}(y)$ is the unit vector of the outward normal to the curve $\partial\Pi_i^{(\varepsilon)}$ at the point $y$. Since $\partial\Pi_i^{(\varepsilon)} = \partial\mathcal{D}_i \cup \partial\mathcal{D}_i^{(\varepsilon)}$ and $g_i^{(\varepsilon)}(y) = 0$ for $y \in \partial\mathcal{D}_i$,

$g_i^{(\varepsilon)}(y) = 1$ for $y \in \partial\mathcal{D}_i^{(\varepsilon)}$, it follows that the integrals over $\partial\Pi_i^{(\varepsilon)}$ are simplified as follows

$$X_{2,\varepsilon}(r) = \sum_{i=1}^{q} \Big\{ - \int_{\Pi_i^{(\varepsilon)}} g_i^{(\varepsilon)}(y) \frac{\partial}{\partial y_k} \Big( \frac{\chi_i(y, (y-r)/|y-r|)}{|r-y|} Q^{(\varepsilon)}(r,y) \Big) \, dy$$

$$+ \int_{\partial\mathcal{D}_i^{(\varepsilon)}} \frac{(n_i^{(\varepsilon)}(y) \cdot e_k)\chi_i(y, (y-r)/|y-r|)}{|r-y|} Q^{(\varepsilon)}(r,y) \, d\sigma_y \Big\}. \quad (7)$$

Each integral over $\partial\mathcal{D}_i^{(\varepsilon)}$ in the right-hand side of (7) converges to the limit

$$\int_{\partial\mathcal{D}_i} \frac{(n_i(y) \cdot e_k)\chi_i(y, (y-r)/|y-r|)}{|r-y|} Q(r,y) \, d\sigma_y.$$

uniformly with respect to $r \in \overline{V}$ as $\varepsilon \to 0$ because of the restrictions imposed on the domains $\mathcal{D}_i, \mathcal{D}_i^{(\varepsilon)}$.

Now we consider the integrals in (7) taken over $\Pi_i^{(\varepsilon)}$ and prove that they uniformly converge to zero as $\varepsilon \to 0$. We write the corresponding integrands more explicitly

$$g_i^{(\varepsilon)}(y) \frac{\partial}{\partial y_k} \Big( \frac{1}{|r-y|} \chi_i\Big(y, \frac{y-r}{|y-r|}\Big) Q^{(\varepsilon)}(r,y) \Big)$$

$$= g_i^{(\varepsilon)}(y) \Big( \frac{\partial}{\partial y_k} \frac{1}{|r-y|} \Big) \cdot \chi_i\Big(y, \frac{y-r}{|y-r|}\Big) Q^{(\varepsilon)}(r,y)$$

$$+ \frac{g_i^{(\varepsilon)}(y)}{|r-y|} \Big( \frac{\partial}{\partial y_k} \chi_i\Big(y, \frac{y-r}{|y-r|}\Big) \Big) Q^{(\varepsilon)}(r,y)$$

$$+ \frac{g_i^{(\varepsilon)}(y)}{|r-y|} \chi_i\Big(y, \frac{y-r}{|y-r|}\Big) \frac{\partial}{\partial y_k} Q^{(\varepsilon)}(r,y). \quad (8)$$

As $|r-y| \geq \text{const} > 0$ for $r \in \overline{V}$, and $y \in \Pi_i^{(\varepsilon)}$, the absolute values of the derivatives of $|r-y|^{-1}$ with respect to $y_k$ are bounded. The absolute values of the derivatives of $\chi_i$ are not greater than the integrable function $\text{const} \cdot |\ln \rho(y, \partial\mathcal{D}_0)|$. Therefore, since $\text{mes}_2(\Pi_i^{(\varepsilon)}) \leq \text{const} \cdot \varepsilon$, the integrals of the first two terms in the right-hand side of (7) uniformly converge to zero as $\varepsilon \to 0$.

It remains to establish that the integrals over $\Pi_i^{(\varepsilon)}$ of the last terms in (8) converge to zero. Evidently,

$$\Big|\int_{\Pi_i^{(\varepsilon)}} \frac{g_i^{(\varepsilon)}(y)}{|r-y|}\,\chi_i\Big(y,\frac{y-r}{|y-r|}\Big)\Big(\frac{\partial}{\partial y_k}\,Q^{(\varepsilon)}(r,y)\Big)\,dy\Big|$$
$$\le \text{const}\cdot\int_{\Pi_i^{(\varepsilon)}}\Big|\frac{\partial}{\partial y_k}\,Q^{(\varepsilon)}(r,y)\Big|\,dy. \quad (9)$$

The right-hand side of (9) converges to zero as $\varepsilon\to 0$ uniformly with respect to $r\in\overline{V}$, which follows from the estimate $mes_2(\Pi_i^{(\varepsilon)})\le \text{const}\cdot\varepsilon$, the inequality (4) and the condition (1.2.5).

Thus, we have proved that the integrals over $\Pi_i^{(\varepsilon)}$ in (7) converge to zero as $\varepsilon\to 0$, uniformly with respect to $r\in\overline{V}$. This means that $X_{2,\varepsilon}(r)$, $r\in\overline{V}$ uniformly converges to

$$\sum_{i=1}^{q}\int_{\partial\mathcal{D}_i}\frac{n_i(y)\cdot e_k}{|r-y|}\,\chi_i\Big(y,\frac{y-r}{|y-r|}\Big)\,Q(r,y)\,d\sigma_y.$$

This statement together with the equality (6) implies the assertion of the lemma. □

Suppose that a point $z\in\mathcal{D}$ belongs to the boundaries of two domains $\mathcal{D}_l$ and $\mathcal{D}_j$ only, $1\le l<j\le q$. Assume that the curves $\partial\mathcal{D}_l$ and $\partial\mathcal{D}_j$ are of the class $C^2$ in the neighborhood of the point $z$. Such point $z$ will be called a contact point for the domains $\mathcal{D}_l$ and $\mathcal{D}_j$.

We consider an arbitrary Cartesian coordinate system in $\mathcal{E}^2$ with the center at the point $z$ such that its first coordinate axis is located on the straight line tangent to $\partial\mathcal{D}_l$ at the point $z$. The direction of the second axis coincides with that of the inward normal $n_l(z)$ to $\partial\mathcal{D}_l$. Such a system will be called local coordinate system associated with the point $z\in\partial\mathcal{D}_l$. From here and up to the end of the proof of Lemma 5 we will use the representation of vectors in this system, in particular $y=(y_1,y_2,y_3)$, $z=(0,0,0)$ and $n_l(z)=(0,0,1)$.

By $\mathrm{C}_z$ we denote the set

$$\mathrm{C}_z=\{y\in\mathcal{E}^2\mid y=(y_1,y_2),\ |y_1|\le\delta<1,\ |y_2|\le\delta_1<1\},$$

By our assumptions, there exist sufficiently small positive numbers $\delta,\delta_1$ such that the curve $\partial\mathcal{D}_{l,z}=\partial\mathcal{D}_l\cap\mathrm{C}_z=\partial\mathcal{D}_j\cap\mathrm{C}_z=\partial\mathcal{D}_{j,z}$ can be represented as the graph of a smooth function $y_2=q(y_1)$:

$$\partial\mathcal{D}_{l,z}=\{y\in\mathcal{E}^2\mid y=(y_1,q(y_1)),\ |y_1|\le\delta\}, \quad (10)$$

where $C_z^+ = \{y \in C_z \mid y_2 - q(y_1) > 0\}$ is a subset of $\mathcal{D}_l$ and $C_z^- = \{y \in C_z \mid y_2 - q(y_1) < 0\}$ in a subset of $\mathcal{D}_j$. The function $q(y_1)$ has the following properties:

$$|q(y_1)| \leq \text{const} \cdot y_1^2, \qquad \left|\frac{dq}{dy_1}(y_1)\right| \leq \text{const} \cdot |y_1|, \quad |y_1| \leq \delta. \tag{11}$$

We consider the set $Z = \{r \in \mathcal{E}^2 \mid r = z + tn_l(z),\ 0 < t < \delta_1\}$, where $\delta_1$ is small enough that $\rho(r, \partial\mathcal{D}_0) = |r - z|$. Let $m_0(r, \omega)$: $Z \times \Omega_1 \to \mathcal{E}^1$ be a continuous and bounded function. We introduce the expression

$$I(r) = \int_{\partial\mathcal{D}_{l,z}} \frac{m_0(r, (y - r)/|y - r|)}{|r - y|}\, d\sigma_y, \tag{12}$$

where the integral is a curvilinear integral of the first kind. We define the function $\mathcal{M}(r, y_1', y_1'')$, $r \in Z$, $y_1' \in [-\delta, 0]$, $y_2'' \in [0, \delta]$ by the formula

$$\mathcal{M}(r, y_1', y_1'') = m_0\Big(r, \frac{y(y_1') - r}{|y(y_1') - r|}\Big) + m_0\Big(r, \frac{y(y_1'') - r}{|y(y_1'') - r|}\Big). \tag{13}$$

If the function $m_0(r, \omega)$ is defined for $r = z$, $\omega = \pm s$, where $s$ is the unit vector of the axis $Oy_1$, then we also define the function $M$:

$$M(z) = m_0(z, s) + m_0(z, -s). \tag{14}$$

In these designations the following statement holds.

**Lemma 5.** *There exist the functions $t_1(r) : Z \to [-\delta, 0]$, $t_2(r) : Z \to [0, \delta]$, such that*

$$I(r) = \mathcal{M}(r, t_1(r), t_2(r))\, |\ln \rho(r, \partial\mathcal{D}_0)| + O(1), \tag{15}$$

*where $O(1)$ is a function bounded for $0 < |t| < \delta_1$. If the function $m_0$ is defined also for the points $(z, s)$ and $(z, -s)$ and satisfies the Holder condition*

$$|m_0(r, \omega) - m_0(z, s_0)| \leq \text{const} \cdot \{|r - z|^\gamma + |\omega - s_0|^\gamma\},$$
$$\gamma \in (0, 1), \qquad s_0 = \pm s. \tag{16}$$

*then*

$$I(r) = M(z)\, |\ln \rho(r, \partial\mathcal{D}_0)| + O(1). \tag{17}$$

**Proof.** Taking into account the representation (10), we write the integral $I(r)$ as follows:

$$I(r) = \int_{-\delta}^{\delta} \frac{m_0(r,(y-r)/|y-r|)}{|r-y|} \sqrt{1+q'^2(y_1))}\, dy_1 = A_1(r) + A_2(r),$$

where

$$A_1(r) = \int_{-\delta}^{\delta} \frac{m_0(r,(y-r)/|y-r|)}{|r-y|}\, dy_1,$$

$$A_2(r) = \int_{-\delta}^{\delta} \frac{m_0(r,(y-r)/|y-r|)}{|r-y|} [\sqrt{1+q'^2(y_1)} - 1]\, dy_1.$$

It is easy to see that

$$\sqrt{1+q'^2(y_1)} - 1 = \frac{q'^2(y_1)}{\sqrt{1+q'^2(y_1)}+1} \le q'^2(y_1) \le \text{const} \cdot y_1^2.$$

Since $r = (0,t)$, $y = (y_1, y_2)$ and $|y_1| < 1$, then

$$|r-y| = \sqrt{y_1^2 + (y_2-t)^2} \ge |y_1| > |y_1|^2.$$

Therefore taking into account the boundedness of $m_0(r,\omega)$ and the inequality $|r-y|^{-1}y_1^2 \le 1$, we obtain that $|A_2(r)| \le$ const and, hence, $I(r) = A_1(r) + O(1)$.

To calculate the integral

$$A_1(r) = \int_{-\delta}^{\delta} \frac{m_0(r,(y-r)/|y-r|)}{\sqrt{y_1^2+(y_2-t)^2}}\, dy_1,$$

we make certain transformations. It is evidently that

$$\frac{1}{\sqrt{y_1^2+(y_2-t^2)}} = \frac{1}{\sqrt{y_1^2+t^2}} + \frac{1}{\sqrt{y_1^2+(y_2-t)^2}} - \frac{1}{\sqrt{y_1^2+t^2}}$$

We denote the sum of the last two terms by $B_1$ and have

$$B_1 = \frac{\sqrt{y_1^2+t^2} - \sqrt{y_1^2+(y_2-t)^2}}{\sqrt{y_1^2+(y_2-t)^2}\,\sqrt{y_1^2+t^2}} = \Big[\sqrt{\frac{y_1^2+t^2}{y_1^2+(y_2-t)^2}} - 1\Big]\sqrt{y_1^2+t^2}$$

$$= \Big[\frac{y_1^2+t^2}{y_1^2+(y_2-t)^2} - 1\Big](y_1^2+t^2)^{-1}\Big[1+\sqrt{\frac{y_1^2+t^2}{y_1^2+(y_2-t)^2}}\Big]^{-1}.$$

This implies that

$$|B_1| \le \frac{|y_1^2+t^2-y_1^2-(y_2-t)^2|}{\sqrt{y_1^2+t^2}[y_1^2+(y_2-t)^2]} = \left|\frac{y_2(2t-y_2)}{y_1^2\sqrt{y_1^2+t^2}}\right|\left[1+\left(\frac{y_2-t}{y_1}\right)^2\right]^{-1}$$

$$\le \text{const}\cdot\frac{|2t-y_2|}{\sqrt{y_1^2+t^2}} \le \text{const}\cdot\frac{|t|}{\sqrt{y_1^2+t^2}} + \text{const}\cdot|y_1|.$$

Thus, $A_1(r) = A_3(r) + A_4(r)$, where

$$A_3(r) = \int_{-\delta}^{\delta} \frac{m_0(r,(y-r)/|y-r|)}{\sqrt{y_1^2+t^2}}\,dy_1, \tag{18}$$

$$A_4(r) = \int_{-\delta}^{\delta} m_0\Big(r,\frac{y-r}{|y-r|}\Big)\Big[\frac{1}{\sqrt{y_1^2+(y_2-t)^2}} - \frac{1}{\sqrt{y_1^2+t^2}}\Big]\,dy_1. \tag{19}$$

The inequality pointed above and the boundedness of $m_0(r,\omega)$ provide

$$|A_4(r)| \le \text{const}\cdot\int_{-\delta}^{\delta}\frac{dy_1}{\sqrt{y_1^2+t^2}} + \text{const}\cdot\int_{-\delta}^{\delta}|y_1|\,dy_1$$

$$= \text{const}\cdot|t|\ln\left|\frac{\sqrt{\delta^2+t^2}+\delta}{\sqrt{\delta^2+t^2}-\delta}\right| + O(1),$$

therefore, $I(r) = A_3(r) + O(1)$. It remains to evaluate $A_3(r)$. The representation (18) yields

$$A_3(r) = \int_{-\delta}^{0}\frac{m_0(r,(y-r)/|y-r|)}{\sqrt{y_1^2+t^2}}\,dy_1 + \int_{0}^{\delta}\frac{m_0(r,(y-r)/|y-r|)}{\sqrt{y_1^2+t^2}}\,dy_1.$$

Since the function $m_0(r,\omega)$ is continuous and the function $(y_1^2+t^2)^{1/2}$ is nonnegative for $y_1 \in [-\delta,\delta]$ by the Integral Mean Value Theorem (see Zorich, 1981) for any $r \in Z$ there exist point $t_1(r) \in [-\delta, 0]$ and $t_2(r) \in [0,\delta]$ such that

$$A_3(r) = m_0\Big(r,\frac{y(t_1(r))-r}{|y(t_1(r))-r|}\Big)\int_{-\delta}^{0}\frac{dy_1}{\sqrt{y_1^2+t^2}}\,dy_1$$

$$+\, m_0\Big(r,\frac{y(t_2(r))-r}{|y(t_2(r))-r|}\Big)\int_{0}^{\delta}\frac{dy_1}{\sqrt{y_1^2+t^2}}\,dy_1$$

$$= \Big[m_0\Big(r,\frac{y(t_1(r))-r}{|y(t_1(r))-r|}\Big) + m_0\Big(r,\frac{y(t_2(r))-r}{|y(t_2(r))-r|}\Big)\Big]\int_{0}^{\delta}\frac{dy_1}{\sqrt{y_1^2+t^2}}\,dy_1$$

$$= \mathcal{M}(r,t_1(r),t_2(r))\ln\left|\frac{\sqrt{\delta^2+t^2}+\delta}{t}\right| = \mathcal{M}(r,t_1(r),t_2(r))|\ln|t|| + O(1).$$

Since $|t| = \rho(r,\partial\mathcal{D}_0)$ the formula (15) is proved.

We make the following evaluation before starting the proof of the second part of the lemma. It is easy to see that

$$\frac{1}{y_1^2+(y_2-t)^2}-\frac{1}{y_1^2+t^2}=\frac{2y_2t-y_2^2}{(y_1^2+(y_2-t)^2)(y_1^2+t^2)}.$$

Since $|y_2|\le \text{const}\cdot y_1^2$, then

$$\frac{|2y_2t|}{(y_1^2+(y_2-t)^2)(y_1^2+t^2)}\le\frac{\text{const}\cdot y_1^2}{y_1^2+(y_2-t)^2}\cdot\frac{|t|}{y_1^2+t^2}\le\frac{\text{const}}{\sqrt{y_1^2+t^2}},$$

$$\frac{y_2^2}{(y_1^2+(y_2-t)^2)(y_1^2+t^2)}\le\frac{\text{const}\cdot y_1^4}{(y_1^2+(y_2-t)^2)(y_1^2+t^2)}\le\text{const}\,.$$

Therefore

$$\left|\frac{1}{y_1^2+(y_2-t)^2}-\frac{1}{y_1^2+t^2}\right|\le\frac{\text{const}}{\sqrt{y_1^2+t^2}}.\tag{20}$$

Now let the conditions (16) be satisfied. Therefore, for $\omega=(y-r)\cdot|y-r|^{-1}$ we have

$$\left|m_0\Big(r,\frac{y-r}{|y-r|}\Big)-m_0(z,s_0)\right|\le\text{const}\cdot\Big\{|t|^\gamma+\left|\frac{y-r}{|y-r|}-s_0\right|^\gamma\Big\},\tag{21}$$

where $s_0=\pm s$. We estimate

$$\left|\frac{y-r}{|y-r|}-s_0\right|^2=2\,\frac{|y-r|-(y-r)\cdot s_0}{|y-r|}.$$

Since $y=(y_1,y_2)$, $r=(0,t)$, then $|y-r|=(y_1^2+(y_2-t)^2)^{1/2}$, $(y-r)\cdot s_0=y_1$. Consequently, by virtue of the inequality $\sqrt{t_1}-\sqrt{t_2}\le\sqrt{t_1-t_2}$, where $t_1\ge t_2\ge 0$, we get

$$\left|\frac{y-r}{|y-r|}-s_0\right|^2=\frac{2}{|y-r|}\,\Big(\sqrt{y_1^2+(y_2-t)^2}-\sqrt{y_1^2}\Big)\le\frac{2}{|y-r|}\,|y_2-t|.$$

Using the inequality $|t_1-t_2|^\gamma\le|t_1|^\gamma+|t_2|^\gamma$, where $t_1\ge t_2$, we obtain

$$\left|\frac{y-r}{|y-r|}-s_0\right|^\gamma\le\text{const}\cdot\frac{|y_2|^{\gamma/2}+|t|^{\gamma/2}}{(y_1^2+(y_2-t)^2)^{\gamma/4}}.\tag{22}$$

We write the evident equality

$$\frac{1}{y_1^2+(y_2-t)^2}=\frac{1}{y_1^2+t^2}+\Big(\frac{1}{y_1^2+(y_2-t)^2}-\frac{1}{y_1^2+t^2}\Big).$$

The estimate (20) applied to the expression in parentheses yields

$$\frac{1}{y_1^2+(y_2-t)^2} \le \frac{1}{y_1^2+t^2} + \frac{\text{const}}{\sqrt{y_1^2+t^2}} \le \frac{\text{const}}{y_1^2+t^2},$$

therefore

$$\left|\frac{y-r}{|y-r|} - s_0\right|^\gamma \le \text{const}\cdot\frac{|y_2|^{\gamma/2}+|t|^{\gamma/2}}{(y_1^2+(y_2-t)^2)^{\gamma/4}} \le \text{const}\cdot\frac{|y_2|^{\gamma/2}+|t|^{\gamma/2}}{(y_1^2+t^2)^{\gamma/4}}.$$

The last inequality and (21) imply

$$\begin{aligned}\left|m_0\Big(r,\frac{y-r}{|y-r|}\Big) - m_0(z,s)\right| &\le \text{const}\cdot\Big\{|t|^\gamma + \frac{|y_2|^{\gamma/2}+|t|^{\gamma/2}}{(y_1^2+t^2)^{\gamma/4}}\Big\}\\ &\le \text{const}\cdot\Big\{|t|^\gamma + \frac{|y_1|^{\gamma}+|t|^{\gamma/2}}{(y_1^2+t^2)^{\gamma/4}}\Big\}. \end{aligned} \tag{23}$$

We represented the integrals $A_3(r)$ in the form $A_3(r) = A_5(r) + A_6(r) + A_7(r)$, where

$$\begin{aligned} A_5(r) &= \int_{-\delta}^{0} \frac{m_0(r,-s)}{\sqrt{y_1^2+t^2}}\,dy_1 + \int_0^\delta \frac{m_0(r,s)}{\sqrt{y_1^2+t^2}}\,dy_1,\\ A_6(r) &= \int_{-\delta}^{0} \frac{1}{\sqrt{y_1^2+t^2}}\Big[m_0\Big(r,\frac{y-r}{|y-r|}\Big) - m_0(r,-s)\Big]\,dy_1,\\ A_7(r) &= \int_0^\delta \frac{1}{\sqrt{y_1^2+t^2}}\Big[m_0\Big(r,\frac{y-r}{|y-r|}\Big) - m_0(r,s)\Big]\,dy_1. \end{aligned}$$

By virtue of (23) we obtain

$$|A_7(r)| \le \text{const}\cdot\Big\{\int_0^\delta \frac{|t|^\gamma}{\sqrt{y_1^2+t^2}}\,dy_1 + \int_0^\delta \frac{|y_1|^\gamma+|t|^{\gamma/2}}{(y_1^2+t^2)^{1/2+\gamma/4}}\,dy_1\Big\}.$$

Using simply calculation, we see that

$$\int_0^\delta \frac{|t|^\gamma}{\sqrt{y_1^2+t^2}}\,dy_1 = |t|^\gamma[\ln|\delta+\sqrt{\delta^2+t^2}| - \ln|t|] \le \text{const},$$

$$\int_0^\delta \frac{|y_1|^\gamma}{(y_1^2+t^2)^{1/2+\gamma/4}}\,dy_1 \le \int_0^\delta \frac{|y_1|^\gamma}{|y_1|^{1+\gamma/2}}\,dy_1 = \int_0^\delta \frac{dy_1}{y_1^{1-\gamma/2}} = \frac{2\delta^{\gamma/2}}{\gamma} \le \text{const}\,.$$

The evident inequality $(a+b)^2 \le 2(a^2+b^2)$; $a, b, \in \mathcal{E}^1$ yields that

$$\int_0^\delta \frac{|t|^{\gamma/2}\,dy_1}{(y_1^2+t^2)^{1/2+\gamma/4}} \le 2^{1/2+\gamma/4}|t|^{\gamma/2}\int_0^\delta \frac{dy_1}{(y_1+|t|)^{1+\gamma/2}}$$
$$- \frac{2^{3/2+\gamma/4}}{\gamma}|t|^{\gamma/2}\big[(\delta+|t|)^{-\gamma/2}-|t|^{-\gamma/2}\big] \le \text{const}\,.$$

Thus, $|A_7(r)| \le \text{const}$. By the same way it can be proved that $|A_6(r)| \le \text{const}$. Hence,

$$|I(r)| = A_5(r) + O(1) = \int_0^\delta \frac{m_0(z,-s)+m_0(z,s)}{\sqrt{y_1^2+t^2}}\,dy_1 + O(1)$$
$$= M(z)\int_0^\delta \frac{dy_1}{\sqrt{y_1^2+t^2}} + O(1) = M(z)\ln\left|\frac{\sqrt{\delta^2+t^2}+\delta}{t}\right| + O(1)$$
$$= M(z)\,|\ln|t|| + O(1).$$

Thus $|t| = \rho(r, \partial\mathcal{D}_0)$, then the formula (17) is proved. This means that the lemma is proved. □

**Remark 2.** It is easy to see that $\mathcal{M}(z, y_1', y_1'') \to M(z)$ as $y_1', y_1'' \to 0$ if the condition (16) holds.

We recall that $P(r,\omega) = N(r,\omega) + J(r,\omega)$, $P_\varepsilon(r,\omega) = N_\varepsilon(r,\omega) + J_\varepsilon(r,\omega)$. Let $a(r)$, $r \in \mathcal{E}^2$ be an arbitrary function vanishing outside of $\overline{\mathcal{D}}$ and having uniformly continuous partial derivatives up to the second order in $\mathcal{D}_i$, $i = 1, \ldots, q$. In particular, $a(r)$ may be equal to $\mu(r)$. We consider the set of functions

$$U^{(\varepsilon)}(r) = \int_{\Omega_1} \exp\Big(-\int_0^{d(r,\omega)} a_\varepsilon(r+t\omega)\,dt\Big) D_k f^{(\varepsilon)}(r,\omega)\,d\omega, \quad r \in \mathcal{D}, \quad (24)$$

where $k = 1, 2$, $\varepsilon \in (0, \varepsilon_0]$, and the functions $f^{(\varepsilon)}(r,\omega)$ are defined by (3).

**Lemma 6.** *The functions $U^{(\varepsilon)}(r)$ are continuous in $\mathcal{D}$ and converge to the limit $U(r)$, as $\varepsilon \to 0$ uniformly with respect to $r \in \overline{V}$ ($\overline{V} \subset \mathcal{D}_0$), where*

$$U(r) = \sum_{i=1}^q \int_{\partial\mathcal{D}_i} \frac{n_i(y)\cdot e_k}{|r-y|} \exp\Big(-\int_0^{d(r,(r-y)/|r-y|)} a\Big(r + t\frac{r-y}{|r-y|}\Big)\,dt\Big) \times$$

$$\times \Big\{ -\mu_i(y) f\Big(r, \frac{r-y}{|r-y|}\Big) + P_i\Big(y, \frac{r-y}{|r-y|}\Big)\Big\}\, d\sigma_y + U_0(r) + O(1), \qquad r \in \mathcal{D}_0. \quad (25)$$

*Here $U_0(r)$ is a function continuous in $\mathcal{D}_0$ and bounded in every set $\mathcal{D}_0 \cup \mathcal{D}'$; $\mathcal{D}'$ is a domain such that $\overline{\mathcal{D}'} \subset \mathcal{D}$; $O(1)$ is a bounded function in $\mathcal{D}_0$.*

**Proof.** Suppose $\mathcal{D}'$ is a domain such that $\overline{\mathcal{D}'} \subset \mathcal{D}$. By Lemma 1 $d(r,\omega) \in C(\overline{\mathcal{D}'} \times \Omega_1)$. For any $\varepsilon \in (0, \varepsilon_0]$, the functions $a_\varepsilon(r)$ and $D_k f^{(\varepsilon)}(r,\omega)$ belong to $C(\overline{\mathcal{D}} \times \Omega_1)$ and hence to $C(\overline{\mathcal{D}'} \times \Omega_1)$. Therefore, taking into account (24), we have $U^{(\varepsilon)}(r) \in C(\overline{\mathcal{D}'})$. Since $\mathcal{D}'$ is arbitrary, $U^{(\varepsilon)}(r) \in C(\mathcal{D})$.

We now analyze the convergence of $U^{(\varepsilon)}(r)$ as $\varepsilon \to 0$. We will write $D_k f^{(\varepsilon)}(r,\omega)$ more explicitly taking into account (3). Note that, by Lemma 1, the function $d(r,\omega)$ has the derivative $D_k d(r,\omega)$ continuous in $\mathcal{D} \times \Omega_1$ and possibly unbounded only for $r \to \partial\mathcal{D}$. Note that the functions $\mu_\varepsilon(r)$ and $P_\varepsilon(r,\omega)$ are equal to zero for $r \in \partial\mathcal{D}$. Thus, we have

$$D_k f^{(\varepsilon)}(r,\omega) = I_{0,\varepsilon}(r,\omega) + I_{1,\varepsilon}(r,\omega) + I_{2,\varepsilon}(r,\omega) + I_{3,\varepsilon}(r,\omega), \qquad (26)$$

where

$$I_{0,\varepsilon}(r,\omega) = \exp\Big(-\int_0^{d(r,-\omega)} \mu_\varepsilon(r - t'\omega)\, dt'\Big) D_k \tilde{h}(r,\omega),$$

$$I_{1,\varepsilon}(r,\omega) = -\tilde{h}(r,\omega) \exp\Big(-\int_0^{d(r,-\omega)} \mu_\varepsilon(r - \nu\omega)\, d\nu\Big) \times \int_0^{d(r,-\omega)} D_k \mu_\varepsilon(r - t'\omega)\, dt',$$

$$I_{2,\varepsilon}(r,\omega) = -\int_0^{d(r,-\omega)} \exp\Big(-\int_0^t \mu_\varepsilon(r - \nu\omega)\, d\nu\Big) \times \int_0^t D_k \mu_\varepsilon(r - t'\omega)\, dt' \cdot P_\varepsilon(r - t\omega, \omega)\, dt,$$

$$I_{3,\varepsilon}(r,\omega) = \int_0^{d(r,-\omega)} \exp\Big(-\int_0^t \mu_\varepsilon(r - t'\omega)\, dt'\Big) D_k P_\varepsilon(r - t\omega, \omega)\, dt.$$

We replace $t'$ by $\nu$ wherever needed for convenience. A similar change will be used bellow. The relations (24) and (26) yield

$$U^{(\varepsilon)}(r) = U_{0,\varepsilon}(r) + U_{1,\varepsilon}(r) + U_{2,\varepsilon}(r) + U_{3,\varepsilon}(r),$$

$$U_{j,\varepsilon}(r) = \int_{\Omega_1} \exp\Big(-\int_0^{d(r,\omega)} a_\varepsilon(r + t'\omega) dt'\Big)\, I_{j,\varepsilon}(r,\omega)\, d\omega, \quad j = 0,1,2,3.$$

In particular

$$U_{0,\varepsilon}(r) = \int_{\Omega_1} \exp\Big(-\int_0^{d(r,\omega)} a_\varepsilon(r+\nu\omega)\,d\nu\Big) \times \exp\Big(-\int_0^{d(r,-\omega)} \mu_\varepsilon(r-t'\omega)\,dt'\Big)\cdot D_k\tilde{h}(r,\omega)d\omega.$$

As follows from Remark 1, $U_{0,\varepsilon}(r)$ converge to $U_0(r)$ as $\varepsilon \to 0$ uniformly with respect to $r \in \overline{V}$, where

$$U_0(r) = \int_{\Omega_1} \exp\Big(-\int_0^{d(r,\omega)} a(r+\nu\omega)\,d\nu\Big) \times \exp\Big(-\int_0^{d(r,-\omega)} \mu(r-t'\omega)\,dt'\Big) D_k\tilde{h}(r,\omega)\,d\omega. \quad (27)$$

It is clear that the function $U_0(r)$ is continuous for $r \in \overline{V}$. As $V$ is arbitrary, $U_0(r)$ may be unbounded only in the neighborhood of $\partial\mathcal{D}$, i.e. where the function $D_k\tilde{h}(r,\omega)$ may be unbounded.

Now consider $U_{1,\varepsilon}(r)$

$$U_{1,\varepsilon}(r) = -\int_{\Omega_1} \exp\Big(-\int_0^{d(r,\omega)} a_\varepsilon(r+t'\omega)\,dt'\Big)\tilde{h}(r,\omega) \times \exp\Big(-\int_0^{d(r,-\omega)} \mu_\varepsilon(r-\nu\omega)\,d\nu\Big)\int_0^{d(r,-\omega)} D_k\mu_\varepsilon(r-t'\omega)\,dt'\,d\omega.$$

Making the change $y = r - t'\omega$, we obtain

$$U_{1,\varepsilon}(r) = -\int_{\mathcal{D}} \frac{D_k\mu_\varepsilon(y)}{|r-y|} Q_{1,\varepsilon}(r,y)\,dy,$$

where

$$Q_{1,\varepsilon}(r,y) = \exp\Big(-\int_0^{d(r,(r-y)/|r-y|)} a_\varepsilon\Big(r+t'\frac{r-y}{|r-y|}\Big)\,dt'\Big) \times \exp\Big(-\int_0^{d(r,(y-r)/|y-r|)} \mu_\varepsilon\Big(r-\nu\frac{r-y}{|r-y|}\Big)\,d\nu\Big)\tilde{h}\Big(r,\frac{r-y}{|r-y|}\Big).$$

It is easy to verify that every $Q_{1,\varepsilon}(r,y)$ satisfies all the conditions of Lemma 4 for the function $Q^{(\varepsilon)}(r,y)$. Therefore, $U_{1,\varepsilon}(r)$ tend to $U_1(r)$ as

$\varepsilon \to 0$ uniformly with respect to $r \in \overline{V}$, where

$$U_1(r) = -\sum_{i=1}^{q} \int_{\mathcal{D}_i} \frac{D_k\mu_i(y)}{|r-y|}\, Q_1(r,y)\, dy - \sum_{i=1}^{q} \int_{\partial\mathcal{D}_i} \frac{n_i(y)\cdot e_k}{|r-y|}\, \mu_i(y) Q_1(r,y)\, d\sigma_y, \tag{28}$$

$$Q_1(r,y) = \exp\Big(-\int_0^{d(r,(r-y)/|r-y|)} a\Big(r + t'\,\frac{r-y}{|r-y|}\Big)\, dt'\Big)$$
$$\times \exp\Big(-\int_0^{d(r,(y-r)/|y-r|)} \mu\Big(r-\nu\,\frac{r-y}{|r-y|}\Big)\, d\nu\Big) \tilde{h}\Big(r, \frac{r-y}{|r-y|}\Big).$$

We now transform $U_{2,\varepsilon}(r)$. To this end, we change the order of integration in the expression for $I_{2,\varepsilon}(r,\omega)$. Instead of integration first by $t'$ ($t' \in (0,t)$) and then by $t$ ($t \in (0, d(r,-\omega))$), we integrate first by $t$ ($t \in (t', d(r,-\omega))$) and then by $t'$ ($t' \in (0, d(r,-\omega))$). As a result, we obtain

$$I_{2,\varepsilon}(r,\omega) = -\int_0^{d(r,-\omega)} D_k\mu_\varepsilon(r - t'\omega)$$
$$\Big(\int_{t'}^{d(r,-\omega)} \exp\Big(-\int_0^t \mu_\varepsilon(r-\nu\omega)\, d\nu\Big) P_\varepsilon(r - t\omega, \omega)\, dt\Big)\, dt'.$$

The change of variables $y = r - t'\omega$ leads to the equality

$$U_{2,\varepsilon}(r) = -\int_G \frac{D_k\mu_\varepsilon(y)}{|r-y|}\, Q_{2,\varepsilon}(r,y)\, dy,$$

where

$$Q_{2,\varepsilon}(r,y) = \int_{|r-y|}^{d(r,(y-r)/|y-r|)} \exp\Big(-\int_0^t \mu_\varepsilon\Big(r-\nu\,\frac{r-y}{|r-y|}\Big)\, d\nu$$
$$\times P_\varepsilon\Big(r - t\frac{r-y}{|r-y|}, \frac{r-y}{|r-y|}\Big)\, dt \cdot \exp\Big(-\int_0^{d(r,(r-y)/|r-y|)} a_\varepsilon\Big(r + t'\,\frac{r-y}{|r-y|}\Big)\, dt'\Big).$$

Using Lemma 4, we can show that $U_{2,\varepsilon}(r)$ converge to $U_2(r)$ as $\varepsilon \to 0$ uniformly with respect to $r \in \overline{V}$, where

$$U_2(r) = -\sum_{i=1}^{q} \int_{\mathcal{D}_i} \frac{D_k\mu_i(y)}{|r-y|}\, Q_2(r,y)\, dy$$
$$-\sum_{i=1}^{q} \int_{\partial\mathcal{D}_i} \frac{n_i(y)\cdot e_k}{|r-y|}\, \mu_i(y) Q_2(r,y)\, d_y\sigma, \tag{29}$$

$$Q_2(r,y) = \exp\Big(-\int_0^{d(r,(r-y)/|r-y|)} a\Big(r + t'\,\frac{r-y}{|r-y|}\Big)\,dt'\Big) \times \int_{|r-y|}^{d(r,(r-y)/|r-y|)} \exp\Big(-\int_0^t \mu\Big(r - \nu\,\frac{r-y}{|r-y|}\Big)\,d\nu\Big) \times P\Big(r - t\,\frac{r-y}{|r-y|}, \frac{r-y}{|r-y|}\Big)\,dt.$$

It remains to analyze $U_{3,\varepsilon}(r)$. We have

$$U_{3,\varepsilon}(r) = \int_{\Omega_1} \exp\Big(-\int_0^{d(r,\omega)} a_\varepsilon(r+\nu\omega)\,d\nu\Big) \times \int_0^{d(r,-\omega)} \exp\Big(-\int_0^t \mu_\varepsilon(r - t'\omega)\,dt'\Big) D_k P_\varepsilon(r - t\omega, \omega)\,dt\,d\omega.$$

Making the change of variables $y = r - t\omega$, we obtain

$$U_{3,\varepsilon}(r) = \int_{\mathcal{D}} \frac{D_k P_\varepsilon(y,(r-y)/|r-y|)}{|r-y|}\,Q_{3,\varepsilon}(r,y)\,dy,$$

where

$$Q_{3,\varepsilon}(r,y) = \exp\Big(-\int_0^{d(r,(r-y)/|r-y|)} a_\varepsilon\Big(r + \nu\,\frac{r-y}{|r-y|}\Big)\,d\nu\Big) \times \exp\Big(-\int_0^{|r-y|} \mu_\varepsilon\Big(r - t'\,\frac{r-y}{|r-y|}\Big)\,dt'\Big).$$

Applying Lemma 4 to $U_{3,\varepsilon}(r)$, we see that $U_{3,\varepsilon}(r)$ converge to $U_3(r)$ as $\varepsilon \to 0$ uniformly with respect to $r \in \overline{V}$, where

$$U_3(r) = \sum_{i=1}^{q} \int_{\mathcal{D}_i} \frac{D_k P_i(y,(r-y)/|r-y|)}{|r-y|}\,Q_3(r,y)\,dy + \sum_{i=1}^{q} \int_{\partial\mathcal{D}_i} \frac{n_i(y)\cdot e_k}{|r-y|}\,P_i\Big(y, \frac{r-y}{|r-y|}\Big) Q_3(r,y)\,d\sigma_y, \tag{30}$$

$$Q_3(r,y) = \exp\Big(-\int_0^{d(r,(r-y)/|r-y|)} a\Big(r + \nu\,\frac{r-y}{|r-y|}\Big)\,d\nu\Big) \times \exp\Big(-\int_0^{|r-y|} \mu\Big(r - t'\,\frac{r-y}{|r-y|}\Big)\,dt'\Big).$$

The next part of the proof will consist in the summation of $U_j(r)$, $j = 0, 1, 2, 3$, and the transformation of the resulting sum. Taking into account the equalities (27)–(30), we see that $U(r) = U_0(r) + \ldots + U_3(r)$ has the form

$$U(r) = \sum_{i=1}^{q} \int_{\mathcal{D}_i} \frac{1}{|r-y|} \Big\{ - D_k \mu_i(y)(Q_1(r,y) + (Q_2(r,y)) + \Big( D_k P_i\Big(y, \frac{r-y}{|r-y|}\Big)\Big) Q_3(r,y) \Big\}\, dy$$
$$+ \sum_{i=1}^{q} \int_{\partial\mathcal{D}_i} \frac{n_i(y)\cdot e_k}{|r-y|} \Big\{ - \mu_i(y)\Big(Q_1(r,y) + Q_2(r,y)\Big) + P_i\Big(y, \frac{r-y}{|r-y|}\Big) Q_3(r,y) \Big\}\, d\sigma_y + U_0(r). \quad (31)$$

From general properties of the potential-type integrals with weak singularity it follows that the integrals over $\mathcal{D}_i$ in (31) are bounded functions in $\mathcal{D}_0$ and their sum can be replaced by $O(1)$. The integrals over $\partial\mathcal{D}_i$ are of major interest here.

We set

$$\Phi_i(r,y) = -\mu_i(y)(Q_1(r,y) + Q_2(r,y)) + P_i\Big(y, \frac{r-y}{|r-y|}\Big) Q_3(r,y), \quad i = 1, \ldots, q. \quad (32)$$

and transform these functions. First, we note that

$$Q_2(r,y) = \exp\Big( - \int_0^{d(r,(r-y)/|r-y|)} a\Big(r + t' \frac{r-y}{|r-y|}\Big)\, dt' \Big) \times \int_0^{d(r,(y-r)/|y-r|)} \exp\Big( - \int_0^t \mu\Big(r - \nu \frac{r-y}{|r-y|}\Big)\, d\nu \Big) \times P\Big(r - t\frac{r-y}{|r-y|}, \frac{r-y}{|r-y|}\Big)\, dt + Q_4(r,y),$$

$$Q_4(r,y) = -\exp\Big( - \int_0^{d(r,(r-y)/|r-y|)} a\Big(r + t' \frac{r-y}{|r-y|}\Big)\, dt' \Big) \times \int_0^{|r-y|} \exp\Big( - \int_0^t \mu\Big(r - \nu \frac{r-y}{|r-y|}\Big)\, d\nu \Big) \times P\Big(r - t\frac{r-y}{|r-y|}, \frac{r-y}{|r-y|}\Big)\, dt. \quad (33)$$

It is easy to see that $|Q_4(r,y)| \le \text{const} \cdot |r-y|$.

For $Q_3(r,y)$ we make the similar transformation:

$$Q_3(r,y) = \exp\Big(-\int_0^{d\left(r,(r-y)/|r-y|\right)} a\Big(r+\nu\,\frac{r-y}{|r-y|}\Big)\,d\nu\Big) + Q_5(r,y), \quad (34)$$

$$Q_5(r,y) = \exp\Big(-\int_0^{d(r,(r-y)/|r-y|)} a\Big(r+\nu\,\frac{r-y}{|r-y|}\Big)\,d\nu\Big) \times \Big(\exp\Big(-\int_0^{|r-y|} \mu\Big(r-t'\,\frac{r-y}{|r-y|}\Big)\,dt'\Big)-1\Big).$$

Evidently, $|Q_5(r,y)| \le \mathrm{const}\cdot|r-y|$.

Taking into account the equalities (33), (34) we transform the equality (32) as follows

$$\Phi_i(r,y) = \exp\Big(-\int_0^{d(r,(r-y)/|r-y|)} a\Big(r+t'\,\frac{r-y}{|r-y|}\Big)\,dt'\Big)$$
$$\times\Big\{-\mu_i(y)\Big(\tilde h\Big(r,\frac{r-y}{|r-y|}\Big)\cdot\exp\Big(-\int_0^{d(r,(y-r)/|y-r|)} \mu\Big(r-t'\,\frac{r-y}{|r-y|}\Big)\,dt'\Big)$$
$$+\int_0^{d(r,(y-r)/|y-r|)} \exp\Big(-\int_0^t \mu\Big(r-\nu\,\frac{r-y}{|r-y|}\Big)\,d\nu\Big)\cdot P\Big(r-t\,\frac{r-y}{|r-y|},\frac{r-y}{|r-y|}\Big)\,dt\Big)$$
$$+P_i\Big(y,\frac{r-y}{|r-y|}\Big)\Big\} - \mu_i(y)Q_4(r,y) + P_i\Big(y,\frac{r-y}{|r-y|}\Big)Q_5(r,y). \quad (35)$$

The estimates for $Q_4(r,y)$ and $Q_5(r,y)$ yield

$$\Big|-\mu_i(y)Q_4(r,y)+P_i\Big(y,\frac{r-y}{|r-y|}\Big)Q_5(r,y)\Big| \le \mathrm{const}\cdot|r-y|, \quad i=1,\dots,q.$$

Comparing the expression in braces at (35) with the representation (1.1.12) for $f(r,\omega)$, we see that it is equal to

$$-\mu_i(y)f\Big(r,\frac{r-y}{|r-y|}\Big)+P_i\Big(y,\frac{r-y}{|r-y|}\Big).$$

Therefore the equality (35) can be rewritten as follows

$$\Phi_i(r,y) = \exp\Big(-\int_0^{d(r(r-y)/|r-y|)} a\Big(r+t'\,\frac{r-y}{|r-y|}\Big)\Big)dt'$$
$$\times\Big\{-\mu_i(y)f\Big(r,\frac{r-y}{|r-y|}\Big)+P_i\Big(y,\frac{r-y}{|r-y|}\Big)\Big\}+Q_6(r,y), \quad (36)$$

where

$$|Q_6(r,y)| \leq \text{const} \cdot |r-y|. \tag{37}$$

Taking into account (36) and (37), we rewrite (31) in the form

$$U(r) = \sum_{i=1}^{q} \int_{\partial\mathcal{D}_i} \frac{n_i(y)\cdot e_k}{|r-y|} \exp\Big( - \int_0^{d(r,(r-y)/|r-y|)} a\Big(r + t'\,\frac{r-y}{|r-y|}\Big)\,dt'\Big)$$
$$\times \Big\{ -\mu_i(y) f\Big(r, \frac{r-y}{|r-y|}\Big) + P_i\Big(y, \frac{r-y}{|r-y|}\Big)\Big\}\, d\sigma_y + U_0(r) + O(1).$$

This equality coincides with (25), which completes the proof of Lemma 6. □

The following very simple statement will be often used bellow.

**Lemma 7.** *Suppose that the vector-functions $A(r)\colon \mathcal{D}_0 \to \mathcal{E}^2$, $B(r)\colon \mathcal{D}_0 \to \mathcal{E}^2$, then*

$$|A(r) + B(r)| = |A(r)| + \varphi(r), \qquad r \in \mathcal{D}_0, \tag{38}$$

*where $|\varphi(r)| \leq |B(r)|$. In the case where $|B(r)| \leq \text{const}$, then*

$$|A(r) + B(r)| = |A(r)| + O(1), \tag{39}$$

*where $O(1)$ is a function bounded for $r \in \mathcal{D}_0$.*

**Proof.** We define the function $\varphi$ by the formula $\varphi = |A(r) - B(r)| - |A(r)|$. From the inequality $|A(r) + B(r)| \leq |A(r)| + |B(r)|$ it follows that $|A(r)+B(r)| - |A(r)| \leq |B(r)|$. On the other hand $|A(r)| = |A(r)+B(r) - B(r)| \leq |A(r) + B(r)| + |B(r)|$. Therefore $|A(r)| - |A(r) + B(r)| \leq |B(r)|$. Thus, we obtain $|\varphi| = ||A(r) - B(r)| - |A(r)|| \leq |B(r)|$. Since $|B(r)| \leq \text{const}$, then $\varphi(r) = O(1)$. Thus the equality (39) is proved, which completes the proof of this lemma. □

## 1.4. MODIFICATION OF THE INDICATOR OF HETEROGENEITY AND ITS PROPERTIES

We introduce the functions $F(r,\omega) = f(r + d(r,\omega)\omega, \omega)$, $(r,\omega) \in \mathcal{D}_0 \times \Omega_1$ and $F^{(\varepsilon)}(r,\omega) = f^{(\varepsilon)}(r + d(r,\omega)\omega, \omega)$, $(r,\omega) \in \overline{\mathcal{D}} \times \Omega_1$, where $f^{(\varepsilon)}(r,\omega)$ are defined by (1.3.3). In these designations the equalities (1.1.12) and (1.3.3) for $\eta = r + d(r,\omega)\omega$, $(r,\omega) \in \mathcal{D}_0 \times \Omega_1$ can be rewritten as follows

$$F(r,\omega) = \tilde{h}(r,\omega)\exp\Big(-\int_0^{d(\eta,-\omega)} \mu(\eta - t'\omega)\,dt'\Big) + \int_0^{d(\eta,-\omega)} \exp\Big(-\int_0^t \mu(\eta - t'\omega)\,dt'\Big) P(\eta - t\omega,\omega)\,dt, \quad (1)$$

$$F^{(\varepsilon)}(r,\omega) = \tilde{h}(r,\omega)\exp\Big(-\int_0^{d(\eta,-\omega)} \mu_\varepsilon(\eta - t'\omega)\,dt'\Big) + \int_0^{d(\eta,-\omega)} \exp\Big(-\int_0^t \mu_\varepsilon(\eta - t'\omega)\,dt'\Big) P_\varepsilon(\eta - t\omega,\omega)\,dt. \quad (2)$$

We remind that $\tilde{h}(r,\omega) = h(r - d(r,-\omega)\omega,\omega)$.

Consider the functions

$$v^{(\varepsilon)}(r) = \int_{\Omega_1} F^{(\varepsilon)}(r,\omega)\,d\omega, \qquad r \in \mathcal{D}_0, \quad \varepsilon \in (0,\varepsilon_0], \quad (3)$$

$$v(r) = \int_{\Omega_1} F(r,\omega)\,d\omega, \qquad r \in \mathcal{D}_0. \quad (4)$$

**Theorem 1.** *For any neighborhood $V$ such that $\overline{V} \subset \mathcal{D}_0$, the continuous functions $v^{(\varepsilon)}(r)$ converge to $v(r)$ as $\varepsilon \to 0$ uniformly with respect to $r \in \overline{V}$. For each $k = 1, 2$, the continuous derivations $D_k v^{(\varepsilon)}(r)$ converge to $D_k v(r)$ uniformly in $\overline{V}$ as $\varepsilon \to 0$. For all $r \in \mathcal{D}_0$ we have*

$$D_k v(r) = \sum_{i=1}^{q} \int_{\partial \mathcal{D}_i} \frac{n_i(y)\cdot e_k}{|r-y|} R_i(r,y)d\sigma_y + U_0(r) + O(1), \quad (5)$$

*where*

$$R_i(r,y) = \exp\Big(-\int_0^{d(r,(r-y)/|r-y|)} \mu\Big(r + \nu\frac{r-y}{|r-y|}\Big)\,d\nu\Big)\Big\{-\mu_i(y) f\Big(r, \frac{r-y}{|r-y|}\Big) + P_i\Big(y, \frac{r-y}{|r-y|}\Big)\Big\} + \exp\Big(-\int_0^{d(r,(y-r)/|y-r|)} \mu\Big(r + \nu\frac{y-r}{|y-r|}\Big)\,d\nu\Big) \times \Big\{-\mu_i(y) f\Big(r, \frac{y-r}{|y-r|}\Big) + P_i\Big(y, \frac{y-r}{|y-r|}\Big)\Big\}, \quad y \in \partial\mathcal{D}_0. \quad (6)$$

*Here a function $O(1)$ is bounded in $\mathcal{D}_0$ and the continuous function $U_0(r)$ is defined by the equality (1.3.27) for $a(r) = \mu(r)$.*

**Proof.** The continuity of $v^{(\varepsilon)}(r)$ follows easily from the fact that the integrands and the functions $d(r,\omega)$, $\tilde{h}(r,\omega)$ in (2) and (3) are continuous in $\mathcal{D}\times\Omega_1$.

We now rewrite the formula (2). From integration along the ray $L_{\eta,-\omega}$ we pass to integration along $L_{r,\omega}$ and $L_{r,-\omega}$. Using the equality $\eta = r + d(r,\omega)\omega$ and making a shift-type change of variables, we obtain

$$F^{(\varepsilon)}(r,\omega) = \exp\Big(-\int_0^{d(r,\omega)} \mu_\varepsilon(r+t'\omega)\,dt'\Big) f^{(\varepsilon)}(r,\omega) + \int_0^{d(r,\omega)} \exp\Big(-\int_t^{d(r,\omega)} \mu_\varepsilon(r+t'\omega)\,dt'\Big) P_\varepsilon(r+t\omega,\omega)\,dt. \quad (7)$$

Note that we can obtain the analogous equality for the function $F(r,\omega)$, but without $\varepsilon$. Lemmas 1.3.2, 1.3.3 and Remark 1.3.1 imply that $F^{(\varepsilon)}(r,\omega)$ uniformly converge to $F(r,\omega)$ as $\varepsilon\to 0$, $(r,\omega)\in\overline{V}\times\Omega_1$.

We now prove that $D_k v^{(\varepsilon)}(r)$ converge to $D_k v(r)$. The function $F^{\varepsilon}(r,\omega)$ has the first continuous derivatives with respect to $r_k$, $k=1,2$, therefore

$$D_k v^{(\varepsilon)}(r) = \int_{\Omega_1} D_k F^{(\varepsilon)}(r,\omega)\,d\omega, \qquad r\in\mathcal{D}_0. \quad (8)$$

We represent this expression as the sum of four other terms

$$D_k v^{(\varepsilon)}(r) = w_{1,\varepsilon}(r) + w_{2,\varepsilon}(r) + w_{3,\varepsilon}(r) + w_{4,\varepsilon}(r), \quad (9)$$

where

$$w_{1,\varepsilon}(r) = \int_{\Omega_1} \exp\Big(-\int_0^{d(r,\omega)} \mu_\varepsilon(r+\tau\omega)\,d\tau\Big) D_k f^{(\varepsilon)}(r,\omega)\,d\omega, \quad (10)$$

$$w_{2,\varepsilon}(r) = -\int_{\Omega_1} \exp\Big(-\int_0^{d(r,\omega)} \mu_\varepsilon(r+\nu\omega)\,d\nu\Big) \times \int_0^{d(r,\omega)} (D_k\mu_\varepsilon(r+t'\omega)\,dt') f^{(\varepsilon)}(r,\omega)\,d\omega, \quad (11)$$

$$w_{3,\varepsilon}(r) = -\int_{\Omega_1}\int_0^{d(r,\omega)} \exp\Big(-\int_t^{d(r,\omega)} \mu_\varepsilon(r+\nu\omega)\,d\nu\Big) \times \Big(\int_t^{d(r,\omega)} D_k\mu_\varepsilon(r+t'\omega)\,dt'\Big) P_\varepsilon(r+t\omega,\omega)\,dt\,d\omega, \quad (12)$$

$$w_{4,\varepsilon}(r) = \int_{\Omega_1} \int_0^{d(r,\omega)} \exp\Big( - \int_t^{d(r,\omega)} \mu_\varepsilon(r + t'\omega)\, dt'\Big) D_k P_\varepsilon(r + t\omega, \omega)\, dt\, d\omega. \tag{13}$$

In doing so we took into account the equality $\mu_\varepsilon(r + d(r,\omega)\omega) = P_\varepsilon(r + d(r,\omega)\omega) = 0$ for $r \in \partial\mathcal{D}_0$, $\omega \in \Omega_1$.

Transform the expressions (10)–(13). The expression (10) coincides with the expression (1.3.24) if we set $a_\varepsilon(r) = \mu_\varepsilon(r)$ in (1.3.24). Therefore, using Lemma 1.3.6 for $a(r) = \mu(r)$, we prove that the expressions $w_{1,\varepsilon}(r) = U^{(\varepsilon)}(r)$ uniformly in $\overline{V}$ converge to the following expression as $\varepsilon \to 0$

$$\sum_{i=1}^{p} \int_{\partial\mathcal{D}_i} \frac{n_i(y) \cdot e_k}{|r-y|} \Big\{ \exp\Big( - \int_0^{d(r,(r-y)/|r-y|)} \mu\Big(r + \nu\frac{r-y}{|r-y|}\Big)\, d\nu\Big) \times \Big( - \mu_i(y) f\Big(r, \frac{r-y}{|r-y|}\Big) + P_i\Big(y, \frac{r-y}{|r-y|}\Big)\Big)\Big\}\, d\sigma_y + U_0(r) + O(1) \tag{14}$$

Making the change of variables $y = r + t'\omega$, we rewrite (11) in the form

$$w_{2,\varepsilon}(r) = - \int_{\mathcal{D}} \frac{D_k\mu_\varepsilon(y)}{|r-y|} Q_{2,\varepsilon}(r,y)\, dy, \tag{15}$$

where

$$Q_{2,\varepsilon}(r,y) = \exp\Big( - \int_0^{d(r,(y-r)/|r-y|)} \mu_\varepsilon\Big(r + \nu\frac{y-r}{|y-r|}\Big)\, d\nu\Big) f^{(\varepsilon)}\Big(r, \frac{y-r}{|y-r|}\Big).$$

To transform $w_{3,\varepsilon}(r)$, we change the order of integration in (12). Instead of integration first with respect to $t'$ ($t' \in (t, d(r,\omega))$), and then with respect to $t$ ($t \in (0, d(r,\omega))$), we integrate first with respect to $t$ ($t \in (0,t')$) and then with respect to $t'$ ($t' \in (0, d(r,\omega))$). As a result, we obtain

$$w_{3,\varepsilon}(r) = - \int_{\Omega_1} \int_0^{d(r,\omega)} \Big\{ \int_0^{t'} \exp\Big(- \int_t^{d(r,\omega)} \mu_\varepsilon(r+\nu\omega)\, d\nu\Big) P_\varepsilon(r+t\omega,\omega)\, dt\Big\} \times D_k\mu_\varepsilon(r + t'\omega)\, dt'\, d\omega.$$

Making the change of variables $y = r + t'\omega$, we obtain

$$w_{3,\varepsilon}(r) = - \int_{\mathcal{D}} \frac{D_k\mu_\varepsilon(y)}{|r-y|} Q_{3,\varepsilon}(r,y)\, dy, \tag{16}$$

where

$$Q_{3,\varepsilon}(r,y) = \int_0^{|r-y|} \exp\Big( - \int_t^{d(r,(y-r)/|y-r|)} \mu_\varepsilon\Big(r + \nu\frac{y-r}{|y-r|}\Big)\, d\nu\Big) \times P_\varepsilon\Big(r + t\frac{y-r}{|y-r|}, \frac{y-r}{|y-r|}\Big)\, dt.$$

Making the change of variables $y = r + t\omega$ in the equality (13), we have

$$w_{4,\varepsilon}(r) = \int_{\mathcal{D}} \frac{D_k P_\varepsilon(y, (y-r)/|y-r|)}{|r-y|} \, Q_{4,\varepsilon}(r,y)\, dy, \tag{17}$$

where

$$Q_{4,\varepsilon}(r,y) = \exp\Big( - \int_{|r-y|}^{d(r,(y-r)/|y-r|)} \mu_\varepsilon\Big(r + t' \frac{y-r}{|y-r|}\Big)\, dt'\Big).$$

The next equality is obtained by summing (15),(16) and (17)

$$\begin{aligned} w_{2,\varepsilon}(r) + w_{3,\varepsilon}(r) + w_{4,\varepsilon}(r) = &- \int_{\mathcal{D}} \frac{D_k \mu_\varepsilon(y)}{|r-y|} \Big( Q_{2,\varepsilon}(r,y) + Q_{3,\varepsilon}(r,y)\Big)\, dy \\ &+ \int_{\mathcal{D}} \frac{D_k P_\varepsilon(y, (y-r)/|y-r|\Big)}{|r-y|} \, Q_{4,\varepsilon}(r,y)\, dy. \end{aligned}$$

Applying Lemma 1.3.4 to the right-hand side of this equality, we see that $w_{2,\varepsilon}(r) + w_{3,\varepsilon}(r) + w_{4,\varepsilon}(r)$ converge to the following limit uniformly in $\overline{V}$ as $\varepsilon \to 0$

$$\begin{aligned} &- \sum_{i=1}^{q} \int_{\mathcal{D}_i} \frac{D_k \mu_i(y)}{|r-y|} \Big( Q_2(r,y) + Q_3(r,y)\Big)\, dy \\ &\quad - \sum_{i=1}^{q} \int_{\partial\mathcal{D}_i} \frac{n_i(y)\cdot e_k}{|r-y|} \, \mu_i(y) \Big( Q_2(r,y) + Q_3(r,y)\Big)\, d\sigma_y \\ &\quad\quad + \sum_{i=1}^{q} \int_{\mathcal{D}_i} \frac{D_k P_i(y, (y-r)/|y-r|)}{|r-y|} \, Q_4(r,y)\, dy \\ &\quad\quad\quad + \sum_{i=1}^{q} \int_{\partial\mathcal{D}_i} \frac{n_i(y)\cdot e_k}{|r-y|} \, P_i\Big(y, \frac{y-r}{|y-r|}\Big) Q_4(r,y)\, d\sigma_y, \end{aligned} \tag{18}$$

where

$$Q_2(r,y) = \exp\Big( - \int_0^{d(r,(y-r)/|y-r|)} \mu\Big(r + \nu \frac{y-r}{|y-r|}\Big)\, d\nu\Big) f\Big(r, \frac{y-r}{|y-r|}\Big), \tag{19}$$

$$\begin{aligned} Q_3(r,y) = \int_0^{|r-y|} &\exp\Big( - \int_t^{d(r,(y-r)/|y-r|)} \mu\Big(r + \nu \frac{y-r}{|y-r|}\Big)\, d\nu\Big) \\ &\times P\Big(r + t\frac{y-r}{|y-r|}, \frac{y-r}{|y-r|}\Big)\, dt, \end{aligned}$$

$$Q_4(r,y) = \exp\Big( - \int_{|r-y|}^{d(r,(y-r)/|y-r|)} \mu\Big(r + t' \frac{y-r}{|y-r|}\Big)\, dt'\Big).$$

We will not change the expression for $Q_2(r,y)$; $Q_3(r,y)$ satisfies the estimate $|Q_3(r,y)| \le \mathrm{const}\cdot|r-y|$, $r \in \mathcal{D}_0$, $y \in \partial\mathcal{D}_0$ and $Q_4(r,y)$ is represented as follows

$$Q_4(r,y) = Q_5(r,y) + Q_6(r,y),$$

where

$$Q_5(r,y) = \exp\Big( - \int_0^{d(r,(y-r)/|y-r|)} \mu\Big(r + \nu \frac{y-r}{|y-r|}\Big)\, d\nu\Big), \tag{20}$$

$$Q_6(r,y) = \exp\Big( - \int_{|r-y|}^{d(r,(y-r)/|y-r|)} \mu\Big(r + t' \frac{y-r}{|y-r|}\Big)\, dt'\Big) - \exp\Big( - \int_0^{d(r,(y-r)/|y-r|)} \mu\Big(r + t' \frac{y-r}{|y-r|}\Big)\, dt'\Big). \tag{21}$$

It is easy to obtain the following estimate from (21): $|Q_6(r,y)| \le \mathrm{const}\cdot |r-y|$, $r \in \mathcal{D}_0$, $y \in \partial\mathcal{D}_0$. The expression (18) becomes as follows

$$\sum_{i=1}^{q} \int_{\partial\mathcal{D}_i} \frac{n_i(y)\cdot e_k}{|r-y|}\Big\{ - \mu_i(y) Q_2(r,y) + P_i\Big(y, \frac{y-r}{|y-r|}\Big) Q_5(r,y)\Big\}\, d\sigma_y + O(1). \tag{22}$$

We replace all the integrals in (18) by $O(1)$ except those selected in (22), since they are bounded for $r \in \mathcal{D}_0$, $y \in \partial\mathcal{D}_0$, having weak singularities.

Using (19) and (20), we represent the expression in braces in (22) as

$$\Big\{ \exp\Big( - \int_0^{d(y,(y-r)/|y-r|)} \mu\Big(r + \nu \frac{y-r}{|y-r|}\Big)\, d\nu\Big) \times \Big( - \mu_i(y) f\Big(r, \frac{y-r}{|y-r|}\Big) + P_i\Big(y, \frac{y-r}{|y-r|}\Big)\Big)\Big\}.$$

Thus, we have proved that the uniform limit for $w_{2,\varepsilon}(r) + w_{3,\varepsilon}(r) + w_{4,\varepsilon}(r)$, $r \in \overline{V}$, as $\varepsilon \to 0$ is given by the expression

$$\sum_{i=1}^{q} \int_{\partial\mathcal{D}_i} \frac{n_i(y)\cdot e_k}{|r-y|}\Big\{ \exp\Big( - \int_0^{d(r,(y-r)/|y-r|)} \mu\Big(r + \nu \frac{y-r}{|y-r|}\Big)\, d\nu\Big) \times \Big( - \mu_i(y) f\Big(r, \frac{y-r}{|y-r|}\Big) + P_i\Big(y, \frac{y-r}{|y-r|}\Big)\Big)\Big\}\, d\sigma_y + O(1). \tag{23}$$

Summing (14) and (23), we set that $D_k v^{(\varepsilon)}(r) = w_{1,\varepsilon}(r) + w_{2,\varepsilon}(r) + w_{3,\varepsilon}(r) + w_{4,\varepsilon}(r)$ converge to the right-hand side of (5) as $\varepsilon \to 0$ uniformly with respect to $r \in \overline{V}$. This means that $v(r)$ has the derivative $D_k v(r)$ satisfying the equality (5). As the neighborhood $V$ is arbitrary, the formula (5) holds for all $r \in \mathcal{D}_0$. Theorem 1 is proved. □

We consider the function $\mathrm{Ind}^*(r)$ defined by the formula

$$\mathrm{Ind}^*(r) = |\nabla_r^* v(r)| = \left| e_1 \cdot \frac{\partial v}{\partial r_1}(r) + e_2 \cdot \frac{\partial v}{\partial r_2}(r) \right|, \qquad r \in \mathcal{D}_0, \tag{24}$$

where $v(r)$ is given by the equality (4).

**Theorem 2.** *For $r \in \mathcal{D}_0$ we have*

$$\mathrm{Ind}^*(r) = \Big\{ \sum_{k=1}^{2} \Big( \sum_{i=1}^{q} \int_{\partial \mathcal{D}_i} \frac{n_i(y) \cdot e_k}{|r-y|} R_i(r,y)\, d\sigma_y \Big)^2 \Big\}^{1/2} + \varphi(r), \tag{25}$$

*where the functions $R_i(r,y)$ are defined by (6) and $\varphi(r)$ is a function which may be unbounded only for $\rho(r, \partial\mathcal{D}) \to 0$.*

**Proof.** We use the formula (5) for $D_k v(r)$. Using the formula successively for $k = 1, k = 2$, we denote the sum of the integrals in the right-hand side of (5) by $A_1(r), A_2(r)$. Similarly the sum of the functions $U_0(r) + O(1)$ for $k = 1, 2$ is denoted by $B_1(r), B_2(r)$ respectively. With this notation, the equality (5) takes the form

$$D_k v(r) = A_k(r) + B_k(r), \qquad k - 1, 2, \quad r \in \mathcal{D}_0,$$

where each of the functions $B_k(r)$ is bounded everywhere in $\mathcal{D}_0$

Now let us consider the vector-functions $A(r) = (A_1(r), A_2(r))$, $B(r) = (B_1(r), B_2(r))$. We have $\nabla_r^* v(r) = A(r) + B(r)$, $\mathrm{Ind}^*(r) = |A(r) + B(r)|$. The equality $\mathrm{Ind}^*(r) = |A(r)| + \varphi(r)$ follows from Lemma 3.7, where

$$|A(r)| = \Big\{ \sum_{k=1}^{2} \Big( \sum_{i=1}^{q} \int_{\partial \mathcal{D}_i} \frac{n_i(y) \cdot e_k}{|r-y|} R_i(r,y)\, d\sigma_y \Big)^2 \Big\}^{1/2},$$

which proves Theorem 2. □

We return to the notation introduced before Lemma 1.2.5. Fix a point $z \in \mathcal{D} \cap \partial\mathcal{D}_0$, which is a contact point for the domains $\mathcal{D}_l$ and $D_j$, $1 \leq l <$

$j \le q$. For the points $r = z + tn_l(z)$, $0 < t \le \delta_1$, $\omega \in \Omega_1$ we define the function

$$m(r,\omega) = \exp\Big(-\int_0^{d(r,\omega)} \mu(r+\nu\omega)\,d\nu\Big)\{-[\![\mu(z)]\!]f(r,\omega) + [\![P(z,\omega)]\!]\}. \quad (26)$$

Here $[\![\mu(z)]\!]$, $[\![P(z,\omega)]\!]$ are the jumps of functions described above. Note that in some cases $m(r,\omega)$ can be defined also for $r = z$, $\omega = \pm s$.

In this section $\mathcal{M}(r, y_1', y_1'')$ will denote the function defined also by the equality (1.3.13) for $m_0(r,\omega) = (m(r,\omega) + m(r,-\omega))/2$ and $M(z)$ is given by (1.3.14) for $m_0(z,s) = (m(z,s)+m(z,-s))/2$, if the function $m$ is defined for $r = z$, $\omega = \pm s$. With this notation, the following theorem holds.

**Theorem 3.** *For any contact point $z$, $z \in \mathcal{D}\cap\partial\mathcal{D}_l\cap\partial\mathcal{D}_j$, $1 \le l < j \le p$, there exist the function $t_1(r)$, $-\delta \le t_1(r) \le 0$, and the function $t_2(r)$, $0 \le t_2(r) \le \delta$, such that the following equality holds for $r = z + tn_l(z)$, $0 < |t| \le \delta_1$*

$$\mathrm{Ind}^*(r) = 2|\mathcal{M}(r, t_1(r), t_2(r))|\,|\ln \rho(r, \partial\mathcal{D}_0)| + O(1). \quad (27)$$

*If, in addition, every surface $\partial G_i$, $i = 1,\dots,p$, consists of a finite number of algebraic surfaces and intersects every straight line at a finite number of points, then the function $m(r,\omega)$ is defined for $r = z$, $\omega = \pm s$, and the following equality holds*

$$\mathrm{Ind}^*(r) = 2|M(z)|\,|\ln \rho(r, \partial\mathcal{D}_0)| + O(1). \quad (28)$$

*Here $O(1)$ is a function depending on $r$ and bounded for $0 < |t| \le \delta_1$.*

**Proof.** Consider the equality (25). Since the points $z$ and $r$ are separated from the curve $\partial\mathcal{D}$, the function $\varphi(r)$ is bounded. For each $k = 1, 2$ we select two terms in the interior sum. The first of them is the sum $A_k^*(r)$ of the integrals over $\partial\mathcal{D}_l$ and $\partial\mathcal{D}_j$. The second term $B_k^*(r)$ is the sum of the remaining integrals over $\partial\mathcal{D}_i$, $i = 1,\dots,q$, $i \ne l, j$. Then (25) can be written in the form

$$\mathrm{Ind}^*(r) = \Big\{\sum_{k=1}^{2}\Big(A_k^*(r) + B_k^*(r)\Big)^2\Big\}^{1/2} + O(1),$$

or $\mathrm{Ind}^*(r) = |A^*(r) + B^*(r)| + O(1)$, where $A^*(r) = (A_1^*(r), A_2^*(r))$, $B^*(r) = (B_1^*(r), B_2^*(r))$. Since $z$ is a contact point for two domains $\mathcal{D}_l$ and $\mathcal{D}_j$ and the numbers $\delta$, $\delta_1$ are small enough, the inequality $|r - y| \ge \text{const} > 0$ holds for all $y \in \partial\mathcal{D}_i$, $i \ne l, j$. This means that $|B(r)| \le \text{const}$. Using the equality (1.3.39) from Lemma 1.3.7 for $A(r) = A^*(r)$, $B(r) = B^*(r)$, we obtain

$$\operatorname{Ind}^*(r) = \Big\{ \sum_{k=1}^{2} \Big( \int_{\partial\mathcal{D}_l} \frac{n_l(y)\cdot e_k}{|r-y|} R_l(r,y)\, d\sigma_y + \int_{\partial\mathcal{D}_j} \frac{n_j(y)\cdot e_k}{|r-y|} R_j(r,y)\, d\sigma_y \Big)^2 \Big\}^{1/2} + O(1). \quad (29)$$

We select the common part $\partial\mathcal{D}_{l,z} = \partial\mathcal{D}_{j,z}$ of the curves $\partial\mathcal{D}_l$ and $\partial\mathcal{D}_j$ in the small enough neighborhood of $z$. We represent each of the integrals in (29) as a sum. The first term is the integral over $\partial\mathcal{D}_{l,z} = \partial\mathcal{D}_{j,z}$. The second term is the integral over the remaining set. As a result, we obtain

$$\operatorname{Ind}^*(r) = \Big\{ \sum_{k=1}^{2} \Big( \int_{\partial\mathcal{D}_{l,z}} \frac{n_l(y)\cdot e_k}{|r-y|} R_l(r,y)\, d\sigma_y + \int_{\partial\mathcal{D}_{j,z}} \frac{n_j(y)\cdot e_k}{|r-y|} R_j(r,y)\, d\sigma_y + \int_{\partial\mathcal{D}_l\setminus\partial\mathcal{D}_{l,z}} \frac{n_l(y)\cdot e_k}{|r-y|} R_l(r,y)\, d\sigma_y + \int_{\partial\mathcal{D}_j\setminus\partial\mathcal{D}_{j,z}} \frac{n_j(y)\cdot e_k}{|r-y|} R_j(r,y)\, d\sigma_y \Big)^2 \Big\}^{1/2} + O(1). \quad (30)$$

Taking into account the inequality $|r-y| \geq \delta > 0$ for $y \in \partial\mathcal{D}_l\setminus\partial\mathcal{D}_{l,z}$, $y \in \partial\mathcal{D}_j\setminus\partial\mathcal{D}_{j,z}$, we see that the absolute values of the last two integrals in (30) are bounded. For $k = 1, 2$, we denoted their sum by $B_k^{**}(r)$ and the sum of the first two integrals is denoted by $A_k^{**}(r)$. Then, by Lemma 1.3.7 for the vectors $A(r) = A^{**}(r) = (A_1^{**}(r), A_2^{**}(r))$ and $B(r) = B^{**}(r) = (B_1^{**}(r), B_2^{**}(r))$, the equality (30) can be rewritten as follows

$$\operatorname{Ind}^*(r) = |A^{**}(r)| + O(1), \quad (31)$$

where

$$A_k^{**}(r) = \int_{\partial\mathcal{D}_{l,z}} \frac{n_l(y)\cdot e_k}{|r-y|} R_l(r,y)\, d\sigma_y + \int_{\partial\mathcal{D}_{j,z}} \frac{n_j(y)\cdot e_k}{|r-y|} R_j(r,y)\, d\sigma_y.$$

Since $\partial\mathcal{D}_{l,z} = \partial\mathcal{D}_{j,z}$ and $n_j(y) = -n_l(y)$, the foregoing equality can be rewritten in the form

$$A_k^{**}(r) = \int_{\partial\mathcal{D}_{l,z}} \frac{n_l(y)\cdot e_k}{|r-y|} \big(R_l(r,y) - R_j(r,y)\big)\, d\sigma_y. \quad (32)$$

Since $\partial\mathcal{D}_{l,z}$ is a curve of the class $C^2$, we have $|n_l(y)\cdot e_k - n_l(z)\cdot e_k| \leq \mathrm{const}\cdot|y-z|$, $y \in \partial\mathcal{D}_{l,z}$. By the assumption, $|\mu_i(y) - \mu_i(z)| \leq \mathrm{const}\cdot$

$|y-z|$, $y \in \partial\mathcal{D}_{l,z}$, $i = l, j$. The function $P(r,\omega)$ belongs to the class $W$ (see Section 1.2); therefore $|P_i(y,\omega) - P_i(z,\omega)| \le \text{const}\cdot|y-z|^\gamma$, $y \in \partial\mathcal{D}_{l,z}$, $i = l,j$, $0 < \gamma < 1$. In the local coordinates associated with the point $z$, we have $|y-z|^2 = y_1^2 + (q(y_1))^2$, $|r-y|^2 = y_1^2 + (t - q(y_1))^2$. Recall that by virtue of (1.3.11), we have $|q(y_1)| \le \text{const}\cdot(y_1^2)$. Therefore

$$
\begin{aligned}
|y-z|^2 = y_1^2 + (q(y_1))^2 \le y_1^2 + \text{const}\cdot y_1^4 \le \text{const}\cdot y_1^2 \\
\le \text{const}\cdot(y_1^2 + (t-q(y_1))^2) = \text{const}\cdot|r-y|^2.
\end{aligned}
$$

Hence $|y-z| \le \text{const}\cdot|r-y|$ and therefore

$$
\begin{aligned}
|\mu_i(y) - \mu_i(z)| \le \text{const}\cdot|r-y|, \qquad |P_i(y,\omega) - P_i(z,\omega)| \le \text{const}\cdot|r-y|^\gamma, \\
|n_l(y)\cdot e_k - n_l(z)\cdot e_k| \le \text{const}\cdot|r-y|, \qquad \gamma \in (0,1), \quad i = l,j; \qquad (33)
\end{aligned}
$$

We represent the expression $R_l(r,y) - R_j(r,y)$ in the form

$$
\begin{aligned}
R_l(r,y) - R_j(r,y) = \Phi_l(r,y) - \Phi_j(r,y) + R_l(r,y) \\
- \Phi_l(r,y) + \Phi_j(r,y) - R_j(r,y), \quad (34)
\end{aligned}
$$

where for $i = l,j$, we have

$$
\begin{aligned}
\Phi_i(r,y) = \exp\Big(-\int_0^{d(r,(r-y)/|r-y|)} \mu\Big(r + \nu\frac{r-y}{|r-y|}\Big)\,d\nu\Big) \\
\times\Big\{-\mu_i(z) f\Big(r, \frac{r-y}{|r-y|}\Big) + P_i\Big(z, \frac{r-y}{|r-y|}\Big)\Big\} \\
+ \exp\Big(-\int_0^{d(r,(y-r)/|y-r|)} \mu\Big(r + \nu\frac{y-r}{|y-r|}\Big)\,d\nu\Big) \\
\times\Big\{-\mu_i(z) f\Big(r, \frac{y-r}{|y-r|}\Big) + P_i\Big(z, \frac{y-r}{|y-r|}\Big)\Big\}. \quad (35)
\end{aligned}
$$

Comparing (6) and (35), we see that $\Phi_i(r,y)$ and $R_i(r,y)$ differ so that the expression for $R_i(r,y)$ contains $\mu_i(y)$ and $P_i(y,\omega)$, whereas the expression $\Phi_i(r,y)$ contains $\mu_i(z)$ and $P_i(z,\omega)$ at the corresponding positions. Therefore, taking into account (33), we obtain the inequalities

$$
|R_i(r,y) - \Phi_i(r,y)| + |n_i(y)\cdot e_k - n_i(z)\cdot e_k| \le \text{const}\cdot|r-y|^\gamma, \quad i = l,j, \ \gamma \in (0,1).
$$

Thus, from (34) it follows that the equality (32) can be rewritten in the form

$$
A_k^{**}(r) = \int_{\partial\mathcal{D}_{l,z}} \frac{n_l(z)\cdot e_k}{|r-y|}\big(\Phi_l(r,y) - \Phi_j(r,y)\big)\,d\sigma_y + O(1). \qquad (36)
$$

Here we have used the fact that the integrals over $\partial\mathcal{D}_{l,z}$ with the singularity $|r-y|^{-1+\gamma}$ are the values of $O(1)$ type.

We now consider the difference $\Phi_l(r,y) - \Phi_j(r,y)$. Using the equality (35), we obtain

$$\begin{aligned}\Phi_l(r,y) - \Phi_j(r,y) &= \exp\Big(-\int_0^{d(r,(r-y)/|r-y|)} \mu\Big(r+\nu\,\frac{r-y}{|r-y|}\Big)\,d\nu\Big)\\ &\quad\times\Big\{-[\![\mu(z)]\!]_{lj} f\Big(r,\frac{r-y}{|r-y|}\Big) + [\![P\Big(z,\frac{r-y}{|r-y|}\Big)]\!]_{lj}\Big\}\\ &+\exp\Big(-\int_0^{d(r,(y-r)/|y-r|)} \mu\Big(r+\nu\,\frac{y-r}{|y-r|}\Big)\,d\nu\Big)\\ &\quad\times\Big\{-[\![\mu(z)]\!]_{lj} f\Big(r,\frac{y-r}{|y-r|}\Big) + [\![P\Big(z,\frac{y-r}{|y-r|}\Big)]\!]_{lj}\Big\}.\end{aligned}$$

By virtue of (26), it is easy to see that

$$\Phi_l(r,y) - \Phi_j(r,y) = m\Big(r,\frac{r-y}{|r-y|}\Big) + m\Big(r,\frac{y-r}{|y-r|}\Big).$$

Therefore, (36) may be rewritten as follows:

$$A_k^{**}(r) = (n_l(z)\cdot e_k)\int_{\partial\mathcal{D}_{l,z}} \frac{1}{|r-y|}\Big(m\Big(r,\frac{r-y}{|r-y|}\Big)+m\Big(r,\frac{y-r}{|y-r|}\Big)\Big)\,d\sigma_y + O(1).$$

Then, applying Lemma 1.3.7, from (32) we obtain

$$\begin{aligned}\mathrm{Ind}^*(r) &= \Big\{\sum_{k=1}^{2}\Big((n_l(z)\cdot e_k)\\ &\times\int_{\partial\mathcal{D}_{l,z}} \frac{1}{|r-y|}\Big(m\Big(r,\frac{r-y}{|r-y|}\Big)+m\Big(r,\frac{y-r}{|y-r|}\Big)\Big)\,d\sigma_y\Big)^2\Big\}^{1/2} + O(1).\end{aligned}$$

Since $(n_l(z)\cdot e_1)^2 + (n_l(z)\cdot e_2)^2 = |n_l(z)|^2 = 1$, then

$$\mathrm{Ind}^*(r) = \Big|\int_{\partial\mathcal{D}_{l,z}} \frac{1}{|r-y|}\Big(m\Big(r,\frac{r-y}{|r-y|}\Big)+m\Big(r,\frac{y-r}{|y-r|}\Big)\Big)\,d\sigma_y\Big| + O(1). \quad (37)$$

Define the function $m_0(r,\omega)$ by the equality

$$m_0(r,\omega) = (m(r,\omega) + m(r,-\omega))/2. \quad (38)$$

By virtue of (26), we see that $m_0(r,\omega)$ satisfies all the conditions formulated before Lemma 1.3.5. Therefore there exist the functions $t_1(r)$ and $t_2(r)$ such that

$$I(r) = \int_{\partial\mathcal{D}_{l,z}} \frac{1}{|r-y|} m_0\Big(r, \frac{y-r}{|y-r|}\Big)\, d\sigma_y \\ = \mathcal{M}(r, t_1(r), t_2(r))\, |\ln(r, \partial\mathcal{D}_0)| + O(1). \quad (39)$$

Thus, using the equalities (37)–(39), we obtain the equality

$$\mathrm{Ind}^*(r) = 2\Big|\int_{\partial\mathcal{D}_{l,z}} \frac{1}{|r-y|} m_0\Big(r, \frac{y-r}{|y-r|}\Big)\, d\sigma_y\Big| + O(1) \\ = 2|I(r)| + O(1) = 2|\mathcal{M}(r, t_1(r), t_2(r))|\, |\ln(r, \partial\mathcal{D}_0)| + O(1), \quad (40)$$

which completes the proof of the equality (37).

If each of the surfaces $\partial G_i$, $i = 1, \dots, p$, consists of a finite number of algebraic surfaces and intersects any straight line at a finite number of points, then, as shown in Germogenova (1986), all the factors in $m(r,\omega)$ are defined for $r = z$, $\omega = \pm s$ and the Holder condition holds:

$$|m(r,\omega) - m(z, s_0)| \le \mathrm{const} \cdot \{|r-z|^\gamma + |\omega - s_0|^\gamma\}, \\ \omega \in \Omega_1, \qquad s_0 = \pm s, \qquad \gamma \in (0,1).$$

In this case it is easy to see that the function $m_0(r,\omega)$ is also defined for $r = z$, $\omega = \pm s$ and satisfies the Holder condition. Therefore the equalities (1.3.12), (1.3.14) and (1.3.17) yield:

$$I(r) = \int_{\partial\mathcal{D}_{l,z}} \frac{1}{|r-y|} m_0\Big(r, \frac{y-r}{|y-r|}\Big)\, d\sigma_y = M(z)\, |\ln(\rho, \partial\mathcal{D}_0)| + O(1). \quad (41)$$

Therefore

$$\mathrm{Ind}^*(r) = 2|M(z)|\, |\ln(\rho, \partial\mathcal{D}_0)| + O(1). \quad (42)$$

Thus, the theorem is proved. □

**Remark 1.** The equality (38) implies that $m_0(z,s) = m_0(z,-s)$. Therefore, taking into account (1.3.14), we see that

$$M(z) = 2m_0(z,s) = 2m_0(z,-s) = m(z,s) + m(z,-s), \quad (43)$$

where

$$m(z,s) = \exp\Big(-\int_0^{d(z,s)} \mu(z+\nu s)\, d\nu\Big)\{-[\![\mu(z)]\!] f(z,s) + [\![P(z,s)]\!]\}. \quad (44)$$

For brevity, a point $z \in \partial\mathcal{D}_0$ will be called a smoothness point if the curve $\partial\mathcal{D}_0$ is smooth in the neighborhood of this point.

**Theorem 4.** *The function* $\mathrm{Ind}^*(r)$ *is continuous in* $\mathcal{D}_0$. *Let* $z$ *be a smoothness point at the curve* $\partial\mathcal{D}_0$, *and* $n(z)$ *be the unit normal to* $\partial\mathcal{D}_0$ *at* $z$. *Consider the points* $r = z + tn(z)$, *where* $0 < |t| \le \delta_1$. *If*

$$|\mathcal{M}(r, t_1, t_2)| \ge \mathrm{const} > 0, \qquad -\delta \le t_1 \le 0, \quad 0 \le t_2 \le \delta, \tag{45}$$

*then* $\mathrm{Ind}^*(r) \to \infty$ *as* $\rho(r, \partial\mathcal{D}_0) \to 0$.

**Proof.** As follows from Theorem 3, for any neighborhood $V$, $(\overline{V} \subset \mathcal{D}_0)$, the continuous functions $D_k v^{(\varepsilon)}$, $k = 1, 2$, converge to $D_k v(r)$ as $\varepsilon \to 0$ uniformly with respect to $\overline{V}$. Therefore $D_k v(r) \in C(\overline{V})$, $k = 1, 2$. Since $V$ is arbitrary, the functions $D_k v(r)$ are continuous in $\mathcal{D}_0$. Since $\mathrm{Ind}^*(r) = |\nabla_r^* v(r)|$, then $\mathrm{Ind}^*(r)$ is also continuous in $\mathcal{D}_0$.

The smoothness of $\partial\mathcal{D}_0$ in the neighborhood of $z$ means that there exist positive numbers $\delta, \delta_1$, such that the intersection of the set $\mathrm{C}_z = \{y = (y_1, y_2) \in \mathcal{E}^2 \mid |y_1| \le \delta,\ |y_2| \le \delta_1\}$ and the set $\partial\mathcal{D}_0$ is represented as a graph: $\partial\mathcal{D}_{0,z} = \{y = (y_1, y_2) \in \mathcal{E}^2 \mid |y_1| \le \delta,\ y_2 = q(y_1)\}$ (here we use the local coordinate system associated with $z$). The function $q(y_1)$ belongs to $C^2[-\delta, \delta]$ and satisfies the condition (1.3.11). It is clear that $\mathrm{C}_z \backslash \partial\mathcal{D}_{0,z} \subset \mathcal{D}_0$. Decreasing the number $\delta > 0$ if necessary, we may assume that $|q(y_1)| < \delta_1$ for $|y_1| \le \delta$.

It is clear that $z$ belongs to the boundaries of the certain domains $\mathcal{D}_l$ and $\mathcal{D}_j$, $1 \le l < j \le q$. We show that there are no elements of the other domains $\mathcal{D}_i$, $i \ne l, j$, in the neighborhood of $z$. Assume the contrary, i. e. in every ball centered at $z$ there are elements of at least three domains $\mathcal{D}_{i1}$, $\mathcal{D}_{i2}$ and $\mathcal{D}_{i3}$. Choosing the ball with sufficiently small radius, we may assume that these elements belong to $\mathrm{C}_z$. At least two of them belong to the set $\mathrm{C}_z^+ = \{y = (y_1, y_2) \in \mathrm{C}_z \mid y_2 - q(y_1) > 0\}$ or $\mathrm{C}_z^- = \{y = (y_1, y_2) \in \mathrm{C}_z \mid y_2 - q(y_1) < 0\}$. For definiteness, suppose $x = (x_1, x_2) \in \mathcal{D}_{i1}$, $u = (u_1, u_2) \in \mathcal{D}_{i2}$, $x \in \mathrm{C}_z^+$, $u \in \mathrm{C}_z^+$. It is clear that $\mathrm{C}_z^+ \subset \mathcal{D}_0$ and the segment $L_1 = \{(x_1, t) \mid x_2 \le t \le \delta_1\}$ lies in $\mathcal{D}_{i1}$ completely. The open sets $\mathcal{D}_i$ have empty intersections, therefore $L_1 \subset \mathcal{D}_{i1}$. Analogously, the segment $L_2 = \{(u_1, t) \mid u_2 \le t \le \delta_1\}$ lies in $\mathcal{D}_{i2}$. The segment $L_3$ of the straight line connecting the points $(x_1, \delta_1) \in \mathcal{D}_{i1}$ and $(u_1, \delta_1) \in \mathcal{D}_{i2}$, lies in $\mathrm{C}_z^+$ because of $|q(y_1)| < \delta_1$ for $|y_1| \le \delta$. But this fact cannot take place because $L_3$ is a connected set and $\mathrm{C}_z^+$ has no points from $\partial\mathcal{D}_0$. This contradiction shows that there are points of only two domains $\mathcal{D}_l$ and $\mathcal{D}_j$, in the neighborhood of $z$, i. e. $z$ is a contact point.

Without loss of generality, we may take $n_l(z)$ for the normal $n(z)$. We now use Theorem 3. In particular, the condition (45) and the formula (27) yields that $\mathrm{Ind}^*(r) \to \infty$ as $\rho(r, \partial\mathcal{D}_0) \to 0$. The theorem is proved. □

**Corollary 1.** *Suppose, in addition, that each surface $\partial G_i$, $i = 1, \dots, p$ consists of a finite number of algebraic surfaces and intersects any straight line in a finite number of points. If the condition* (45) *holds, then $M(z)$ is the limit of $\mathcal{M}(z, t_1, t_2)$ as $t_1 \to 0$, $t_2 \to 0$ and*

$$M(z) \neq 0. \tag{46}$$

*From the condition* (46) *it follows that* $\mathrm{Ind}^*(r) \to \infty$ *for* $\rho(r, \partial\mathcal{D}_0) \to 0$.

**Proof.** By Theorem 3, the assumptions of this corollary guarantee the existence of $M(z)$. Using Remark 3.2, we have $\mathcal{M}(z, t_1, t_2) \to M(z)$ as $t_1, t_2 \to 0$. By the condition (45) $M(z) \neq 0$. Consequently, from the formula (28) for $\mathrm{Ind}^*(r)$ we see that $\mathrm{Ind}^*(r) \to \infty$ as $\rho(r, \partial\mathcal{D}_0) \to 0$. The corollary is proved. □

We select the cases where the conditions (45) and (46) are satisfied. The function $\mathcal{M}(r, t_1, t_2)$ is defined by the formula (1.3.13) where $m_0(r, \omega) = (m(r, \omega) + m(r, -\omega))/2$ and $m(r, \omega)$ is defined by (26). Since $f(r, \omega) > 0$ then the equality (26) yields the following property. If the values $[\![\mu(z)]\!]$ and $[\![P(z, \omega)]\!]$ have the different signs for any $\omega \in \Omega_1$, then $m(r, \omega)$ does not change the sign. Hence, $m_0(r, \omega)$ also does not change the sign. This means that the condition (45) holds for the point $z$.

Now we consider the condition (46). Again suppose that each surface $\partial G_i$, $i = 1, \dots, p$ consists of a finite number of algebraic surfaces and intersects any straight line at a finite number of points. The function $M(z)$ is defined by (43), and $m(z, s)$ is defined by (44). Since $P = N + J$, then $[\![P(z, s)]\!] = [\![N(z, s)]\!] + [\![J(z, s)]\!]$. Under these conditions the function $f(r, \omega)$ is continuous in $G \times \Omega$ (see Prokhorov, 1996). Therefore

$$[\![N(z, s)]\!] = \int_\Omega [\![k(z, s \cdot \omega)]\!] f(z, \omega)\, d\omega.$$

Since $f(z, \omega) > 0$, the sign of $[\![N(z, s)]\!]$ coincides with the sign of $[\![k(z, s \cdot \omega)]\!]$, if $[\![k(z, s \cdot \omega)]\!] \neq 0$. From (44) it follows that if the sign of $[\![k(z, s \cdot \omega)]\!]$ and $[\![J(z, s)]\!]$ is opposite to the sign of $[\![\mu(z)]\!]$, then $m(z, s)$ does not change the sign and the condition (46) holds.

We now show that the condition (45) of Theorem 4 guarantees the uniqueness of a solution of the tomography problem formulated above.

We use the following notation for the exact formulation of the uniqueness theorem. Take two systems of the functions $\{\mu_k(r), k_k(r,\omega,\omega'), J_k(r,\omega), h_k(\xi,\omega)\}$, $k = 1,2$, as the coefficients for the transport equation and the distribution of input radiation. Each of this system has its own curve of the coefficient discontinuities $\partial\mathcal{D}_0^{(k)}$, and the set $\mathcal{D}_0^{(k)}$, $k = 1,2$. Suppose $f_1^*(r,\omega)$ and $f_2^*(r,\omega)$ are the traces of the solutions of the boundary value problem (1.1.1), (1.1.2) for the first and the second system, respectively both in the same domain $G$.

For any smoothness point $z \in \partial\mathcal{D}_0^{(k)} \cap \mathcal{D}$, we consider $r = z + tn^{(k)}(z)$, $0 < |t| \le \delta_1^{(k)}$, where $n^{(k)}(z)$ is the unit normal to the curve $\partial\mathcal{D}_0^{(k)}$ at the point $z$. The functions $\mathcal{M}_k(r,t_1,t_2)$, $-\delta^{(k)} \le t_1 \le 0$, $0 \le t_2 \le \delta^{(k)}$, $k = 1,2$ are defined by these two systems, respectively. With this notation, we prove the following theorem.

**Theorem 5.** *Assume that for any smoothness point* $z \in \partial\mathcal{D}_0^{(k)}$, $z \in \mathcal{D}$ *we have* $|\mathcal{M}_k(r,t_1,t_2)| \ge \text{const} > 0$, $r = z + tn^{(k)}(z)$, $0 < |t| \le \delta_1^{(k)}$, $-\delta^{(k)} \le t_1 \le 0$, $0 \le t_2 \le \delta^{(k)}$, $k = 1,2$, *and* $f_1^*(r + d(r,\omega)\omega,\omega) = f_2^*(r + d(r,\omega)\omega,\omega)$ *for all* $r \in \mathcal{D}_0^{(1)} \cap \mathcal{D}_0^{(2)}$, $\omega \in \Omega_1$. *Then the curves* $\partial\mathcal{D}_0^{(1)}$ *and* $\partial\mathcal{D}_0^{(2)}$ *coincide.*

**Proof.** First, we note that $\partial\mathcal{D} \cap \partial\mathcal{D}_0^{(1)} = \partial\mathcal{D} \cap \partial\mathcal{D}_0^{(2)}$. Therefore we consider only the point $z$ belonging to $\mathcal{D}$. Take an arbitrary point $z \in \mathcal{D} \cap \partial\mathcal{D}_0^{(1)}$ such that the curve $\partial\mathcal{D}_0^{(1)}$ is smooth in the neighborhood of $z$. Assume the contrary, i.e. it does not belong to $\partial\mathcal{D}_0^{(2)}$. Then there exists a neighborhood $V_2$ of the point $z$ separated from $\partial\mathcal{D}_0^{(2)}$ ($\overline{V}_2 \subset \mathcal{D}_0^{(2)}$). It is clear that for sufficiently small $\tilde{\delta}_1 > 0$ the point $r = z + tn^{(1)}(z)$ belongs to $V_2$. Since $\partial\mathcal{D}_0^{(1)}$ is smooth at $z$, decreasing the number $\tilde{\delta}_1$ if necessary, we make sure that the points $r = z + tn^{(1)}(z)$, $0 < |t| \le \tilde{\delta}_1$ belong to $\mathcal{D}_0^{(1)}$. Suppose $\tilde{\delta}_1 < \delta_1^{(1)}$. The points that belong to $V_2$ also belong to $\mathcal{D}_0^{(2)}$. Therefore $r \in \mathcal{D}_0^{(1)} \cap \mathcal{D}_0^{(2)}$. By the assumption of the theorem for such $r$, we have $f_1^*(r + d(r,\omega)\omega,\omega) = f_2^*(r + d(r,\omega)\omega,\omega)$, $\omega \in \Omega_1$. Consequently, the corresponding functions $\text{Ind}_1^*(r)$ and $\text{Ind}_2^*(r)$ coincide for $r = z + tn^{(1)}(z)$, $0 < |t| \le \tilde{\delta}_1$. By Theorem 4, $\text{Ind}_1^*(r) \to \infty$ as $\rho(r,\partial\mathcal{D}_0^{(1)}) \to 0$, i.e. as $t \to 0$. The function $\text{Ind}_2^*(r)$ is bounded for all $r \in \overline{V}_2$, since $\overline{V}_2 \subset \mathcal{D}_0^{(2)}$. In particular, it is bounded for $r = z + tn^{(1)}(z)$, $0 < |t| \le \tilde{\delta}_1$. Hence, $\text{Ind}_1^*(r)$ and $\text{Ind}_2^*(r)$ do not coincide. Therefore, the assumption is false and every smooth point $z \in \partial\mathcal{D}_0^{(1)} \cap \mathcal{D}$ also belongs to $\partial\mathcal{D}_0^{(2)}$. Since every point of $\partial\mathcal{D}_0^{(1)}$ is a limit point of the set of smooth points $z \in \partial\mathcal{D}_0^{(1)}$, every point of $\partial\mathcal{D}_0^{(1)}$ belongs to $\partial\mathcal{D}_0^{(2)}$ because the sets $\partial\mathcal{D}_0^{(1)}$ and $\partial\mathcal{D}_0^{(2)}$ are closed.

By symmetry, all points of $\partial\mathcal{D}_0^{(2)}$ are the elements of $\partial\mathcal{D}_0^{(1)}$. This means that $\partial\mathcal{D}_0^{(1)}$ and $\partial\mathcal{D}_0^{(2)}$ coincide. The theorem is proved. □

**Remark 2.** According to Corollary 1, the condition $M(z) \neq 0$ yields $\text{Ind}^*(r) \to \infty$ as $\rho(r, \partial\mathcal{D}_0) \to 0$. Therefore, under the assumptions of Corollary 1, we may replace the condition (45) for (46) to prove Theorem 5.

## 1.5. INVISIBLE AND POORLY VISIBLE MEDIA IN X-RAY TOMOGRAPHY

In Sections 1.3, 1.4 we have explained how to solve the tomography problem which was formulated in Section 1.2. It has been implemented by using the indicators of heterogeneity which require the special inequalities (see Section 1.4 and below). Here, we are going to check the necessity of these inequalities not only for the indicators, but for any tomography method. As a result, notions of invisible and poorly visible media are in the focus of our attention.

For convenience of a reader, we remind and make more precise some previous notations. The indicatrix of scattering has the form

$$k(r, \omega \cdot \omega') = \sum_{i=1}^{M} \sigma_i(r) S_i(\omega \cdot \omega'),$$

where each item in the sum corresponds to a certain kind of scattering. We can take the following condition of normalization without loss of generality

$$\int_\Omega S_i(\omega \cdot \omega')\, d\omega' = \int_\Omega S_i(\omega \cdot \omega')\, d\omega = 1, \qquad i = 1, \ldots, M. \tag{1}$$

It is easy to see that the coefficient of scattering $\mu_s$ (defined as the integral of $k(r, \omega \cdot \omega')$ over $\omega \in \Omega$) is given by the formula

$$\mu_s(r) = \sum_{i=1}^{M} \sigma_i(r). \tag{2}$$

The function $\mu_a(r) = \mu(r) - \mu_s(r)$ is called the coefficient of absorption.

Let $z \in \partial G_0$ be a common point of the boundaries of two and only two domains $G_l$ and $G_j$, $1 \leq l < j \leq p$. Then

$$[\![J(z, \omega)]\!] = \lim_{r' \to z} J(r', \omega) - \lim_{r'' \to z} J(r'', \omega), \qquad r' \in G_l, \quad r'' \in G_j.$$

The jumps $[\![\sigma_i(z)]\!]$, $[\![\mu(z)]\!]$, $[\![\mu_s(z)]\!]$ and $[\![\mu_a(z)]\!]$ are defined in the similar way.

The restrictions in this section are not so strong as ones in Sections 1.2–1.4. Firstly, we assume that the functions $\sigma_i(r)$, $i = 1, \dots, M$, and $\mu(r)$ are uniformly continuous in each domain $G_i$, $i = 1, \dots, p$, and the functions $S_i(\nu)$, $i = 1, \dots, M$ belong to the class $C^2[-1, 1]$.

Secondly, we assume that other restrictions for the functions $\mu$, $k$, $J$, $h$ and the domains $G_i$, $i = 1, \dots, p$, are such that they provide continuity and positiveness of the corresponding solution of the direct problem (1.1.1), (1.1.2) $f(r, \omega)$ for all $(r, \omega) \in \overline{G} \times \Omega$. In particular, these properties can be provided by restrictions of Sections 1.2–1.4 together with the conditions of Corollary 1.4.1, although they seem to be too strong for such purpose. Generally, the question of minimization of needed conditions is not studied carefully in this book.

Consider the following function

$$\begin{aligned} m_1(z, \omega) &= [\![\mu(z)]\!] f(z, \omega) \\ &- \sum_{i=1}^{M} [\![\sigma_i(r)]\!] \int_\Omega S_i(\omega \cdot \omega') f(z, \omega')\, d\omega' + [\![J(r, \omega)]\!], \quad z \in \partial G_l \cap \partial G_j. \end{aligned} \tag{3}$$

As we have seen from Sections 1.2–1.4, the inequality $m_1(z, \omega) \neq 0$ for all $z \in \partial G_0$, $\omega \in \Omega$ provides uniqueness of solving the tomography problem by using the indicator $\mathrm{Ind}(r)$ and particularly by $\mathrm{Ind}^*(r)$.

Now we study the contrary condition.

**Theorem 1.** *Assume that there exist functions $\mu(r)$, $k(r, \omega \cdot \omega')$, $J(r, \omega)$, $h(\xi, \omega)$ and the corresponding solution to the direct problem $f(r, \omega)$ such that:*

*a) $[\![\mu(z)]\!] \neq 0$ or $[\![\mu_s(z)]\!] \neq 0$ for all $z \in \partial G_j$, where $j$ is a fixed index $1 \leq j \leq p$;*

*b) $J(r, \omega) = 0$ for all $(r, \omega) \in G_j \times \Omega$ and $[\![J(z, \omega)]\!] = 0$, $(z, \omega) \in \partial G_j \times \Omega$;*

*c) $[\![\sigma_i(z)]\!][\![\sigma_k(z)]\!] \geq 0$, $i, k = 1, \dots, M$, $z \in \partial G_j$;*

*d) for all $(z, \omega) \in \partial G_j \times \Omega$*

$$m_1(z, \omega) = 0; \tag{4}$$

*Then:*

$$[\![\mu_a(z)]\!] = [\![\mu(z)]\!] - [\![\mu_s(z)]\!] = 0, \qquad z \in \partial G_j$$

*and there are infinitely many different functions $\tilde{\mu}$, $\tilde{\mu}_s$ and domains $\tilde{G}_j$ that stand for $\mu, \mu_s$ and $G_j$, respectively, so that the corresponding solutions $\tilde{f}(r,\omega)$ to the direct problems are the same everywhere in $\overline{G} \times \Omega$, coinciding with $f(r,\omega)$.*

**Proof.** We rewrite the condition (4) in the form

$$[\![\mu(z)]\!] f(z,\omega) = \sum_{i=1}^{M} [\![\sigma_i(r)]\!] \int_{\Omega} S_i(\omega \cdot \omega') f(z,\omega')\, d\omega', \qquad z \in \partial G_j. \tag{5}$$

Integrating both sides of the latter equality with respect to $\omega \in \Omega$ and changing the order of integration in the right-hand side, we obtain

$$[\![\mu(z)]\!] \int_{\Omega} f(z,\omega)\, d\omega = \sum_{i=1}^{M} [\![\sigma_i(r)]\!] \int_{\Omega} \Big( \int_{\Omega} S_i(\omega \cdot \omega')\, d\omega \Big) f(z,\omega')\, d\omega'$$

Taking into account the relation (2) and the condition (1) of normalization for $S_i(\omega \cdot \omega')$, we have

$$[\![\mu(z)]\!] \int_{\Omega} f(z,\omega)\, d\omega = [\![\mu_s(z)]\!] \int_{\Omega} f(z,\omega')\, d\omega'.$$

Since the positive integrals in the both sides coincide, then

$$[\![\mu(z)]\!] = [\![\mu_s(z)]\!] \tag{6}$$

and the equivalent conditions $[\![\mu(z)]\!] \neq 0$ and $[\![\mu_s(z)]\!] \neq 0$ hold simultaneously.

The condition $[\![\mu_s(z)]\!] \neq 0$ and the formula (2) easily imply that there exists the index $k$, $1 \le k \le M$ such that $[\![\sigma_k(r)]\!] \neq 0$, $z \in \partial G_j$. Multiplying the equality (5) by the value $[\![\sigma_k(r)]\!]$, we obtain

$$[\![\mu(z)]\!][\![\sigma_k(r)]\!] f(z,\omega) = \sum_{i=1}^{M} [\![\sigma_i(r)]\!][\![\sigma_k(r)]\!] \int_{\Omega} S_i(\omega \cdot \omega') f(z,\omega')\, d\omega',$$
$$(z,\omega) \in \partial G_j \times \Omega. \tag{7}$$

Now we prove that $f(z,\omega)$, $(z,\omega) \in \partial G_j \times \Omega$, actually does not depend on $\omega$. Suppose the contrary. By continuity, the function $f(z,\omega)$ achieves its greatest value with respect to $\omega$ at a point $\omega = \omega_0$. By supposition, there exists a point $\omega^*$ such that $f(z,\omega_0) > f(z,\omega^*)$. By continuity, the inequality

$f(z,\omega_0) > f(z,\omega')$ holds for $\omega'$ from a certain neighborhood of the point $\omega^*$ in $\Omega$.

We consider the equality (7) for $\omega = \omega_0$, and obtain

$$[\![\mu(z)]\!][\![\sigma_k(r)]\!]f(z,\omega_0) = \sum_{i=1}^{M}[\![\sigma_i(r)]\!][\![\sigma_k(r)]\!]\int_\Omega S_i(\omega_0\cdot\omega')f(z,\omega')\,d\omega'. \quad (8)$$

In view of the condition c) of the theorem and pointed inequality $f(z,\omega_0) > f(z,\omega')$, we see that

$$\sum_{i=1}^{M}[\![\sigma_i(r)]\!][\![\sigma_k(r)]\!]\int_\Omega S_i(\omega_0\cdot\omega')f(z,\omega')\,d\omega' < \sum_{i=1}^{M}[\![\sigma_i(r)]\!][\![\sigma_k(r)]\!]f(z,\omega_0).$$

Here it has been taken into account that $[\![\sigma_i(z)]\!][\![\sigma_k(z)]\!] > 0$, at least for $i = k$.

Comparing the last inequality and (8), we obtain

$$[\![\mu(z)]\!][\![\sigma_k(r)]\!]f(z,\omega_0) < \sum_{i=1}^{M}[\![\sigma_i(r)]\!][\![\sigma_k(r)]\!]f(z,\omega_0).$$

This inequality is equivalent to each of the following inequalities

$$[\![\mu(z)]\!][\![\sigma_k(r)]\!] < \sum_{i=1}^{M}[\![\sigma_i(r)]\!][\![\sigma_k(r)]\!],$$

$$[\![\mu(z)]\!] < \sum_{i=1}^{M}[\![\sigma_i(r)]\!], \qquad [\![\mu_s(z)]\!] < \sum_{i=1}^{M}[\![\sigma_i(r)]\!].$$

The last inequality contradicts to the relation (2). This means that indeed $f(z,\omega) = g(z)$, $z \in \partial G_j$.

Note, that $f(r,\omega)$ is the solution of the direct problem not only for $(r,\omega) \in G \times \Omega$, but also for $(r,\omega) \in \overline{G}_j \times \Omega$. Therefore, we can use the Maximum Principle for $(r,\omega) \in \overline{G}_j \times \Omega$ (see Germogenova, 1986). According to this theorem

$$f(r,\omega) \le \sup_{z\in\partial G_j} g(z) = g(z_0), \qquad z_0 \in \partial G_j, \quad (r,\omega) \in \overline{G}_j \times \Omega.$$

Since $f(z,\omega)$, for $z \in \partial G_j$ does not depend on $\omega$, the value $g(z_0)$ is the greatest for the input and output radiation distribution with respect to the set $\overline{G}_j \times \Omega$. We have assumed that $J(r,\omega) = 0$, $(r,\omega) \in \overline{G}_j \times \Omega$. In this case the third item of the Maximum Principle implies the equalities: $\mu(r) = \mu_s(r)$, $f(r,\omega) = \text{const}$ for $(r,\omega) \in \overline{G}_j \times \Omega$. It is evident that $f(r,\omega) = g(z_0)$.

Now we prove that the same function $f(r,\omega)$ for $(r,\omega) \in \overline{G}_j \times \Omega$ satisfies the same boundary condition and the transport equation in which the functions $\mu(r)$ and $\mu_s(r)$ are replaced by $\tilde{\mu}(r) = \mu(r) + \alpha(r)$ and $\tilde{\mu}_s(r) = \mu_s(r)+\alpha(r)$, respectively, where $\alpha(r)$ is an arbitrary function $r \in G_j$. Naturally, $\alpha(r)$ must have the same general properties as the functions $\mu(r)$ and $\mu_s(r)$ have. It is also necessary that $\tilde{\mu}(r) > 0$, $r \in \overline{G}_j$. The last inequality is equivalent to $\alpha(r) > -\mu(r)$, $r \in \overline{G}_j$.

Since $f(r,\omega) = g(z_0)$, $(r,\omega) \in \overline{G}_j \times \Omega$, $z_0 \in \partial G_j$ the transport equation (1.1.1) proves to be equivalent to the equations

$$\mu(r)g(z_0) = \mu_s(r)g(z_0), \qquad \mu(r) = \mu_s(r), \quad r \in \overline{G}_j.$$

Adding a function $\alpha(r)$ to the both sides of the last equality, we obtain

$$\mu(r) + \alpha(r) = \mu_s(r) + \alpha(r), \qquad \tilde{\mu}(r) = \tilde{\mu}_s(r).$$

It is easy to see that the last equality is equivalent to the each of the following ones

$$\omega \cdot \nabla_r g(z_0) + \tilde{\mu}(r)g(z_0) = \tilde{\mu}_s(r)g(z_0),$$

$$\omega \cdot \nabla_r f(r,\omega) + \tilde{\mu}(r)f(r,\omega) = \int_\Omega \sum_{i=1}^{M} \tilde{\sigma}_i(r)S_i(\omega\cdot\omega')f(r,\omega')\,d\omega',$$
$$(r,\omega) \in G_j \times \Omega,$$

where $\tilde{\sigma}_i(r) = \sigma_i(r) + \alpha(r)/M$. This means that a function $\alpha(r)$ being added to $\mu(r)$ and $\mu_s(r)$ does not change the solution of the direct problem in $\overline{G}_j \times \Omega$.

We now prove that the solution of the direct problem (1.1.1), (1.1.2) does not change in $\overline{G} \times \Omega$ if the functions $\mu(r)$ and $\mu_s(r)$ are replaced by $\mu(r) + \alpha(r)$, and $\mu_s(r) + \alpha(r)$ respectively, where $\alpha(r) = 0$, $r \notin \overline{G}_j$. Indeed, $\tilde{\mu}(r) = \mu(r)$ and $\tilde{\mu}_s(r) = \mu_s(r)$ for $r \notin \overline{G}_j$ Therefore, the transport equations (1.1.1) for $\mu, \mu_s$ and for $\tilde{\mu}(r), \tilde{\mu}_s(r)$ coincide outside of $\overline{G}_j$ and the same function $f(r,\omega)$ is the solution of the equations. As noted before, the solution of the direct problem in $\overline{G}_j \times \Omega$ does not change when $\mu$ and $\mu_s$ are replaced by $\tilde{\mu}(r)$ and $\tilde{\mu}_s(r)$, respectively. This means that there are infinitely many different coefficients $\tilde{\mu}(r)$, $\tilde{\mu}_s(r)$ preserving the function $f(r,\omega)$.

It remains to prove that there are infinitely many different $G_j$ also preserving the solution of the direct problem. To this end, we take a function $\alpha(r)$ with the property $[\![\alpha(z)]\!] = -[\![\mu(z)]\!]$, $z \in \partial G_j$. In this case the following equalities hold:

$$[\![\tilde{\mu}(z)]\!] = [\![\mu(z)]\!] + [\![\alpha(z)]\!] = 0, \quad [\![\tilde{\mu}_s(z)]\!] = [\![\mu_s(z)]\!] + [\![\alpha(z)]\!] = 0, \quad z \in \partial G_j.$$

Suppose that $\alpha(r)$ has an additional property: it has nonzero jump of the first kind on the boundary of $\tilde{G}_j$, where $G_j$ contains the closure of $\tilde{G}_j$. Certainly, $\partial\tilde{G}_j$ is as smooth as $\partial G_j$. It is easy to understand that there exist infinitely many domains $\tilde{G}_j$ and the functions $\alpha(r)$ with these needed properties. For example, one can take an arbitrary ball within $G_j$ as a domain $\tilde{G}_j$. Since $[\![\tilde{\mu}(z)]\!] = [\![\tilde{\mu}_s(z)]\!] = 0$ for $z \in \partial G_j$, it follows that $\tilde{\mu}(r)$ and $\tilde{\mu}_s(r)$ are continuous on the surface $\partial G_j$ and have nonzero jumps on $\partial\tilde{G}_j$. We also note that for $r \in \overline{G}_j$

$$\mu(r) = \mu_s(r) = \sum_{i=1}^{M} \sigma_i(r), \qquad \tilde{\mu}(r) = \tilde{\mu}_s(r) = \sum_{i=1}^{M} \tilde{\sigma}_i(r),$$

$$[\![\mu(z)]\!] = [\![\mu_s(z)]\!] = \sum_{i=1}^{M} [\![\sigma_i(z)]\!], \quad [\![\tilde{\mu}(z)]\!] = [\![\tilde{\mu}_s(z)]\!] = \sum_{i=1}^{M} [\![\tilde{\sigma}_i(z)]\!], \quad z \in \partial G_j.$$

The assumption *c*) of this theorem means that the values $[\![\sigma_i(z)]\!]$, $z \in \partial G_j$ have the same sign. In view of $[\![\tilde{\sigma}_i(z)]\!] = [\![\sigma_i(z)]\!]$, the equality $[\![\tilde{\mu}_s(z)]\!] \equiv 0$, $z \in \partial G_j$ implies the equalities $[\![\tilde{\sigma}_i(z)]\!] \equiv 0$, $z \in \partial G_j$, $i = 1, \ldots, M$. This means that all functions $\tilde{\sigma}_i(r)$ are continuous on $\partial G_j$ as well as $\tilde{\mu}(r)$ and $\tilde{\mu}_s(r)$. At the same time the functions $\tilde{\mu}(r)$, $\tilde{\mu}_s(r)$ and at least one function $\tilde{\sigma}_i(r)$ have nonzero jumps on $\partial\tilde{G}_j$. Therefore, the domain $\tilde{G}_j$ can be viewed as a new inclusion instead of $G_j$. As shown above, changing $G_j$ for $\tilde{G}_j$ preserves the solution of the direct problem (1.1.1), (1.1.2), which is equal to $f(r, \omega)$, $(r, \omega) \in \overline{G}_j \times \Omega$. The theorem is proved. □

Note that it is not yet clear whether the assumptions of the theorem can be satisfied. To clarify this issue, we will represent some examples in the next section. While, we give comments to the theorem and introduce the important notions.

The assumption *a*) of the theorem means that at least one inclusion $(G_j)$ really exists. The point b) explains the feature of the internal sources. In particular, the case $J \equiv 0$ is allowed. The inequality c) can be treated as predominance of scattering in one of neighboring domains over scattering in another, for example each cross-section $\sigma_i(r)$, $i = 1, \ldots, M$ in $G_l$ is greater or equal to $\sigma_i(r)$ in $G_j$. Also that the condition c) is satisfied in the case $M = 1$, i. e. when we consider only one kind of scattering. The assumption d) seems to be the most important in the theorem and it is the base for the following notations.

Consider the function

$$mv(z,\omega) = m_1(z,\omega)\exp\Big(-\int_0^{d(z,\omega)} \mu(z+t\omega)\,dt\Big),$$
$$z \in \partial G_0, \qquad \omega \in \Omega, \tag{9}$$

where $m_1(z,\omega)$ is defined by (3).

It is evident that the equalities $mv(z,\omega) = 0$ and $m_1(z,\omega) = 0$ are equivalent.

**Definition 1.** The value $|mv(z,\omega)|$ is called the measure of visibility of the medium $G$ at the point $z \in \partial G_0$ in the direction $\omega$ under radiography of this medium by X-ray radiation.

The condition $|mv(z,\omega)| > 0$, $z \in \partial G_0$, $\omega \in \Omega$ guarantees the uniqueness of solving the tomography problems (see Section 1.4). At the same time the condition $|mv(z,\omega)| = 0$, $z \in \partial G_j$, $\omega \in \Omega$ (together with other not so important conditions) excludes successful solving the tomography problems by any method described in frameworks of our mathematical model (see Theorem 1).

Note that the exponential multiplier in (9) explains the well-known fact in tomography: the more optical thickness of the medium, the more difficult is to determine its structure.

**Definition 2.** The medium $G$ with the property

$$mv(z,\omega) = 0, \qquad z \in \partial G_0, \quad \omega \in \Omega \tag{10}$$

is called invisible under its radio-diagnostics by the given X-ray radiation.

The last definition depends on all parameters of the process, in particular, it depends on the distribution of the external sources $h(\xi,\omega)$. Therefore, this notation seems to be too complicate for its practical application.

Now we try to approximate (10) by a more simple relation for the case $J \equiv 0$, when the internal sources of radiation are absent.

We rewrite the function $mv(z,\omega)$ in another form. Firstly, we transform $m_1(z,\omega)$

$$m_1(z,\omega) = [\![\mu(z)]\!] f(z,\omega) - \sum_{i=1}^{M} [\![\sigma_i(r)]\!] \int_\Omega S_i(\omega\cdot\omega') f(z,\omega)\, d\omega'$$
$$+ \sum_{i=1}^{M} [\![\sigma_i(r)]\!] \int_\Omega S_i(\omega\cdot\omega')(f(z,\omega) - f(z,\omega'))\, d\omega'$$
$$= f(z,\omega)\Big([\![\mu(z)]\!] - \sum_{i=1}^{M} [\![\sigma_i(r)]\!]\Big) + \sum_{i=1}^{M} [\![\sigma_i(r)]\!] \int_\Omega S_i(\omega\cdot\omega')(f(z,\omega) - f(z,\omega'))\, d\omega'$$
$$= f(z,\omega)[\![\mu_a(z)]\!] + \sum_{i=1}^{M} [\![\sigma_i(r)]\!] \int_\Omega S_i(\omega\cdot\omega')(f(z,\omega) - f(z,\omega'))\, d\omega'.$$

Thus, we have

$$mv(z,\omega) = \exp\Big(-\int_0^{d(z,\omega)} \mu(z+t\omega)\, dt\Big)$$
$$\times \Big(f(z,\omega)[\![\mu_a(z)]\!] + \sum_{i=1}^{M} [\![\sigma_i(r)]\!] \int_\Omega S_i(\omega\cdot\omega')(f(z,\omega) - f(z,\omega'))\, d\omega'\Big).$$

Note, that the positiveness of $f(r,\omega)$ and $f(r,\omega')$ leads to partial vanishing of the sum in the right-hand side of the last equality. Therefore the equality $mv(z,\omega) = 0$ is close to $[\![\mu_a(z)]\!] = 0$.

**Definition 3.** The medium $G$ with the property

$$[\![\mu_a(z)]\!] = 0, \qquad z \in \partial G_0 \tag{11}$$

is called poorly visible under its radio-diagnostics by X-ray radiation.

Is other words, the equality (11) is obtained from (10) by using the approximation $f(z,\omega) \simeq f(z,\omega')$ which becomes rather exact in certain difficult tomography conditions.

Suppose that the traditional difficulties in tomography are increasing: the optical distance from $G_j$ to $\partial G$ is large. In addition, the optical thickness of $G_j$ is decreasing and the level of scattering in the medium $G$ is increasing. Then, as it is shown in Fano, Spenser and Berger (1963), the function $f(r,\omega)$ for $(r,\omega) \in \overline{G}_j \times \Omega$ becomes more and more isotropic. In particular, the approximate equality $f(z,\omega) \simeq f(z,\omega')$, $z \in \partial G_j$ tends to the exact one.

It is clear that the condition (11) is much simpler than the condition (10). The equality (11) means continuity of the coefficient of absorption on the boundary of the inclusion $G_j$.

Thus, using the known tables (see Hubbell and Seltzer, 1995) we can compare the values of $\mu_a$ for various substances and for various levels of energy.

We call two different substances a poorly visible pair, if they have the same value of $\mu_a$ for a certain level of energy. The set of such pairs is represented in the second part of this book.

Perhaps, the determination of the contact boundary between the substances within a poorly visible pair appears to be a difficult problem for tomography methods. These theoretical conclusions are confirmed by means of the following numerical experiments.

The main part of the method of determination of $\partial G_0$ is the calculation of the indicator $\mathrm{Ind}^*(r)$. The surface $\partial G_0$ is determined approximately as consisting of the points $r$ where successfully computed $\mathrm{Ind}^*(r)$ has greater values than in other points. The simplicity of the formulas (1.4.4) and (1.4.24) allows us to construct easily and test the algorithm.

The main steps for testing the algorithm are as follows.

1. A choice of domain $G$, a partition $G_0$ and functions $\mu, k, J, h$.
2. Numerical solving of the direct problem (1.1.1), (1.1.2) and calculation of the function $H^*(\eta,\omega) = f^*(r + d(r,\omega)\omega, \omega)$, $\eta = r + d(r,\omega)\omega$.
3. Calculation of the function $\mathrm{Ind}^*(r)$ using formula (1.4.24).
4. Graphical representation of the values of $\mathrm{Ind}^*(r)$ in a certain section using shades of grey.

In the description of tests below, the domain $G$ is a ball of a radius $a$ centered at the origin, and the functions $k(r,\omega\cdot\omega') = \mu_s(r)S(\omega\cdot\omega')$, $h(\xi,\omega) \equiv 1$ and internal sources are absent. In these numerical experiments, the function $S$ is Thompson's type function (see Fano, Berger and Spencer, 1963). In the latter case, we have

$$S(\omega\cdot\omega') = 3(1 + (\omega\cdot\omega')^2)/(16\pi).$$

In all numerical experiments, using the Monte-Carlo method (see Ermakov, Mikhailov, 1982), the function $H^*(\eta,\omega)$ is calculated at the points

$$\eta_{ij} = \rho_i \omega_{\perp j} + \sqrt{a^2 - \rho_i^2}\,\omega_j,$$

$$\omega_j = (-\sin\gamma_j, \cos\gamma_j, 0), \qquad \omega_{\perp j} = (\cos\gamma_j, \sin\gamma_j, 0),$$

$$\rho_i = i\cdot a/60, \quad i = -60,\dots,60, \qquad \gamma_j = j\cdot 2\pi/180, \quad j = 1,\dots,180.$$

The function $\mathrm{Ind}^*(r)$ is calculated at the points $r_{ij} = (i \cdot a/200, j \cdot a/200, 0)$, $i, j = -200, \ldots, 200$.

We present the results of three experiments which use the parameters of certain real substances (see Chapter 2).

In the experiments the energy level $E$ is in the interval 1–15 keV. In these cases, radiation in substances is characterized by considerable attenuation. The coefficient $\mu$ may achieve the values about $10^5$ cm$^{-1}$ (see Henke, Gullikson, and Davis 1993; Hubbell and Seltzer, 1995). These conditions correspond to microtomography.

**Test 3.** In this numerical experiment the medium $G$ consists of three substances:

1) polyethylene terephthalate, "mylar" (number 137, see Section 2.3);

2) blood, whole (number 107);

3) brain, grey/white matter (number 109).

The domain $G$ is the ball of the radius $a = 10^{-2}$ cm. The inclusion $G_1$ is the ball of the radius $0.2a$, centered at the point $(0.1a; 0; 0)$. The inclusion $G_1$ is assumed to be "mylar". Inclusion $G_2$ which is a cylindrical body defined as follows

$$G_2 = \{r \in G \mid ((r_1 + 0.5a)/(0.1a))^2 + (r_3/(0.2a))^2 < 1\},$$

and $G_3 = G \setminus \overline{G_1 \cup G_2}$. The inclusion $G_2$ is assumed to be blood and $G_3$ represents brain.

The numerical experiment involves three energy levels: $E = 3.644$ keV, $E = 6.209$ keV and $E = 5$ keV. Bellow we give the values of the coefficients $\mu$ and $\mu_a$ ($\mu_s = \mu - \mu_a$) within $G_i$, $i = 1, 2, 3$ (see Section 2.1).

| $E$, keV | $\mu_1$, cm$^{-1}$ | $\mu_{a1}$, cm$^{-1}$ | $\mu_2$, cm$^{-1}$ | $\mu_{a2}$, cm$^{-1}$ | $\mu_3$, cm$^{-1}$ | $\mu_{a3}$, cm$^{-1}$ |
|---|---|---|---|---|---|---|
| 3.644 | 111.7 | 110.7 | 114.6 | 113.1 | 112.5 | 110.7 |
| 6.209 | 20.84 | 20.21 | 24.10 | 23.44 | 24.12 | 23.44 |
| 5 | 38.53 | 37.77 | 44.86 | 43.96 | 44.12 | 43.18 |

For the first energy level we have $[\![\mu_a(z)]\!] = 0$ at the boundary of $G_1$, and $|[\![\mu_a(z)]\!]| = 2.4$ at the boundary of $G_2$. For the second energy level we have $[\![\mu_a(z)]\!] = 0$ at the boundary of $G_2$, and $|[\![\mu_a(z)]\!]| = 3.23$ at the boundary of $G_1$.

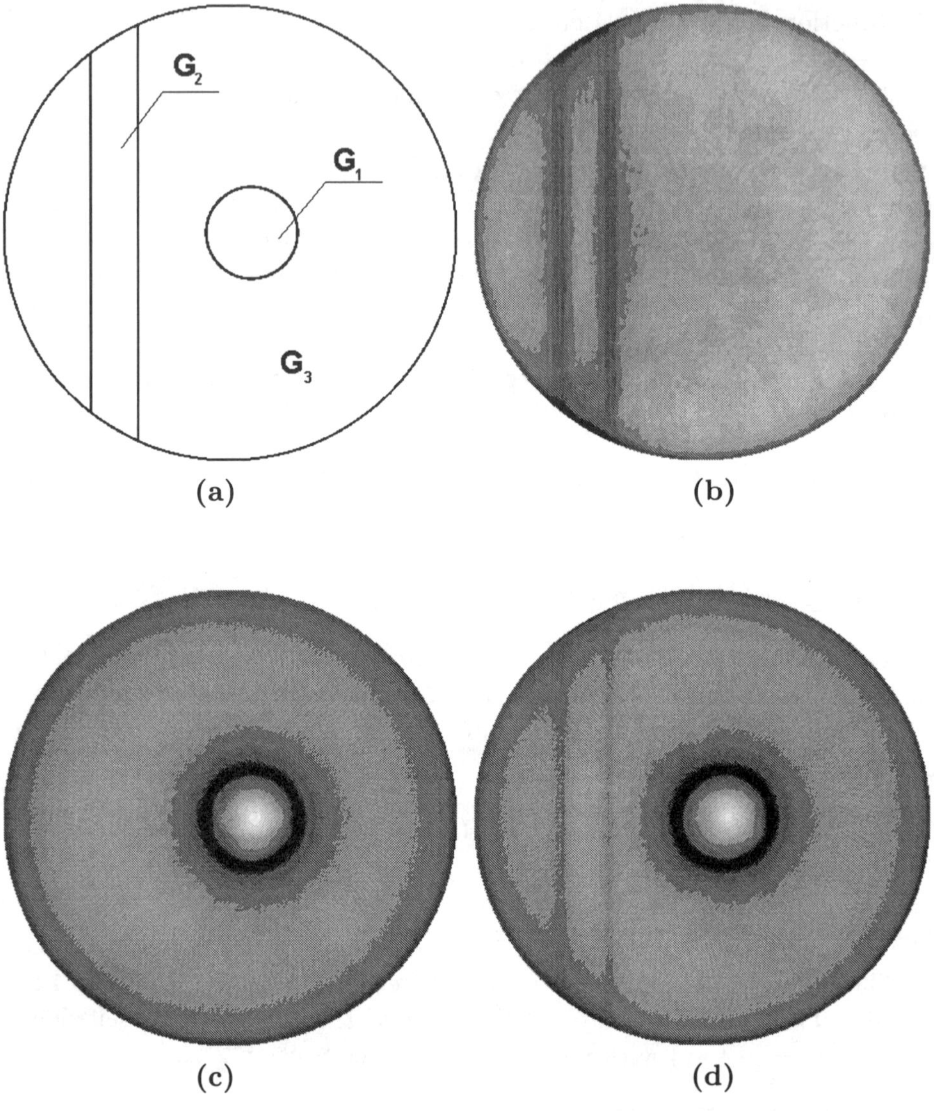


**Figure 1:** There are four sections (**a**,**b**,**c**,**d**) of the domain $G$ by the plane $r_3 = 0$. The original is shown in **a** and the boundaries of the inclusions $G_1$ and $G_2$ are assumed to be unknown. Other parts of the figure illustrate the algorithm based on the indicator $\mathrm{Ind}^*(r)$ for various levels of energy. The first reconstruction is represented in **b**, where the medium state proves to be poorly visible for $G_1$ on the energy level $E = 3.644$ keV. The second reconstruction **c** for $E = 6.209$ keV corresponds to poorly visible medium state for $G_2$. The last reconstruction **d** for $E = 5$ keV is appropriate for $G_1$ and $G_2$ simultaneously.

According to our definition, the inclusion $G_1$ is a poor visible medium at the first energy level, and $G_2$ is a poor visible medium at the second level. Thus, successful reconstruction of $\partial G_1$ and $\partial G_2$ using the indicator or other methods, is not guaranteed, for $E = 3.644$ and $6.209$ keV, respectively. For the third energy level we have $|[\![\mu_a(z)]\!]| = 6.19$ at the boundary of $G_1$, and $|[\![\mu_a(z)]\!]| = 0.78$ at the boundary of $G_2$.

In Figures 1b,c,d, the distribution of values of $\mathrm{Ind}^*(r)$ in the section $r_3 = 0$ is shown using shades of grey. Larger values of $\mathrm{Ind}^*(r)$ correspond to the darker shades of grey.

The boundary of $G_0$ is shown in Figure 1a; Figure 1b represents the reconstruction of $\partial G_0$ for $E = 3.644$ keV; Figure 1c represents the reconstruction of $\partial G_0$ for $E = 6.209$ keV; Figure 1d represents the reconstruction of $\partial G_0$ for $E = 6$ keV. As expected, the boundary between brain and blood is not visible in the first case, and the boundary between brain and "mylar" is not visible in the second case.

It is important to note that the disadvantage of the test consists in a very small difference between the values of the total attenuation coefficients for brain and "mylar" in the case $E = 3.644$ keV, and for brain and blood in the case $E = 6.209$ keV. But the basic reason for unsuccessful reconstruction is different, namely, it is coincidence of the absorption coefficients. A more interesting case would be provided by a larger difference between the values of the coefficient $\mu$ (see the following test).

**Test 3.** In this numerical experiment the medium $G$ consists of three substances: niobium (number 41), vanadium (23) and selenium (34).

The domain $G$ is the ball of the radius $a = 10^{-3}$cm with the center in the origin. The inclusion $G_1$ is the ball of the radius $0.2a$, centered at the point $(-0.6a; 0; 0)$. The inclusion $G_2$ is an ellipsoid defined as follows

$$G_2 = \{r \in G \mid (r_1/(0.4a))^2 + (r_2/(0.3a))^2 + (r_3/(0.3a))^2 < 1\}.$$

and $G_3 = G \setminus \overline{G_1 \cup G_2}$. The inclusions $G_1$, $G_2$ and $G_3$ are assumed to be niobium, vanadium and selenium, respectively.

The numerical experiment involves two energy levels: $E = 13.58$ keV, and $E = 15$ keV. Bellow we give the values of the coefficients $\mu$ and $\mu_a$ within $G_i$, $i = 1, 2, 3$ (see Section 2.1).

| $E$, keV | $\mu_1$, cm$^{-1}$ | $\mu_{a1}$, cm$^{-1}$ | $\mu_2$, cm$^{-1}$ | $\mu_{a2}$, cm$^{-1}$ | $\mu_3$, cm$^{-1}$ | $\mu_{a3}$, cm$^{-1}$ |
|---|---|---|---|---|---|---|
| 13.58 | 359.9 | 342.9 | 385.9 | 345.8 | 616.8 | 345.8 |
| 15 | 229 | 214.9 | 243.4 | 221.6 | 464.9 | 282.2 |

For the first energy level, except the point $z = (-0.4a, 0, 0)$, we have $[\![\mu_a(z)]\!] = 0$ at the boundary of $G_2$, and $|[\![\mu_a(z)]\!]| = 2.9$ at the boundary of $G_1$. For the second energy level, except the point $z = (-0.4a, 0, 0)$, we have $|[\![\mu_a(z)]\!]| = 67.3$ at the boundary of $G_1$, and $|[\![\mu_a(z)]\!]| = 60.6$ at the boundary of $G_2$.

In Figures 2b and 2c the distribution of the values of $\mathrm{Ind}^*(r)$ in the section $r_3 = 0$ is shown using shades of grey.

The boundary of $G_0$ is shown in Figure 2a; Figure 2b represents the reconstruction of $\partial G_0$ for the $E = 13.58$ keV; Figure 1c represents the reconstruction of $\partial G_0$ for $E = 15$ keV. As expected, the boundary between selenium and vanadium is not visible at the energy $E = 13.58$ keV.

Remind that in Corollary 1.4.1 and Remark 1.4.2 we assume that $\partial G_0$ is a Lipshitz surface and does not contain any linear parts. It was assumed for simplification of the corresponding proofs. At the same time, in Test 1 the surface $\partial G_2$ contains linear parts and in Test 2 $\partial G_0$ is not a Lipshitz surface at the common point of $\partial G_1$ and $\partial G_2$. Nevertheless, the indicator $\mathrm{Ind}^*(r)$ (based on Corollary 1.4.1 and Remark 1.4.2, in particular) appears to be able to reconstruct the internal structure of $G$. This circumstance shows that our tomography methods can have more extensive application than it is proved in this book.

**Test 3.** Not rarely in practice we can know substances of possible inclusions and a surrounding medium and need only to determine the shapes and locations of these inclusions. In such cases the difficulty of reconstruction connected with poor visibility of the inclusions can be overcome. For this, we find the energy levels of good visibility for each inclusion separately, using tables of the values of the absorption coefficients. After that, a certain tomography method is used for each selected energy level. Therefore a rather good reconstruction of the corresponding inclusion appears separately. Simultaneously the images of other inclusions may be arbitrary, particularly poorly visible. Adding the results of these reconstructions, it is possible to obtain a good reconstruction of the medium in whole.

We explain this general idea more explicitly in the following test, where the inclusions $G_1$ and $G_2$ consist of beryllium and copper, respectively. The medium $G$ consists of selenium and the inclusions $G_1$ and $G_2$. The domain $G$ is the ball of the radius $a = 10^{-3}$cm. The ellipsoids $G_1$ and $G_2$ are defined by the inequalities

$$((r_1 - 0.2a)/(0.1a))^2 + ((r_2 - 0.2a)/(0.05a))^2 + (r_3/(0.05a))^2 < 1,$$
$$((r_1 + 0.05a)/(0.05a))^2 + (r_2/(0.2a))^2 + (r_3/(0.05a))^2 < 1.$$

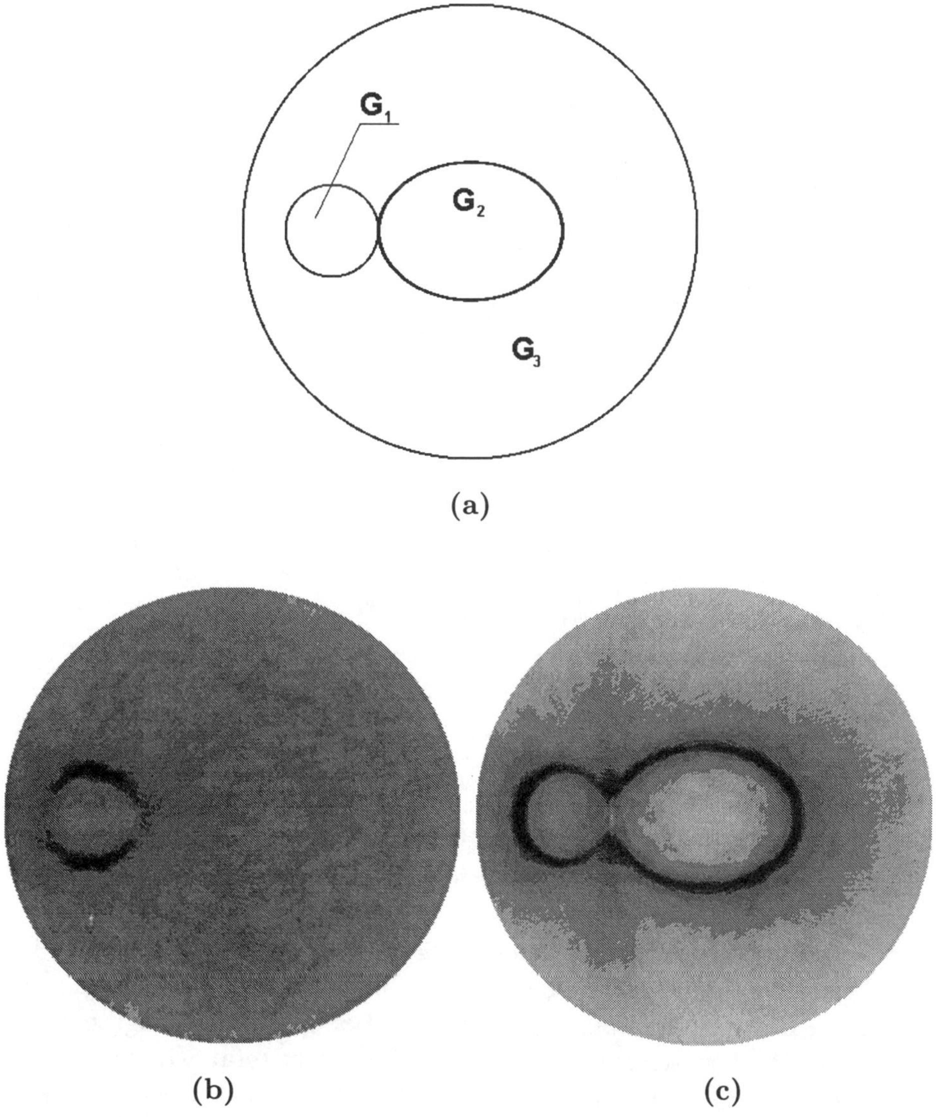


**Figure 2:** There are three sections (**a**,**b**,**c**) of the domain $G$ by the plane $r_3 = 0$. The original is shown in **a**, where the boundaries of the inclusions $G_1$ and $G_2$ are sought for. The first reconstruction for $E = 13.58$ keV is given in **b** where $G_2$ is not shown due to its poor visibility. The second reconstruction for $E = 15$ keV appears to be successful for both inclusions. Note, that the conditions of Test 2 do not satisfy all assumptions required for the indicator $\text{Ind}^*(r)$, as well as the conditions of Test 1. Nevertheless, the image **c** seems to be appropriate (see the corresponding remark after the test 2).

We apply the indicator $\mathrm{Ind}^*(r)$ choosing the energy level $\tilde{E}_1$ and $\tilde{E}_2$ such that the quantities

$$|\mu_{a1}(E)-\mu_{a3}(E)|\cdot\exp(-\mu_3(E)\cdot a), \quad |\mu_{a2}(E)-\mu_{a3}(E)|\cdot\exp(-\mu_3(E)\cdot a) \quad (12)$$

becomes close to their greatest values respectively. Here $\mu_{a1}$ and $\mu_{a2}$ are the coefficients of absorption for $G_1$ and $G_2$ respectively; $\mu_3$ is the total attenuation coefficient of the surrounding medium $G_3$ ($G_3 = G \setminus \overline{G_1 \cup G_2}$); $\mu_{a3}$ is the absorption coefficient of the medium $G_3$. The exponential multiplier in (12) makes these quantities similar with respect to measure of visibility (see the definition in this section). In our case we select $\tilde{E}_1 = 6$ keV and $\tilde{E}_2 = 8.99$ keV.

| $E$, keV | $\mu_1$, cm$^{-1}$ | $\mu_{a1}$, cm$^{-1}$ | $\mu_2$, cm$^{-1}$ | $\mu_{a2}$, cm$^{-1}$ | $\mu_3$, cm$^{-1}$ | $\mu_{a3}$, cm$^{-1}$ |
|---|---|---|---|---|---|---|
| $\tilde{E}_1$ | 4.67 | 4.176 | 1035 | 1011 | 797.9 | 781.7 |
| $\tilde{E}_2$ | 1.645 | 1.219 | 2494 | 1634 | 283.7 | 273.7 |

It what follows we consequently use the indicator $\mathrm{Ind}^*(r)$ for $E = \tilde{E}_1$ and for $E = \tilde{E}_2$.

The boundary of $G_0$ is shown in Figure 3a; Figure 3b represents the reconstruction of $\partial G_0$ for the $E = \tilde{E}_1$; Figure 3c represents the reconstruction of $\partial G_0$ for $E = \tilde{E}_2$.

Summing two obtained normalized values $\mathrm{Ind}^*(r)$, we have the appropriate final result (see Figure 3d), although the reconstruction 3b is proved to be not so successful for the inclusion $G_2$, as well as the image of $G_1$ in the reconstruction 3c.

Now we try to explain (in general) the definition of poor visibility from the physical point of view. This definition means that the coefficient of absorption $\mu_a$ is more important characteristic for X-ray tomography than the coefficient of scattering $\mu_s$ and the coefficient of total attenuation $\mu$.

In fact, (in the framework of the admitted mathematical model) many tomography methods (including the indicators $\mathrm{Ind}(r)$, $\mathrm{Ind}^*(r)$) are based on using a difference between values of the distribution $H(\eta,\omega)$ with respect to different values of the variables $(\eta,\omega) \in \Gamma^+$. Just the coefficient of absorption describes decreasing of the distribution of the particle flux. The coefficient of scattering has not the similar sense because it describes both decreasing and increasing of the distribution at the same point of the medium. By the similar reason, such complex characteristic as the coefficient of total attenuation cannot influence explicitly on the formation of the difference between the various values of $H(\eta,\omega)$.

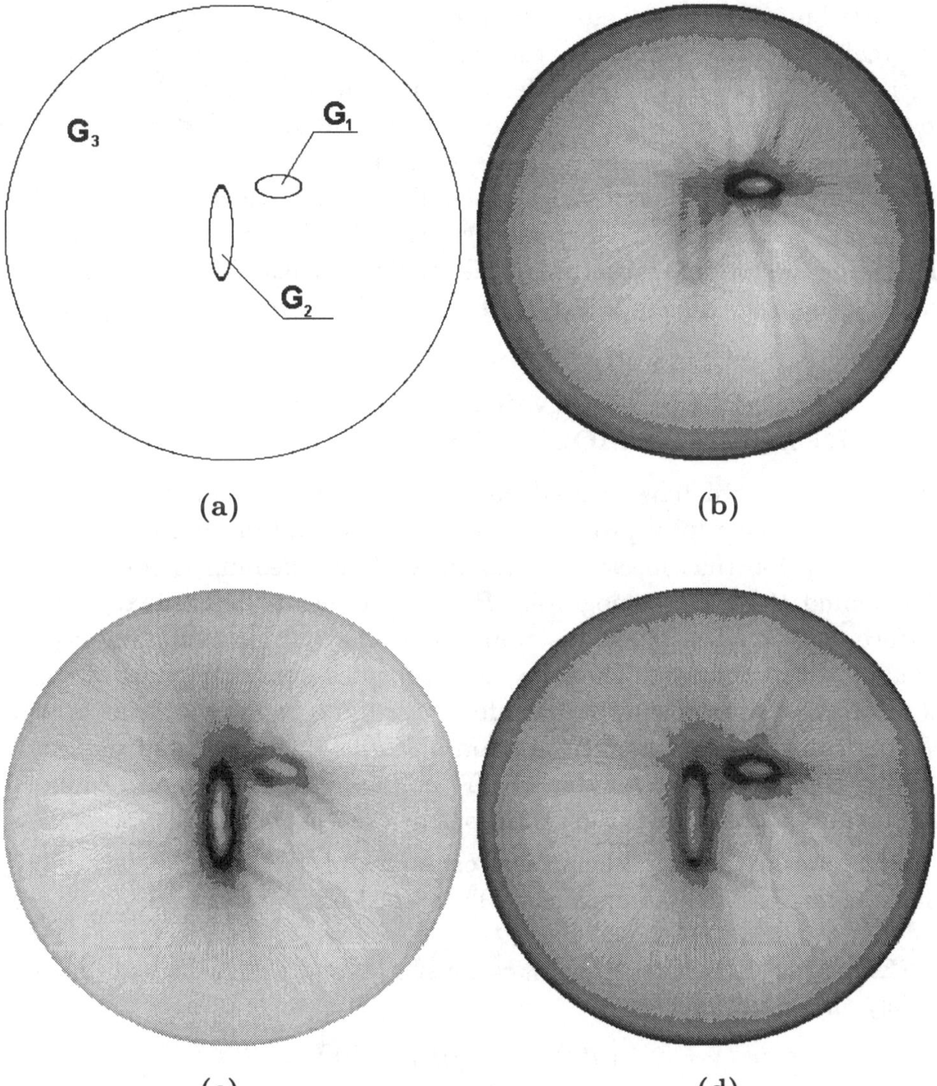


(a) (b)

(c) (d)

**Figure 3:** There are four sections (**a**,**b**,**c**,**d**) of the domain $G$ by the plane $r_3 = 0$. The original is shown in **a**, where the boundaries of the inclusions $G_1$ and $G_2$ are sought for. The first reconstruction for energy level $\tilde{E}_1 = 6$ keV is represented in **b** which appears to be better for $G_2$ than for $G_1$. The second reconstruction **c** for $\tilde{E} = 8.99$ keV is better for $G_1$. The final appropriate result obtained by summing the previous values of the indicator is given in **d**.

At last, we make the important remark. It is meant in our theory that the distribution $H(\eta,\omega)$ is measured for a fixed level of energy $\tilde{E}$. However, the real detectors respond to the particles having energy from a certain interval $[E^*, E^{**}]$. Let us consider the case when the value $\tilde{E}$ corresponds to the state of poor visibility in the medium and $E^* < \tilde{E} < E^{**}$. We have established the fact that the particles with the energy $\tilde{E}$ (and close to them) almost do not form the difference of the distribution which is the base of the tomography methods. Therefore these particles decrease the possibility to determine the internal structure of the medium. Thus, the condition of poor visibility on a fixed energy level $\tilde{E}$ is to be taken into account in practice.

## 1.6. EXAMPLES OF INVISIBLE MEDIA IN X-RAY TOMOGRAPHY

In Section 1.5 we have proved the theorem on non-uniqueness of solving of the tomography problems. The main condition of this theorem is the assumption that measure of visibility of the medium is equal to zero. We remind that the Tomography Problem 1 means determination of the surface $\partial G_0$ by the given distribution of the output radiation $H(\eta,\omega)$, $(\eta,\omega) \in \Gamma^+$. However, Theorem 1.5.1 provides non-uniqueness of solving not only for this problem, but also for other tomography problems in which the distribution of the input radiation $h(\xi,\omega)$, $(\xi,\omega) \in \Gamma^-$ is given in addition to $H(\eta,\omega)$. It is clear that the Tomography Problem 2 also cannot be successfully solved under the conditions of this theorem.

Here we give the mathematical examples of such cases. Naturally, in these examples the assumptions of Theorem 1.5.1 are satisfied.

**Example 1.** Let $h = h_0$, $h_0 = \text{const} > 0$ and the coefficients $\mu$, $\mu_s$, $J$ satisfy the condition

$$(\mu(r) - \mu_s(r))h_0 = J(r). \tag{1}$$

It is easy to see that the unique solution to the direct problem for this case is the function $f(r,\omega) = h_0$ for any system of the domains $G_1, G_2, \ldots, G_p$. It is also evident that there are infinitely many different functions $\mu, \mu_s, J$ satisfying the equality (1). In these cases any reasonable tomography problem cannot be successfully solved.

Moreover, we note that

$$[\![\mu(z)]\!]h_0 - [\![\mu_s(z)]\!]h_0 = [\![J(z)]\!], \qquad z \in \partial G_0, \tag{2}$$

and consequently

$$m_1(z,\omega) = -[\![\mu(z)]\!]f(z,\omega) + [\![N(z,\omega) + J(z)]\!] \\ = -[\![\mu(z)]\!]h_0 + [\![\mu_s(z)]\!]h_0 + [\![J(z)]\!] = 0. \quad (3)$$

Therefore the measure of visibility is equal to zero, i. e.

$$mv(z,\omega) = \exp\Big(-\int_0^{d(z,\omega)} \mu(z+t\omega)\,dt\Big) m_1(z,\omega) = 0. \quad (4)$$

It remains to assume that $[\![J(z)]\!] = 0$ for $z \in \partial G_i$ at least for one index $j$ to satisfy all assumptions of Theorem 1.5.1.

Thus, in this example we see that the structure of the medium cannot be determined by tomography methods and at the same time all assumptions of the Theorem 1.5.1 are satisfied.

In the following two similar examples the function $f(r,\omega)$ has more complicate form.

Consider the well-known case of spherical symmetry which is a partial case of the relations (1.1.1), (1.1.2). Let $G$ be a ball in $\mathcal{E}^3$, $\rho$ is the distance from the center of this ball to the point $r$, and let $\theta$ be the angle between the direction $\omega$ and the vector $r$. We suppose that the functions $\mu, k, J$ depend only on $\rho$ instead of the variable $r$, and $k, J, h$ depend only on $\theta, \theta'$ instead of the direction variables $\omega, \omega'$. Then the function $f$ also depends on $\rho$ and $\theta$ only. Hereafter we change the variable $\theta$ for $\nu = \cos\theta$, $\nu \in [-1,1]$.

We consider the case of isotropic scattering:

$$k(r, \omega\cdot\omega') = \mu_s(r)/(4\pi).$$

Then the transport equation can be written in the following form (see Anikonov, Kovtanyuk and Prokhorov, 2002)

$$\nu\,\frac{\partial f(\rho,\nu)}{\partial\rho} + \frac{1-\nu^2}{\rho}\,\frac{\partial f(\rho,\nu)}{\partial\nu} + \mu(\rho)f(\rho,\nu) = \frac{\mu_s(\rho)}{2}\int_{-1}^{1} f(\rho,\nu')\,d\nu' + J(\rho,\nu), \quad (5)$$

**Example 2.** Suppose that $G_0 = G_1 \cup G_2$, $G_1 = \{0 \le \rho < \rho_1\}$, $G_2 = \{\rho_1 < \rho < \rho_2\}$, $J \equiv 0$, where $\rho_1, \rho_2$ are the given positive numbers, and

$$\mu(\rho) = \begin{cases} \rho^2 - \rho_1^2, & \rho \in G_2, \\ \alpha(\rho), & \rho \in G_1, \end{cases} \qquad \mu_s(\rho) = \begin{cases} 0, & \rho \in G_2, \\ \alpha(\rho), & \rho \in G_1. \end{cases}$$

Here an arbitrary function $\alpha(\rho)$ is taken such that all assumptions of Section 1.5 for the functions $\mu$ and $\mu_s$ are satisfied. It is not difficult to verify that the following function is the solution of the equation (5)

$$f(\rho,\nu) = \begin{cases} C\exp\{\rho^3\nu^3/3 - \rho\nu(\rho_1^2 - \rho^2(1-\nu^2)) \\ \qquad + 2/3 \cdot (\rho_1^2 - \rho^2(1-\nu^2))^{3/2}\}, & |\nu| \geq \nu_1, \\ C\exp\{\rho^3\nu^3/3 - \rho\nu(\rho_1^2 - \rho^2(1-\nu^2))\}, & |\nu| < \nu_1, \end{cases} \tag{6}$$

for $\rho \in G_2$, and $f(\rho,\nu) \equiv C$ ($C = \text{const}$) for $\rho \in G_1$. The value $\nu_1$ in (6) is equal to $\sqrt{1-\rho_1^2/\rho^2}$. The function $h$ has the form:

$$h(\nu) = \begin{cases} C\exp\{\rho_2^3\nu^3/3 - \rho_2\nu(\rho_1^2 - \rho_2^2(1-\nu^2)) \\ \qquad + 2/3 \cdot (\rho_1^2 - \rho_2^2(1-\nu^2))^{3/2}\}, & -1 \leq \nu \leq -\sqrt{1-\rho_1^2/\rho_2^2}, \\ C\exp\{\rho_2^3\nu^3/3 - \rho_2\nu(\rho_1^2 - \rho_2^2(1-\nu^2))\}, & -\sqrt{1-\rho_1^2/\rho_2^2} < \nu \leq 0. \end{cases}$$

Since $\alpha(r)$ is an arbitrary function, then there are infinitely many complexes $\tilde{\mu}$, $\tilde{\mu}_s$ preserving the function $f$ everywhere in $\overline{G} \times \Omega$. In particular, there are such functions $\tilde{\mu}$, $\tilde{\mu}_s$ which appear to be continuous for $\rho = \rho_1$.

We can easy verify that $f(\rho,\nu) \in C(\overline{G} \times [-1,1])$, $h \in C([-1,1])$ and

$$\begin{aligned} m_1(\rho_1,\nu) &= -[\![\mu(z)]\!] f(\rho_1,\nu) + \frac{[\![\mu_s(\rho_1)]\!]}{2} \int_{-1}^{1} f(\rho_1,\nu')\,d\nu' + [\![J(\rho_1,\nu)]\!] \\ &= -C\alpha(\rho_1) + C\alpha(\rho_1) = 0. \end{aligned} \tag{7}$$

**Example 3.** Suppose that $G_0 = G_1 \cup G_2$, $G_1 = \{0 \leq \rho < \rho_1\}$, $G_2 = \{\rho_1 < \rho < \rho_2\}$ and

$$\mu(\rho) = \begin{cases} \rho, & \rho \in G_2, \\ \rho_1 + \alpha(\rho), & \rho \in G_1, \end{cases} \qquad \mu_s(\rho) = \begin{cases} \rho_1, & \rho \in G_2, \\ \rho_1 + \alpha(\rho), & \rho \in G_1, \end{cases}$$

$$J(\rho,\nu) = 2\nu(\rho - \rho_1) + \mu_a(\rho)(2 + (\rho - \rho_1)),$$

where $\alpha(\rho)$ is an arbitrary function providing the property:

$$\mu_a(\rho) = \mu(\rho) - \mu_s(\rho) = \begin{cases} \rho - \rho_1, & \rho \in G_2, \\ 0, & \rho \in G_1. \end{cases}$$

It is not difficult to see that $J \geq 0$, $[\![J(\rho_1,\nu)]\!] = 0$ and the solution of the equation (5) is the following function

$$f(\rho,\nu) = \begin{cases} 2 + (\rho - \rho_1)^2, & \rho \in G_2, \quad \nu \in [-1,1], \\ 2, & \rho \in G_1, \quad \nu \in [-1,1]. \end{cases} \tag{8}$$

The respective function $h$ has the form $h(\nu) = 2 + (\rho_2 - \rho_1)^2$. We see that

$$m_1(\rho_1, \nu) = -2\alpha(\rho_1) + 2\alpha(\rho_1) + 0 = 0.$$

Thus, we have the situation similar to Example 2.

These three examples show that the conditions of Theorem 1.5.1 can be satisfied and invisible media really exist, at least, theoretically.

## 1.7. CONSIDERATION OF THE CASE WITH ENERGY DEPENDENCE

Accordingly to descriptions of passing soft X-ray radiation through a substance the loss of photon energy in the Rayleigh and Compton scattering is negligible. However, similar loss of energy is to be taken into account for higher energy for the better adequacy to natural conditions. Therefore, in this section we consider a mathematical model based on a transport equation with energy dependence and proper boundary conditions (see Leypunskii, Novozhilov and Sakharov, 1960; Fano, Berger and Spencer, 1963).

We use the same notations for the same physical quantities adding a new scalar variable $E$ that stands for energy measured in the electron-volts. Thus, we write

$$\omega \cdot \nabla_r f(r, \omega, E) + \mu(r, E) f(r, \omega, E) = \int_\Omega \int_E^{E_2} k(r, \omega \cdot \omega', E, E') f(r, \omega', E')\, dE'\, d\omega' + J(r, \omega, E), \quad (1)$$

$$f(\xi, \omega, E) = h(\xi, \omega, E), \qquad (\xi, \omega) \in \Gamma^-, \quad E_1 \le E \le E_2, \quad (2)$$

$$f(\eta, \omega, E) = H(\eta, \omega, E), \qquad (\eta, \omega) \in \Gamma^+, \quad E_1 \le E \le E_2. \quad (3)$$

The collision integral in the right-hand side of (1) is designated by $N(r, \omega, E)$. The coefficient of scattering $\mu_s$ is defined by the formula

$$\mu_s(r, E') = \int_\Omega \int_{E_1}^{E'} k(r, \omega \cdot \omega', E, E')\, dE\, d\omega. \quad (4)$$

Since $k$ depends on the scalar product $\omega \cdot \omega'$, the integral (4) does not depend on $\omega'$. Hereinafter the symbols $(\omega', E')$ and $(\omega, E)$ stand for the states of a photon before and after an act of interaction, respectively.

The boundary value problem (direct problem) consists in determining $f(r, \omega, E)$ from the relations (1), (2), where all other functions are known. Under various restrictions, this problem has been investigated in papers of several authors, particularly, in Anikonov, Kovtanyuk and Prokhorov (2002). The last paper also contains the results of investigation of a certain tomography problem based on the relations (1)–(3), where only the functions $h$ and $H$ are known. However, the notion of invisibility was not introduced for this case. Now we intend to represent such definition.

Accordingly to the conditions of generalized convexity from Section 1.1, a ray $L_{r,\omega} = \{r + t\omega \mid t \geq 0\}$, $(r,\omega) \in G_0 \times \Omega$ intersects $G_0$ by the intervals $\{r + t\omega \mid t_{i-1}(r,\omega) < t < t_i(r,\omega)\}$, $i = 1, \dots, l(r,\omega)$, $t_0(r,\omega) = 0$. It is clear that the points $z_i = r + t_i(r,\omega)\omega$ belong to $\partial G_0$. Under rather general assumptions the solution of the direct problem (1), (2) $f(r,\omega,E)$ appears to be continuous along each ray $L_{r,\omega}$. Moreover, we are able to establish the following property: *"the function $f(r + t\omega, \omega, E)$ has the continuous derivative with respect to $t$, $t \in (t_{i-1}(r,\omega), t_i(r,\omega))$"*. Note that the first term in the left-hand side of the equation (1) is treated as follows

$$\omega \cdot \nabla_r f(r,\omega,E) = \frac{df(r + t\omega, \omega, E)}{dt}\Big|_{t=0}.$$

We emphasize that, generally speaking, this derivative is not obliged to be continuous for $t = t_i(r,\omega)$, $i = 1, \dots, l(r,\omega)$ and the corresponding jumps can be given by the formula

$$[\![\omega \cdot \nabla_r f(z_i,\omega,E)]\!] = \lim_{t \to t_i(r,\omega)+0} \frac{df(r + t\omega, \omega, E)}{dt} - \lim_{t \to t_i(r,\omega)-0} \frac{df(r + t\omega, \omega, E)}{dt}.$$

Now we are ready to formulate our definitions.

*The equality*

$$[\![\omega \cdot \nabla_r f(z,\omega,E)]\!] = 0, \qquad z \in \partial G_0, \quad \omega \in \Omega, \quad E_1 \leq E \leq E_2 \tag{5}$$

*is the condition of invisibility of the medium $G$ under radiography.*

*The measure of visibility of the medium $G$ is defined as follows*

$$mv(r,\omega) = |[\![\omega \cdot \nabla_r f(r,\omega,E)]\!]| \exp\Big( - \int_0^{d(r,\omega)} \mu(r + t\omega, E)\, dt \Big). \tag{6}$$

*(The positiveness of the exponential multiplier provides the equivalency of* (5) *and the equality $mv(z,\omega,E) = 0$). In case of the continuous function $f(r,\omega,E)$, for $(r,\omega) \in G \times \Omega$ and absence of internal sources ($J \equiv 0$), the condition of poor visibility has the form*

$$[\![\mu(r,\omega,E)]\!] = [\![\mu_s^*(r,\omega,E)]\!], \qquad z \in \partial G_0, \quad E_1 \leq E \leq E_2, \tag{7}$$

*where the function $\mu_s^*$, which may be called the dual coefficient of scattering, is given by the equality*

$$\mu_s^*(r,E) = \int_\Omega \int_E^{E_2} k(r, \omega\cdot\omega', E, E')\, dE'\, d\omega', \tag{8}$$

From the formal point of view, definitions do not need of proofs. However, it is desirable to justify that the definitions useful and fruitful. While, we can justify our definitions by the following three ideas.

1. It is evidently that the equality $[\![\omega\cdot\nabla_r f(r,\omega,E)]\!] = 0$ is valid for all $r\in G_0$, i.e. at the point $r$ where the medium $G$ has not contact boundaries between various substances in $G$. Thus, the condition (5) really corresponds to the absence of heterogeneity at the point $r$.

2. In the monoenergetic case the left-hand side of (5) is equal to $\pm m_1(z,\omega)$ that was explained in Section 1.5. In fact, replacing the second term in the equation (1.1.1) from the left into the right and taking the jumps from obtained both sides, we become sure that

$$m_1(z,\omega) = \pm[\![\omega\cdot\nabla_r f(z,\omega)]\!] = 0, \qquad z\in\partial G_0, \quad \omega\in\Omega. \tag{9}$$

The sign in the right-hand side of (9) depends on the numeration of the domains $G_i$, $i=1,\dots,p$ and does not influence on the previous condition of invisibility: $m_1(z,\omega) = 0$ the significance of which has been carefully substantiated in Section 1.5. Thus, the condition of invisibility (5) is a direct generalization of the corresponding previous condition and both these definitions have the same foundation in essence.

3. Now we explain the condition of poor visibility (7). Taking the jumps in (1) we obtain the following equality for the case $J\equiv 0$:

$$[\![\omega\cdot\nabla_r f(r,\omega,E)]\!] = -[\![\mu(r,E)]\!] f(r,\omega,E) + [\![N(r,\omega,E)]\!].$$

Therefore, the equality (5) can be rewritten as follows

$$-[\![\mu(z,E)]\!] f(z,\omega,E) + \left[\!\!\left[\int_\Omega\int_E^{E_2} k(z,\omega\cdot\omega',E,E') f(z,\omega',E')\, dE'\, d\omega'\right]\!\!\right] = 0,$$
$$z\in\partial G_0, \qquad \omega\in\Omega. \tag{10}$$

Remind that a condition of poor visibility appears to be a simple approximation of the condition (5) or (10). Therefore, dividing (10) by $f(z,\omega,E)$

and using the approximation $f(z,\omega,E) \simeq f(z,\omega',E')$, we can obtain the equality

$$[\![\mu(z,E)]\!] = \left[\!\!\left[ \int_\Omega \int_E^{E_2} k(z,\omega\cdot\omega',E,E')\,dE'\,d\omega' \right]\!\!\right], \qquad z \in \partial G_0, \quad \omega \in \Omega,$$

which coincides with the condition of poor visibility (7).

Naturally, there are many various ways for approximation of (5). Perhaps, the equality (7) is one of the simplest of such definitions, and it coincides with the same definition in the monoenergetic case when $\mu_s = \mu_s^*$.

We can represent the condition of poor visibility (7) in more familiar form: $[\![\mu_a^*(z,E)]\!] = 0$, $z \in \partial G_0$, $E_1 \le E \le E_2$, which means continuity of the function $\mu_a^*(r,E)$ at the point $r = z$, where the dual coefficient of absorption is defined by the equality $\mu_a^* = \mu - \mu_s^*$.

Thus we complete the justifications of our definitions which we have at present.

Our main hypotheses consists in the following statements which have to be established in future.

1. *The indicators similar to* $\mathrm{Ind}(r)$ *and* $\mathrm{Ind}^*(r)$, *but depending on energy, also guarantee the uniqueness of solving the tomography problems, if the measure of visibility* $mv(r,\omega,E)$ *is positive for* $z \in \partial G_0$, $\omega \in \Omega$, $E_1 \le E \le E_2$.

2. *Similarly to Theorem 1.5.1 the condition of invisibility* $mv(r,\omega,E) = 0$, $z \in \partial G_j$, $\omega \in \Omega$, $E_1 \le E \le E_2$ *excludes any successful solving the tomography problems.*

At present, these statements are not still proved and we can to limit foundations of our approach by the points 1,2,3 after the definitions (see above), and the following consideration.

It is important to notice that the indicatrix $k(r,\omega\cdot\omega',E,E')$ considered here and in Anikonov, Kovtanyuk and Prokhorov (2002) is an ordinary scalar function, which can be unbounded on a set of zero measure. As we have remarked (see Anikonov, Kovtanyuk and Prokhorov, 2002, p.6) such a function, describing the Rayleigh scattering, can be an approximation of the Compton indicatrix which contains Dirac's delta-function (see Fano, Berger and Spencer, 1963).

We consider the distribution $f(r,\omega,E)$ as the density or intensity of the particle flux. Note, that we understand the density as a number of photons per unit measure of its arguments and per unit time. The intensity is equal to the density multiplied by the corresponding value $E$ of photon energy (see Case and Zweifel, 1972).

In what follows, these different interpretation are to be studied separately. Firstly, let us consider the case when $f(r, \omega, E)$ is the density of the photon flux. In this case we dare to call $\mu_a$ the coefficient of absorption of photons and $\mu_a^*$ the dual coefficient of absorption of photons.

Now we explain some aspects of the Rayleigh and the Compton scattering (see Leypunskii, Novozhilov and Sakharov, 1960; Fano, Berger and Spencer, 1963). The following case is studied in this book:

$$k(r, \omega \cdot \omega', E, E') = k_R(r, \omega \cdot \omega', E, E') + k_C(r, \omega \cdot \omega', E, E'), \qquad (11)$$

where $k_R$ and $k_C$ are the indicatrices of the Rayleigh and Compton scattering respectively. These functions have the following forms:

$$k_R(r, \omega \cdot \omega', E, E') = \chi_R(r, \omega \cdot \omega', E, E')\delta(E - E'), \qquad (12)$$

$$k_C(r, \omega \cdot \omega', E, E') = \chi_C(r, \omega \cdot \omega', E, E') \times \delta(1 - \omega \cdot \omega' - E_0/E + E_0/E'), \qquad (13)$$

where $E_0$ is the value of energy of an electron at rest and $\chi_R, \chi_C$ are ordinary scalar functions. The exact form of $\chi_R$ does not influence on the following consideration and $k_C$ is given by the formula of Klein—Nishina:

$$k_C(r, \omega \cdot \omega', E, E') = n_0(r)\sigma(\omega \cdot \omega', \alpha, \alpha'), \qquad (14)$$

where $n_0(r)$ is the concentration of electrons in a given substance, and for simplicity energy $\alpha$ is traditionally expressed in the unit $E_0$, i. e. $\alpha = E/E_0$, $\alpha' = E'/E_0$ ($\alpha_1 = E_1/E_0$, $\alpha_2 = E_2/E_0$, $E_0 = 0.511$ MeV). The function $\sigma$ has the form:

$$\sigma(\omega \cdot \omega', \alpha, \alpha') = \frac{r_0^2}{2}\Big(\frac{1}{\alpha'}\Big)^2\Big[\frac{\alpha}{\alpha'} + \frac{\alpha'}{\alpha} + 2\Big(\frac{1}{\alpha'} - \frac{1}{\alpha}\Big) + \Big(\frac{1}{\alpha'} - \frac{1}{\alpha}\Big)^2\Big] \times \delta\Big(1 - \omega \cdot \omega' - \frac{1}{\alpha} + \frac{1}{\alpha'}\Big), \qquad (15)$$

where $r_0$ is the classical radius of an electron.

It is clear that

$$\mu_s(r, \alpha') = \int_\Omega \int_{\alpha_1}^{\alpha'} k(r, \omega \cdot \omega', \alpha, \alpha')\, d\alpha\, d\omega'$$
$$= \int_\Omega \int_{\alpha_1}^{\alpha'} k_R(r, \omega \cdot \omega', \alpha, \alpha')\, d\alpha\, d\omega' + \int_\Omega \int_{\alpha_1}^{\alpha'} k_C(r, \omega \cdot \omega', \alpha, \alpha')\, d\alpha\, d\omega'$$
$$= \mu_R(r, \alpha') + \mu_C(r, \alpha'),$$

where $\mu_R$ is a coefficient of the Rayleigh scattering and $\mu_C$ is the coefficient of the Compton scattering. Consider the latter coefficient

$$\begin{aligned}\mu_C(r,\alpha') &= \int_\Omega \int_{\alpha_1}^{\alpha'} k_C(r,\omega\cdot\omega',\alpha,\alpha')\,d\alpha\,d\omega \\ &= \int_\Omega \int_{\alpha_1}^{\alpha'} \frac{\alpha}{\alpha'} k_C(r,\omega\cdot\omega',\alpha,\alpha')\,d\alpha\,d\omega \\ &\quad + \int_\Omega \int_{\alpha_1}^{\alpha'} \Big(1-\frac{\alpha}{\alpha'}\Big) k_C(r,\omega\cdot\omega',\alpha,\alpha')\,d\alpha\,d\omega. \qquad (16)\end{aligned}$$

In the right-hand side of (16) we denote the first item $\mu_{ac}$ and the second $\mu_{sc}$ (see Leypunskii, Novozhilov and Sakharov, 1960), i.e.

$$\mu_C(r,\alpha') = \mu_{ac}(r,\alpha') + \mu_{sc}(r,\alpha'). \qquad (17)$$

Now we consider the dual quantities:

$$\begin{aligned}\mu_s^*(r,\alpha) &= \int_\Omega \int_{\alpha}^{\alpha_2} k(r,\omega\cdot\omega',\alpha,\alpha')\,d\alpha'\,d\omega' \\ &= \int_\Omega \int_{\alpha}^{\alpha_2} k_R(r,\omega\cdot\omega',\alpha,\alpha')\,d\alpha'\,d\omega' \\ &\quad + \int_\Omega \int_{\alpha}^{\alpha_2} k_C(r,\omega\cdot\omega',\alpha,\alpha')\,d\alpha'\,d\omega'. \qquad (18)\end{aligned}$$

The first item in the right-hand side of (18) is denoted as $\mu_R^*(r,\alpha)$, the second as $\mu_C^*(r,\alpha)$. It is easy to see that $\mu_R^*(r,\tilde\alpha) = \mu_R(r,\tilde\alpha)$. Hereinafter we use the new energy variables $\tilde\alpha$, $\tilde E$ ($\tilde\alpha = \tilde E/E_0$) instead of $\alpha'$, $E'$ and $\alpha$, $E$ connected with the state of photons before and after the interaction respectively.

The dual coefficient of absorption $\mu_a^*(r,\tilde\alpha)$ is given as follows

$$\mu_a^*(r,\tilde\alpha) = \mu(r,\tilde\alpha) - \mu_R(r,\tilde\alpha) + \mu_C^*(r,\tilde\alpha). \qquad (19)$$

Just this coefficient ($\mu_a^*(r,\tilde\alpha)$) is to be used for creation of the tables of poorly visible pairs of substances from the part 2 of this book. However, we have the tables of the similar coefficient of energy absorption $\mu_{en}(r,\tilde\alpha)$ and intend to use it instead of $\mu_a^*(r,\tilde\alpha)$. In our terms $\mu_{en}(r,\tilde\alpha)$ has the following form

$$\mu_{en}(r,\tilde\alpha) = \mu(r,\tilde\alpha) - \mu_R(r,\tilde\alpha) + \mu_{sc}(r,\tilde\alpha). \qquad (20)$$

Comparing (19) and (20), we introduced the relative difference $\Lambda(r,\tilde\alpha)$ of these quantities

$$\Lambda(r,\tilde\alpha) = |\mu_{sc}(r,\tilde\alpha) - \mu_C^*(r,\tilde\alpha)|/\mu_{en}(r,\tilde\alpha). \qquad (21)$$

It is necessary to evaluate $\Lambda(r,\tilde\alpha)$.

It remains to study the case when the distribution $f(r, \omega, E)$ is the intensity of the photon flux. Firstly, note that the transport equation (1) with respect to the density can be easily transformed into the transport equation with respect to the intensity. It is enough to multiply the first version of (1) by energy $E$ and put the factor $E/E'$ under the collision integral (see Leypunskii, Novozhilov and Sakharov, 1960). It is not difficult to see that the coefficient of total attenuation $\mu(r, \alpha)$ is the same in this transformation as well as the coefficient of Rayleigh scattering $\mu_R$, and the new indicatrix of scattering $k_I$ takes the form

$$k_I(r, \omega \cdot \omega', \alpha, \alpha') = (\alpha/\alpha')k(r, \omega \cdot \omega', \alpha, \alpha'), \tag{22}$$

where $k$ is given by (11). For this case we designate $\mu^*_{ia}(r, \tilde{\alpha})$ as follows

$$\mu^*_{ia}(r, \tilde{\alpha}) = \mu(r, \tilde{\alpha}) - \mu_R(r, \tilde{\alpha}) + \mu^*_{ic}(r, \tilde{\alpha}),$$

where

$$\mu^*_{ic} = \int_\Omega \int_\alpha^{\alpha_2} \frac{\alpha}{\alpha'} k_C(r, \omega \cdot \omega', \alpha, \alpha')\, d\alpha'\, d\omega',$$

We dare to call the quality $\mu^*_{ia}(r, \tilde{\alpha})$ the dual intensity coefficient of absorption. Accordingly to our approach this coefficient must be used for creation of the tables from Part 2 for the last interpretation of $f(r, \omega, E)$. Thus, we have to compare the values of $\mu_{en}(r, \tilde{\alpha})$ and $\mu^*_{ia}(r, \tilde{\alpha})$, i.e. to evaluate the following quantity

$$\Lambda_I(r, \tilde{\alpha}) = |\mu_{sc}(r, \tilde{\alpha}) - \mu^*_{ic}(r, \tilde{\alpha})| / \mu_{en}(r, \alpha). \tag{23}$$

(Remind that we use $\mu_{en}(r, \tilde{\alpha})$ instead of $\mu^*_{ic}(r, \tilde{\alpha})$).

To estimate the relative difference $\Lambda$ and $\Lambda_I$ we calculate the following integrals by analytical and computer methods which have been implemented by V. G. Nazarov with a help of D. S. Konovalova. We omit these bulky calculations and represent the results

$$\begin{aligned}\sigma_{sc}(\alpha') &= \int_\Omega \int_{\alpha_1}^{\alpha'} \frac{\alpha}{\alpha'} \sigma(\omega \cdot \omega', \alpha, \alpha')\, d\alpha\, d\omega \\ &= \pi r_0^2 \Big[\frac{\ln(1+2\alpha')}{\alpha'^3} + \frac{32\alpha'^4 + 12\alpha'^3 - 36\alpha'^2 - 30\alpha' - 6}{3\alpha'^2(1+2\alpha')^3}\Big],\end{aligned} \tag{24}$$

$$\sigma_C^*(\alpha) = \int_\Omega \int_\alpha^{\alpha_2} \sigma(\omega\cdot\omega',\alpha,\alpha')\,d\alpha'\,d\omega'$$

$$= \pi r_0^2 \cdot \begin{cases} \dfrac{2}{3} - 2\alpha - \dfrac{1}{\alpha}\ln(1-2\alpha), & \alpha \le \dfrac{\alpha_2}{1+2\alpha_2}, \\ \left(\dfrac{1}{\alpha} - \dfrac{1}{\alpha_2}\right) - \left(1+\dfrac{\alpha}{2}\right)\left(\dfrac{1}{\alpha} - \dfrac{1}{\alpha_2}\right)^2 & \\ \qquad + \dfrac{1}{3}\left(\dfrac{1}{\alpha} - \dfrac{1}{\alpha_2}\right)^3 - \dfrac{1}{\alpha}\ln\dfrac{\alpha}{\alpha_2}, & \alpha \ge \dfrac{\alpha_2}{1+2\alpha_2}, \end{cases} \tag{25}$$

$$\sigma_{ic}^*(\alpha) = \int_\Omega \int_\alpha^{\alpha_2} \frac{\alpha}{\alpha'}\sigma(\omega\cdot\omega',\alpha,\alpha')\,d\alpha'\,d\omega'$$

$$= \pi r_0^2 \cdot \begin{cases} 8(\alpha^2-\alpha+1)/3, & \alpha \le 1/2, \\ (16\alpha^2 - 4\alpha + 1)/(12\alpha^3), & \alpha \ge 1/2, \end{cases} \tag{26}$$

All this quantities have been calculated for interaction of photons per unit electron. The needed coefficients can be obtained as follows

$$\mu_{sc}(r,\alpha') = n_0(r)\sigma_{sc}(\alpha'),$$
$$\mu_C^*(r,\alpha) = n_0(r)\sigma_C^*(\alpha), \qquad \mu_{ic}^*(r,\alpha) = n_0(r)\sigma_{ic}^*(\alpha). \tag{27}$$

It is not improbably that the formulas (24)–(27) have scientific importance not only for our investigation. We tabulate the functions $\sigma_{sc}(\tilde\alpha)$, $\sigma_{sc}^*(\tilde\alpha)$, $\sigma_{ic}^*(\tilde\alpha)$ and represent their plots at Figure 1. It is shown that the difference between $\sigma_{sc}(\tilde\alpha)$ and $\sigma_C^*(\tilde\alpha)$ increases when the level of energy increases, as well as the difference between $\sigma_{sc}(\tilde\alpha)$ and $\sigma_{ic}^*(\tilde\alpha)$ up to the level of energy $\tilde E_0 = 48$ keV. The formulas (27) imply that the same behavior have the functions $|\mu_{sc}(r,\tilde\alpha) - \mu_C^*(r,\tilde\alpha)|$ and $|\mu_{sc}(r,\tilde\alpha) - \mu_{ic}^*(r,\tilde\alpha)|$ corresponding to any substance.

For the level of energy between 48 keV and 60 keV the function $\sigma_C^*$ fast tends to zero as energy tends to $E_2 = 60$ keV. This fact easily follows from the formula (18) and needs in the subsequent study. We interpret this circumstance as follows. The inequalities $E \le E' \le E_2$, in particular, means that the sources of photons produce no photons having energy greater than $E_2$. From the physical point of view it seems reasonable that the sources produce small number of photons with energy $\tilde E$ ($\tilde E \le E_2$) close to $E_2$, such that these photons cannot essentially influence on the process of passing radiation through the medium. Thus, we don't take into account

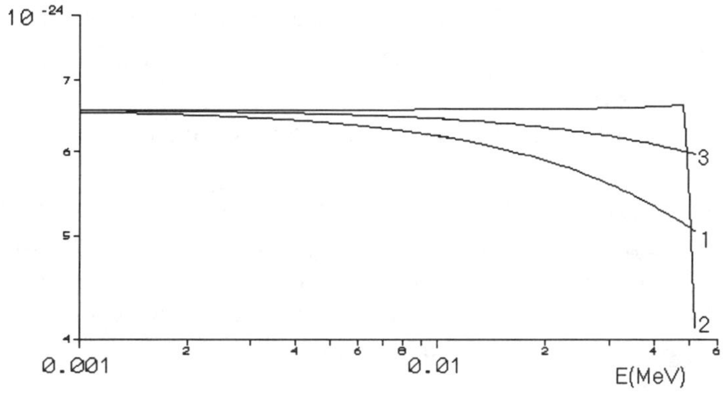


**Figure 1:** Plots of the functions: 1 — $\sigma_{sc}$, 2 — $\sigma^*_{sc}$, 3 — $\sigma^*_{ic}$, depending on energy are presented

the singular energy band 48–60 keV and consider only the band 1–48 keV in our evaluations.

Since $\mu_{en}(r, \tilde{E})$ is a monotone decreasing function for considered energy and $|\mu_{sc}(r, \tilde{E}) - \mu^*_C(r, \tilde{E})|$, $|\mu_{sc}(r, \tilde{E}) - \mu^*_{ic}(r, \tilde{E})|$ are monotone increasing functions, then the quantities $\Lambda(r, \tilde{E})$ and $\Lambda_I(r, \tilde{E})$ achieve their greatest values when $\tilde{E} = \tilde{E}_0$ ($\tilde{E}_0 = 48$ keV). These upper estimates $\Lambda(r, \tilde{E}_0)$ and $\Lambda_I(r, \tilde{E}_0)$ depend on a chemical element. We study this dependence in detail and become sure that the values $\Lambda(r, \tilde{E}_0)$ and $\Lambda_I(r, \tilde{E}_0)$ decrease as their atomic number $Z$ increases.

We represent the following table illustrating the pointed dependence for four chemical elements.

| The estimates | C ($Z = 6$) | Fe ($Z = 26$) | Ag ($Z = 47$) | Pb ($Z = 82$) |
|---|---|---|---|---|
| $\Lambda(r, \tilde{E}_0) \cdot 100\%$ | 183% | 2.2% | 0.5% | 0.4% |
| $\Lambda_I(r, \tilde{E}_0) \cdot 100\%$ | 106% | 1.3% | 0.3% | 0.2% |

As shown in this table the upper estimates for heavy elements seem to be sufficiently small, but these estimates for light elements may occur too large, that we see for carbon. However, the estimates $\Lambda(r, \tilde{E})$ and $\Lambda_I(r, \tilde{E})$ even for light elements fast decrease as $\tilde{E} \to E_1$. In particular, for carbon $\Lambda(r, \tilde{E}) \cdot 100\% = 44\%$ and $\Lambda_I(r, \tilde{E}) \cdot 100\% = 27\%$ for $\tilde{E} = 30$ keV and $\Lambda(r, \tilde{E}) \cdot 100\% = 0.5\%$ and $\Lambda_I(r, \tilde{E}) \cdot 100\% = 0.3\%$ for $\tilde{E} = 10$ keV.

It is useful to add that our estimates are rather rough and can be proved to be significantly greater than the evaluated quantities. Also note that our approach is not very sensitive with respect to errors (see the remark at the end of Section 1.5).

Although the pointed disadvantages take place we dare to form the tables of poorly visible pairs of substances in the part 2 using the coefficient $\mu_{en}(r, \tilde{E})$ as the base.

Finally we give the short conclusions of this section.

1. The investigation shows that there are many difficult cases in X-ray tomography, when the values of $\mu_a^*(r, \tilde{E})$ for various substances coincide at certain levels of energy. Such big number of poorly visible cases appears to be unexpected even for the authors, and it is the main reason of the appearance of this work.

2. The tables from the part 2 of this book are justified better for heavy substances and for low energy levels than for other cases. Interpretation of $f(r, \omega, E)$ as the intensity of the photon flux turns out more suitable (for our purpose) than for another interpretations.

3. Due to the pointed disadvantages, this investigation may be considered as a preliminary one in this interesting scientific direction. It is desirable to continue and improve this research.

# Chapter 2.

# The tables of poorly visible pairs of substances in soft X-ray tomography

## 2.1. THE TABLES OF POORLY VISIBLE PAIRS AT THE POINTS OF THEIR COEFFICIENTS CONTINUITY

Let us consider a case when a reader knows *a priori* the enumeration of possible substances in the unknown medium whose internal structure is to be determined. In such a case one can look over the represented tables (see below) to verify weather a poorly visible pair of the substances appears to be in the proposed determination.

The list of pairs of substances whose contact boundaries are poorly visible from the tomography point of view for some values of photon energy has been composed on the basis of data taken from the tables of Hubbell and Seltzer (1995). These tables in their main part contain energy dependence of the mass attenuation coefficient $\mu(E)/\rho$ and the mass energy-absorption coefficient $\mu_{en}(E)/\rho$ for 92 elements from hydrogen to uranium inclusive and 48 additional substances of complex chemical composition which are of dosimetric interest. Such data are presented as tabulated functions. To compose our list of pairs a computer program was created. The program forms all possible pairs from 140 substances and for each pair finds all energy values $E$ when the energy-absorption coefficients are equal

$\mu_{1en}(E) = \mu_{2en}(E)$. To find these values $E$ the linear interpolation of the tabulated functions has been used. As the calculations showed the number of different poorly visible pairs and energy values corresponding to them proved to be quite large. Results of these calculations covering the energy range from 1 to 60 keV are presented in the tables of this and the next sections.

First tables contain the list of all those pairs of substances and energy values $E$ for which functions $\mu_{1en}, \mu_{2en}$ are continuous at point $E$ and the equality $\mu_{1en}(E) = \mu_{2en}(E)$ takes place (it would be desirable to look to the remark about fixed level of energy at the end of Section 1.5).

Name of the first substance forming a pair is printed in a bold face as the title of the proper sub-table.

The first column of every sub-table contains a list of substances (the second substances) which form a poorly visible pair with the first substance. For a chemical element the second substance is indicated as the ordinal number of the element and its symbol in the standard chemical notation. For substances of complex chemical composition it is a conventional number attributed to it (from 101 for A-100 tissue equivalent plastic to 148 for water). Full titles of the substances and their corresponding numbers are listed in the table of Section 2.3.

The second column of a sub-table lists values of energy $E$ for which the equality $\mu_{1en}(E) = \mu_{2en}(E)$ is valid. The third column contains corresponding values $\mu_{1en}(E)$, the fourth and fifth contains values of total attenuation coefficients $\mu_1(E)$ and $\mu_2(E)$ respectively. The last column lists values $R(E)$, which are defined by equality:

$$R(E) = \frac{|\mu_1(E) - \mu_2(E)|}{\min\{\mu_1(E), \mu_2(E)\}} \cdot 100.$$

This value is the relative difference of the attenuation coefficients at point $E$ in per cent.

The term $R(E)$ is of interest in the following aspect. If $R(E) = 0$, then $\mu_1(E) = \mu_2(E)$ and inasmuch as $\mu_{1en}(E) = \mu_{2en}(E)$ then the coefficients of scattering for such energy coincide, i. e. $\mu_{1s}(E) = \mu_{2s}(E)$. Hence, the attenuation coefficients and the coefficients of scattering, which enter the transport equation are the same for both substances. As an example of such situation one can adduce the pair manganese—thallium for $E = 1.131$ keV, $R = 4.66 \cdot 10^{-5}$ % or pair astatine—francium for $E = 1.0741$ keV, $R = 7.29 \cdot 10^{-6}$ %. Note that in these cases the values $R$ are very close to zero. For such pairs the tomography invisibility of their contact boundary is clear (in the context of a chosen mathematical model). In the case when $R(E) \neq 0$ we have two inequalities: $\mu_1(E) \neq \mu_2(E)$ and $\mu_{1s}(E) \neq \mu_{2s}(E)$, then the invisibility of the contact boundary is by no means obvious, but we consider such case as a poorly visible case. As one can see from the table of this section the value $R(E)$ exceeds 1000 % at some cases; for example see pair lithium—chlorine for $E = 30.693$ keV, $R = 1151$ % or pair lithium—argon for $E = 26.129$ keV, $R = 1011$ %.

| Material | $E$, MeV | $\mu_{1en}$, cm$^{-1}$ | $\mu_1$, cm$^{-1}$ | $\mu_2$, cm$^{-1}$ | $R$, % |
|---|---|---|---|---|---|
| | | | 3.LITHIUM | | |
| 17.Cl | 2.9742E−03 | 4.1393E+00 | 4.3002E+00 | 4.4830E+00 | 4.2514E+00 |
| | 3.0693E−02 | 6.0743E−03 | 8.7445E−02 | 6.9913E−03 | 1.1508E+03 |
| 18.Ar | 5.9020E−03 | 4.3151E−01 | 5.6036E−01 | 4.5753E−01 | 2.2476E+01 |
| | 2.6129E−02 | 7.6212E−03 | 9.2172E−02 | 8.2991E−03 | 1.0106E+03 |
| 36.Kr | 2.7624E−03 | 6.3417E+00 | 6.5082E+00 | 6.4347E+00 | 1.1428E+00 |
| 54.Xe | 2.8893E−03 | 5.0222E+00 | 5.1854E+00 | 5.0629E+00 | 2.4186E+00 |
| 86.Rn | 2.4318E−03 | 9.7784E+00 | 9.9538E+00 | 9.8820E+00 | 7.2700E−01 |
| | | | 4.BERYLLIUM | | |
| 35.Br | 4.9160E−02 | 2.5948E−02 | 2.8851E−01 | 3.2314E−02 | 7.9285E+02 |
| 36.Kr | 1.4985E−02 | 2.1296E−01 | 5.6922E−01 | 4.0736E−01 | 3.9737E+01 |
| | 3.7638E−02 | 2.8582E−02 | 3.0971E−01 | 3.7517E−02 | 7.2551E+02 |
| 54.Xe | 8.7688E−03 | 1.3078E+00 | 1.7380E+00 | 1.3801E+00 | 2.5934E+01 |
| | 3.3760E−02 | 3.1879E−02 | 3.2060E−01 | 3.6318E−02 | 7.8275E+02 |
| | 5.8180E−02 | 2.6903E−02 | 2.7796E−01 | 4.7807E−02 | 4.8141E+02 |
| 86.Rn | 5.4477E−03 | 6.0351E+00 | 6.5500E+00 | 6.2142E+00 | 5.4033E+00 |
| 102. | 5.5548E−02 | 2.6577E−02 | 2.8093E−01 | 1.9383E−01 | 4.4932E+01 |
| 135. | 4.8893E−02 | 2.5966E−02 | 2.8894E−01 | 2.0834E−01 | 3.8685E+01 |
| 136. | 4.4975E−02 | 2.6234E−02 | 2.9516E−01 | 2.0274E−01 | 4.5590E+01 |
| 139. | 4.9724E−02 | 2.5909E−02 | 2.8762E−01 | 2.1109E−01 | 3.6252E+01 |
| 142. | 5.7849E−02 | 2.6862E−02 | 2.7833E−01 | 2.1222E−01 | 3.1150E+01 |
| | | | 5.BORON | | |
| 6.C | 4.9468E−02 | 4.1604E−02 | 3.9622E−01 | 3.1992E−01 | 2.3848E+01 |
| 35.Br | 2.4607E−02 | 1.7683E−01 | 6.1048E−01 | 2.5795E−01 | 1.3666E+02 |
| | 3.6810E−02 | 6.0142E−02 | 4.4535E−01 | 7.7595E−02 | 4.7395E+02 |
| 54.Xe | 3.9041E−02 | 5.2624E−02 | 4.3108E−01 | 1.3463E−01 | 2.2020E+02 |
| | 4.2480E−02 | 4.7352E−02 | 4.1742E−01 | 1.1094E−01 | 2.7627E+02 |
| 101. | 3.7082E−03 | 6.3582E+01 | 6.4616E+01 | 6.4311E+01 | 4.7445E−01 |
| | 5.4547E−02 | 4.0553E−02 | 3.8577E−01 | 2.3798E−01 | 6.2103E+01 |
| 102. | 2.9827E−03 | 1.1404E+02 | 1.1523E+02 | 1.1500E+02 | 1.9988E−01 |
| | 3.5453E−02 | 6.4714E−02 | 4.5404E−01 | 2.5643E−01 | 7.7060E+01 |
| 104. | 5.7150E−02 | 4.0201E−02 | 3.8071E−01 | 2.8250E−01 | 3.4762E+01 |
| 106. | 4.0638E−02 | 4.8866E−02 | 4.2301E−01 | 2.7820E−01 | 5.2049E+01 |
| 107. | 5.5831E−02 | 4.0379E−02 | 3.8327E−01 | 2.2781E−01 | 6.8244E+01 |
| 109. | 5.4459E−02 | 4.0565E−02 | 3.8594E−01 | 2.2654E−01 | 7.0364E+01 |
| 110. | 4.7197E−02 | 4.3472E−02 | 4.0311E−01 | 2.3281E−01 | 7.3151E+01 |
| 119. | 5.1421E−02 | 4.0975E−02 | 3.9184E−01 | 2.3338E−01 | 6.7897E+01 |
| 120. | 5.5839E−02 | 4.0378E−02 | 3.8326E−01 | 2.2304E−01 | 7.1834E+01 |

| Material | $E$, MeV | $\mu_{1en}$, cm$^{-1}$ | $\mu_1$, cm$^{-1}$ | $\mu_2$, cm$^{-1}$ | $R$, % |
|---|---|---|---|---|---|
| 122. | 4.6316E−02 | 4.4196E−02 | 4.0578E−01 | 2.8084E−01 | 4.4488E+01 |
| 128. | 5.4808E−02 | 4.0517E−02 | 3.8526E−01 | 2.2739E−01 | 6.9424E+01 |
| 131. | 5.4451E−02 | 4.0566E−02 | 3.8595E−01 | 2.2751E−01 | 6.9644E+01 |
| 132. | 5.4451E−02 | 4.0566E−02 | 3.8595E−01 | 2.2820E−01 | 6.9132E+01 |
| 137. | 5.2077E−02 | 4.0886E−02 | 3.9057E−01 | 2.7440E−01 | 4.2334E+01 |
| 138. | 4.5334E−02 | 4.5004E−02 | 4.0876E−01 | 2.6213E−01 | 5.5937E+01 |
| 142. | 2.6061E−03 | 2.1484E+02 | 2.1612E+02 | 2.1583E+02 | 1.3286E−01 |
| | 3.4251E−02 | 6.8765E−02 | 4.6173E−01 | 2.8558E−01 | 6.1679E+01 |
| 143. | 5.3774E−02 | 4.0657E−02 | 3.8727E−01 | 2.2730E−01 | 7.0375E+01 |
| 144. | 5.4918E−02 | 4.0503E−02 | 3.8505E−01 | 2.2872E−01 | 6.8346E+01 |
| 145. | 4.9221E−02 | 4.1808E−02 | 3.9697E−01 | 2.2531E−01 | 7.6190E+01 |
| 148. | 5.1184E−02 | 4.1007E−02 | 3.9230E−01 | 2.2441E−01 | 7.4813E+01 |
| | | | 6.CARBON, GRAPHITE | | |
| 5.B | 4.9468E−02 | 4.1604E−02 | 3.1992E−01 | 3.9622E−01 | 2.3848E+01 |
| 14.Si | 1.3297E−03 | 2.0627E+03 | 2.0652E+03 | 2.0687E+03 | 1.7261E−01 |
| | 1.7647E−03 | 8.3062E+02 | 8.3248E+02 | 8.3585E+02 | 4.0458E−01 |
| 19.K | 1.4464E−03 | 1.4636E+03 | 1.4658E+03 | 1.4664E+03 | 3.9915E−02 |
| 101. | 4.6920E−03 | 4.1445E+01 | 4.2274E+01 | 4.3826E+01 | 3.6698E+00 |
| | 5.8524E−02 | 3.6416E−02 | 3.0097E−01 | 2.2946E−01 | 3.1163E+01 |
| 107. | 1.0618E−03 | 3.4381E+03 | 3.4413E+03 | 3.4482E+03 | 2.0062E−01 |
| | 1.1399E−03 | 3.0373E+03 | 3.0403E+03 | 3.0460E+03 | 1.8686E−01 |
| | 2.3463E−03 | 3.8791E+02 | 3.8944E+02 | 3.8966E+02 | 5.7573E−02 |
| | 2.6855E−03 | 2.6572E+02 | 2.6707E+02 | 2.6728E+02 | 8.0045E−02 |
| | 5.9508E−02 | 3.5916E−02 | 2.9900E−01 | 2.1919E−01 | 3.6407E+01 |
| 109. | 1.0180E−03 | 3.6631E+03 | 3.6664E+03 | 3.6740E+03 | 2.0624E−01 |
| | 1.3451E−03 | 1.9836E+03 | 1.9861E+03 | 1.9890E+03 | 1.4690E−01 |
| | 2.2543E−03 | 4.2110E+02 | 4.2267E+02 | 4.2317E+02 | 1.1882E−01 |
| | 2.7677E−03 | 2.3608E+02 | 2.3739E+02 | 2.3770E+02 | 1.3244E−01 |
| | 5.7696E−02 | 3.6837E−02 | 3.0263E−01 | 2.1923E−01 | 3.8042E+01 |
| 110. | 2.9789E−03 | 1.5998E+02 | 1.6118E+02 | 1.6132E+02 | 8.5221E−02 |
| | 4.4011E−02 | 5.0381E−02 | 3.3894E−01 | 2.4399E−01 | 3.8918E+01 |
| 115. | 1.1138E−03 | 3.1708E+03 | 3.1739E+03 | 3.1806E+03 | 2.1030E−01 |
| | 1.3921E−03 | 1.7424E+03 | 1.7447E+03 | 1.7475E+03 | 1.6142E−01 |
| 119. | 1.0191E−03 | 3.6570E+03 | 3.6604E+03 | 3.6677E+03 | 1.9849E−01 |
| | 1.3519E−03 | 1.9485E+03 | 1.9510E+03 | 1.9540E+03 | 1.5319E−01 |
| | 2.2085E−03 | 4.3760E+02 | 4.3919E+02 | 4.3944E+02 | 5.6186E−02 |
| | 2.8063E−03 | 2.2216E+02 | 2.2345E+02 | 2.2378E+02 | 1.4577E−01 |
| | 5.3386E−02 | 3.9028E−02 | 3.1128E−01 | 2.2926E−01 | 3.5774E+01 |
| 120. | 5.9315E−02 | 3.6014E−02 | 2.9938E−01 | 2.1482E−01 | 3.9367E+01 |

| Material | $E$, MeV | $\mu_{1en}$, cm$^{-1}$ | $\mu_1$, cm$^{-1}$ | $\mu_2$, cm$^{-1}$ | $R$, % |
|---|---|---|---|---|---|
| 122. | 9.3908E−03 | 4.6532E+00 | 5.1749E+00 | 5.0923E+00 | 1.6236E+00 |
| | 3.4044E−02 | 8.9952E−02 | 4.0213E−01 | 3.4995E−01 | 1.4913E+01 |
| 128. | 1.0518E−03 | 3.4893E+03 | 3.4926E+03 | 3.4993E+03 | 1.9388E−01 |
| | 1.1908E−03 | 2.7756E+03 | 2.7785E+03 | 2.7833E+03 | 1.7350E−01 |
| | 2.3310E−03 | 3.9344E+02 | 3.9497E+02 | 3.9530E+02 | 8.2017E−02 |
| | 2.6774E−03 | 2.6863E+02 | 2.6999E+02 | 2.7046E+02 | 1.7512E−01 |
| | 5.8169E−02 | 3.6596E−02 | 3.0168E−01 | 2.1974E−01 | 3.7293E+01 |
| 131. | 1.0307E−03 | 3.5976E+03 | 3.6009E+03 | 3.6081E+03 | 1.9948E−01 |
| | 1.3013E−03 | 2.2086E+03 | 2.2112E+03 | 2.2152E+03 | 1.8351E−01 |
| | 2.2608E−03 | 4.1874E+02 | 4.2031E+02 | 4.2038E+02 | 1.7056E−02 |
| | 2.7495E−03 | 2.4264E+02 | 2.4396E+02 | 2.4434E+02 | 1.5744E−01 |
| 131. | 5.7714E−02 | 3.6828E−02 | 3.0260E−01 | 2.2018E−01 | 3.7433E+01 |
| 132. | 1.0600E−03 | 3.4470E+03 | 3.4502E+03 | 3.4568E+03 | 1.9008E−01 |
| | 1.1398E−03 | 3.0375E+03 | 3.0406E+03 | 3.0461E+03 | 1.8416E−01 |
| | 2.3749E−03 | 3.7761E+02 | 3.7912E+02 | 3.7941E+02 | 7.6962E−02 |
| | 2.6665E−03 | 2.7253E+02 | 2.7389E+02 | 2.7429E+02 | 1.4449E−01 |
| | 5.7714E−02 | 3.6828E−02 | 3.0260E−01 | 2.2083E−01 | 3.7026E+01 |
| 137. | 5.6281E−02 | 3.7557E−02 | 3.0547E−01 | 2.6559E−01 | 1.5018E+01 |
| 138. | 7.1765E−03 | 1.1620E+01 | 1.2241E+01 | 1.2116E+01 | 1.0292E+00 |
| | 3.5264E−02 | 8.3165E−02 | 3.9205E−01 | 3.1809E−01 | 2.3252E+01 |
| 141. | 1.8961E−03 | 6.5312E+02 | 6.5489E+02 | 6.5574E+02 | 1.2946E−01 |
| | 2.2653E−03 | 4.1711E+02 | 4.1868E+02 | 4.1955E+02 | 2.0909E−01 |
| 143. | 1.0480E−03 | 3.5087E+03 | 3.5119E+03 | 3.5187E+03 | 1.9284E−01 |
| | 1.2124E−03 | 2.6648E+03 | 2.6676E+03 | 2.6728E+03 | 1.9457E−01 |
| | 2.2989E−03 | 4.0500E+02 | 4.0654E+02 | 4.0677E+02 | 5.5534E−02 |
| | 2.7168E−03 | 2.5443E+02 | 2.5576E+02 | 2.5605E+02 | 1.1192E−01 |
| | 5.6769E−02 | 3.7308E−02 | 3.0449E−01 | 2.2067E−01 | 3.7985E+01 |
| 144. | 1.0369E−03 | 3.5659E+03 | 3.5692E+03 | 3.5764E+03 | 2.0214E−01 |
| | 1.2651E−03 | 2.3941E+03 | 2.3968E+03 | 2.4013E+03 | 1.8650E−01 |
| | 2.2903E−03 | 4.0810E+02 | 4.0965E+02 | 4.1004E+02 | 9.3150E−02 |
| | 2.7107E−03 | 2.5662E+02 | 2.5796E+02 | 2.5845E+02 | 1.8968E−01 |
| | 5.8366E−02 | 3.6496E−02 | 3.0129E−01 | 2.2083E−01 | 3.6435E+01 |
| 145. | 4.9000E−02 | 4.2358E−02 | 3.2156E−01 | 2.2616E−01 | 4.2180E+01 |
| 148. | 5.2823E−02 | 3.9314E−02 | 3.1241E−01 | 2.2097E−01 | 4.1379E+01 |
| 8.OXYGEN | | | | | |
| 147. | 5.4610E−02 | 5.1383E−05 | 2.7017E−04 | 3.7165E−04 | 3.7563E+01 |
| 10.NEON | | | | | |
| 147. | 5.8652E−02 | 4.7604E−05 | 1.8593E−04 | 3.6065E−04 | 9.3976E+01 |

| Material | $E$, MeV | $\mu_{1en}$, cm$^{-1}$ | $\mu_1$, cm$^{-1}$ | $\mu_2$, cm$^{-1}$ | $R$, % |
|---|---|---|---|---|---|
| | | | 11.SODIUM | | |
| 20.Ca | 1.3412E−03 | 4.2013E+03 | 4.2690E+03 | 4.2085E+03 | 1.4378E+00 |
| 108. | 2.1842E−03 | 1.2812E+03 | 1.2956E+03 | 1.3094E+03 | 1.0685E+00 |
| | 2.7365E−03 | 7.4403E+02 | 7.5174E+02 | 7.5996E+02 | 1.0931E+00 |
| 117. | 1.1737E−03 | 5.4061E+03 | 5.5011E+03 | 5.4227E+03 | 1.4457E+00 |
| 124. | 1.1343E−03 | 5.6894E+03 | 5.7909E+03 | 5.7097E+03 | 1.4212E+00 |
| 127. | 1.4151E−03 | 3.6700E+03 | 3.7257E+03 | 3.6823E+03 | 1.1780E+00 |
| | 5.9638E−02 | 6.5736E−02 | 2.2211E−01 | 4.3732E−01 | 9.6897E+01 |
| 129. | 1.1930E−03 | 5.2673E+03 | 5.3592E+03 | 5.2817E+03 | 1.4677E+00 |
| 140. | 9.1808E−03 | 2.0290E+01 | 2.0929E+01 | 2.1269E+01 | 1.6255E+00 |
| | 4.2036E−02 | 1.7807E−01 | 3.6236E−01 | 5.7198E−01 | 5.7850E+01 |
| | | | 12.MAGNESIUM | | |
| 21.Sc | 1.3355E−03 | 8.8607E+03 | 9.0808E+03 | 8.8776E+03 | 2.2888E+00 |
| 37.Rb | 1.8372E−03 | 4.4482E+03 | 4.5356E+03 | 4.5304E+03 | 1.1529E−01 |
| 39.Y | 1.4804E−03 | 7.0610E+03 | 7.2191E+03 | 7.0880E+03 | 1.8490E+00 |
| 113. | 1.3930E−03 | 8.1458E+03 | 8.3412E+03 | 8.1769E+03 | 2.0099E+00 |
| 114. | 2.4924E−03 | 2.2341E+03 | 2.2706E+03 | 2.3313E+03 | 2.6719E+00 |
| 124. | 3.9818E−03 | 5.2232E+02 | 5.2891E+02 | 5.3321E+02 | 8.1240E−01 |
| 141. | 2.9976E−03 | 1.1361E+03 | 1.1511E+03 | 1.2254E+03 | 6.4526E+00 |
| | | | 13.ALUMINUM | | |
| 14.Si | 1.9374E−03 | 6.5717E+03 | 6.7574E+03 | 6.8459E+03 | 1.3106E+00 |
| 15.P | 2.5359E−03 | 3.8791E+03 | 3.9744E+03 | 4.0787E+03 | 2.6230E+00 |
| 16.S | 2.6653E−03 | 3.3795E+03 | 3.4594E+03 | 3.6048E+03 | 4.2050E+00 |
| 19.K | 1.4741E−02 | 2.2711E+01 | 2.4021E+01 | 2.3984E+01 | 1.5189E−01 |
| 37.Rb | 2.8476E−03 | 2.6753E+03 | 2.7334E+03 | 2.7187E+03 | 5.4124E−01 |
| 110. | 1.0313E−03 | 3.0608E+03 | 3.0662E+03 | 3.0689E+03 | 8.9529E−02 |
| | 1.4244E−03 | 1.3993E+03 | 1.4050E+03 | 1.4031E+03 | 1.3159E−01 |
| 118. | 2.9134E−03 | 2.4212E+03 | 2.4715E+03 | 2.4669E+03 | 1.8481E−01 |
| 133. | 3.7107E−03 | 1.2837E+03 | 1.3068E+03 | 1.3284E+03 | 1.6496E+00 |
| 134. | 1.5711E−03 | 1.0220E+04 | 1.0561E+04 | 1.0312E+04 | 2.4069E+00 |
| | | | 14.SILICON | | |
| 6.C | 1.3297E−03 | 2.0627E+03 | 2.0687E+03 | 2.0652E+03 | 1.7261E−01 |
| | 1.7647E−03 | 8.3062E+02 | 8.3585E+02 | 8.3248E+02 | 4.0458E−01 |
| 13.Al | 1.9374E−03 | 6.5717E+03 | 6.8459E+03 | 6.7574E+03 | 1.3106E+00 |
| 15.P | 2.8018E−03 | 3.0104E+03 | 3.1104E+03 | 3.1511E+03 | 1.3099E+00 |
| 16.S | 2.7863E−03 | 3.0723E+03 | 3.1752E+03 | 3.2697E+03 | 2.9763E+00 |
| 19.K | 1.5909E−03 | 1.1009E+03 | 1.1064E+03 | 1.1035E+03 | 2.6251E−01 |
| 23.V | 3.9976E−03 | 1.0343E+03 | 1.0582E+03 | 1.0490E+03 | 8.7565E−01 |

| Material | $E$, MeV | $\mu_{1en}$, cm$^{-1}$ | $\mu_1$, cm$^{-1}$ | $\mu_2$, cm$^{-1}$ | $R$, % |
|---|---|---|---|---|---|
| 37.Rb | 4.7272E−03 | 6.8802E+02 | 7.0298E+02 | 6.9911E+02 | 5.5335E−01 |
| 109. | 1.0402E−03 | 3.4575E+03 | 3.4643E+03 | 3.4676E+03 | 9.3876E−02 |
| | 1.3587E−03 | 1.9230E+03 | 1.9289E+03 | 1.9281E+03 | 4.1816E−02 |
| 115. | 1.1451E−03 | 2.9522E+03 | 2.9588E+03 | 2.9613E+03 | 8.5007E−02 |
| | 1.4057E−03 | 1.6965E+03 | 1.7024E+03 | 1.7017E+03 | 4.1477E−02 |
| 118. | 3.5188E−03 | 1.6021E+03 | 1.6444E+03 | 1.6332E+03 | 6.8979E−01 |
| 119. | 1.0414E−03 | 3.4516E+03 | 3.4585E+03 | 3.4610E+03 | 7.4637E−02 |
| | 1.3719E−03 | 1.8594E+03 | 1.8653E+03 | 1.8645E+03 | 4.3878E−02 |
| 131. | 1.0547E−03 | 3.3874E+03 | 3.3943E+03 | 3.3974E+03 | 9.1636E−02 |
| | 1.2706E−03 | 2.3473E+03 | 2.3535E+03 | 2.3543E+03 | 3.3185E−02 |
| 134. | 2.4655E−03 | 4.3560E+03 | 4.5196E+03 | 4.4022E+03 | 2.6661E+00 |
| | 2.4767E−03 | 4.3113E+03 | 4.4727E+03 | 4.3607E+03 | 2.5687E+00 |
| 141. | 1.8032E−03 | 7.7074E+02 | 7.7592E+02 | 7.7344E+02 | 3.2042E−01 |
| 143. | 1.0711E−03 | 3.3085E+03 | 3.3153E+03 | 3.3179E+03 | 7.8324E−02 |
| 144. | 1.0615E−03 | 3.3549E+03 | 3.3617E+03 | 3.3640E+03 | 6.7700E−02 |
| | 1.1843E−03 | 2.7630E+03 | 2.7695E+03 | 2.7712E+03 | 6.0500E−02 |
| | | | 15.PHOSPHORUS | | |
| 13.Al | 2.5359E−03 | 3.8791E+03 | 4.0787E+03 | 3.9744E+03 | 2.6230E+00 |
| 14.Si | 2.8018E−03 | 3.0104E+03 | 3.1511E+03 | 3.1104E+03 | 1.3099E+00 |
| 16.S | 2.7707E−03 | 3.1118E+03 | 3.2594E+03 | 3.3128E+03 | 1.6387E+00 |
| 23.V | 2.9214E−03 | 2.6197E+03 | 2.7339E+03 | 2.6385E+03 | 3.6157E+00 |
| 37.Rb | 1.2419E−02 | 5.6979E+01 | 5.9015E+01 | 5.9752E+01 | 1.2490E+00 |
| 104. | 1.4971E−03 | 1.4507E+03 | 1.4562E+03 | 1.4550E+03 | 8.2587E−02 |
| | 2.0701E−03 | 6.0367E+02 | 6.0841E+02 | 6.0562E+02 | 4.6073E−01 |
| 115. | 2.1289E−03 | 5.5720E+02 | 5.6185E+02 | 5.5922E+02 | 4.6899E−01 |
| 133. | 3.8882E−03 | 1.2566E+03 | 1.2993E+03 | 1.2997E+03 | 2.9181E−02 |
| 148. | 2.1196E−03 | 5.6456E+02 | 5.6922E+02 | 5.6655E+02 | 4.7071E−01 |
| | | | 16.SULFUR | | |
| 13.Al | 2.6653E−03 | 3.3795E+03 | 3.6048E+03 | 3.4594E+03 | 4.2050E+00 |
| 14.Si | 2.7863E−03 | 3.0723E+03 | 3.2697E+03 | 3.1752E+03 | 2.9763E+00 |
| 15.P | 2.7707E−03 | 3.1118E+03 | 3.3128E+03 | 3.2594E+03 | 1.6387E+00 |
| 23.V | 2.8643E−03 | 2.8743E+03 | 3.0536E+03 | 2.8934E+03 | 5.5362E+00 |
| 37.Rb | 2.5997E−03 | 3.5459E+03 | 3.7864E+03 | 3.6076E+03 | 4.9563E+00 |
| 105. | 2.2649E−03 | 5.7668E+02 | 5.8145E+02 | 5.7916E+02 | 3.9530E−01 |
| 133. | 6.6514E−03 | 3.3566E+02 | 3.4702E+02 | 3.4622E+02 | 2.2902E−01 |
| | 1.1817E−02 | 7.2444E+01 | 7.5075E+01 | 7.5883E+01 | 1.0764E+00 |
| 134. | 3.2070E−03 | 2.2575E+03 | 2.3861E+03 | 2.2862E+03 | 4.3722E+00 |

| Material | $E$, MeV | $\mu_{1en}$, cm$^{-1}$ | $\mu_1$, cm$^{-1}$ | $\mu_2$, cm$^{-1}$ | $R$, % |
|---|---|---|---|---|---|
| | | 17.CLORINE | | | |
| 3.Li | 2.9742E−03 | 4.1393E+00 | 4.4830E+00 | 4.3002E+00 | 4.2514E+00 |
| | 3.0693E−02 | 6.0743E−03 | 6.9913E−03 | 8.7445E−02 | 1.1508E+03 |
| 36.Kr | 1.3501E−02 | 8.5119E−02 | 8.8811E−02 | 9.0332E−02 | 1.7120E+00 |
| 54.Xe | 4.6722E−03 | 1.3977E+00 | 1.4763E+00 | 1.4272E+00 | 3.4383E+00 |
| | | 18.ARGONE | | | |
| 3.Li | 5.9020E−03 | 4.3151E−01 | 4.5753E−01 | 5.6036E−01 | 2.2476E+01 |
| | 2.6129E−02 | 7.6212E−03 | 8.2991E−03 | 9.2172E−02 | 1.0106E+03 |
| | | 19.POTASSIUM | | | |
| 6.C | 1.4464E−03 | 1.4636E+03 | 1.4664E+03 | 1.4658E+03 | 3.9915E−02 |
| 13.Al | 1.4741E−02 | 2.2711E+01 | 2.3984E+01 | 2.4021E+01 | 1.5189E−01 |
| 14.Si | 1.5909E−03 | 1.1009E+03 | 1.1035E+03 | 1.1064E+03 | 2.6251E−01 |
| 22.Ti | 3.8760E−03 | 7.7970E+02 | 8.7287E+02 | 7.9042E+02 | 1.0431E+01 |
| 107. | 2.1073E−03 | 5.2515E+02 | 5.2760E+02 | 5.2708E+02 | 9.8231E−02 |
| | 2.9503E−03 | 2.0621E+02 | 2.0830E+02 | 2.0797E+02 | 1.6103E−01 |
| 109. | 2.0357E−03 | 5.5222E+02 | 5.5470E+02 | 5.5414E+02 | 1.0098E−01 |
| | 2.9868E−03 | 1.9241E+02 | 1.9449E+02 | 1.9429E+02 | 1.0024E−01 |
| | 3.3308E−03 | 1.4665E+02 | 1.4858E+02 | 1.4824E+02 | 2.2879E−01 |
| 114. | 3.7518E−03 | 8.4367E+02 | 9.4797E+02 | 8.7387E+02 | 8.4786E+00 |
| 115. | 1.2049E−03 | 2.5617E+03 | 2.5653E+03 | 2.5695E+03 | 1.6248E−01 |
| | 1.3651E−03 | 1.8333E+03 | 1.8364E+03 | 1.8385E+03 | 1.1429E−01 |
| | 2.3019E−03 | 4.5150E+02 | 4.5387E+02 | 4.5333E+02 | 1.1827E−01 |
| | 2.6497E−03 | 3.1991E+02 | 3.2213E+02 | 3.2300E+02 | 2.6888E−01 |
| 119. | 2.0255E−03 | 5.5607E+02 | 5.5856E+02 | 5.5798E+02 | 1.0422E−01 |
| | 3.1933E−03 | 1.6358E+02 | 1.6557E+02 | 1.6499E+02 | 3.5501E−01 |
| 120. | 2.2780E−03 | 4.6054E+02 | 4.6292E+02 | 4.6233E+02 | 1.2794E−01 |
| | 2.8474E−03 | 2.4512E+02 | 2.4725E+02 | 2.4753E+02 | 1.1314E−01 |
| 128. | 2.0962E−03 | 5.2933E+02 | 5.3178E+02 | 5.3118E+02 | 1.1336E−01 |
| | 2.9461E−03 | 2.0779E+02 | 2.0988E+02 | 2.0971E+02 | 8.1143E−02 |
| 131. | 2.0557E−03 | 5.4464E+02 | 5.4712E+02 | 5.4662E+02 | 9.0835E−02 |
| | 2.9932E−03 | 1.8998E+02 | 1.9205E+02 | 1.9166E+02 | 2.0230E−01 |
| | 3.1826E−03 | 1.6490E+02 | 1.6689E+02 | 1.6642E+02 | 2.8176E−01 |
| 132. | 2.1093E−03 | 5.2436E+02 | 5.2682E+02 | 5.2630E+02 | 9.6985E−02 |
| | 2.9499E−03 | 2.0635E+02 | 2.0844E+02 | 2.0806E+02 | 1.8302E−01 |
| 137. | 2.5395E−03 | 3.6163E+02 | 3.6389E+02 | 3.6319E+02 | 1.9482E−01 |
| | 3.5146E−03 | 1.2400E+02 | 1.2585E+02 | 1.2509E+02 | 6.1071E−01 |
| 143. | 2.0914E−03 | 5.3116E+02 | 5.3362E+02 | 5.3310E+02 | 9.5874E−02 |
| | 2.9712E−03 | 1.9831E+02 | 2.0039E+02 | 1.9990E+02 | 2.4387E−01 |

| Material | $E$, MeV | $\mu_{1en}$, cm$^{-1}$ | $\mu_1$, cm$^{-1}$ | $\mu_2$, cm$^{-1}$ | $R$, % |
|---|---|---|---|---|---|
| | 3.5442E−03 | 1.2037E+02 | 1.2221E+02 | 1.2156E+02 | 5.3458E−01 |
| 144. | 2.0710E−03 | 5.3887E+02 | 5.4134E+02 | 5.4078E+02 | 1.0332E−01 |
| | 2.9680E−03 | 1.9949E+02 | 2.0157E+02 | 2.0133E+02 | 1.2041E−01 |
| | 3.5952E−03 | 1.1408E+02 | 1.1590E+02 | 1.1537E+02 | 4.6178E−01 |
| 145. | 2.4584E−03 | 3.9231E+02 | 3.9462E+02 | 3.9385E+02 | 1.9524E−01 |
| | 3.4415E−03 | 1.3302E+02 | 1.3490E+02 | 1.3400E+02 | 6.7168E−01 |
| 20.CALSIUM | | | | | |
| 11.Na | 1.3412E−03 | 4.2013E+03 | 4.2085E+03 | 4.2690E+03 | 1.4378E+00 |
| 24.Cr | 4.1079E−03 | 1.3379E+03 | 1.5383E+03 | 1.3570E+03 | 1.3362E+01 |
| 25.Mn | 6.0958E−03 | 5.1172E+02 | 5.6342E+02 | 5.2639E+02 | 7.0354E+00 |
| 56.Ba | 4.9100E−03 | 8.8380E+02 | 9.9502E+02 | 9.0263E+02 | 1.0236E+01 |
| 117. | 1.0447E−03 | 7.0976E+03 | 7.1066E+03 | 7.1165E+03 | 1.4018E−01 |
| | 1.4501E−03 | 3.1375E+03 | 3.1440E+03 | 3.1479E+03 | 1.2300E−01 |
| 127. | 1.9463E−03 | 1.3867E+03 | 1.3919E+03 | 1.3917E+03 | 1.8920E−02 |
| 129. | 1.0989E−03 | 6.5683E+03 | 6.5769E+03 | 6.5858E+03 | 1.3395E−01 |
| 21.SCANDIUM | | | | | |
| 12.Mg | 1.3355E−03 | 8.8607E+03 | 8.8776E+03 | 9.0808E+03 | 2.2888E+00 |
| 28.Ni | 4.8732E−03 | 1.7350E+03 | 2.0223E+03 | 1.7642E+03 | 1.4629E+01 |
| 29.Cu | 5.6298E−03 | 1.2555E+03 | 1.4380E+03 | 1.2822E+03 | 1.2152E+01 |
| 30.Zn | 4.6228E−03 | 1.9527E+03 | 2.2942E+03 | 1.9808E+03 | 1.5824E+01 |
| 33.As | 4.7513E−03 | 1.8410E+03 | 2.1547E+03 | 1.8674E+03 | 1.5387E+01 |
| 39.Y | 1.6436E−02 | 7.4917E+01 | 8.0317E+01 | 8.0851E+01 | 6.6487E−01 |
| 57.La | 4.7813E−03 | 1.8150E+03 | 2.1221E+03 | 1.8494E+03 | 1.4747E+01 |
| 62.Sm | 1.0011E−03 | 1.5612E+04 | 1.5633E+04 | 1.5687E+04 | 3.4343E−01 |
| 63.Eu | 1.1315E−03 | 1.2980E+04 | 1.2999E+04 | 1.3060E+04 | 4.6782E−01 |
| | 6.9541E−03 | 7.7987E+02 | 8.7543E+02 | 8.0671E+02 | 8.5189E+00 |
| 113. | 3.7403E−03 | 5.1489E+02 | 5.2156E+02 | 5.2071E+02 | 1.6250E−01 |
| 118. | 5.9787E−03 | 1.0509E+03 | 1.1907E+03 | 1.1284E+03 | 5.5230E+00 |
| 133. | 2.6056E−02 | 2.2650E+01 | 2.4591E+01 | 4.8359E+01 | 9.6655E+01 |
| 134. | 1.0086E−02 | 2.7107E+02 | 2.9401E+02 | 2.8199E+02 | 4.2608E+00 |
| 22.TITANIUM | | | | | |
| 19.K | 3.8760E−03 | 7.7970E+02 | 7.9042E+02 | 8.7287E+02 | 1.0431E+01 |
| 37.Rb | 2.8777E−02 | 2.6020E+01 | 2.8615E+01 | 3.8221E+01 | 3.3569E+01 |
| 40.Zr | 1.4926E−02 | 1.5482E+02 | 1.6787E+02 | 1.6501E+02 | 1.7360E+00 |
| 55.Cs | 2.8644E−03 | 1.8978E+03 | 1.9110E+03 | 1.9122E+03 | 6.0396E−02 |
| 61.Pm | 1.0354E−03 | 2.5394E+04 | 2.5434E+04 | 2.5525E+04 | 3.5974E−01 |
| 62.Sm | 1.0861E−03 | 2.3658E+04 | 2.3695E+04 | 2.3790E+04 | 4.0003E−01 |
| 63.Eu | 1.1498E−03 | 2.1476E+04 | 2.1512E+04 | 2.1609E+04 | 4.5362E−01 |

| Material | $E$, MeV | $\mu_{1en}$, cm$^{-1}$ | $\mu_1$, cm$^{-1}$ | $\mu_2$, cm$^{-1}$ | $R$, % |
|---|---|---|---|---|---|
| 64.Gd | 1.2008E−03 | 1.9734E+04 | 1.9767E+04 | 1.9867E+04 | 5.0557E−01 |
| | 6.8200E−03 | 1.3224E+03 | 1.5345E+03 | 1.3643E+03 | 1.2473E+01 |
| 68.Er | 1.4031E−03 | 1.2810E+04 | 1.2836E+04 | 1.2909E+04 | 5.7265E−01 |
| 69.Tm | 1.0560E−03 | 2.4688E+04 | 2.4727E+04 | 2.4791E+04 | 2.5763E−01 |
| | 1.2893E−03 | 1.6704E+04 | 1.6734E+04 | 1.6804E+04 | 4.1442E−01 |
| 118. | 1.4833E−03 | 1.0064E+04 | 1.0087E+04 | 1.0095E+04 | 7.6386E−02 |
| | 1.5561E−03 | 8.9288E+03 | 8.9508E+03 | 8.9590E+03 | 9.1188E−02 |
| | 1.5779E−03 | 8.7095E+03 | 8.7312E+03 | 8.7392E+03 | 9.1424E−02 |
| | 2.3736E−03 | 3.3527E+03 | 3.3677E+03 | 3.3734E+03 | 1.6968E−01 |
| 121. | 1.2037E−03 | 1.9634E+04 | 1.9667E+04 | 1.9755E+04 | 4.4618E−01 |
| 123. | 1.0799E−02 | 4.0586E+02 | 4.4829E+02 | 6.0545E+02 | 3.5055E+01 |
| 133. | 3.7305E−02 | 1.1806E+01 | 1.3426E+01 | 2.0261E+01 | 5.0911E+01 |
| 134. | 1.4886E−02 | 1.5724E+02 | 1.7058E+02 | 2.2825E+02 | 3.3809E+01 |

23.VANADIUM

| Material | $E$, MeV | $\mu_{1en}$, cm$^{-1}$ | $\mu_1$, cm$^{-1}$ | $\mu_2$, cm$^{-1}$ | $R$, % |
|---|---|---|---|---|---|
| 14.Si | 3.9976E−03 | 1.0343E+03 | 1.0490E+03 | 1.0582E+03 | 8.7565E−01 |
| 15.P | 2.9214E−03 | 2.6197E+03 | 2.6385E+03 | 2.7339E+03 | 3.6157E+00 |
| 16.S | 2.8643E−03 | 2.8743E+03 | 2.8934E+03 | 3.0536E+03 | 5.5362E+00 |
| 30.Zn | 1.0333E−03 | 3.7922E+04 | 3.7993E+04 | 3.8226E+04 | 6.1286E−01 |
| 31.Ga | 1.1404E−03 | 3.2495E+04 | 3.2558E+04 | 3.2802E+04 | 7.4738E−01 |
| 34.Se | 1.3577E−02 | 3.4583E+02 | 3.8591E+02 | 6.1687E+02 | 5.9848E+01 |
| 37.Rb | 4.5959E−03 | 7.4771E+02 | 7.6099E+02 | 7.5956E+02 | 1.8821E−01 |
| 38.Sr | 2.5071E−02 | 6.4325E+01 | 7.0483E+01 | 1.0773E+02 | 5.2847E+01 |
| 41.Nb | 1.1040E−03 | 3.4343E+04 | 3.4408E+04 | 3.4408E+04 | 2.0322E−03 |
| | 2.3238E−03 | 5.2875E+03 | 5.3100E+03 | 5.3375E+03 | 5.1920E−01 |
| | 1.2461E−02 | 4.4320E+02 | 4.9765E+02 | 4.6248E+02 | 7.6053E+00 |
| 55.Cs | 3.6818E−02 | 1.8666E+01 | 2.1116E+01 | 5.5908E+01 | 1.6476E+02 |
| 56.Ba | 1.4324E−03 | 1.7697E+04 | 1.7739E+04 | 1.7751E+04 | 6.7384E−02 |
| | 2.8908E−02 | 3.8107E+01 | 4.2082E+01 | 4.2110E+01 | 6.5512E−02 |
| | 3.2401E−02 | 2.6424E+01 | 2.9460E+01 | 2.9688E+01 | 7.7311E−01 |
| 61.Pm | 1.0473E−03 | 3.7212E+04 | 3.7282E+04 | 3.7399E+04 | 3.1578E−01 |
| 62.Sm | 1.0991E−03 | 3.4591E+04 | 3.4658E+04 | 3.4783E+04 | 3.6157E−01 |
| 64.Gd | 1.2139E−03 | 2.8772E+04 | 2.8829E+04 | 2.8969E+04 | 4.8380E−01 |
| 65.Tb | 1.2545E−03 | 2.6713E+04 | 2.6768E+04 | 2.6917E+04 | 5.5574E−01 |
| 66.Dy | 1.3061E−03 | 2.4101E+04 | 2.4152E+04 | 2.4303E+04 | 6.2387E−01 |
| 67.Ho | 1.3579E−03 | 2.1474E+04 | 2.1521E+04 | 2.1658E+04 | 6.3617E−01 |
| | 5.7433E−03 | 2.6037E+03 | 3.2107E+03 | 2.6647E+03 | 2.0488E+01 |
| 68.Er | 1.4098E−03 | 1.8842E+04 | 1.8885E+04 | 1.9008E+04 | 6.5200E−01 |
| | 7.8529E−03 | 1.2527E+03 | 1.4656E+03 | 1.3009E+03 | 1.2657E+01 |
| 70.Yb | 1.5305E−03 | 1.3813E+04 | 1.3849E+04 | 1.3965E+04 | 8.3727E−01 |

| Material | $E$, MeV | $\mu_{1en}$, cm$^{-1}$ | $\mu_1$, cm$^{-1}$ | $\mu_2$, cm$^{-1}$ | $R$, % |
|---|---|---|---|---|---|
| 88.Ra | 1.4827E−03 | 1.5149E+04 | 1.5187E+04 | 1.5214E+04 | 1.8022E−01 |
| 118. | 3.8119E−03 | 1.2641E+03 | 1.2795E+03 | 1.2894E+03 | 7.7124E−01 |
| | 3.8675E−02 | 1.5403E+01 | 1.7607E+01 | 4.3548E+01 | 1.4733E+02 |
| 125. | 5.6478E−03 | 2.6993E+03 | 3.3397E+03 | 2.7737E+03 | 2.0408E+01 |
| 134. | 1.8634E−03 | 8.7931E+03 | 8.8208E+03 | 8.8885E+03 | 7.6688E−01 |
| | 2.3072E−03 | 5.3616E+03 | 5.3842E+03 | 5.4181E+03 | 6.2911E−01 |
| | 2.7061E−03 | 3.5808E+03 | 3.6009E+03 | 3.6226E+03 | 6.0232E−01 |
| | | | 24.CROMIUM | | |
| 20.Ca | 4.1079E−03 | 1.3379E+03 | 1.3570E+03 | 1.5383E+03 | 1.3362E+01 |
| 31.Ga | 1.1455E−03 | 4.3222E+04 | 4.3323E+04 | 4.3651E+04 | 7.5841E−01 |
| | 1.1486E−02 | 6.8932E+02 | 7.9690E+02 | 1.1131E+03 | 3.9684E+01 |
| 32.Ge | 1.2716E−03 | 3.4710E+04 | 3.4793E+04 | 3.5103E+04 | 8.9239E−01 |
| | 1.4021E−02 | 4.0410E+02 | 4.5884E+02 | 6.2975E+02 | 3.7247E+01 |
| 33.As | 1.3408E−02 | 4.7304E+02 | 5.4056E+02 | 7.9952E+02 | 4.7907E+01 |
| 34.Se | 1.6953E−02 | 2.3086E+02 | 2.5716E+02 | 3.6797E+02 | 4.3088E+01 |
| 38.Sr | 3.8102E−02 | 2.2314E+01 | 2.5381E+01 | 3.0602E+01 | 2.0571E+01 |
| 39.Y | 1.8217E−02 | 1.9009E+02 | 2.1120E+02 | 3.9879E+02 | 8.8823E+01 |
| 42.Mo | 1.4470E−03 | 2.2869E+04 | 2.2927E+04 | 2.2940E+04 | 5.9633E−02 |
| | 2.2818E−03 | 7.4302E+03 | 7.4629E+03 | 7.4908E+03 | 3.7431E−01 |
| | 9.6798E−03 | 9.5934E+02 | 1.1247E+03 | 9.9222E+02 | 1.3352E+01 |
| 48.Cd | 2.5773E−02 | 7.9987E+01 | 8.8525E+01 | 8.8768E+01 | 2.7354E−01 |
| 49.In | 2.3850E−02 | 9.7490E+01 | 1.0778E+02 | 1.0644E+02 | 1.2548E+00 |
| 52.Te | 3.1654E−02 | 3.7583E+01 | 4.1946E+01 | 4.2671E+01 | 1.7273E+00 |
| 53.I | 1.5189E−03 | 1.8909E+04 | 1.8959E+04 | 1.8963E+04 | 2.1840E−02 |
| 55.Cs | 4.1609E−02 | 1.6430E+01 | 1.8997E+01 | 4.1459E+01 | 1.1824E+02 |
| 56.Ba | 3.5651E−03 | 2.1399E+03 | 2.1615E+03 | 2.1634E+03 | 9.0439E−02 |
| 57.La | 1.0604E−03 | 4.8965E+04 | 4.9079E+04 | 4.9107E+04 | 5.7171E−02 |
| 63.Eu | 1.2986E−03 | 3.2890E+04 | 3.2969E+04 | 3.3090E+04 | 3.6933E−01 |
| 64.Gd | 1.2306E−03 | 3.7479E+04 | 3.7568E+04 | 3.7739E+04 | 4.5720E−01 |
| 65.Tb | 1.2667E−03 | 3.5039E+04 | 3.5123E+04 | 3.5312E+04 | 5.3892E−01 |
| 66.Dy | 1.3191E−03 | 3.1506E+04 | 3.1582E+04 | 3.1777E+04 | 6.1934E−01 |
| 67.Ho | 1.3715E−03 | 2.7965E+04 | 2.8033E+04 | 2.8221E+04 | 6.7000E−01 |
| 68.Er | 1.4224E−03 | 2.4528E+04 | 2.4590E+04 | 2.4768E+04 | 7.2467E−01 |
| 69.Tm | 1.4735E−03 | 2.1078E+04 | 2.1132E+04 | 2.1292E+04 | 7.5362E−01 |
| 70.Yb | 1.5472E−03 | 1.8335E+04 | 1.8383E+04 | 1.8552E+04 | 9.1497E−01 |
| 71.Lu | 1.5952E−03 | 1.7359E+04 | 1.7406E+04 | 1.7550E+04 | 8.2599E−01 |
| | 7.2551E−03 | 2.0173E+03 | 2.5122E+03 | 2.0811E+03 | 2.0718E+01 |
| 72.Hf | 1.4793E−03 | 2.0688E+04 | 2.0741E+04 | 2.0834E+04 | 4.4928E−01 |
| | 1.6178E−03 | 1.6899E+04 | 1.6946E+04 | 1.7046E+04 | 5.8735E−01 |

| Material | $E$, MeV | $\mu_{1en}$, cm$^{-1}$ | $\mu_1$, cm$^{-1}$ | $\mu_2$, cm$^{-1}$ | $R$, % |
|---|---|---|---|---|---|
| 83.Bi | 1.0156E−03 | 5.1996E+04 | 5.2116E+04 | 5.2132E+04 | 3.1331E−02 |
| 88.Ra | 2.8542E−03 | 3.9717E+03 | 3.9978E+03 | 4.0270E+03 | 7.3078E−01 |
| 112. | 1.3731E−03 | 2.7862E+04 | 2.7931E+04 | 2.7929E+04 | 6.1260E−03 |
| | 7.8641E−03 | 1.5931E+03 | 1.9335E+03 | 1.6627E+03 | 1.6282E+01 |
| 114. | 4.8907E−03 | 8.2989E+02 | 8.4672E+02 | 9.0453E+02 | 6.8279E+00 |
| 116. | 1.8332E−03 | 1.2522E+04 | 1.2562E+04 | 1.2570E+04 | 5.9064E−02 |
| 118. | 4.6535E−02 | 1.2171E+01 | 1.4378E+01 | 2.8359E+01 | 9.7240E+01 |
| 121. | 1.3110E−03 | 3.2053E+04 | 3.2130E+04 | 3.2269E+04 | 4.3062E−01 |
| 123. | 1.4173E−02 | 3.8695E+02 | 4.3851E+02 | 5.9652E+02 | 3.6032E+01 |
| 130. | 1.4645E−03 | 2.1690E+04 | 2.1745E+04 | 2.1768E+04 | 1.0367E−01 |
| | 1.0421E−02 | 8.0924E+02 | 9.3904E+02 | 8.4989E+02 | 1.0490E+01 |
| 134. | 2.8863E−02 | 5.1852E+01 | 5.7581E+01 | 1.0194E+02 | 7.7032E+01 |
| | | | 25.MANGANESE | | |
| 20.Ca | 6.0958E−03 | 5.1172E+02 | 5.2639E+02 | 5.6342E+02 | 7.0354E+00 |
| 31.Ga | 1.3835E−02 | 4.7069E+02 | 5.4936E+02 | 7.0603E+02 | 2.8518E+01 |
| 32.Ge | 1.3915E−03 | 3.0358E+04 | 3.0449E+04 | 3.0686E+04 | 7.7838E−01 |
| | 1.4907E−02 | 3.3976E+02 | 3.8800E+02 | 5.0070E+02 | 2.9045E+01 |
| 33.As | 1.4325E−02 | 4.1087E+02 | 4.7564E+02 | 6.6434E+02 | 3.9674E+01 |
| 34.Se | 1.4852E−03 | 2.3256E+04 | 2.3326E+04 | 2.3592E+04 | 1.1410E+00 |
| | 1.9902E−02 | 1.5341E+02 | 1.7167E+02 | 2.2167E+02 | 2.9128E+01 |
| 38.Sr | 2.8496E−03 | 4.6271E+03 | 4.6566E+03 | 4.7101E+03 | 1.1496E+00 |
| | 5.4654E−02 | 8.5397E+00 | 1.0488E+01 | 1.1004E+01 | 4.9260E+00 |
| 39.Y | 1.9402E−02 | 1.7128E+02 | 1.9232E+02 | 3.3737E+02 | 7.5417E+01 |
| 42.Mo | 7.7670E−03 | 1.7666E+03 | 2.2460E+03 | 1.8147E+03 | 2.3768E+01 |
| 43.Tc | 2.6489E−03 | 6.0207E+03 | 6.0537E+03 | 6.0879E+03 | 5.6523E−01 |
| | 1.8783E−02 | 1.9336E+02 | 2.1785E+02 | 2.0878E+02 | 4.3463E+00 |
| 47.Ag | 2.4852E−02 | 1.0021E+02 | 1.1207E+02 | 1.1116E+02 | 8.1259E−01 |
| 48.Cd | 2.1476E−02 | 1.3480E+02 | 1.5073E+02 | 1.4632E+02 | 3.0147E+00 |
| 49.In | 1.4077E−03 | 2.9132E+04 | 2.9219E+04 | 2.9202E+04 | 6.0710E−02 |
| | 9.6934E−03 | 1.0433E+03 | 1.2656E+03 | 1.0856E+03 | 1.6582E+01 |
| 50.Sn | 1.1045E−03 | 5.2109E+04 | 5.2264E+04 | 5.2198E+04 | 1.2704E−01 |
| | 1.4213E−02 | 4.2450E+02 | 4.9244E+02 | 4.4652E+02 | 1.0284E+01 |
| 51.Sb | 1.3502E−03 | 3.3491E+04 | 3.3591E+04 | 3.3566E+04 | 7.5888E−02 |
| | 9.8610E−03 | 9.8625E+02 | 1.1895E+03 | 1.0307E+03 | 1.5405E+01 |
| 52.Te | 1.4730E−03 | 2.4181E+04 | 2.4254E+04 | 2.4246E+04 | 3.5227E−02 |
| | 7.9572E−03 | 1.6467E+03 | 2.0731E+03 | 1.7264E+03 | 2.0080E+01 |
| 53.I | 2.9458E−03 | 3.9591E+03 | 3.9868E+03 | 3.9937E+03 | 1.7121E−01 |
| 55.Cs | 4.6485E−02 | 1.4086E+01 | 1.6557E+01 | 3.1952E+01 | 9.2977E+01 |
| 58.Ce | 1.0833E−03 | 5.3720E+04 | 5.3880E+04 | 5.3902E+04 | 4.0491E−02 |

| Material | $E$, MeV | $\mu_{1en}$, cm$^{-1}$ | $\mu_1$, cm$^{-1}$ | $\mu_2$, cm$^{-1}$ | $R$, % |
|---|---|---|---|---|---|
| 60.Nd | 1.0382E−03 | 5.7140E+04 | 5.7310E+04 | 5.7392E+04 | 1.4330E−01 |
| 61.Pm | 1.1060E−03 | 5.1995E+04 | 5.2150E+04 | 5.2260E+04 | 2.0996E−01 |
| 62.Sm | 1.1239E−03 | 5.0643E+04 | 5.0794E+04 | 5.0925E+04 | 2.5743E−01 |
| 63.Eu | 1.4101E−03 | 2.8945E+04 | 2.9032E+04 | 2.9120E+04 | 3.0202E−01 |
| 64.Gd | 1.2914E−03 | 3.7949E+04 | 3.8062E+04 | 3.8209E+04 | 3.8665E−01 |
| 65.Tb | 1.2727E−03 | 3.9362E+04 | 3.9479E+04 | 3.9669E+04 | 4.8134E−01 |
| 66.Dy | 1.3251E−03 | 3.5393E+04 | 3.5499E+04 | 3.5700E+04 | 5.6603E−01 |
| 67.Ho | 1.3775E−03 | 3.1416E+04 | 3.1511E+04 | 3.1709E+04 | 6.3099E−01 |
| 68.Er | 1.4291E−03 | 2.7512E+04 | 2.7594E+04 | 2.7790E+04 | 7.0751E−01 |
| 69.Tm | 1.4783E−03 | 2.3782E+04 | 2.3854E+04 | 2.4032E+04 | 7.4689E−01 |
| 70.Yb | 1.5565E−03 | 2.0822E+04 | 2.0887E+04 | 2.1076E+04 | 9.0511E−01 |
| 71.Lu | 1.6039E−03 | 1.9721E+04 | 1.9784E+04 | 1.9957E+04 | 8.7625E−01 |
| | 6.7882E−03 | 2.3837E+03 | 3.1362E+03 | 2.4523E+03 | 2.7891E+01 |
| 73.Ta | 1.1615E−03 | 4.7795E+04 | 4.7938E+04 | 4.7990E+04 | 1.0826E−01 |
| 81.Tl | 1.1310E−03 | 5.0101E+04 | 5.0250E+04 | 5.0250E+04 | 4.6642E−05 |
| 82.Pb | 1.0949E−03 | 5.2839E+04 | 5.2997E+04 | 5.2985E+04 | 2.2611E−02 |
| 83.Bi | 1.3995E−03 | 2.9750E+04 | 2.9840E+04 | 2.9879E+04 | 1.3164E−01 |
| 84.Po | 1.3860E−03 | 3.0779E+04 | 3.0871E+04 | 3.0902E+04 | 1.0000E−01 |
| 85.At | 1.1460E−03 | 4.8965E+04 | 4.9111E+04 | 4.9105E+04 | 1.2163E−02 |
| 87.Fr | 1.0504E−03 | 5.6210E+04 | 5.6377E+04 | 5.6350E+04 | 4.8456E−02 |
| | 1.1951E−03 | 4.5243E+04 | 4.5378E+04 | 4.5382E+04 | 8.3242E−03 |
| 112. | 2.5801E−03 | 6.4986E+03 | 6.5329E+03 | 6.5424E+03 | 1.4639E−01 |
| | 3.4169E−03 | 2.7716E+03 | 2.7959E+03 | 2.8094E+03 | 4.8119E−01 |
| | 7.2832E−03 | 2.0716E+03 | 2.6860E+03 | 2.1659E+03 | 2.4015E+01 |
| 116. | 3.4804E−03 | 2.6480E+03 | 2.6720E+03 | 2.6777E+03 | 2.1381E−01 |
| | 4.5424E−03 | 1.2288E+03 | 1.2480E+03 | 1.2541E+03 | 4.8765E−01 |
| 118. | 4.9761E−02 | 1.0839E+01 | 1.3011E+01 | 2.2762E+01 | 7.4950E+01 |
| 121. | 1.3676E−03 | 3.2171E+04 | 3.2267E+04 | 3.2386E+04 | 3.6956E−01 |
| 123. | 1.4931E−02 | 3.3679E+02 | 3.8435E+02 | 4.9847E+02 | 2.9691E+01 |
| 130. | 2.3200E−03 | 8.3051E+03 | 8.3441E+03 | 8.3966E+03 | 6.2951E−01 |
| | 7.7583E−03 | 1.7721E+03 | 2.2539E+03 | 1.8548E+03 | 2.1519E+01 |
| 134. | 2.9936E−02 | 4.8138E+01 | 5.3862E+01 | 9.0704E+01 | 6.8401E+01 |
| | | | 26.IRON | | |
| 30.Zn | 1.0850E−02 | 9.6028E+02 | 1.1914E+03 | 1.4785E+03 | 2.4100E+01 |
| 31.Ga | 1.3894E−03 | 3.6541E+04 | 3.6666E+04 | 3.6873E+04 | 5.6292E−01 |
| | 1.9489E−02 | 1.9915E+02 | 2.2746E+02 | 2.5971E+02 | 1.4176E+01 |
| 32.Ge | 1.4449E−03 | 3.1592E+04 | 3.1698E+04 | 3.1923E+04 | 7.0890E−01 |
| | 2.7556E−02 | 8.6634E+01 | 9.8065E+01 | 1.1063E+02 | 1.2817E+01 |
| 33.As | 1.4468E−03 | 3.1426E+04 | 3.1531E+04 | 3.1819E+04 | 9.1433E−01 |

| Material | $E$, MeV | $\mu_{1en}$, cm$^{-1}$ | $\mu_1$, cm$^{-1}$ | $\mu_2$, cm$^{-1}$ | $R$, % |
|---|---|---|---|---|---|
| | 1.8180E−02 | 2.5352E+02 | 2.9223E+02 | 3.7192E+02 | 2.7273E+01 |
| 34.Se | 1.7780E−03 | 1.8938E+04 | 1.9003E+04 | 1.9187E+04 | 9.6765E−01 |
| | 3.5108E−02 | 4.0619E+01 | 4.6089E+01 | 5.1647E+01 | 1.2059E+01 |
| 38.Sr | 6.5554E−03 | 5.2761E+02 | 5.4356E+02 | 5.3904E+02 | 8.3776E−01 |
| 39.Y | 2.5634E−02 | 1.0986E+02 | 1.2455E+02 | 1.9241E+02 | 5.4487E+01 |
| 42.Mo | 7.1595E−03 | 2.3170E+03 | 3.1665E+03 | 2.3760E+03 | 3.3271E+01 |
| 43.Tc | 9.0281E−03 | 1.4403E+03 | 1.8598E+03 | 1.4862E+03 | 2.5140E+01 |
| 44.Ru | 1.1460E−03 | 5.8250E+04 | 5.8459E+04 | 5.8354E+04 | 1.7960E−01 |
| | 1.4864E−02 | 4.0429E+02 | 4.7368E+02 | 4.2778E+02 | 1.0731E+01 |
| 45.Rh | 2.0819E−02 | 1.6806E+02 | 1.9092E+02 | 1.8332E+02 | 4.1449E+00 |
| 46.Pd | 2.1698E−02 | 1.5743E+02 | 1.7881E+02 | 1.7194E+02 | 3.9938E+00 |
| 47.Ag | 2.0006E−02 | 1.7788E+02 | 2.0213E+02 | 1.9268E+02 | 4.9001E+00 |
| 48.Cd | 2.2177E−03 | 1.0928E+04 | 1.0972E+04 | 1.0987E+04 | 1.4065E−01 |
| | 3.4580E−03 | 3.2768E+03 | 3.3055E+03 | 3.3277E+03 | 6.7345E−01 |
| | 9.1443E−03 | 1.3970E+03 | 1.7981E+03 | 1.4499E+03 | 2.4020E+01 |
| 49.In | 7.5981E−03 | 2.0595E+03 | 2.7698E+03 | 2.1416E+03 | 2.9331E+01 |
| 50.Sn | 2.8845E−03 | 5.3286E+03 | 5.3626E+03 | 5.3780E+03 | 2.8748E−01 |
| | 7.8212E−03 | 1.9286E+03 | 2.5680E+03 | 2.0101E+03 | 2.7755E+01 |
| 51.Sb | 3.2575E−03 | 3.7501E+03 | 3.7804E+03 | 3.7931E+03 | 3.3537E−01 |
| | 7.5981E−03 | 2.0596E+03 | 2.7698E+03 | 2.1555E+03 | 2.8502E+01 |
| 52.Te | 3.8662E−03 | 2.3129E+03 | 2.3384E+03 | 2.3492E+03 | 4.6428E−01 |
| | 4.1200E−03 | 1.8868E+03 | 1.9108E+03 | 1.9215E+03 | 5.6278E−01 |
| | 7.2850E−03 | 2.2433E+03 | 3.0529E+03 | 2.3595E+03 | 2.9390E+01 |
| 55.Cs | 5.2965E−02 | 1.1304E+01 | 1.3659E+01 | 2.2237E+01 | 6.2798E+01 |
| 56.Ba | 3.7593E−02 | 3.2606E+01 | 3.7193E+01 | 1.0120E+02 | 1.7210E+02 |
| 57.La | 1.4337E−03 | 3.2587E+04 | 3.2697E+04 | 3.2698E+04 | 2.8254E−03 |
| | 3.6979E−02 | 3.4587E+01 | 3.9392E+01 | 3.9481E+01 | 2.2578E−01 |
| 58.Ce | 1.3449E−03 | 4.0510E+04 | 4.0650E+04 | 4.0651E+04 | 3.1711E−03 |
| 61.Pm | 1.2888E−03 | 4.5514E+04 | 4.5673E+04 | 4.5736E+04 | 1.3662E−01 |
| 62.Sm | 1.2458E−03 | 4.9351E+04 | 4.9526E+04 | 4.9620E+04 | 1.9105E−01 |
| 64.Gd | 1.3671E−03 | 3.8535E+04 | 3.8667E+04 | 3.8795E+04 | 3.3111E−01 |
| 67.Ho | 1.3868E−03 | 3.6770E+04 | 3.6896E+04 | 3.7120E+04 | 6.0715E−01 |
| 68.Er | 1.4389E−03 | 3.2126E+04 | 3.2234E+04 | 3.2460E+04 | 7.0398E−01 |
| 69.Tm | 1.4855E−03 | 2.7967E+04 | 2.8059E+04 | 2.8274E+04 | 7.6678E−01 |
| 70.Yb | 1.5714E−03 | 2.4690E+04 | 2.4771E+04 | 2.5001E+04 | 9.2767E−01 |
| 71.Lu | 1.6162E−03 | 2.3441E+04 | 2.3518E+04 | 2.3742E+04 | 9.5312E−01 |
| 72.Hf | 1.6683E−03 | 2.1991E+04 | 2.2065E+04 | 2.2246E+04 | 8.2351E−01 |
| 74.W | 1.0405E−03 | 6.7661E+04 | 6.7907E+04 | 6.7891E+04 | 2.3222E−02 |
| 80.Hg | 1.3487E−03 | 4.0168E+04 | 4.0307E+04 | 4.0345E+04 | 9.2124E−02 |

| Material | $E$, MeV | $\mu_{1en}$, cm$^{-1}$ | $\mu_1$, cm$^{-1}$ | $\mu_2$, cm$^{-1}$ | $R$, % |
|---|---|---|---|---|---|
| 81.Tl | 1.5914E−03 | 2.4133E+04 | 2.4213E+04 | 2.4274E+04 | 2.5285E−01 |
| 82.Pb | 1.5205E−03 | 2.6107E+04 | 2.6192E+04 | 2.6243E+04 | 1.9369E−01 |
| 83.Bi | 1.9559E−03 | 1.3985E+04 | 1.4036E+04 | 1.4103E+04 | 4.7811E−01 |
| | 2.2098E−03 | 1.0994E+04 | 1.1039E+04 | 1.1109E+04 | 6.3448E−01 |
| 83.Bi | 1.3189E−02 | 6.3627E+02 | 7.7314E+02 | 6.7915E+02 | 1.3840E+01 |
| 84.Po | 1.9325E−03 | 1.4635E+04 | 1.4688E+04 | 1.4748E+04 | 4.1219E−01 |
| | 2.4927E−03 | 8.6182E+03 | 8.6580E+03 | 8.7253E+03 | 7.7686E−01 |
| 85.At | 1.4822E−03 | 2.8269E+04 | 2.8361E+04 | 2.8409E+04 | 1.6643E−01 |
| 87.Fr | 1.4510E−03 | 3.1049E+04 | 3.1153E+04 | 3.1181E+04 | 8.9290E−02 |
| 89.Ac | 1.3846E−03 | 3.6974E+04 | 3.7100E+04 | 3.7110E+04 | 2.5153E−02 |
| 112. | 2.8338E−02 | 7.7179E+01 | 8.7282E+01 | 1.5912E+02 | 8.2311E+01 |
| 113. | 6.6849E−03 | 4.9889E+02 | 5.1454E+02 | 5.4411E+02 | 5.7481E+00 |
| 118. | 5.9697E−02 | 7.6866E+00 | 9.6680E+00 | 1.4136E+01 | 4.6213E+01 |
| 121. | 1.4368E−03 | 3.2314E+04 | 3.2423E+04 | 3.2530E+04 | 3.3077E−01 |
| 123. | 1.4910E−03 | 2.7483E+04 | 2.7573E+04 | 2.7770E+04 | 7.1489E−01 |
| | 2.7408E−02 | 8.8421E+01 | 1.0010E+02 | 1.1356E+02 | 1.3442E+01 |
| 125. | 2.5136E−03 | 8.4426E+03 | 8.4822E+03 | 8.6498E+03 | 1.9757E+00 |
| | 1.3917E−02 | 5.3551E+02 | 6.4308E+02 | 6.6539E+02 | 3.4688E+00 |
| 130. | 2.3645E−03 | 9.6946E+03 | 9.7364E+03 | 9.8343E+03 | 1.0058E+00 |
| 134. | 3.8850E−02 | 2.8552E+01 | 3.2693E+01 | 4.6648E+01 | 4.2683E+01 |
| | | | 27.COBALT | | |
| 28.Ni | 1.0039E−03 | 8.6354E+04 | 8.6761E+04 | 8.6853E+04 | 1.0591E−01 |
| 29.Cu | 1.0599E−03 | 8.0301E+04 | 8.0677E+04 | 8.0868E+04 | 2.3717E−01 |
| | 9.3209E−03 | 1.5323E+03 | 2.0637E+03 | 2.3069E+03 | 1.1786E+01 |
| 30.Zn | 1.4453E−03 | 3.8679E+04 | 3.8843E+04 | 3.8965E+04 | 3.1443E−01 |
| | 2.4934E−02 | 1.4373E+02 | 1.6574E+02 | 1.7687E+02 | 6.7179E+00 |
| 31.Ga | 6.7377E−03 | 6.3624E+02 | 6.5489E+02 | 6.5221E+02 | 4.1096E−01 |
| 32.Ge | 7.1217E−03 | 5.4410E+02 | 5.6171E+02 | 5.5845E+02 | 5.8440E−01 |
| 33.As | 3.5822E−02 | 4.7151E+01 | 5.3951E+01 | 5.8604E+01 | 8.6236E+00 |
| 34.Se | 7.2109E−03 | 5.2269E+02 | 5.4006E+02 | 5.3592E+02 | 7.7220E−01 |
| 39.Y | 2.1784E−03 | 1.3916E+04 | 1.3981E+04 | 1.4250E+04 | 1.9225E+00 |
| | 3.0973E−02 | 6.6241E+01 | 7.5450E+01 | 9.8629E+01 | 3.0721E+01 |
| 40.Zr | 1.9460E−02 | 2.4198E+02 | 2.8214E+02 | 5.1003E+02 | 8.0773E+01 |
| 44.Ru | 9.0000E−03 | 1.6621E+03 | 2.2646E+03 | 1.7157E+03 | 3.1994E+01 |
| 45.Rh | 2.9711E−03 | 5.7138E+03 | 5.7547E+03 | 5.7874E+03 | 5.6759E−01 |
| | 1.0202E−02 | 1.2254E+03 | 1.5946E+03 | 1.2716E+03 | 2.5399E+01 |
| 46.Pd | 2.6171E−03 | 9.3764E+03 | 9.4284E+03 | 9.4546E+03 | 2.7820E−01 |
| | 3.1421E−03 | 4.9990E+03 | 5.0377E+03 | 5.0706E+03 | 6.5325E−01 |
| | 1.2120E−02 | 9.1980E+02 | 1.1778E+03 | 9.5789E+02 | 2.2960E+01 |

| Material | $E$, MeV | $\mu_{1en}$, cm$^{-1}$ | $\mu_1$, cm$^{-1}$ | $\mu_2$, cm$^{-1}$ | $R$, % |
|---|---|---|---|---|---|
| 47.Ag | 9.4356E−03 | 1.4859E+03 | 1.9919E+03 | 1.5404E+03 | 2.9311E+01 |
| 56.Ba | 3.9925E−02 | 3.0998E+01 | 3.5761E+01 | 8.6466E+01 | 1.4179E+02 |
| 57.La | 2.7345E−03 | 8.1617E+03 | 8.2101E+03 | 8.2145E+03 | 5.4287E−02 |
| | 7.8945E−03 | 2.1262E+03 | 2.9897E+03 | 2.2836E+03 | 3.0918E+01 |
| 58.Ce | 1.4890E−03 | 3.3960E+04 | 3.4099E+04 | 3.4082E+04 | 5.1175E−02 |
| | 1.3531E−02 | 6.9498E+02 | 8.7121E+02 | 7.4307E+02 | 1.7244E+01 |
| 59.Pr | 1.4749E−03 | 3.5483E+04 | 3.5630E+04 | 3.5629E+04 | 3.5632E−03 |
| 60.Nd | 1.4310E−03 | 4.0221E+04 | 4.0393E+04 | 4.0399E+04 | 1.6634E−02 |
| 61.Pm | 1.3891E−03 | 4.4751E+04 | 4.4946E+04 | 4.4966E+04 | 4.6341E−02 |
| 63.Eu | 1.8811E−03 | 1.9805E+04 | 1.9891E+04 | 1.9929E+04 | 1.8876E−01 |
| | 9.7200E−03 | 1.3708E+03 | 1.8138E+03 | 1.5212E+03 | 1.9235E+01 |
| 64.Gd | 1.4413E−03 | 3.9109E+04 | 3.9275E+04 | 3.9370E+04 | 2.4141E−01 |
| 65.Tb | 1.3761E−03 | 4.6150E+04 | 4.6352E+04 | 4.6511E+04 | 3.4306E−01 |
| 66.Dy | 1.3678E−03 | 4.7044E+04 | 4.7250E+04 | 4.7459E+04 | 4.4216E−01 |
| 68.Er | 1.4514E−03 | 3.8020E+04 | 3.8180E+04 | 3.8426E+04 | 6.4373E−01 |
| 69.Tm | 1.4949E−03 | 3.3325E+04 | 3.3461E+04 | 3.3704E+04 | 7.2633E−01 |
| 70.Yb | 1.5768E−03 | 3.0158E+04 | 3.0281E+04 | 3.0548E+04 | 8.7953E−01 |
| 71.Lu | 1.6278E−03 | 2.8422E+04 | 2.8540E+04 | 2.8799E+04 | 9.0918E−01 |
| 72.Hf | 1.6822E−03 | 2.6572E+04 | 2.6682E+04 | 2.6915E+04 | 8.7328E−01 |
| | 7.8986E−03 | 2.1239E+03 | 2.9859E+03 | 2.2039E+03 | 3.5483E+01 |
| 73.Ta | 1.7388E−03 | 2.4648E+04 | 2.4752E+04 | 2.4942E+04 | 7.6847E−01 |
| 75.Re | 1.3146E−03 | 5.2791E+04 | 5.3027E+04 | 5.3044E+04 | 3.1035E−02 |
| 80.Hg | 1.9835E−03 | 1.6322E+04 | 1.6395E+04 | 1.6485E+04 | 5.4769E−01 |
| | 2.0320E−03 | 1.5431E+04 | 1.5501E+04 | 1.5593E+04 | 5.8942E−01 |
| 81.Tl | 1.1818E−02 | 9.6793E+02 | 1.2435E+03 | 1.0244E+03 | 2.1390E+01 |
| 82.Pb | 1.2176E−02 | 9.1080E+02 | 1.1656E+03 | 9.6483E+02 | 2.0805E+01 |
| 83.Bi | 1.0201E−02 | 1.2256E+03 | 1.5949E+03 | 1.2849E+03 | 2.4123E+01 |
| 84.Po | 1.0435E−02 | 1.1883E+03 | 1.5440E+03 | 1.2457E+03 | 2.3949E+01 |
| 85.At | 1.3920E−02 | 6.3287E+02 | 7.8650E+02 | 6.7698E+02 | 1.6178E+01 |
| 87.Fr | 2.2339E−03 | 1.3341E+04 | 1.3405E+04 | 1.3466E+04 | 4.5460E−01 |
| 89.Ac | 1.8056E−03 | 2.2373E+04 | 2.2468E+04 | 2.2504E+04 | 1.5796E−01 |
| 90.Th | 1.4162E−03 | 4.1818E+04 | 4.1998E+04 | 4.1976E+04 | 5.1462E−02 |
| 123. | 6.9351E−03 | 5.8886E+02 | 6.0697E+02 | 6.0367E+02 | 5.4803E−01 |
| 125. | 2.5768E−03 | 9.7934E+03 | 9.8467E+03 | 1.0044E+04 | 2.0061E+00 |
| 130. | 2.5351E−03 | 1.0225E+04 | 1.0280E+04 | 1.0406E+04 | 1.2216E+00 |
| | 1.4364E−02 | 5.6219E+02 | 6.9011E+02 | 6.7583E+02 | 2.1135E+00 |
| 134. | 3.6822E−03 | 3.4183E+03 | 3.4517E+03 | 3.5374E+03 | 2.4825E+00 |
| | 5.3760E−02 | 1.3511E+01 | 1.6304E+01 | 1.9681E+01 | 2.0710E+01 |

| Material | $E$, MeV | $\mu_{1en}$, cm$^{-1}$ | $\mu_1$, cm$^{-1}$ | $\mu_2$, cm$^{-1}$ | $R$, % |
|---|---|---|---|---|---|
| 28.NICKEL | | | | | |
| 21.Sc | 4.8732E−03 | 1.7350E+03 | 1.7642E+03 | 2.0223E+03 | 1.4629E+01 |
| 27.Co | 1.0039E−03 | 8.6354E+04 | 8.6853E+04 | 8.6761E+04 | 1.0591E−01 |
| 29.Cu | 1.3587E−03 | 5.4681E+04 | 5.4962E+04 | 5.5031E+04 | 1.2563E−01 |
| | 1.3839E−02 | 7.0690E+02 | 9.1595E+02 | 9.5857E+02 | 4.6522E+00 |
| 33.As | 8.0875E−03 | 4.1148E+02 | 4.2856E+02 | 4.2527E+02 | 7.7578E−01 |
| 39.Y | 2.6496E−03 | 1.0433E+04 | 1.0494E+04 | 1.0656E+04 | 1.5450E+00 |
| | 4.3106E−02 | 3.0092E+01 | 3.5072E+01 | 4.0814E+01 | 1.6372E+01 |
| 40.Zr | 2.3135E−02 | 1.9141E+02 | 2.2563E+02 | 3.7391E+02 | 6.5715E+01 |
| 45.Rh | 9.3075E−03 | 1.6214E+03 | 2.3057E+03 | 1.6771E+03 | 3.7476E+01 |
| 46.Pd | 9.5247E−03 | 1.5384E+03 | 2.1661E+03 | 1.5933E+03 | 3.5948E+01 |
| 47.Ag | 8.6679E−03 | 1.8659E+03 | 2.7169E+03 | 1.9317E+03 | 4.0646E+01 |
| 53.I | 3.5727E−02 | 5.4388E+01 | 6.2781E+01 | 1.5126E+02 | 1.4094E+02 |
| 55.Cs | 5.4989E−03 | 1.2581E+03 | 1.2839E+03 | 1.3590E+03 | 5.8492E+00 |
| 56.Ba | 4.4998E−02 | 2.6910E+01 | 3.1490E+01 | 6.7137E+01 | 1.1320E+02 |
| 58.Ce | 2.7856E−03 | 8.8160E+03 | 8.8714E+03 | 8.8755E+03 | 4.5507E−02 |
| | 9.4899E−03 | 1.5517E+03 | 2.1885E+03 | 1.6662E+03 | 3.1349E+01 |
| 59.Pr | 1.9328E−03 | 2.0754E+04 | 2.0855E+04 | 2.0849E+04 | 3.0605E−02 |
| | 1.1850E−02 | 1.0435E+03 | 1.4053E+03 | 1.1224E+03 | 2.5207E+01 |
| 60.Nd | 1.6888E−03 | 3.0204E+04 | 3.0348E+04 | 3.0341E+04 | 2.4320E−02 |
| | 1.4933E−02 | 5.2184E+02 | 6.4693E+02 | 5.6084E+02 | 1.5349E+01 |
| 62.Sm | 1.4596E−03 | 4.2421E+04 | 4.2629E+04 | 4.2653E+04 | 5.6529E−02 |
| 63.Eu | 2.8052E−03 | 8.5835E+03 | 8.6382E+03 | 8.6504E+03 | 1.4182E−01 |
| 64.Gd | 1.4841E−03 | 3.9440E+04 | 3.9630E+04 | 3.9701E+04 | 1.7961E−01 |
| 65.Tb | 1.4407E−03 | 4.4715E+04 | 4.4936E+04 | 4.5060E+04 | 2.7461E−01 |
| 66.Dy | 1.4216E−03 | 4.7047E+04 | 4.7281E+04 | 4.7457E+04 | 3.7021E−01 |
| 67.Ho | 1.4213E−03 | 4.7077E+04 | 4.7312E+04 | 4.7546E+04 | 4.9550E−01 |
| 69.Tm | 1.5073E−03 | 3.7232E+04 | 3.7409E+04 | 3.7661E+04 | 6.7356E−01 |
| 70.Yb | 1.7457E−03 | 2.7997E+04 | 2.8131E+04 | 2.8362E+04 | 8.1850E−01 |
| 71.Lu | 1.6366E−03 | 3.2222E+04 | 3.2376E+04 | 3.2657E+04 | 8.6744E−01 |
| 72.Hf | 1.6915E−03 | 3.0099E+04 | 3.0243E+04 | 3.0509E+04 | 8.7999E−01 |
| 73.Ta | 1.7478E−03 | 2.7916E+04 | 2.8049E+04 | 2.8278E+04 | 8.1370E−01 |
| 74.W | 1.8098E−03 | 2.5516E+04 | 2.5639E+04 | 2.5830E+04 | 7.4266E−01 |
| 75.Re | 1.8372E−03 | 2.4455E+04 | 2.4573E+04 | 2.4711E+04 | 5.6269E−01 |
| 76.Os | 1.3620E−03 | 5.4285E+04 | 5.4563E+04 | 5.4545E+04 | 3.1532E−02 |
| 77.Ir | 1.2097E−03 | 7.2795E+04 | 7.3183E+04 | 7.3077E+04 | 1.4521E−01 |
| 78.Pt | 1.2085E−03 | 7.2948E+04 | 7.3337E+04 | 7.3205E+04 | 1.7989E−01 |
| 79.Au | 1.3847E−03 | 5.1528E+04 | 5.1790E+04 | 5.1780E+04 | 1.9999E−02 |
| 80.Hg | 2.3054E−03 | 1.4523E+04 | 1.4599E+04 | 1.4767E+04 | 1.1558E+00 |

| Material | $E$, MeV | $\mu_{1en}$, cm$^{-1}$ | $\mu_1$, cm$^{-1}$ | $\mu_2$, cm$^{-1}$ | $R$, % |
|---|---|---|---|---|---|
| | 1.1891E−02 | 1.0367E+03 | 1.3954E+03 | 1.0999E+03 | 2.6863E+01 |
| 81.Tl | 2.3932E−03 | 1.3479E+04 | 1.3552E+04 | 1.3740E+04 | 1.3890E+00 |
| | 1.0711E−02 | 1.2364E+03 | 1.6856E+03 | 1.2998E+03 | 2.9682E+01 |
| 82.Pb | 1.0937E−02 | 1.1980E+03 | 1.6299E+03 | 1.2594E+03 | 2.9417E+01 |
| 83.Bi | 9.1166E−03 | 1.6944E+03 | 2.4284E+03 | 1.7639E+03 | 3.7677E+01 |
| 84.Po | 9.1676E−03 | 1.6749E+03 | 2.3957E+03 | 1.7439E+03 | 3.7377E+01 |
| 85.At | 1.2054E−02 | 1.0091E+03 | 1.3552E+03 | 1.0641E+03 | 2.7360E+01 |
| 87.Fr | 2.9865E−03 | 6.4287E+03 | 6.4755E+03 | 6.5369E+03 | 9.4862E−01 |
| 89.Ac | 2.6495E−03 | 1.0433E+04 | 1.0494E+04 | 1.0552E+04 | 5.4521E−01 |
| 90.Th | 1.6132E−03 | 3.3129E+04 | 3.3286E+04 | 3.3281E+04 | 1.6585E−02 |
| 116. | 3.7740E−02 | 4.5405E+01 | 5.2499E+01 | 1.2213E+02 | 1.3263E+02 |
| 121. | 1.7936E−03 | 2.6143E+04 | 2.6268E+04 | 2.6312E+04 | 1.6598E−01 |
| 130. | 2.7614E−03 | 9.1043E+03 | 9.1608E+03 | 9.2742E+03 | 1.2378E+00 |
| 134. | 3.8616E−03 | 3.3556E+03 | 3.3912E+03 | 3.4744E+03 | 2.4542E+00 |
| **29.COPPER** | | | | | |
| 21.Sc | 5.6298E−03 | 1.2555E+03 | 1.2822E+03 | 1.4380E+03 | 1.2152E+01 |
| 27.Co | 1.0599E−03 | 8.0301E+04 | 8.0868E+04 | 8.0677E+04 | 2.3717E−01 |
| | 9.3209E−03 | 1.5323E+03 | 2.3069E+03 | 2.0637E+03 | 1.1786E+01 |
| 28.Ni | 1.3587E−03 | 5.4681E+04 | 5.5031E+04 | 5.4962E+04 | 1.2563E−01 |
| | 1.3839E−02 | 7.0690E+02 | 9.5857E+02 | 9.1595E+02 | 4.6522E+00 |
| 39.Y | 2.8279E−03 | 8.8151E+03 | 8.8766E+03 | 8.9953E+03 | 1.3371E+00 |
| | 5.0569E−02 | 1.9181E+01 | 2.2893E+01 | 2.5182E+01 | 1.0001E+01 |
| 40.Zr | 2.4767E−02 | 1.7066E+02 | 2.0508E+02 | 3.2347E+02 | 5.7727E+01 |
| 44.Ru | 9.1791E−03 | 1.5746E+03 | 2.3847E+03 | 1.6262E+03 | 4.6638E+01 |
| 45.Rh | 9.6874E−03 | 1.4229E+03 | 2.1059E+03 | 1.4740E+03 | 4.2873E+01 |
| 46.Pd | 9.8127E−03 | 1.3856E+03 | 2.0372E+03 | 1.4363E+03 | 4.1833E+01 |
| 47.Ag | 9.3737E−03 | 1.5165E+03 | 2.2779E+03 | 1.5719E+03 | 4.4914E+01 |
| 53.I | 3.6645E−02 | 5.2889E+01 | 6.1773E+01 | 1.4217E+02 | 1.3015E+02 |
| 56.Ba | 4.6631E−02 | 2.5591E+01 | 3.0202E+01 | 6.0978E+01 | 1.0190E+02 |
| 58.Ce | 3.6410E−03 | 4.3611E+03 | 4.4033E+03 | 4.4086E+03 | 1.2075E−01 |
| | 9.8301E−03 | 1.3804E+03 | 2.0277E+03 | 1.4793E+03 | 3.7068E+01 |
| 59.Pr | 2.6965E−03 | 1.0461E+04 | 1.0530E+04 | 1.0530E+04 | 2.7730E−03 |
| | 1.2629E−02 | 9.0323E+02 | 1.2662E+03 | 9.7093E+02 | 3.0412E+01 |
| 60.Nd | 1.9161E−03 | 2.2575E+04 | 2.2702E+04 | 2.2683E+04 | 8.6210E−02 |
| | 1.4670E−02 | 5.7218E+02 | 7.4745E+02 | 6.1554E+02 | 2.1430E+01 |
| 61.Pm | 1.4886E−03 | 4.0603E+04 | 4.0837E+04 | 4.0804E+04 | 8.1947E−02 |
| | 1.5576E−03 | 3.7036E+04 | 3.7246E+04 | 3.7220E+04 | 7.1219E−02 |
| | 4.3672E−02 | 3.0816E+01 | 3.6165E+01 | 3.5985E+01 | 5.0045E−01 |
| 62.Sm | 1.4907E−03 | 4.0366E+04 | 4.0599E+04 | 4.0586E+04 | 3.0635E−02 |

| Material | $E$, MeV | $\mu_{1en}$, cm$^{-1}$ | $\mu_1$, cm$^{-1}$ | $\mu_2$, cm$^{-1}$ | $R$, % |
|---|---|---|---|---|---|
| | 1.5236E−03 | 3.8410E+04 | 3.8628E+04 | 3.8622E+04 | 1.6789E−02 |
| 63.Eu | 3.5016E−03 | 4.8605E+03 | 4.9048E+03 | 4.9108E+03 | 1.2195E−01 |
| | 9.4271E−03 | 1.5006E+03 | 2.2486E+03 | 1.6706E+03 | 3.4603E+01 |
| 64.Gd | 1.4983E−03 | 3.9550E+04 | 3.9775E+04 | 3.9810E+04 | 8.8417E−02 |
| | 1.5099E−03 | 3.8961E+04 | 3.9183E+04 | 3.9218E+04 | 9.0482E−02 |
| 65.Tb | 1.4532E−03 | 4.4439E+04 | 4.4705E+04 | 4.4780E+04 | 1.6911E−01 |
| 66.Dy | 1.4291E−03 | 4.7047E+04 | 4.7334E+04 | 4.7456E+04 | 2.5818E−01 |
| 67.Ho | 1.4265E−03 | 4.7331E+04 | 4.7620E+04 | 4.7803E+04 | 3.8286E−01 |
| 68.Er | 1.4534E−03 | 4.4419E+04 | 4.4685E+04 | 4.4909E+04 | 5.0202E−01 |
| 70.Yb | 1.8282E−03 | 2.6122E+04 | 2.6270E+04 | 2.6455E+04 | 7.0442E−01 |
| 72.Hf | 1.6942E−03 | 3.1526E+04 | 3.1705E+04 | 3.1962E+04 | 8.0980E−01 |
| 73.Ta | 1.7515E−03 | 2.9218E+04 | 2.9383E+04 | 2.9607E+04 | 7.6196E−01 |
| 74.W | 1.8132E−03 | 2.6728E+04 | 2.6879E+04 | 2.7066E+04 | 6.9825E−01 |
| 75.Re | 1.8553E−03 | 2.5029E+04 | 2.5170E+04 | 2.5316E+04 | 5.7843E−01 |
| 76.Os | 1.0238E−03 | 8.8312E+04 | 8.8965E+04 | 8.8603E+04 | 4.0843E−01 |
| | 1.3675E−03 | 5.3736E+04 | 5.4078E+04 | 5.3997E+04 | 1.5070E−01 |
| 79.Au | 1.0313E−03 | 8.6523E+04 | 8.7156E+04 | 8.6774E+04 | 4.4015E−01 |
| | 1.4207E−03 | 4.7961E+04 | 4.8255E+04 | 4.8212E+04 | 8.9595E−02 |
| 80.Hg | 2.3116E−03 | 1.5286E+04 | 1.5376E+04 | 1.5558E+04 | 1.1821E+00 |
| | 1.2001E−02 | 1.0050E+03 | 1.4257E+03 | 1.0674E+03 | 3.3568E+01 |
| 81.Tl | 2.3998E−03 | 1.4181E+04 | 1.4267E+04 | 1.4466E+04 | 1.3988E+00 |
| 81.Tl | 1.0985E−02 | 1.1699E+03 | 1.6841E+03 | 1.2316E+03 | 3.6739E+01 |
| 82.Pb | 1.1230E−02 | 1.1301E+03 | 1.6217E+03 | 1.1897E+03 | 3.6309E+01 |
| 83.Bi | 9.6561E−03 | 1.4323E+03 | 2.1231E+03 | 1.4962E+03 | 4.1896E+01 |
| 84.Po | 9.6838E−03 | 1.4240E+03 | 2.1079E+03 | 1.4872E+03 | 4.1736E+01 |
| 85.At | 1.2373E−02 | 9.4472E+02 | 1.3312E+03 | 9.9786E+02 | 3.3408E+01 |
| 87.Fr | 1.4958E−02 | 5.2546E+02 | 6.7423E+02 | 5.6560E+02 | 1.9207E+01 |
| 89.Ac | 2.8959E−03 | 7.9622E+03 | 8.0200E+03 | 8.0760E+03 | 6.9848E−01 |
| 90.Th | 1.8486E−03 | 2.5300E+04 | 2.5443E+04 | 2.5453E+04 | 3.7591E−02 |
| 112. | 3.6617E−03 | 4.2868E+03 | 4.3287E+03 | 4.4347E+03 | 2.4492E+00 |
| 116. | 4.7080E−03 | 2.0816E+03 | 2.1133E+03 | 2.1819E+03 | 3.2478E+00 |
| | 3.8465E−02 | 4.4431E+01 | 5.1893E+01 | 1.1618E+02 | 1.2388E+02 |
| 118. | 5.8474E−03 | 1.1116E+03 | 1.1373E+03 | 1.1947E+03 | 5.0474E+00 |
| 121. | 2.4069E−03 | 1.4092E+04 | 1.4177E+04 | 1.4196E+04 | 1.3395E−01 |
| | 2.9533E−02 | 9.1515E+01 | 1.0741E+02 | 1.0175E+02 | 5.5566E+00 |
| | 3.1133E−02 | 7.8501E+01 | 9.1691E+01 | 8.7660E+01 | 4.5991E+00 |
| 130. | 2.8337E−03 | 8.7423E+03 | 8.8035E+03 | 8.9084E+03 | 1.1911E+00 |
| 134. | 3.9996E−03 | 3.0764E+03 | 3.1131E+03 | 3.1833E+03 | 2.2521E+00 |
| | 4.0037E−03 | 3.0699E+03 | 3.1066E+03 | 3.1765E+03 | 2.2493E+00 |

| Material | $E$, MeV | $\mu_{1en}$, cm$^{-1}$ | $\mu_1$, cm$^{-1}$ | $\mu_2$, cm$^{-1}$ | $R$, % |
|---|---|---|---|---|---|
| | | | 30.ZINK | | |
| 21.Sc | 4.6228E−03 | 1.9527E+03 | 1.9808E+03 | 2.2942E+03 | 1.5824E+01 |
| 23.V | 1.0333E−03 | 3.7922E+04 | 3.8226E+04 | 3.7993E+04 | 6.1286E−01 |
| 26.Fe | 1.0850E−02 | 9.6028E+02 | 1.4785E+03 | 1.1914E+03 | 2.4100E+01 |
| 27.Co | 1.4453E−03 | 3.8679E+04 | 3.8965E+04 | 3.8843E+04 | 3.1443E−01 |
| | 2.4934E−02 | 1.4373E+02 | 1.7687E+02 | 1.6574E+02 | 6.7179E+00 |
| 33.As | 2.7308E−03 | 8.8267E+03 | 8.8924E+03 | 8.9133E+03 | 2.3567E−01 |
| | 5.8733E−02 | 1.1088E+01 | 1.3578E+01 | 1.3663E+01 | 6.3111E−01 |
| 39.Y | 3.5741E−02 | 4.9640E+01 | 5.8715E+01 | 7.1671E+01 | 2.2066E+01 |
| 40.Zr | 1.9257E−02 | 2.4599E+02 | 3.1190E+02 | 5.2475E+02 | 6.8244E+01 |
| 41.Nb | 1.0331E−03 | 3.7756E+04 | 3.8058E+04 | 3.7824E+04 | 6.2032E−01 |
| 43.Tc | 9.7980E−03 | 1.1109E+03 | 1.7492E+03 | 1.1498E+03 | 5.2129E+01 |
| 44.Ru | 1.3347E−02 | 6.4424E+02 | 9.3727E+02 | 6.7372E+02 | 3.9118E+01 |
| 45.Rh | 1.4469E−02 | 5.0222E+02 | 6.9404E+02 | 5.2897E+02 | 3.1206E+01 |
| 46.Pd | 1.2446E−03 | 5.5200E+04 | 5.5645E+04 | 5.5303E+04 | 6.1902E−01 |
| | 1.4719E−02 | 4.7065E+02 | 6.3997E+02 | 4.9650E+02 | 2.8897E+01 |
| 47.Ag | 1.3921E−02 | 5.7157E+02 | 8.1280E+02 | 5.9948E+02 | 3.5584E+01 |
| 48.Cd | 1.0610E−03 | 5.8826E+04 | 5.9336E+04 | 5.8912E+04 | 7.2068E−01 |
| | 9.8453E−03 | 1.1008E+03 | 1.7290E+03 | 1.1436E+03 | 5.1181E+01 |
| 53.I | 1.0375E−03 | 4.1484E+04 | 4.1824E+04 | 4.1568E+04 | 6.1493E−01 |
| | 3.3745E−02 | 5.7628E+01 | 6.8235E+01 | 1.7089E+02 | 1.5045E+02 |
| 56.Ba | 1.0216E−03 | 2.8460E+04 | 2.8668E+04 | 2.8535E+04 | 4.6795E−01 |
| | 4.2272E−02 | 2.9111E+01 | 3.4365E+01 | 7.7422E+01 | 1.2529E+02 |
| 57.La | 3.9007E−03 | 3.0382E+03 | 3.0719E+03 | 3.0778E+03 | 1.9431E−01 |
| 57.La | 1.2996E−02 | 6.8867E+02 | 1.0134E+03 | 7.3339E+02 | 3.8176E+01 |
| 58.Ce | 1.0457E−03 | 5.8556E+04 | 5.9069E+04 | 5.8752E+04 | 5.3976E−01 |
| | 1.8189E−03 | 2.3109E+04 | 2.3270E+04 | 2.3204E+04 | 2.8563E−01 |
| | 1.7752E−02 | 3.1282E+02 | 4.0631E+02 | 3.3513E+02 | 2.1238E+01 |
| 59.Pr | 1.0805E−03 | 5.9170E+04 | 5.9676E+04 | 5.9396E+04 | 4.7182E−01 |
| | 2.9012E−02 | 8.6490E+01 | 1.0381E+02 | 9.5464E+01 | 8.7395E+00 |
| 60.Nd | 1.4160E−03 | 4.1091E+04 | 4.1400E+04 | 4.1273E+04 | 3.0638E−01 |
| 63.Eu | 1.9784E−03 | 1.7577E+04 | 1.7697E+04 | 1.7686E+04 | 6.4583E−02 |
| | 1.6227E−02 | 3.8056E+02 | 5.0201E+02 | 4.1410E+02 | 2.1229E+01 |
| 64.Gd | 1.4402E−03 | 3.9100E+04 | 3.9390E+04 | 3.9361E+04 | 7.4094E−02 |
| 65.Tb | 1.3466E−03 | 4.6805E+04 | 4.7169E+04 | 4.7174E+04 | 9.5236E−03 |
| 66.Dy | 1.3437E−03 | 4.7043E+04 | 4.7409E+04 | 4.7460E+04 | 1.0879E−01 |
| 68.Er | 1.4517E−03 | 3.8153E+04 | 3.8434E+04 | 3.8561E+04 | 3.3044E−01 |
| 69.Tm | 1.4968E−03 | 3.4438E+04 | 3.4683E+04 | 3.4832E+04 | 4.3082E−01 |
| 70.Yb | 1.6385E−03 | 2.9368E+04 | 2.9575E+04 | 2.9749E+04 | 5.8806E−01 |

| Material | $E$, MeV | $\mu_{1en}$, cm$^{-1}$ | $\mu_1$, cm$^{-1}$ | $\mu_2$, cm$^{-1}$ | $R$, % |
|---|---|---|---|---|---|
| 71.Lu | 1.0241E−03 | 3.0408E+04 | 3.0635E+04 | 3.0525E+04 | 3.6102E−01 |
| | 1.6306E−03 | 2.9642E+04 | 2.9851E+04 | 3.0037E+04 | 6.2478E−01 |
| 72.Hf | 1.0385E−03 | 4.2353E+04 | 4.2700E+04 | 4.2499E+04 | 4.7382E−01 |
| | 1.6857E−03 | 2.7730E+04 | 2.7925E+04 | 2.8096E+04 | 6.1385E−01 |
| 73.Ta | 1.7419E−03 | 2.5781E+04 | 2.5961E+04 | 2.6099E+04 | 5.2857E−01 |
| 80.Hg | 1.0839E−03 | 5.9230E+04 | 5.9735E+04 | 5.9406E+04 | 5.5446E−01 |
| | 2.2975E−03 | 1.3570E+04 | 1.3664E+04 | 1.3780E+04 | 8.5074E−01 |
| 83.Bi | 1.2794E−02 | 7.1422E+02 | 1.0571E+03 | 7.5927E+02 | 3.9227E+01 |
| 84.Po | 1.3261E−02 | 6.5515E+02 | 9.5596E+02 | 6.9783E+02 | 3.6991E+01 |
| 87.Fr | 2.7589E−03 | 8.5194E+03 | 8.5832E+03 | 8.6327E+03 | 5.7693E−01 |
| 88.Ra | 1.0232E−03 | 2.9687E+04 | 2.9908E+04 | 2.9758E+04 | 5.0553E−01 |
| 89.Ac | 1.0575E−03 | 5.8764E+04 | 5.9274E+04 | 5.8905E+04 | 6.2766E−01 |
| | 1.9821E−03 | 1.7446E+04 | 1.7565E+04 | 1.7577E+04 | 6.9441E−02 |
| 90.Th | 1.3846E−03 | 4.3678E+04 | 4.4012E+04 | 4.3838E+04 | 3.9596E−01 |
| 116. | 1.0343E−03 | 3.8760E+04 | 3.9072E+04 | 3.8850E+04 | 5.7286E−01 |
| | 3.6325E−02 | 4.7304E+01 | 5.5931E+01 | 1.3373E+02 | 1.3909E+02 |
| 125. | 1.0220E−03 | 2.8790E+04 | 2.9001E+04 | 2.8864E+04 | 4.7370E−01 |
| 126. | 1.0037E−03 | 1.0949E+04 | 1.0985E+04 | 1.1014E+04 | 2.7187E−01 |
| 130. | 1.0385E−03 | 4.2418E+04 | 4.2767E+04 | 4.2513E+04 | 5.9666E−01 |
| | 2.6584E−03 | 9.6201E+03 | 9.6905E+03 | 9.7954E+03 | 1.0820E+00 |

GALLIUM

| Material | $E$, MeV | $\mu_{1en}$, cm$^{-1}$ | $\mu_1$, cm$^{-1}$ | $\mu_2$, cm$^{-1}$ | $R$, % |
|---|---|---|---|---|---|
| 23.V | 1.1404E−03 | 3.2495E+04 | 3.2802E+04 | 3.2558E+04 | 7.4738E−01 |
| 24.Cr | 1.1455E−03 | 4.3222E+04 | 4.3651E+04 | 4.3323E+04 | 7.5841E−01 |
| | 1.1486E−02 | 6.8932E+02 | 1.1131E+03 | 7.9690E+02 | 3.9684E+01 |
| 25.Mn | 1.3835E−02 | 4.7069E+02 | 7.0603E+02 | 5.4936E+02 | 2.8518E+01 |
| 26.Fe | 1.3894E−03 | 3.6541E+04 | 3.6873E+04 | 3.6666E+04 | 5.6292E−01 |
| | 1.9489E−02 | 1.9915E+02 | 2.5971E+02 | 2.2746E+02 | 1.4176E+01 |
| 27.Co | 6.7377E−03 | 6.3624E+02 | 6.5221E+02 | 6.5489E+02 | 4.1096E−01 |
| 32.Ge | 1.0332E−02 | 1.7514E+02 | 1.8481E+02 | 1.8429E+02 | 2.7908E−01 |
| 33.As | 1.4887E−02 | 3.7270E+02 | 5.2357E+02 | 5.8137E+02 | 1.1041E+01 |
| 34.Se | 1.0122E−02 | 1.8571E+02 | 1.9564E+02 | 1.9429E+02 | 6.9631E−01 |
| 39.Y | 2.7294E−02 | 9.4567E+01 | 1.1793E+02 | 1.5886E+02 | 3.4710E+01 |
| 40.Zr | 1.1157E−03 | 2.3464E+04 | 2.3672E+04 | 2.3508E+04 | 6.9715E−01 |
| 41.Nb | 1.1407E−03 | 3.2574E+04 | 3.2882E+04 | 3.2638E+04 | 7.4582E−01 |
| 42.Mo | 1.0851E−02 | 7.4844E+02 | 1.2232E+03 | 7.7692E+02 | 5.7447E+01 |
| 43.Tc | 1.4359E−02 | 4.2190E+02 | 6.1517E+02 | 4.4451E+02 | 3.8394E+01 |
| 44.Ru | 1.4177E−03 | 3.4811E+04 | 3.5123E+04 | 3.4902E+04 | 6.3191E−01 |
| | 1.8386E−02 | 2.3924E+02 | 3.1977E+02 | 2.5699E+02 | 2.4429E+01 |
| 45.Rh | 2.0452E−02 | 1.7527E+02 | 2.2484E+02 | 1.9087E+02 | 1.7801E+01 |

| Material | $E$, MeV | $\mu_{1en}$, cm$^{-1}$ | $\mu_1$, cm$^{-1}$ | $\mu_2$, cm$^{-1}$ | $R$, % |
|---|---|---|---|---|---|
| 46.Pd | 2.1229E−02 | 1.6611E+02 | 2.1271E+02 | 1.8102E+02 | 1.7503E+01 |
| 47.Ag | 1.4797E−03 | 3.1020E+04 | 3.1288E+04 | 3.1105E+04 | 5.8906E−01 |
| | 2.4367E−03 | 1.0566E+04 | 1.0648E+04 | 1.0642E+04 | 5.9410E−02 |
| | 3.1490E−03 | 4.7714E+03 | 4.8133E+03 | 4.8363E+03 | 4.7593E−01 |
| | 1.9648E−02 | 1.9339E+02 | 2.5107E+02 | 2.0877E+02 | 2.0265E+01 |
| 48.Cd | 1.4554E−02 | 4.0376E+02 | 5.8140E+02 | 4.2520E+02 | 3.6737E+01 |
| 49.In | 1.2510E−03 | 3.9840E+04 | 4.0220E+04 | 3.9917E+04 | 7.5800E−01 |
| | 1.3231E−02 | 5.2693E+02 | 8.1075E+02 | 5.5167E+02 | 4.6964E+01 |
| 50.Sn | 1.3911E−02 | 4.6355E+02 | 6.9273E+02 | 4.8697E+02 | 4.2252E+01 |
| 51.Sb | 1.2865E−03 | 3.7825E+04 | 3.8180E+04 | 3.7903E+04 | 7.3191E−01 |
| | 1.3388E−02 | 5.1225E+02 | 7.8343E+02 | 5.3790E+02 | 4.5645E+01 |
| 52.Te | 1.1899E−03 | 4.2308E+04 | 4.2721E+04 | 4.2394E+04 | 7.6990E−01 |
| | 1.2577E−02 | 5.8781E+02 | 9.2413E+02 | 6.1725E+02 | 4.9716E+01 |
| 56.Ba | 1.1235E−03 | 2.6517E+04 | 2.6759E+04 | 2.6589E+04 | 6.3891E−01 |
| | 3.9068E−02 | 3.1589E+01 | 3.7704E+01 | 9.1882E+01 | 1.4370E+02 |
| 57.La | 1.7951E−03 | 2.0902E+04 | 2.1072E+04 | 2.0985E+04 | 4.1660E−01 |
| | 1.9601E−02 | 1.9509E+02 | 2.5362E+02 | 2.0968E+02 | 2.0957E+01 |
| 63.Eu | 1.6279E−03 | 2.5930E+04 | 2.6148E+04 | 2.6085E+04 | 2.4061E−01 |
| 64.Gd | 1.2852E−03 | 3.7901E+04 | 3.8257E+04 | 3.8162E+04 | 2.5141E−01 |
| | 1.3580E−03 | 3.8464E+04 | 3.8817E+04 | 3.8725E+04 | 2.3926E−01 |
| 65.Tb | 1.2718E−03 | 3.8662E+04 | 3.9028E+04 | 3.8965E+04 | 1.6286E−01 |
| 66.Dy | 1.3322E−03 | 4.0038E+04 | 4.0409E+04 | 4.0387E+04 | 5.5614E−02 |
| 67.Ho | 1.3867E−03 | 3.6705E+04 | 3.7038E+04 | 3.7054E+04 | 4.3051E−02 |
| 68.Er | 1.4415E−03 | 3.3355E+04 | 3.3650E+04 | 3.3705E+04 | 1.6270E−01 |
| 69.Tm | 1.4898E−03 | 3.0405E+04 | 3.0666E+04 | 3.0745E+04 | 2.5694E−01 |
| 71.Lu | 1.1245E−03 | 2.6924E+04 | 2.7171E+04 | 2.7040E+04 | 4.8564E−01 |
| | 1.6224E−03 | 2.6097E+04 | 2.6316E+04 | 2.6439E+04 | 4.6600E−01 |
| 72.Hf | 1.6759E−03 | 2.4488E+04 | 2.4692E+04 | 2.4791E+04 | 4.0260E−01 |
| 80.Hg | 1.4540E−03 | 3.2591E+04 | 3.2877E+04 | 3.2767E+04 | 3.3547E−01 |
| | 1.6517E−03 | 2.5216E+04 | 2.5427E+04 | 2.5388E+04 | 1.5301E−01 |
| 80.Hg | 2.2538E−03 | 1.2312E+04 | 1.2407E+04 | 1.2467E+04 | 4.7949E−01 |
| 83.Bi | 1.1788E−03 | 4.2537E+04 | 4.2954E+04 | 4.2670E+04 | 6.6485E−01 |
| 84.Po | 1.1864E−03 | 4.2382E+04 | 4.2795E+04 | 4.2509E+04 | 6.7443E−01 |
| 85.At | 1.9845E−03 | 1.5203E+04 | 1.5320E+04 | 1.5334E+04 | 8.9656E−02 |
| | 2.3394E−03 | 1.1495E+04 | 1.1584E+04 | 1.1618E+04 | 2.8946E−01 |
| 87.Fr | 1.8290E−03 | 1.9882E+04 | 2.0042E+04 | 2.0012E+04 | 1.5310E−01 |
| 88.Ra | 1.1208E−03 | 2.5466E+04 | 2.5697E+04 | 2.5536E+04 | 6.2853E−01 |
| 89.Ac | 1.3687E−03 | 3.7808E+04 | 3.8154E+04 | 3.7945E+04 | 5.5135E−01 |
| 112. | 2.9051E−02 | 7.3831E+01 | 9.0454E+01 | 1.4889E+02 | 6.4605E+01 |

| Material | $E$, MeV | $\mu_{1en}$, cm$^{-1}$ | $\mu_1$, cm$^{-1}$ | $\mu_2$, cm$^{-1}$ | $R$, % |
|---|---|---|---|---|---|
| 116. | 1.1421E−03 | 3.3059E+04 | 3.3371E+04 | 3.3135E+04 | 7.1078E−01 |
| 121. | 1.4578E−03 | 3.2358E+04 | 3.2642E+04 | 3.2574E+04 | 2.0767E−01 |
| 125. | 1.1172E−03 | 2.4072E+04 | 2.4286E+04 | 2.4146E+04 | 5.8033E−01 |
| | 2.5563E−03 | 9.4228E+03 | 9.4973E+03 | 9.6637E+03 | 1.7522E+00 |
| 130. | 2.4078E−03 | 1.0841E+04 | 1.0925E+04 | 1.1025E+04 | 9.0882E−01 |
| | 1.0725E−02 | 7.6019E+02 | 1.2451E+03 | 7.9896E+02 | 5.5844E+01 |
| 133. | 1.1025E−03 | 7.9472E+03 | 7.9767E+03 | 7.9617E+03 | 1.8870E−01 |
| 134. | 4.7908E−02 | 1.7893E+01 | 2.1433E+01 | 2.7023E+01 | 2.6078E+01 |
| | | | 32.GERMANIUM | | |
| 24.Cr | 1.2716E−03 | 3.4710E+04 | 3.5103E+04 | 3.4793E+04 | 8.9239E−01 |
| | 1.4021E−02 | 4.0410E+02 | 6.2975E+02 | 4.5884E+02 | 3.7247E+01 |
| 25.Mn | 1.3915E−03 | 3.0358E+04 | 3.0686E+04 | 3.0449E+04 | 7.7838E−01 |
| | 1.4907E−02 | 3.3976E+02 | 5.0070E+02 | 3.8800E+02 | 2.9045E+01 |
| 26.Fe | 1.4449E−03 | 3.1592E+04 | 3.1923E+04 | 3.1698E+04 | 7.0890E−01 |
| | 2.7556E−02 | 8.6634E+01 | 1.1063E+02 | 9.8065E+01 | 1.2817E+01 |
| 27.Co | 7.1217E−03 | 5.4410E+02 | 5.5845E+02 | 5.6171E+02 | 5.8440E−01 |
| 31.Ga | 1.0332E−02 | 1.7514E+02 | 1.8429E+02 | 1.8481E+02 | 2.7908E−01 |
| 33.As | 1.4516E−03 | 3.1259E+04 | 3.1585E+04 | 3.1650E+04 | 2.0445E−01 |
| 34.Se | 9.4311E−03 | 2.3659E+02 | 2.4685E+02 | 2.4602E+02 | 3.3934E−01 |
| 38.Sr | 1.1657E−03 | 7.0506E+03 | 7.0796E+03 | 7.0675E+03 | 1.7072E−01 |
| 39.Y | 2.4326E−02 | 1.2192E+02 | 1.5941E+02 | 2.1887E+02 | 3.7300E+01 |
| 42.Mo | 1.3592E−02 | 4.3521E+02 | 6.9214E+02 | 4.5635E+02 | 5.1668E+01 |
| 43.Tc | 1.5062E−02 | 3.3096E+02 | 4.8389E+02 | 3.5135E+02 | 3.7722E+01 |
| 44.Ru | 1.4688E−03 | 3.0402E+04 | 3.0716E+04 | 3.0491E+04 | 7.4007E−01 |
| | 2.0176E−02 | 1.6724E+02 | 2.2208E+02 | 1.8235E+02 | 2.1786E+01 |
| 45.Rh | 2.1714E−02 | 1.5044E+02 | 1.9885E+02 | 1.6489E+02 | 2.0595E+01 |
| 46.Pd | 2.2597E−02 | 1.4079E+02 | 1.8551E+02 | 1.5451E+02 | 2.0063E+01 |
| 47.Ag | 3.2501E−03 | 4.3946E+03 | 4.4358E+03 | 4.4585E+03 | 5.1074E−01 |
| | 2.1726E−02 | 1.5031E+02 | 1.9867E+02 | 1.6374E+02 | 2.1329E+01 |
| 48.Cd | 1.6813E−02 | 2.7360E+02 | 3.9200E+02 | 2.9057E+02 | 3.4907E+01 |
| 49.In | 1.3854E−03 | 3.0655E+04 | 3.0987E+04 | 3.0725E+04 | 8.4997E−01 |
| | 1.4503E−02 | 3.6905E+02 | 5.5945E+02 | 3.8856E+02 | 4.3980E+01 |
| 50.Sn | 1.4817E−02 | 3.4629E+02 | 5.1381E+02 | 3.6550E+02 | 4.0579E+01 |
| 51.Sb | 1.4079E−03 | 2.9561E+04 | 2.9879E+04 | 2.9633E+04 | 8.3078E−01 |
| | 1.4588E−02 | 3.6294E+02 | 5.4720E+02 | 3.8275E+02 | 4.2966E+01 |
| 52.Te | 1.3294E−03 | 3.3374E+04 | 3.3741E+04 | 3.3450E+04 | 8.7095E−01 |
| | 1.4280E−02 | 3.8529E+02 | 5.9201E+02 | 4.0614E+02 | 4.5766E+01 |
| 53.I | 1.2343E−02 | 5.2590E+02 | 8.7403E+02 | 5.5336E+02 | 5.7951E+01 |
| 56.Ba | 1.2209E−03 | 2.3614E+04 | 2.3865E+04 | 2.3683E+04 | 7.6771E−01 |

| Material | $E$, MeV | $\mu_{1en}$, cm$^{-1}$ | $\mu_1$, cm$^{-1}$ | $\mu_2$, cm$^{-1}$ | $R$, % |
|---|---|---|---|---|---|
| | 3.8625E−02 | 3.1895E+01 | 3.8634E+01 | 9.4682E+01 | 1.4508E+02 |
| 57.La | 2.8337E−02 | 7.8103E+01 | 9.8839E+01 | 8.5895E+01 | 1.5069E+01 |
| 63.Eu | 1.5460E−03 | 2.7513E+04 | 2.7790E+04 | 2.7680E+04 | 3.9530E−01 |
| 65.Tb | 1.2665E−03 | 3.4827E+04 | 3.5223E+04 | 3.5098E+04 | 3.5518E−01 |
| 66.Dy | 1.3223E−03 | 3.3563E+04 | 3.3933E+04 | 3.3854E+04 | 2.3539E−01 |
| 67.Ho | 1.3769E−03 | 3.1066E+04 | 3.1403E+04 | 3.1356E+04 | 1.5248E−01 |
| 68.Er | 1.4385E−03 | 3.1912E+04 | 3.2247E+04 | 3.2244E+04 | 8.4317E−03 |
| 69.Tm | 1.4881E−03 | 2.9443E+04 | 2.9743E+04 | 2.9769E+04 | 8.6935E−02 |
| 71.Lu | 1.2207E−03 | 2.3589E+04 | 2.3839E+04 | 2.3702E+04 | 5.7649E−01 |
| | 1.6207E−03 | 2.5341E+04 | 2.5593E+04 | 2.5672E+04 | 3.0762E−01 |
| 72.Hf | 1.6738E−03 | 2.3796E+04 | 2.4030E+04 | 2.4086E+04 | 2.3504E−01 |
| 82.Pb | 1.9684E−03 | 1.5228E+04 | 1.5361E+04 | 1.5354E+04 | 4.9726E−02 |
| | 2.0714E−03 | 1.3649E+04 | 1.3766E+04 | 1.3774E+04 | 5.8555E−02 |
| 83.Bi | 1.3762E−03 | 3.1104E+04 | 3.1441E+04 | 3.1233E+04 | 6.6781E−01 |
| 84.Po | 1.4018E−03 | 2.9858E+04 | 3.0180E+04 | 2.9981E+04 | 6.6317E−01 |
| 85.At | 1.8833E−03 | 1.7703E+04 | 1.7865E+04 | 1.7835E+04 | 1.6741E−01 |
| 87.Fr | 1.6529E−03 | 2.4403E+04 | 2.4644E+04 | 2.4533E+04 | 4.5110E−01 |
| 88.Ra | 1.2465E−02 | 5.1701E+02 | 8.5620E+02 | 5.4478E+02 | 5.7163E+01 |
| 112. | 1.2487E−03 | 3.5228E+04 | 3.5632E+04 | 3.5300E+04 | 9.4240E−01 |
| | 1.3368E−02 | 4.5150E+02 | 7.2481E+02 | 4.7400E+02 | 5.2912E+01 |
| | 2.8484E−02 | 7.6493E+01 | 9.6613E+01 | 1.5703E+02 | 6.2534E+01 |
| 116. | 1.1494E−02 | 5.8747E+02 | 9.9753E+02 | 6.1942E+02 | 6.1043E+01 |
| 121. | 1.3548E−03 | 3.2144E+04 | 3.2495E+04 | 3.2360E+04 | 4.1783E−01 |
| | 1.4306E−03 | 3.2302E+04 | 3.2642E+04 | 3.2517E+04 | 3.8255E−01 |
| 123. | 1.9284E−03 | 1.6390E+04 | 1.6537E+04 | 1.6546E+04 | 5.5723E−02 |
| | 1.0241E−02 | 1.7912E+02 | 1.8836E+02 | 1.8835E+02 | 8.6604E−03 |
| | 1.9082E−02 | 1.9924E+02 | 2.7291E+02 | 2.7447E+02 | 5.7052E−01 |
| 125. | 2.5470E−03 | 9.2553E+03 | 9.3358E+03 | 9.4916E+03 | 1.6690E+00 |
| 130. | 1.2044E−02 | 5.4760E+02 | 9.1757E+02 | 5.7822E+02 | 5.8689E+01 |
| 133. | 1.1101E−03 | 7.8597E+03 | 7.8913E+03 | 7.8742E+03 | 2.1812E−01 |
| 134. | 4.5236E−02 | 2.0755E+01 | 2.5036E+01 | 3.2098E+01 | 2.8209E+01 |

33.ARSENIC

| Material | $E$, MeV | $\mu_{1en}$, cm$^{-1}$ | $\mu_1$, cm$^{-1}$ | $\mu_2$, cm$^{-1}$ | $R$, % |
|---|---|---|---|---|---|
| 21.Sc | 4.7513E−03 | 1.8410E+03 | 1.8674E+03 | 2.1547E+03 | 1.5387E+01 |
| 24.Cr | 1.3408E−02 | 4.7304E+02 | 7.9952E+02 | 5.4056E+02 | 4.7907E+01 |
| 25.Mn | 1.4325E−02 | 4.1087E+02 | 6.6434E+02 | 4.7564E+02 | 3.9674E+01 |
| 26.Fe | 1.4468E−03 | 3.1426E+04 | 3.1819E+04 | 3.1531E+04 | 9.1433E−01 |
| 26.Fe | 1.8180E−02 | 2.5352E+02 | 3.7192E+02 | 2.9223E+02 | 2.7273E+01 |
| 27.Co | 3.5822E−02 | 4.7151E+01 | 5.8604E+01 | 5.3951E+01 | 8.6236E+00 |
| 28.Ni | 8.0875E−03 | 4.1148E+02 | 4.2527E+02 | 4.2856E+02 | 7.7578E−01 |

| Material | $E$, MeV | $\mu_{1en}$, cm$^{-1}$ | $\mu_1$, cm$^{-1}$ | $\mu_2$, cm$^{-1}$ | $R$, % |
|---|---|---|---|---|---|
| 30.Zn | 2.7308E−03 | 8.8267E+03 | 8.9133E+03 | 8.8924E+03 | 2.3567E−01 |
| | 5.8733E−02 | 1.1088E+01 | 1.3663E+01 | 1.3578E+01 | 6.3111E−01 |
| 31.Ga | 1.4887E−02 | 3.7270E+02 | 5.8137E+02 | 5.2357E+02 | 1.1041E+01 |
| 32.Ge | 1.4516E−03 | 3.1259E+04 | 3.1650E+04 | 3.1585E+04 | 2.0445E−01 |
| 39.Y | 2.9660E−02 | 7.2761E+01 | 9.2252E+01 | 1.1100E+02 | 2.0327E+01 |
| 42.Mo | 1.3046E−02 | 4.9757E+02 | 8.5286E+02 | 5.2018E+02 | 6.3955E+01 |
| 43.Tc | 1.3616E−03 | 3.4361E+04 | 3.4806E+04 | 3.4445E+04 | 1.0492E+00 |
| | 1.4548E−02 | 3.9568E+02 | 6.3134E+02 | 4.1766E+02 | 5.1160E+01 |
| 44.Ru | 1.4637E−03 | 3.0840E+04 | 3.1223E+04 | 3.0929E+04 | 9.5172E−01 |
| | 1.7424E−02 | 2.8002E+02 | 4.1772E+02 | 2.9924E+02 | 3.9593E+01 |
| 45.Rh | 1.9478E−02 | 2.0796E+02 | 2.9316E+02 | 2.2484E+02 | 3.0384E+01 |
| 46.Pd | 1.9928E−02 | 1.9218E+02 | 2.6587E+02 | 2.0829E+02 | 2.7644E+01 |
| 47.Ag | 1.4931E−03 | 2.9828E+04 | 3.0194E+04 | 2.9913E+04 | 9.3910E−01 |
| | 1.5192E−03 | 2.8650E+04 | 2.8995E+04 | 2.8734E+04 | 9.0610E−01 |
| | 1.8657E−02 | 2.3676E+02 | 3.4294E+02 | 2.5373E+02 | 3.5156E+01 |
| 48.Cd | 1.3971E−03 | 3.3137E+04 | 3.3560E+04 | 3.3216E+04 | 1.0353E+00 |
| | 1.4673E−02 | 3.8727E+02 | 6.1304E+02 | 4.0820E+02 | 5.0181E+01 |
| 49.In | 1.3975E−02 | 4.3457E+02 | 7.1587E+02 | 4.5625E+02 | 5.6904E+01 |
| 50.Sn | 1.4311E−02 | 4.1177E+02 | 6.6632E+02 | 4.3333E+02 | 5.3765E+01 |
| 51.Sb | 1.4057E−02 | 4.2905E+02 | 7.0387E+02 | 4.5144E+02 | 5.5917E+01 |
| 52.Te | 1.3719E−02 | 4.5192E+02 | 7.5359E+02 | 4.7560E+02 | 5.8453E+01 |
| 56.Ba | 4.1190E−02 | 2.9986E+01 | 3.6605E+01 | 8.1506E+01 | 1.2267E+02 |
| 57.La | 1.4791E−03 | 3.0309E+04 | 3.0683E+04 | 3.0416E+04 | 8.7851E−01 |
| | 1.5159E−03 | 2.8810E+04 | 2.9158E+04 | 2.8914E+04 | 8.4305E−01 |
| | 4.5915E−03 | 2.0419E+03 | 2.0697E+03 | 2.0774E+03 | 3.7122E−01 |
| | 5.2966E−03 | 1.3506E+03 | 1.3733E+03 | 1.3827E+03 | 6.8380E−01 |
| | 1.8389E−02 | 2.4619E+02 | 3.5924E+02 | 2.6358E+02 | 3.6293E+01 |
| 58.Ce | 2.8953E−02 | 8.1311E+01 | 1.0463E+02 | 8.9771E+01 | 1.6555E+01 |
| 59.Pr | 4.0841E−02 | 3.0497E+01 | 3.7230E+01 | 3.5403E+01 | 5.1589E+00 |
| 63.Eu | 1.1217E−03 | 9.3445E+03 | 9.3778E+03 | 9.3969E+03 | 2.0408E−01 |
| | 1.4815E−03 | 3.0226E+04 | 3.0598E+04 | 3.0415E+04 | 6.0488E−01 |
| | 1.9526E−03 | 1.8168E+04 | 1.8357E+04 | 1.8281E+04 | 4.1701E−01 |
| | 2.9511E−02 | 7.4566E+01 | 9.4866E+01 | 8.2736E+01 | 1.4661E+01 |
| 67.Ho | 1.3815E−03 | 3.3677E+04 | 3.4110E+04 | 3.3994E+04 | 3.4126E−01 |
| 68.Er | 1.4381E−03 | 3.1726E+04 | 3.2124E+04 | 3.2055E+04 | 2.1475E−01 |
| 69.Tm | 1.4890E−03 | 2.9968E+04 | 3.0336E+04 | 3.0302E+04 | 1.1158E−01 |
| 70.Yb | 1.5875E−03 | 3.0020E+04 | 3.0381E+04 | 3.0409E+04 | 9.1501E−02 |
| 71.Lu | 1.6284E−03 | 2.8692E+04 | 2.9034E+04 | 2.9074E+04 | 1.3646E−01 |
| 72.Hf | 1.6832E−03 | 2.6913E+04 | 2.7228E+04 | 2.7263E+04 | 1.2760E−01 |

| Material | $E$, MeV | $\mu_{1en}$, cm$^{-1}$ | $\mu_1$, cm$^{-1}$ | $\mu_2$, cm$^{-1}$ | $R$, % |
|---|---|---|---|---|---|
| 73.Ta | 1.3776E−03 | 3.3811E+04 | 3.4247E+04 | 3.3998E+04 | 7.2996E−01 |
| | 1.7399E−03 | 2.5072E+04 | 2.5361E+04 | 2.5375E+04 | 5.4918E−02 |
| 80.Hg | 1.4918E−03 | 2.9873E+04 | 3.0239E+04 | 3.0049E+04 | 6.3175E−01 |
| | 1.5140E−03 | 2.8907E+04 | 2.9256E+04 | 2.9083E+04 | 5.9533E−01 |
| | 2.2966E−03 | 1.3462E+04 | 1.3596E+04 | 1.3669E+04 | 5.3628E−01 |
| 81.Tl | 1.3912E−03 | 3.3340E+04 | 3.3767E+04 | 3.3483E+04 | 8.4791E−01 |
| 82.Pb | 1.4014E−03 | 3.2990E+04 | 3.3411E+04 | 3.3128E+04 | 8.5270E−01 |
| 85.At | 1.4107E−03 | 3.2670E+04 | 3.3086E+04 | 3.2810E+04 | 8.3903E−01 |
| 87.Fr | 1.4400E−03 | 3.1659E+04 | 3.2057E+04 | 3.1791E+04 | 8.3590E−01 |
| | 2.7640E−03 | 8.4724E+03 | 8.5554E+03 | 8.5856E+03 | 3.5299E−01 |
| 89.Ac | 1.9299E−03 | 1.8905E+04 | 1.9105E+04 | 1.9036E+04 | 3.5908E−01 |
| 112. | 1.2782E−02 | 5.1548E+02 | 8.9178E+02 | 5.4043E+02 | 6.5014E+01 |
| | 2.9901E−02 | 6.9842E+01 | 8.8027E+01 | 1.3670E+02 | 5.5297E+01 |
| 121. | 1.4219E−03 | 3.2283E+04 | 3.2692E+04 | 3.2499E+04 | 5.9298E−01 |
| 126. | 1.1317E−03 | 9.1174E+03 | 9.1511E+03 | 9.1708E+03 | 2.1545E−01 |
| 130. | 2.6549E−03 | 9.6375E+03 | 9.7323E+03 | 9.8129E+03 | 8.2835E−01 |
| 140. | 1.2624E−03 | 7.0932E+03 | 7.1238E+03 | 7.1304E+03 | 9.2374E−02 |
| | | | 34.SELENIUM | | |
| 23.V | 1.3577E−02 | 3.4583E+02 | 6.1687E+02 | 3.8591E+02 | 5.9848E+01 |
| 24.Cr | 1.6953E−02 | 2.3086E+02 | 3.6797E+02 | 2.5716E+02 | 4.3088E+01 |
| 25.Mn | 1.4852E−03 | 2.3256E+04 | 2.3592E+04 | 2.3326E+04 | 1.1410E+00 |
| | 1.9902E−02 | 1.5341E+02 | 2.2167E+02 | 1.7167E+02 | 2.9128E+01 |
| 26.Fe | 1.7780E−03 | 1.8938E+04 | 1.9187E+04 | 1.9003E+04 | 9.6765E−01 |
| | 3.5108E−02 | 4.0619E+01 | 5.1647E+01 | 4.6089E+01 | 1.2059E+01 |
| 27.Co | 7.2109E−03 | 5.2269E+02 | 5.3592E+02 | 5.4006E+02 | 7.7220E−01 |
| 31.Ga | 1.0122E−02 | 1.8571E+02 | 1.9429E+02 | 1.9564E+02 | 6.9631E−01 |
| 32.Ge | 9.4311E−03 | 2.3659E+02 | 2.4602E+02 | 2.4685E+02 | 3.3934E−01 |
| 38.Sr | 1.2643E−02 | 9.8315E+01 | 1.0485E+02 | 1.0305E+02 | 1.7529E+00 |
| 39.Y | 1.8947E−02 | 1.7849E+02 | 2.6905E+02 | 3.6093E+02 | 3.4152E+01 |
| 41.Nb | 1.3512E−02 | 3.4873E+02 | 6.2381E+02 | 3.6585E+02 | 7.0509E+01 |
| 42.Mo | 1.4887E−02 | 2.8720E+02 | 4.7690E+02 | 3.0487E+02 | 5.6426E+01 |
| 43.Tc | 1.9768E−02 | 1.5694E+02 | 2.2833E+02 | 1.7105E+02 | 3.3489E+01 |
| 44.Ru | 2.0421E−03 | 1.3408E+04 | 1.3566E+04 | 1.3494E+04 | 5.2862E−01 |
| | 2.1900E−02 | 1.3278E+02 | 1.8926E+02 | 1.4637E+02 | 2.9298E+01 |
| 46.Pd | 2.4225E−02 | 1.1068E+02 | 1.5554E+02 | 1.2298E+02 | 2.6481E+01 |
| 47.Ag | 3.3283E−03 | 4.1033E+03 | 4.1492E+03 | 4.1665E+03 | 4.1768E−01 |
| | 2.4160E−02 | 1.1130E+02 | 1.5649E+02 | 1.2280E+02 | 2.7433E+01 |
| 48.Cd | 2.0856E−02 | 1.4270E+02 | 2.0440E+02 | 1.5462E+02 | 3.2198E+01 |
| 49.In | 1.4912E−03 | 2.3424E+04 | 2.3762E+04 | 2.3490E+04 | 1.1600E+00 |

| Material | $E$, MeV | $\mu_{1en}$, cm$^{-1}$ | $\mu_1$, cm$^{-1}$ | $\mu_2$, cm$^{-1}$ | $R$, % |
|---|---|---|---|---|---|
| | 1.6450E−03 | 1.9531E+04 | 1.9796E+04 | 1.9594E+04 | 1.0309E+00 |
| | 1.8350E−02 | 1.9416E+02 | 2.9865E+02 | 2.0732E+02 | 4.4048E+01 |
| 50.Sn | 1.9414E−02 | 1.6624E+02 | 2.4589E+02 | 1.7845E+02 | 3.7790E+01 |
| 51.Sb | 1.4961E−03 | 2.3560E+04 | 2.3900E+04 | 2.3627E+04 | 1.1571E+00 |
| | 1.5689E−03 | 2.1703E+04 | 2.2009E+04 | 2.1768E+04 | 1.1056E+00 |
| | 1.8733E−02 | 1.8411E+02 | 2.7966E+02 | 1.9676E+02 | 4.2129E+01 |
| 52.Te | 1.4868E−03 | 2.3299E+04 | 2.3636E+04 | 2.3363E+04 | 1.1710E+00 |
| | 1.7682E−02 | 2.1171E+02 | 3.3180E+02 | 2.2525E+02 | 4.7300E+01 |
| 53.I | 1.4551E−02 | 3.0225E+02 | 5.1283E+02 | 3.1935E+02 | 6.0589E+01 |
| 55.Cs | 5.8846E−02 | 9.1399E+00 | 1.1326E+01 | 1.6562E+01 | 4.6238E+01 |
| 56.Ba | 1.2981E−02 | 3.7247E+02 | 6.8047E+02 | 3.9528E+02 | 7.2152E+01 |
| | 3.7869E−02 | 3.2416E+01 | 4.0745E+01 | 9.9461E+01 | 1.4410E+02 |
| 57.La | 3.5794E−02 | 3.8581E+01 | 4.8938E+01 | 4.3768E+01 | 1.1811E+01 |
| 69.Tm | 1.4769E−03 | 2.3025E+04 | 2.3358E+04 | 2.3264E+04 | 4.0204E−01 |
| 70.Yb | 1.5608E−03 | 2.1935E+04 | 2.2245E+04 | 2.2205E+04 | 1.8025E−01 |
| 71.Lu | 1.6072E−03 | 2.0610E+04 | 2.0895E+04 | 2.0862E+04 | 1.5918E−01 |
| 72.Hf | 1.6669E−03 | 2.1519E+04 | 2.1811E+04 | 2.1765E+04 | 2.1142E−01 |
| 81.Tl | 2.1648E−03 | 1.2327E+04 | 1.2471E+04 | 1.2464E+04 | 6.0426E−02 |
| 82.Pb | 2.2669E−03 | 1.1427E+04 | 1.1560E+04 | 1.1552E+04 | 6.6604E−02 |
| 88.Ra | 1.4730E−02 | 2.9425E+02 | 4.9374E+02 | 3.1539E+02 | 5.6547E+01 |
| 112. | 1.4859E−02 | 2.8846E+02 | 4.7991E+02 | 3.0473E+02 | 5.7485E+01 |
| | 2.7177E−02 | 8.2629E+01 | 1.1275E+02 | 1.7578E+02 | 5.5905E+01 |
| 113. | 1.2595E−02 | 9.9956E+01 | 1.0653E+02 | 1.0669E+02 | 1.4881E−01 |
| 116. | 1.4335E−02 | 3.1189E+02 | 5.3585E+02 | 3.2997E+02 | 6.2393E+01 |
| 123. | 1.0082E−02 | 1.8711E+02 | 1.9573E+02 | 1.9652E+02 | 4.0451E−01 |
| 125. | 2.5360E−03 | 9.0562E+03 | 9.1603E+03 | 9.2872E+03 | 1.3849E+00 |
| 130. | 2.3825E−03 | 1.0409E+04 | 1.0530E+04 | 1.0571E+04 | 3.9497E−01 |
| 133. | 1.1879E−03 | 6.9657E+03 | 6.9924E+03 | 6.9794E+03 | 1.8655E−01 |
| | 1.2465E−03 | 6.2922E+03 | 6.3186E+03 | 6.3054E+03 | 2.0967E−01 |
| 134. | 3.9738E−02 | 2.6861E+01 | 3.3363E+01 | 4.3091E+01 | 2.9158E+01 |
| | | | 35.BROMINE | | |
| 4.Be | 4.9160E−02 | 2.5948E−02 | 3.2314E−02 | 2.8851E−01 | 7.9285E+02 |
| 5.B | 2.4607E−02 | 1.7683E−01 | 2.5795E−01 | 6.1048E−01 | 1.3666E+02 |
| | 3.6810E−02 | 6.0142E−02 | 7.7595E−02 | 4.4535E−01 | 4.7395E+02 |
| 54.Xe | 3.8001E−02 | 5.4236E−02 | 6.9484E−02 | 1.4560E−01 | 1.0954E+02 |
| 102. | 2.9428E−02 | 1.0271E−01 | 1.3819E−01 | 3.0520E−01 | 1.2085E+02 |
| | 4.1453E−02 | 4.1405E−02 | 5.2131E−02 | 2.2385E−01 | 3.2940E+02 |
| 135. | 1.8527E−02 | 3.0670E−01 | 4.9583E−01 | 5.5150E−01 | 1.1228E+01 |
| | 4.9345E−02 | 2.5578E−02 | 3.1840E−02 | 2.0742E−01 | 5.5145E+02 |

| Material | $E$, MeV | $\mu_{1en}$, cm$^{-1}$ | $\mu_1$, cm$^{-1}$ | $\mu_2$, cm$^{-1}$ | $R$, % |
|---|---|---|---|---|---|
| 136. | 1.5107E−02 | 4.4379E−01 | 7.8238E−01 | 6.8679E−01 | 1.3919E+01 |
| | 5.2011E−02 | 2.2325E−02 | 2.7762E−02 | 1.9168E−01 | 5.9043E+02 |
| 139. | 1.8941E−02 | 2.9011E−01 | 4.6115E−01 | 5.3825E−01 | 1.6720E+01 |
| | 4.8742E−02 | 2.6786E−02 | 3.3389E−02 | 2.1314E−01 | 5.3836E+02 |
| 142. | 2.8871E−02 | 1.1128E−01 | 1.5203E−01 | 3.3946E−01 | 1.2329E+02 |
| | 4.1404E−02 | 4.1504E−02 | 5.2258E−02 | 2.4604E−01 | 3.7082E+02 |
| | | | 36.KRYPTON | | |
| 3.Li | 2.7624E−03 | 6.3417E+00 | 6.4347E+00 | 6.5082E+00 | 1.1428E+00 |
| 4.Be | 1.4985E−02 | 2.1296E−01 | 4.0736E−01 | 5.6922E−01 | 3.9737E+01 |
| | 3.7638E−02 | 2.8582E−02 | 3.7517E−02 | 3.0971E−01 | 7.2551E+02 |
| 17.Cl | 1.3501E−02 | 8.5119E−02 | 9.0332E−02 | 8.8811E−02 | 1.7120E+00 |
| 54.Xe | 2.7776E−02 | 6.4059E−02 | 9.3057E−02 | 7.0439E−02 | 3.2109E+01 |
| | | | 37.RUBIDIUM | | |
| 12.Mg | 1.8372E−03 | 4.4482E+03 | 4.5304E+03 | 4.5356E+03 | 1.1529E−01 |
| 13.Al | 2.8476E−03 | 2.6753E+03 | 2.7187E+03 | 2.7334E+03 | 5.4124E−01 |
| 14.Si | 4.7272E−03 | 6.8802E+02 | 6.9911E+02 | 7.0298E+02 | 5.5335E−01 |
| 15.P | 1.2419E−02 | 5.6979E+01 | 5.9752E+01 | 5.9015E+01 | 1.2490E+00 |
| 16.S | 2.5997E−03 | 3.5459E+03 | 3.6076E+03 | 3.7864E+03 | 4.9563E+00 |
| 22.Ti | 2.8777E−02 | 2.6020E+01 | 3.8221E+01 | 2.8615E+01 | 3.3569E+01 |
| 23.V | 4.5959E−03 | 7.4771E+02 | 7.5956E+02 | 7.6099E+02 | 1.8821E−01 |
| 39.Y | 1.5570E−02 | 8.7135E+01 | 1.7785E+02 | 9.3506E+01 | 9.0199E+01 |
| 55.Cs | 1.8709E−02 | 6.4270E+01 | 1.1675E+02 | 6.8732E+01 | 6.9867E+01 |
| 118. | 2.9374E−03 | 2.3600E+03 | 2.3968E+03 | 2.4046E+03 | 3.2422E−01 |
| | 1.9261E−02 | 6.0246E+01 | 1.0600E+02 | 6.5078E+01 | 6.2883E+01 |
| 133. | 5.7569E−02 | 4.1608E+00 | 5.2861E+00 | 6.0765E+00 | 1.4952E+01 |
| | | | 38.STRONTIUM | | |
| 23.V | 2.5071E−02 | 6.4325E+01 | 1.0773E+02 | 7.0483E+01 | 5.2847E+01 |
| 24.Cr | 3.8102E−02 | 2.2314E+01 | 3.0602E+01 | 2.5381E+01 | 2.0571E+01 |
| 25.Mn | 2.8496E−03 | 4.6271E+03 | 4.7101E+03 | 4.6566E+03 | 1.1496E+00 |
| | 5.4654E−02 | 8.5397E+00 | 1.1004E+01 | 1.0488E+01 | 4.9260E+00 |
| 26.Fe | 6.5554E−03 | 5.2761E+02 | 5.3904E+02 | 5.4356E+02 | 8.3776E−01 |
| 32.Ge | 1.1657E−03 | 7.0506E+03 | 7.0675E+03 | 7.0796E+03 | 1.7072E−01 |
| 34.Se | 1.2643E−02 | 9.8315E+01 | 1.0305E+02 | 1.0485E+02 | 1.7529E+00 |
| 53.I | 2.7503E−03 | 5.1662E+03 | 5.2621E+03 | 5.2028E+03 | 1.1391E+00 |
| | 2.9864E−02 | 3.8653E+01 | 5.6253E+01 | 4.3340E+01 | 2.9794E+01 |
| 55.Cs | 4.4244E−02 | 1.5163E+01 | 2.0074E+01 | 3.6321E+01 | 8.0937E+01 |
| 56.Ba | 2.3718E−02 | 7.1576E+01 | 1.2227E+02 | 7.7489E+01 | 5.7792E+01 |
| 112. | 2.9632E−03 | 4.0099E+03 | 4.0781E+03 | 4.0499E+03 | 6.9692E−01 |

| Material | $E$, MeV | $\mu_{1en}$, cm$^{-1}$ | $\mu_1$, cm$^{-1}$ | $\mu_2$, cm$^{-1}$ | $R$, % |
|---|---|---|---|---|---|
| | 2.6551E−02 | 5.6396E+01 | 9.1832E+01 | 6.2685E+01 | 4.6498E+01 |
| 113. | 7.8166E−03 | 3.1491E+02 | 3.2346E+02 | 3.3974E+02 | 5.0349E+00 |
| | 1.4791E−02 | 5.3576E+01 | 5.7259E+01 | 5.7210E+01 | 8.6163E−02 |
| | 1.5025E−02 | 4.9026E+01 | 5.2600E+01 | 5.2357E+01 | 4.6456E−01 |
| 116. | 2.4616E−03 | 6.7344E+03 | 6.8677E+03 | 6.7735E+03 | 1.3912E+00 |
| | 2.9327E−02 | 4.1530E+01 | 6.2021E+01 | 4.6204E+01 | 3.4235E+01 |
| 118. | 4.9224E−02 | 1.1060E+01 | 1.4366E+01 | 2.3693E+01 | 6.4926E+01 |
| 130. | 2.2603E−03 | 7.8282E+03 | 7.9876E+03 | 7.8918E+03 | 1.2139E+00 |
| 133. | 1.4544E−03 | 3.9030E+03 | 3.9184E+03 | 3.9144E+03 | 1.0398E−01 |
| | 1.4264E−02 | 6.4542E+01 | 6.8482E+01 | 9.5331E+01 | 3.9205E+01 |
| 134. | 1.7184E−02 | 1.2084E+02 | 2.4840E+02 | 1.7103E+02 | 4.5243E+01 |
| 39.YTTRIUM | | | | | |
| 12.Mg | 1.4804E−03 | 7.0610E+03 | 7.0880E+03 | 7.2191E+03 | 1.8490E+00 |
| 21.Sc | 1.6436E−02 | 7.4917E+01 | 8.0851E+01 | 8.0317E+01 | 6.6487E−01 |
| 24.Cr | 1.8217E−02 | 1.9009E+02 | 3.9879E+02 | 2.1120E+02 | 8.8823E+01 |
| 25.Mn | 1.9402E−02 | 1.7128E+02 | 3.3737E+02 | 1.9232E+02 | 7.5417E+01 |
| 26.Fe | 2.5634E−02 | 1.0986E+02 | 1.9241E+02 | 1.2455E+02 | 5.4487E+01 |
| 27.Co | 2.1784E−03 | 1.3916E+04 | 1.4250E+04 | 1.3981E+04 | 1.9225E+00 |
| | 3.0973E−02 | 6.6241E+01 | 9.8629E+01 | 7.5450E+01 | 3.0721E+01 |
| 28.Ni | 2.6496E−03 | 1.0433E+04 | 1.0656E+04 | 1.0494E+04 | 1.5450E+00 |
| | 4.3106E−02 | 3.0092E+01 | 4.0814E+01 | 3.5072E+01 | 1.6372E+01 |
| 29.Cu | 2.8279E−03 | 8.8151E+03 | 8.9953E+03 | 8.8766E+03 | 1.3371E+00 |
| | 5.0569E−02 | 1.9181E+01 | 2.5182E+01 | 2.2893E+01 | 1.0001E+01 |
| 30.Zn | 3.5741E−02 | 4.9640E+01 | 7.1671E+01 | 5.8715E+01 | 2.2066E+01 |
| 31.Ga | 2.7294E−02 | 9.4567E+01 | 1.5886E+02 | 1.1793E+02 | 3.4710E+01 |
| 32.Ge | 2.4326E−02 | 1.2192E+02 | 2.1887E+02 | 1.5941E+02 | 3.7300E+01 |
| 33.As | 2.9660E−02 | 7.2761E+01 | 1.1100E+02 | 9.2252E+01 | 2.0327E+01 |
| 34.Se | 1.8947E−02 | 1.7849E+02 | 3.6093E+02 | 2.6905E+02 | 3.4152E+01 |
| 37.Rb | 1.5570E−02 | 8.7135E+01 | 9.3506E+01 | 1.7785E+02 | 9.0199E+01 |
| 42.Mo | 1.7270E−02 | 2.0511E+02 | 4.4785E+02 | 2.1993E+02 | 1.0363E+02 |
| 43.Tc | 2.1093E−03 | 1.0931E+04 | 1.1176E+04 | 1.1009E+04 | 1.5162E+00 |
| | 1.9364E−02 | 1.7188E+02 | 3.3932E+02 | 1.8652E+02 | 8.1918E+01 |
| 44.Ru | 2.0834E−02 | 1.5409E+02 | 2.8949E+02 | 1.6862E+02 | 7.1675E+01 |
| 45.Rh | 2.3470E−03 | 1.1668E+04 | 1.1933E+04 | 1.1750E+04 | 1.5562E+00 |
| | 2.2141E−02 | 1.4205E+02 | 2.6306E+02 | 1.5611E+02 | 6.8506E+01 |
| 46.Pd | 2.2292E−03 | 1.3192E+04 | 1.3505E+04 | 1.3274E+04 | 1.7409E+00 |
| | 2.2915E−02 | 1.3491E+02 | 2.4739E+02 | 1.4835E+02 | 6.6760E+01 |
| 47.Ag | 2.2378E−02 | 1.3986E+02 | 2.5826E+02 | 1.5278E+02 | 6.9040E+01 |
| 48.Cd | 1.9625E−02 | 1.6772E+02 | 3.2576E+02 | 1.8071E+02 | 8.0268E+01 |

| Material | $E$, MeV | $\mu_{1en}$, $cm^{-1}$ | $\mu_1$, $cm^{-1}$ | $\mu_2$, $cm^{-1}$ | $R$, % |
|---|---|---|---|---|---|
| 49.In | 2.1405E−03 | 1.0454E+04 | 1.0684E+04 | 1.0511E+04 | 1.6511E+00 |
| | 1.8696E−02 | 1.8248E+02 | 3.7395E+02 | 1.9520E+02 | 9.1576E+01 |
| 50.Sn | 1.9166E−02 | 1.7502E+02 | 3.4959E+02 | 1.8758E+02 | 8.6366E+01 |
| 51.Sb | 2.1071E−03 | 1.0972E+04 | 1.1219E+04 | 1.1025E+04 | 1.7565E+00 |
| | 1.8855E−02 | 1.7996E+02 | 3.6572E+02 | 1.9244E+02 | 9.0037E+01 |
| 52.Te | 2.1524E−03 | 1.0287E+04 | 1.0512E+04 | 1.0336E+04 | 1.7061E+00 |
| | 1.8459E−02 | 1.8624E+02 | 3.8622E+02 | 1.9871E+02 | 9.4362E+01 |
| 53.I | 3.3183E−02 | 5.8546E+01 | 8.6134E+01 | 1.7646E+02 | 1.0487E+02 |
| 55.Cs | 1.0197E−03 | 1.6819E+04 | 1.6850E+04 | 1.6859E+04 | 5.3076E−02 |
| | 1.1173E−03 | 1.4753E+04 | 1.4783E+04 | 1.4790E+04 | 4.7187E−02 |
| | 7.0404E−03 | 8.5707E+02 | 8.7677E+02 | 9.1626E+02 | 4.5037E+00 |
| 56.Ba | 4.5426E−02 | 2.6564E+01 | 3.5746E+01 | 6.5522E+01 | 8.3296E+01 |
| 57.La | 2.2962E−03 | 1.2299E+04 | 1.2585E+04 | 1.2361E+04 | 1.8100E+00 |
| | 2.5892E−02 | 1.0749E+02 | 1.8721E+02 | 1.1700E+02 | 6.0007E+01 |
| 58.Ce | 2.5600E−03 | 1.1246E+04 | 1.1491E+04 | 1.1311E+04 | 1.5891E+00 |
| | 2.9401E−02 | 7.5142E+01 | 1.1623E+02 | 8.3229E+01 | 3.9651E+01 |
| 59.Pr | 2.8823E−03 | 8.3215E+03 | 8.4886E+03 | 8.3851E+03 | 1.2343E+00 |
| 59.Pr | 3.4712E−02 | 5.3221E+01 | 7.7487E+01 | 5.9863E+01 | 2.9440E+01 |
| 60.Nd | 3.9890E−02 | 3.5196E+01 | 4.8216E+01 | 4.0587E+01 | 1.8796E+01 |
| 63.Eu | 1.1349E−03 | 1.4380E+04 | 1.4410E+04 | 1.4468E+04 | 4.0573E−01 |
| | 2.5100E−03 | 1.1699E+04 | 1.1957E+04 | 1.1780E+04 | 1.4974E+00 |
| | 2.9608E−02 | 7.3237E+01 | 1.1205E+02 | 8.1304E+01 | 3.7815E+01 |
| 64.Gd | 1.1033E−03 | 1.5049E+04 | 1.5079E+04 | 1.5135E+04 | 3.6701E−01 |
| 87.Fr | 2.1911E−03 | 1.3734E+04 | 1.4064E+04 | 1.3860E+04 | 1.4667E+00 |
| 89.Ac | 2.6496E−03 | 1.0432E+04 | 1.0656E+04 | 1.0551E+04 | 9.9424E−01 |
| 112. | 1.7265E−02 | 2.0520E+02 | 4.4812E+02 | 2.1816E+02 | 1.0541E+02 |
| 116. | 3.6467E−02 | 4.7114E+01 | 6.7569E+01 | 1.3256E+02 | 9.6191E+01 |
| 118. | 7.4493E−03 | 7.2496E+02 | 7.4274E+02 | 7.8616E+02 | 5.8464E+00 |
| 121. | 1.1332E−03 | 1.4416E+04 | 1.4446E+04 | 1.4487E+04 | 2.8296E−01 |
| 123. | 1.1164E−03 | 1.4771E+04 | 1.4802E+04 | 1.4879E+04 | 5.2377E−01 |
| | 2.4426E−02 | 1.2099E+02 | 2.1684E+02 | 1.5886E+02 | 3.6501E+01 |
| 124. | 2.0251E−03 | 3.1955E+03 | 3.2209E+03 | 3.2897E+03 | 2.1353E+00 |
| 130. | 2.8386E−03 | 8.7176E+03 | 8.8952E+03 | 8.8834E+03 | 1.3296E−01 |
| 134. | 1.0656E−03 | 1.5848E+04 | 1.5879E+04 | 1.5879E+04 | 1.1193E−03 |
| | 1.1472E−03 | 1.4119E+04 | 1.4149E+04 | 1.4148E+04 | 5.5634E−03 |

40.ZIRCONIUM

| Material | $E$, MeV | $\mu_{1en}$, $cm^{-1}$ | $\mu_1$, $cm^{-1}$ | $\mu_2$, $cm^{-1}$ | $R$, % |
|---|---|---|---|---|---|
| 22.Ti | 1.4926E−02 | 1.5482E+02 | 1.6501E+02 | 1.6787E+02 | 1.7360E+00 |
| 27.Co | 1.9460E−02 | 2.4198E+02 | 5.1003E+02 | 2.8214E+02 | 8.0773E+01 |
| 28.Ni | 2.3135E−02 | 1.9141E+02 | 3.7391E+02 | 2.2563E+02 | 6.5715E+01 |

| Material | $E$, MeV | $\mu_{1en}$, cm$^{-1}$ | $\mu_1$, cm$^{-1}$ | $\mu_2$, cm$^{-1}$ | $R$, % |
|---|---|---|---|---|---|
| 29.Cu | 2.4767E−02 | 1.7066E+02 | 3.2347E+02 | 2.0508E+02 | 5.7727E+01 |
| 30.Zn | 1.9257E−02 | 2.4599E+02 | 5.2475E+02 | 3.1190E+02 | 6.8244E+01 |
| 31.Ga | 1.1157E−03 | 2.3464E+04 | 2.3508E+04 | 2.3672E+04 | 6.9715E−01 |
| 45.Rh | 1.8176E−02 | 2.6738E+02 | 6.0319E+02 | 2.8643E+02 | 1.1059E+02 |
| 46.Pd | 1.8419E−02 | 2.6257E+02 | 5.8555E+02 | 2.8126E+02 | 1.0819E+02 |
| 49.In | 2.8900E−02 | 1.1809E+02 | 1.9570E+02 | 3.1929E+02 | 6.3154E+01 |
| 50.Sn | 2.9542E−02 | 1.0992E+02 | 1.7584E+02 | 3.1125E+02 | 7.7009E+01 |
| 51.Sb | 3.4322E−02 | 8.1963E+01 | 1.2382E+02 | 2.1737E+02 | 7.5547E+01 |
| 52.Te | 3.7770E−02 | 6.4305E+01 | 9.3628E+01 | 1.5692E+02 | 6.7600E+01 |
| 53.I | 4.7007E−02 | 3.6895E+01 | 5.0320E+01 | 7.5167E+01 | 4.9380E+01 |
| 56.Ba | 5.7644E−03 | 2.1437E+03 | 2.1885E+03 | 2.3160E+03 | 5.8285E+00 |
| 57.La | 3.9979E−02 | 5.2995E+01 | 7.4287E+01 | 1.5894E+02 | 1.1396E+02 |
| 58.Ce | 2.2473E−03 | 1.4613E+04 | 1.4968E+04 | 1.4686E+04 | 1.9191E+00 |
| | 1.9058E−02 | 2.4992E+02 | 5.3917E+02 | 2.6852E+02 | 1.0079E+02 |
| 59.Pr | 1.9618E−02 | 2.3885E+02 | 4.9858E+02 | 2.5749E+02 | 9.3635E+01 |
| 60.Nd | 2.1242E−02 | 2.1549E+02 | 4.3243E+02 | 2.3330E+02 | 8.5349E+01 |
| 61.Pm | 1.0364E−03 | 2.6123E+04 | 2.6168E+04 | 2.6258E+04 | 3.4318E−01 |
| | 2.6227E−02 | 1.5209E+02 | 2.7833E+02 | 1.6634E+02 | 6.7325E+01 |
| 62.Sm | 1.0872E−03 | 2.4419E+04 | 2.4464E+04 | 2.4556E+04 | 3.7568E−01 |
| | 2.7824E−02 | 1.3177E+02 | 2.2893E+02 | 1.4500E+02 | 5.7886E+01 |
| 63.Eu | 1.1511E−03 | 2.2275E+04 | 2.2319E+04 | 2.2414E+04 | 4.2453E−01 |
| | 2.2584E−03 | 1.4354E+04 | 1.4703E+04 | 1.4447E+04 | 1.7699E+00 |
| | 1.8995E−02 | 2.5117E+02 | 5.4373E+02 | 2.7345E+02 | 9.8841E+01 |
| | 4.9467E−02 | 3.1281E+01 | 4.1971E+01 | 9.9845E+01 | 1.3789E+02 |
| 64.Gd | 1.2021E−03 | 2.0564E+04 | 2.0607E+04 | 2.0703E+04 | 4.6866E−01 |
| | 2.6960E−03 | 1.5052E+04 | 1.5409E+04 | 1.5173E+04 | 1.5540E+00 |
| | 3.1881E−02 | 9.4463E+01 | 1.4520E+02 | 1.0547E+02 | 3.7675E+01 |
| 65.Tb | 1.2415E−03 | 1.9245E+04 | 1.9288E+04 | 1.9378E+04 | 4.6987E−01 |
| | 2.9542E−03 | 1.1850E+04 | 1.2113E+04 | 1.1954E+04 | 1.3364E+00 |
| | 3.9663E−03 | 5.6256E+03 | 5.7364E+03 | 5.7005E+03 | 6.2991E−01 |
| | 7.1970E−03 | 1.2645E+03 | 1.2947E+03 | 1.3075E+03 | 9.9077E−01 |
| | 3.9514E−02 | 5.5374E+01 | 7.8356E+01 | 6.3307E+01 | 2.3772E+01 |
| 66.Dy | 5.1281E−02 | 2.8596E+01 | 3.8137E+01 | 3.4039E+01 | 1.2039E+01 |
| 69.Tm | 1.3780E−03 | 1.4664E+04 | 1.4704E+04 | 1.4760E+04 | 3.7982E−01 |
| 70.Yb | 3.9899E−03 | 5.4875E+03 | 5.5950E+03 | 5.5695E+03 | 4.5785E−01 |
| | 4.0786E−02 | 5.1094E+01 | 7.1436E+01 | 5.8722E+01 | 2.1650E+01 |
| 80.Hg | 2.2980E−03 | 1.3627E+04 | 1.3951E+04 | 1.3839E+04 | 8.0516E−01 |
| | 2.3356E−03 | 1.8205E+04 | 1.8678E+04 | 1.8581E+04 | 5.1811E−01 |
| 81.Tl | 2.4230E−03 | 1.6654E+04 | 1.7080E+04 | 1.7025E+04 | 3.2214E−01 |
| 82.Pb | 2.4864E−03 | 1.5678E+04 | 1.6068E+04 | 1.6037E+04 | 1.9251E−01 |

| Material | $E$, MeV | $\mu_{1en}$, cm$^{-1}$ | $\mu_1$, cm$^{-1}$ | $\mu_2$, cm$^{-1}$ | $R$, % |
|---|---|---|---|---|---|
| 89.Ac | 2.2583E−03 | 1.4357E+04 | 1.4706E+04 | 1.4483E+04 | 1.5361E+00 |
| 91.Pa | 3.1430E−03 | 1.0444E+04 | 1.0671E+04 | 1.0617E+04 | 5.1623E−01 |
| 112. | 3.6867E−02 | 6.8933E+01 | 1.0154E+02 | 1.5673E+02 | 5.4347E+01 |
| 116. | 5.1319E−02 | 2.8553E+01 | 3.8078E+01 | 5.5101E+01 | 4.4705E+01 |
| 121. | 1.2052E−03 | 2.0461E+04 | 2.0504E+04 | 2.0588E+04 | 4.0949E−01 |
| | 2.4937E−02 | 1.6850E+02 | 3.1821E+02 | 1.8503E+02 | 7.1983E+01 |
| 125. | 3.8254E−03 | 6.4506E+03 | 6.5813E+03 | 6.6093E+03 | 4.2429E−01 |
| 130. | 2.8080E−02 | 1.2852E+02 | 2.2104E+02 | 1.5014E+02 | 4.7224E+01 |
| 134. | 1.4889E−02 | 1.5717E+02 | 1.6742E+02 | 2.2814E+02 | 3.6266E+01 |

41.NIOBIUM

| Material | $E$, MeV | $\mu_{1en}$, cm$^{-1}$ | $\mu_1$, cm$^{-1}$ | $\mu_2$, cm$^{-1}$ | $R$, % |
|---|---|---|---|---|---|
| 23.V | 1.1040E−03 | 3.4343E+04 | 3.4408E+04 | 3.4408E+04 | 2.0322E−03 |
| | 2.3238E−03 | 5.2875E+03 | 5.3375E+03 | 5.3100E+03 | 5.1920E−01 |
| | 1.2461E−02 | 4.4320E+02 | 4.6248E+02 | 4.9765E+02 | 7.6053E+00 |
| 30.Zn | 1.0331E−03 | 3.7756E+04 | 3.7824E+04 | 3.8058E+04 | 6.2032E−01 |
| 31.Ga | 1.1407E−03 | 3.2574E+04 | 3.2638E+04 | 3.2882E+04 | 7.4582E−01 |
| 34.Se | 1.3512E−02 | 3.4873E+02 | 3.6585E+02 | 6.2381E+02 | 7.0509E+01 |
| 48.Cd | 3.2193E−02 | 1.2626E+02 | 2.0136E+02 | 2.8798E+02 | 4.3020E+01 |
| 49.In | 4.1111E−02 | 6.9486E+01 | 9.9493E+01 | 1.3007E+02 | 3.0733E+01 |
| 50.Sn | 4.1956E−02 | 6.6860E+01 | 9.5448E+01 | 1.2949E+02 | 3.5669E+01 |
| 51.Sb | 4.8850E−02 | 4.5429E+01 | 6.2442E+01 | 8.1916E+01 | 3.1186E+01 |
| 52.Te | 4.7004E−03 | 5.3206E+03 | 5.4346E+03 | 5.6663E+03 | 4.2627E+00 |
| | 5.7427E−02 | 3.0120E+01 | 4.0315E+01 | 5.1016E+01 | 2.6544E+01 |
| 56.Ba | 1.4762E−03 | 1.6402E+04 | 1.6454E+04 | 1.6453E+04 | 9.8887E−03 |
| | 1.6703E−02 | 1.7038E+02 | 1.8275E+02 | 1.8152E+02 | 6.8098E−01 |
| 57.La | 5.3160E−02 | 3.6862E+01 | 4.9865E+01 | 7.8337E+01 | 5.7097E+01 |
| 58.Ce | 4.9025E−02 | 4.4886E+01 | 6.1606E+01 | 1.0876E+02 | 7.6538E+01 |
| 59.Pr | 4.8921E−02 | 4.5209E+01 | 6.2103E+01 | 1.1560E+02 | 8.6139E+01 |
| 60.Nd | 4.8879E−02 | 4.5340E+01 | 6.2305E+01 | 1.2246E+02 | 9.6550E+01 |
| 61.Pm | 1.0472E−03 | 3.7077E+04 | 3.7144E+04 | 3.7264E+04 | 3.2297E−01 |
| | 1.9016E−02 | 3.2038E+02 | 7.5001E+02 | 3.4658E+02 | 1.1640E+02 |
| | 4.8191E−02 | 4.7478E+01 | 6.5598E+01 | 1.3964E+02 | 1.1287E+02 |
| 62.Sm | 1.0990E−03 | 3.4580E+04 | 3.4645E+04 | 3.4771E+04 | 3.6385E−01 |
| | 2.4075E−03 | 1.7308E+04 | 1.7767E+04 | 1.7418E+04 | 2.0070E+00 |
| | 1.9459E−02 | 3.1092E+02 | 7.0994E+02 | 3.3748E+02 | 1.1037E+02 |
| | 4.8522E−02 | 4.6450E+01 | 6.4015E+01 | 1.4370E+02 | 1.2447E+02 |
| 63.Eu | 7.0437E−03 | 1.9106E+03 | 1.9568E+03 | 2.1156E+03 | 8.1148E+00 |
| 64.Gd | 1.2143E−03 | 2.9027E+04 | 2.9088E+04 | 2.9225E+04 | 4.7320E−01 |
| | 2.3105E−02 | 2.5026E+02 | 5.2666E+02 | 2.7406E+02 | 9.2167E+01 |
| 65.Tb | 1.2551E−03 | 2.7058E+04 | 2.7117E+04 | 2.7264E+04 | 5.4161E−01 |

| Material | $E$, MeV | $\mu_{1en}$, cm$^{-1}$ | $\mu_1$, cm$^{-1}$ | $\mu_2$, cm$^{-1}$ | $R$, % |
|---|---|---|---|---|---|
| | 2.6348E−02 | 1.9898E+02 | 3.8641E+02 | 2.1953E+02 | 7.6016E+01 |
| 66.Dy | 1.3070E−03 | 2.4559E+04 | 2.4617E+04 | 2.4765E+04 | 6.0143E−01 |
| | 2.8085E−02 | 1.7151E+02 | 3.1129E+02 | 1.9035E+02 | 6.3535E+01 |
| 67.Ho | 1.3591E−03 | 2.2045E+04 | 2.2102E+04 | 2.2236E+04 | 6.0704E−01 |
| | 2.4835E−03 | 2.2060E+04 | 2.2689E+04 | 2.2270E+04 | 1.8793E+00 |
| | 2.9284E−02 | 1.5255E+02 | 2.5943E+02 | 1.7025E+02 | 5.2386E+01 |
| 68.Er | 1.4114E−03 | 1.9527E+04 | 1.9581E+04 | 1.9702E+04 | 6.1669E−01 |
| | 3.2757E−02 | 1.2240E+02 | 1.9438E+02 | 1.3767E+02 | 4.1197E+01 |
| 69.Tm | 7.0794E−03 | 1.8850E+03 | 1.9307E+03 | 1.9436E+03 | 6.6500E−01 |
| | 8.3554E−03 | 1.1251E+03 | 1.1576E+03 | 1.1738E+03 | 1.3991E+00 |
| | 3.8754E−02 | 8.1446E+01 | 1.2021E+02 | 9.2965E+01 | 2.9311E+01 |
| 70.Yb | 1.5339E−03 | 1.4734E+04 | 1.4785E+04 | 1.4899E+04 | 7.6881E−01 |
| | 2.3813E−03 | 1.7947E+04 | 1.8421E+04 | 1.8159E+04 | 1.4395E+00 |
| | 2.5958E−02 | 2.0514E+02 | 4.0325E+02 | 2.3055E+02 | 7.4905E+01 |
| 81.Tl | 2.4254E−03 | 1.6913E+04 | 1.7362E+04 | 1.7293E+04 | 3.9484E−01 |
| | 2.4743E−03 | 2.2247E+04 | 2.2883E+04 | 2.2797E+04 | 3.7723E−01 |
| 82.Pb | 2.5628E−03 | 2.0436E+04 | 2.1005E+04 | 2.0967E+04 | 1.8082E−01 |
| 85.At | 2.8648E−03 | 1.8024E+04 | 1.8496E+04 | 1.8582E+04 | 4.6777E−01 |
| 87.Fr | 3.1110E−03 | 1.5016E+04 | 1.5393E+04 | 1.5497E+04 | 6.7639E−01 |
| 88.Ra | 1.7737E−03 | 1.1048E+04 | 1.1099E+04 | 1.1110E+04 | 9.3464E−02 |
| | 5.5471E−03 | 3.4061E+03 | 3.4800E+03 | 3.5149E+03 | 1.0030E+00 |
| | 3.7478E−02 | 9.0161E+01 | 1.3600E+02 | 1.1163E+02 | 2.1824E+01 |
| 89.Ac | 3.3337E−03 | 1.3181E+04 | 1.3505E+04 | 1.3628E+04 | 9.1507E−01 |
| 92.U | 2.7011E−03 | 2.0559E+04 | 2.1114E+04 | 2.0784E+04 | 1.5889E+00 |
| 112. | 4.7054E−03 | 5.3035E+03 | 5.4172E+03 | 5.5864E+03 | 3.1239E+00 |
| 116. | 1.2127E−03 | 2.9104E+04 | 2.9165E+04 | 2.9172E+04 | 2.3706E−02 |
| | 5.8568E−03 | 2.8954E+03 | 2.9592E+03 | 3.0934E+03 | 4.5360E+00 |
| 121. | 5.6769E−02 | 3.1158E+01 | 4.1786E+01 | 8.7146E+01 | 1.0855E+02 |
| 125. | 1.9093E−03 | 8.9628E+03 | 9.0149E+03 | 9.0852E+03 | 7.8028E−01 |
| | 2.5611E−02 | 2.1063E+02 | 4.1828E+02 | 2.5975E+02 | 6.1030E+01 |
| 130. | 1.9175E−02 | 3.1699E+02 | 7.3565E+02 | 3.7604E+02 | 9.5628E+01 |
| | 5.4603E−02 | 3.4581E+01 | 4.6635E+01 | 5.3423E+01 | 1.4555E+01 |
| 134. | 2.3691E−03 | 4.9686E+03 | 5.0184E+03 | 5.0211E+03 | 5.4176E−02 |
| | | | 42.MOLYBDENUM | | |
| 24.Cr | 1.4470E−03 | 2.2869E+04 | 2.2940E+04 | 2.2927E+04 | 5.9633E−02 |
| | 2.2818E−03 | 7.4302E+03 | 7.4908E+03 | 7.4629E+03 | 3.7431E−01 |
| | 9.6798E−03 | 9.5934E+02 | 9.9222E+02 | 1.1247E+03 | 1.3352E+01 |
| 25.Mn | 7.7670E−03 | 1.7666E+03 | 1.8147E+03 | 2.2460E+03 | 2.3768E+01 |
| 26.Fe | 7.1595E−03 | 2.3170E+03 | 2.3760E+03 | 3.1665E+03 | 3.3271E+01 |

| Material | $E$, MeV | $\mu_{1en}$, cm$^{-1}$ | $\mu_1$, cm$^{-1}$ | $\mu_2$, cm$^{-1}$ | $R$, % |
|---|---|---|---|---|---|
| 31.Ga | 1.0851E−02 | 7.4844E+02 | 7.7692E+02 | 1.2232E+03 | 5.7447E+01 |
| 32.Ge | 1.3592E−02 | 4.3521E+02 | 4.5635E+02 | 6.9214E+02 | 5.1668E+01 |
| 33.As | 1.3046E−02 | 4.9757E+02 | 5.2018E+02 | 8.5286E+02 | 6.3955E+01 |
| 34.Se | 1.4887E−02 | 2.8720E+02 | 3.0487E+02 | 4.7690E+02 | 5.6426E+01 |
| 39.Y | 1.7270E−02 | 2.0511E+02 | 2.1993E+02 | 4.4785E+02 | 1.0363E+02 |
| 46.Pd | 2.4564E−02 | 2.6295E+02 | 5.7852E+02 | 6.9788E+02 | 2.0632E+01 |
| 47.Ag | 2.9496E−02 | 1.7868E+02 | 3.1422E+02 | 4.0723E+02 | 2.9602E+01 |
| 48.Cd | 4.8166E−02 | 5.8761E+01 | 8.2985E+01 | 9.7284E+01 | 1.7231E+01 |
| 49.In | 4.5500E−03 | 7.3524E+03 | 7.5259E+03 | 7.7130E+03 | 2.4868E+00 |
| 51.Sb | 4.8720E−03 | 5.9877E+03 | 6.1263E+03 | 6.3288E+03 | 3.3056E+00 |
| 52.Te | 5.9007E−03 | 3.5738E+03 | 3.6580E+03 | 3.7739E+03 | 3.1700E+00 |
| 53.I | 1.9240E−03 | 1.1240E+04 | 1.1305E+04 | 1.1286E+04 | 1.6603E−01 |
| 59.Pr | 5.9196E−02 | 3.4038E+01 | 4.5952E+01 | 7.0191E+01 | 5.2750E+01 |
| 60.Nd | 5.8325E−02 | 3.5726E+01 | 4.8411E+01 | 7.8410E+01 | 6.1966E+01 |
| 61.Pm | 5.6255E−02 | 3.9736E+01 | 5.4255E+01 | 9.6002E+01 | 7.6946E+01 |
| 62.Sm | 5.6232E−02 | 3.9780E+01 | 5.4319E+01 | 1.0133E+02 | 8.6544E+01 |
| 63.Eu | 1.2823E−03 | 3.3029E+04 | 3.3101E+04 | 3.3232E+04 | 3.9785E−01 |
| 64.Gd | 5.6107E−02 | 4.0023E+01 | 5.4674E+01 | 1.1454E+02 | 1.0949E+02 |
| 65.Tb | 1.2654E−03 | 3.4069E+04 | 3.4140E+04 | 3.4334E+04 | 5.6738E−01 |
| | 2.5474E−03 | 1.9009E+04 | 1.9555E+04 | 1.9160E+04 | 2.0622E+00 |
| | 2.0579E−02 | 3.3104E+02 | 7.9208E+02 | 3.6313E+02 | 1.1813E+02 |
| | 5.5412E−02 | 4.1369E+01 | 5.6635E+01 | 1.2677E+02 | 1.2384E+02 |
| 66.Dy | 1.3180E−03 | 3.0823E+04 | 3.0895E+04 | 3.1089E+04 | 6.2834E−01 |
| | 2.3897E−02 | 2.7434E+02 | 6.1424E+02 | 3.0277E+02 | 1.0287E+02 |
| | 5.5312E−02 | 4.1563E+01 | 5.6918E+01 | 1.3455E+02 | 1.3640E+02 |
| 67.Ho | 1.3708E−03 | 2.7572E+04 | 2.7643E+04 | 2.7824E+04 | 6.5362E−01 |
| | 2.6033E−02 | 2.3785E+02 | 4.9979E+02 | 2.6401E+02 | 8.9309E+01 |
| 68.Er | 1.4222E−03 | 2.4402E+04 | 2.4473E+04 | 2.4640E+04 | 6.8002E−01 |
| 68.Er | 2.7622E−02 | 2.1070E+02 | 4.1464E+02 | 2.3520E+02 | 7.6293E+01 |
| 69.Tm | 1.4738E−03 | 2.1218E+04 | 2.1290E+04 | 2.1434E+04 | 6.7498E−01 |
| | 2.8835E−02 | 1.8997E+02 | 3.4964E+02 | 2.1306E+02 | 6.4105E+01 |
| 70.Yb | 1.5483E−03 | 1.8649E+04 | 1.8720E+04 | 1.8871E+04 | 8.0623E−01 |
| | 2.0000E−02 | 3.3733E+02 | 8.2320E+02 | 3.7880E+02 | 1.1732E+02 |
| 71.Lu | 1.5964E−03 | 1.7700E+04 | 1.7770E+04 | 1.7897E+04 | 7.1873E−01 |
| | 3.4238E−02 | 1.3592E+02 | 2.2153E+02 | 1.5421E+02 | 4.3658E+01 |
| 72.Hf | 1.4944E−03 | 1.9948E+04 | 2.0019E+04 | 2.0094E+04 | 3.7401E−01 |
| | 1.5184E−03 | 1.9239E+04 | 1.9311E+04 | 1.9386E+04 | 3.8928E−01 |
| 82.Pb | 2.5376E−03 | 1.9246E+04 | 1.9798E+04 | 1.9749E+04 | 2.4706E−01 |
| 83.Bi | 2.6241E−03 | 1.7424E+04 | 1.7905E+04 | 1.7913E+04 | 4.2586E−02 |

| Material | $E$, MeV | $\mu_{1en}$, cm$^{-1}$ | $\mu_1$, cm$^{-1}$ | $\mu_2$, cm$^{-1}$ | $R$, % |
|---|---|---|---|---|---|
| 84.Po | 2.9339E−03 | 2.1110E+04 | 2.1718E+04 | 2.1780E+04 | 2.8797E−01 |
| 85.At | 2.8293E−03 | 2.0121E+04 | 2.0711E+04 | 2.0761E+04 | 2.4548E−01 |
| 88.Ra | 2.4950E−03 | 5.6827E+03 | 5.7412E+03 | 5.7400E+03 | 2.1343E−02 |
| | 2.5811E−02 | 2.4164E+02 | 5.1169E+02 | 3.2073E+02 | 5.9541E+01 |
| 91.Pa | 2.5580E−03 | 1.8755E+04 | 1.9295E+04 | 1.8941E+04 | 1.8673E+00 |
| 112. | 1.1952E−03 | 3.8398E+04 | 3.8470E+04 | 3.8472E+04 | 5.0364E−03 |
| | 1.7414E−02 | 2.0074E+02 | 2.1540E+02 | 2.1352E+02 | 8.7930E−01 |
| 116. | 2.1128E−03 | 8.8160E+03 | 8.8783E+03 | 8.8597E+03 | 2.1029E−01 |
| 121. | 1.2985E−03 | 3.2027E+04 | 3.2099E+04 | 3.2243E+04 | 4.4931E−01 |
| | 7.3503E−03 | 2.1442E+03 | 2.1997E+03 | 2.3885E+03 | 8.5799E+00 |
| 123. | 1.3539E−03 | 2.8613E+04 | 2.8685E+04 | 2.8908E+04 | 7.7854E−01 |
| | 1.3796E−02 | 4.1187E+02 | 4.3246E+02 | 6.4523E+02 | 4.9199E+01 |
| 130. | 1.4725E−03 | 2.1297E+04 | 2.1369E+04 | 2.1375E+04 | 2.8106E−02 |
| | 7.8016E−03 | 1.7353E+03 | 1.7828E+03 | 1.8162E+03 | 1.8736E+00 |
| | 1.0668E−02 | 7.6939E+02 | 7.9836E+02 | 8.0851E+02 | 1.2708E+00 |

43.TECHNETIUM

| Material | $E$, MeV | $\mu_{1en}$, cm$^{-1}$ | $\mu_1$, cm$^{-1}$ | $\mu_2$, cm$^{-1}$ | $R$, % |
|---|---|---|---|---|---|
| 25.Mn | 2.6489E−03 | 6.0207E+03 | 6.0879E+03 | 6.0537E+03 | 5.6523E−01 |
| | 1.8783E−02 | 1.9336E+02 | 2.0878E+02 | 2.1785E+02 | 4.3463E+00 |
| 26.Fe | 9.0281E−03 | 1.4403E+03 | 1.4862E+03 | 1.8598E+03 | 2.5140E+01 |
| 30.Zn | 9.7980E−03 | 1.1109E+03 | 1.1498E+03 | 1.7492E+03 | 5.2129E+01 |
| 31.Ga | 1.4359E−02 | 4.2190E+02 | 4.4451E+02 | 6.1517E+02 | 3.8394E+01 |
| 32.Ge | 1.5062E−02 | 3.3096E+02 | 3.5135E+02 | 4.8389E+02 | 3.7722E+01 |
| 33.As | 1.3616E−03 | 3.4361E+04 | 3.4445E+04 | 3.4806E+04 | 1.0492E+00 |
| | 1.4548E−02 | 3.9568E+02 | 4.1766E+02 | 6.3134E+02 | 5.1160E+01 |
| 34.Se | 1.9768E−02 | 1.5694E+02 | 1.7105E+02 | 2.2833E+02 | 3.3489E+01 |
| 39.Y | 2.1093E−03 | 1.0931E+04 | 1.1009E+04 | 1.1176E+04 | 1.5162E+00 |
| | 1.9364E−02 | 1.7188E+02 | 1.8652E+02 | 3.3932E+02 | 8.1918E+01 |
| 45.Rh | 3.2251E−03 | 2.0780E+04 | 2.1435E+04 | 2.1596E+04 | 7.5176E−01 |
| | 2.4739E−02 | 2.8393E+02 | 6.4737E+02 | 7.1022E+02 | 9.7083E+00 |
| 46.Pd | 2.8923E−02 | 2.1297E+02 | 4.0627E+02 | 4.7225E+02 | 1.6241E+01 |
| 47.Ag | 4.2208E−02 | 9.4809E+01 | 1.4285E+02 | 1.6262E+02 | 1.3842E+01 |
| 48.Cd | 7.9919E−03 | 1.8891E+03 | 1.9444E+03 | 1.9586E+03 | 7.2709E−01 |
| 49.In | 2.2465E−03 | 9.6827E+03 | 9.7582E+03 | 9.7385E+03 | 2.0226E−01 |
| 50.Sn | 1.4875E−03 | 2.4915E+04 | 2.4996E+04 | 2.4982E+04 | 5.7112E−02 |
| | 2.0331E−02 | 1.4205E+02 | 1.5555E+02 | 1.5327E+02 | 1.4892E+00 |
| 51.Sb | 2.0941E−03 | 1.1069E+04 | 1.1148E+04 | 1.1122E+04 | 2.3262E−01 |
| | 2.0791E−02 | 1.3328E+02 | 1.4639E+02 | 1.4379E+02 | 1.8053E+00 |
| 52.Te | 2.2840E−03 | 9.3414E+03 | 9.4161E+03 | 9.3889E+03 | 2.9046E−01 |
| 57.La | 1.3427E−03 | 3.5784E+04 | 3.5868E+04 | 3.5899E+04 | 8.6155E−02 |

| Material | $E$, MeV | $\mu_{1en}$, cm$^{-1}$ | $\mu_1$, cm$^{-1}$ | $\mu_2$, cm$^{-1}$ | $R$, % |
|---|---|---|---|---|---|
| | 6.8594E−03 | 3.1231E+03 | 3.2052E+03 | 3.3820E+03 | 5.5141E+00 |
| 58.Ce | 1.0547E−03 | 5.7396E+04 | 5.7487E+04 | 5.7589E+04 | 1.7702E−01 |
| 59.Pr | 1.1789E−03 | 4.8074E+04 | 4.8162E+04 | 4.8258E+04 | 2.0024E−01 |
| 60.Nd | 1.0953E−03 | 5.4349E+04 | 5.4439E+04 | 5.4584E+04 | 2.6649E−01 |
| 61.Pm | 1.1268E−03 | 5.1986E+04 | 5.2075E+04 | 5.2249E+04 | 3.3462E−01 |
| 62.Sm | 1.1481E−03 | 5.0386E+04 | 5.0475E+04 | 5.0665E+04 | 3.7765E−01 |
| 63.Eu | 1.4590E−03 | 2.7057E+04 | 2.7138E+04 | 2.7219E+04 | 2.9918E−01 |
| 64.Gd | 1.3117E−03 | 3.8106E+04 | 3.8191E+04 | 3.8367E+04 | 4.6051E−01 |
| 65.Tb | 1.2748E−03 | 4.0878E+04 | 4.0963E+04 | 4.1197E+04 | 5.7165E−01 |
| 66.Dy | 1.3274E−03 | 3.6928E+04 | 3.7013E+04 | 3.7249E+04 | 6.3851E−01 |
| | 5.9744E−02 | 3.9080E+01 | 5.3435E+01 | 1.0911E+02 | 1.0420E+02 |
| 67.Ho | 1.3802E−03 | 3.2966E+04 | 3.3049E+04 | 3.3275E+04 | 6.8454E−01 |
| | 2.3430E−02 | 3.0614E+02 | 7.2281E+02 | 3.3907E+02 | 1.1317E+02 |
| | 5.9567E−02 | 3.9479E+01 | 5.4034E+01 | 1.1758E+02 | 1.1761E+02 |
| 68.Er | 1.4324E−03 | 2.9051E+04 | 2.9133E+04 | 2.9348E+04 | 7.3931E−01 |
| | 2.5429E−02 | 2.7223E+02 | 6.0763E+02 | 3.0328E+02 | 1.0036E+02 |
| | 5.9519E−02 | 3.9589E+01 | 5.4200E+01 | 1.2612E+02 | 1.3269E+02 |
| 69.Tm | 1.4811E−03 | 2.5399E+04 | 2.5479E+04 | 2.5670E+04 | 7.4956E−01 |
| | 2.6957E−02 | 2.4631E+02 | 5.1956E+02 | 2.7580E+02 | 8.8382E+01 |
| 70.Yb | 1.5628E−03 | 2.2463E+04 | 2.2544E+04 | 2.2741E+04 | 8.7514E−01 |
| 71.Lu | 1.6099E−03 | 2.1328E+04 | 2.1409E+04 | 2.1594E+04 | 8.6576E−01 |
| | 2.8891E−02 | 2.1351E+02 | 4.0812E+02 | 2.4118E+02 | 6.9222E+01 |
| 72.Hf | 1.6624E−03 | 2.0062E+04 | 2.0143E+04 | 2.0280E+04 | 6.8102E−01 |
| | 3.9873E−03 | 1.1753E+04 | 1.2070E+04 | 1.1940E+04 | 1.0853E+00 |
| | 5.4577E−02 | 5.0750E+01 | 7.0964E+01 | 6.0375E+01 | 1.7539E+01 |
| 73.Ta | 1.3151E−03 | 3.7855E+04 | 3.7939E+04 | 3.8044E+04 | 2.7557E−01 |
| 81.Tl | 1.2784E−03 | 4.0611E+04 | 4.0697E+04 | 4.0757E+04 | 1.4802E−01 |
| | 2.8551E−03 | 2.3546E+04 | 2.4323E+04 | 2.4153E+04 | 7.0511E−01 |
| | 3.3452E−03 | 1.9358E+04 | 1.9959E+04 | 1.9833E+04 | 6.3688E−01 |
| 82.Pb | 1.2446E−03 | 4.3144E+04 | 4.3231E+04 | 4.3286E+04 | 1.2867E−01 |
| | 2.8454E−03 | 2.3733E+04 | 2.4517E+04 | 2.4391E+04 | 5.1873E−01 |
| | 3.2932E−03 | 1.9974E+04 | 2.0598E+04 | 2.0522E+04 | 3.7356E−01 |
| 83.Bi | 1.5212E−03 | 2.3466E+04 | 2.3546E+04 | 2.3592E+04 | 1.9451E−01 |
| | 3.9560E−03 | 1.2125E+04 | 1.2455E+04 | 1.2450E+04 | 3.6535E−02 |
| 84.Po | 1.4899E−03 | 2.4735E+04 | 2.4815E+04 | 2.4856E+04 | 1.6367E−01 |
| | 3.9595E−03 | 1.2083E+04 | 1.2412E+04 | 1.2417E+04 | 4.3982E−02 |
| | 4.1137E−03 | 1.1029E+04 | 1.1323E+04 | 1.1334E+04 | 9.8564E−02 |
| 85.At | 1.2631E−03 | 4.1756E+04 | 4.1841E+04 | 4.1896E+04 | 1.2918E−01 |
| | 3.5796E−03 | 1.6582E+04 | 1.7079E+04 | 1.7079E+04 | 4.9175E−03 |

| Material | $E$, MeV | $\mu_{1en}$, cm$^{-1}$ | $\mu_1$, cm$^{-1}$ | $\mu_2$, cm$^{-1}$ | $R$, % |
|---|---|---|---|---|---|
| 87.Fr | 1.0166E−03 | 6.0257E+04 | 6.0349E+04 | 6.0397E+04 | 8.0165E−02 |
| | 1.2776E−03 | 4.0666E+04 | 4.0752E+04 | 4.0802E+04 | 1.2464E−01 |
| 88.Ra | 2.1761E−02 | 3.3445E+02 | 8.1901E+02 | 4.5369E+02 | 8.0520E+01 |
| 112. | 2.6371E−03 | 6.1286E+03 | 6.1962E+03 | 6.1719E+03 | 3.9262E−01 |
| 121. | 1.3902E−03 | 3.2218E+04 | 3.2301E+04 | 3.2433E+04 | 4.1092E−01 |
| 123. | 1.4080E−03 | 3.0882E+04 | 3.0965E+04 | 3.1219E+04 | 8.2058E−01 |
| | 1.5232E−02 | 3.2467E+02 | 3.4483E+02 | 4.7733E+02 | 3.8424E+01 |
| 130. | 2.3424E−03 | 8.8101E+03 | 8.8836E+03 | 8.9219E+03 | 4.3068E−01 |
| 44.RUTHENIUM | | | | | |
| 26.Fe | 1.1460E−03 | 5.8250E+04 | 5.8354E+04 | 5.8459E+04 | 1.7960E−01 |
| | 1.4864E−02 | 4.0429E+02 | 4.2778E+02 | 4.7368E+02 | 1.0731E+01 |
| 27.Co | 9.0000E−03 | 1.6621E+03 | 1.7157E+03 | 2.2646E+03 | 3.1994E+01 |
| 29.Cu | 9.1791E−03 | 1.5746E+03 | 1.6262E+03 | 2.3847E+03 | 4.6638E+01 |
| 30.Zn | 1.3347E−02 | 6.4424E+02 | 6.7372E+02 | 9.3727E+02 | 3.9118E+01 |
| 31.Ga | 1.4177E−03 | 3.4811E+04 | 3.4902E+04 | 3.5123E+04 | 6.3191E−01 |
| | 1.8386E−02 | 2.3924E+02 | 2.5699E+02 | 3.1977E+02 | 2.4429E+01 |
| 32.Ge | 1.4688E−03 | 3.0402E+04 | 3.0491E+04 | 3.0716E+04 | 7.4007E−01 |
| | 2.0176E−02 | 1.6724E+02 | 1.8235E+02 | 2.2208E+02 | 2.1786E+01 |
| 33.As | 1.4637E−03 | 3.0840E+04 | 3.0929E+04 | 3.1223E+04 | 9.5172E−01 |
| | 1.7424E−02 | 2.8002E+02 | 2.9924E+02 | 4.1772E+02 | 3.9593E+01 |
| 34.Se | 2.0421E−03 | 1.3408E+04 | 1.3494E+04 | 1.3566E+04 | 5.2862E−01 |
| | 2.1900E−02 | 1.3278E+02 | 1.4637E+02 | 1.8926E+02 | 2.9298E+01 |
| 39.Y | 2.0834E−02 | 1.5409E+02 | 1.6862E+02 | 2.8949E+02 | 7.1675E+01 |
| 45.Rh | 2.9387E−02 | 2.1936E+02 | 4.2562E+02 | 4.4787E+02 | 5.2256E+00 |
| 46.Pd | 3.9259E−02 | 1.2183E+02 | 1.9570E+02 | 2.1048E+02 | 7.5536E+00 |
| 47.Ag | 4.5881E−03 | 9.8128E+03 | 1.0097E+04 | 1.0204E+04 | 1.0660E+00 |
| 48.Cd | 2.7299E−03 | 6.8032E+03 | 6.8771E+03 | 6.8600E+03 | 2.4980E−01 |
| 57.La | 1.4570E−03 | 3.1418E+04 | 3.1507E+04 | 3.1527E+04 | 6.1661E−02 |
| | 1.4285E−02 | 4.9587E+02 | 5.2165E+02 | 5.2806E+02 | 1.2273E+00 |
| 58.Ce | 1.3683E−03 | 3.9073E+04 | 3.9167E+04 | 3.9212E+04 | 1.1518E−01 |
| | 7.3747E−03 | 2.9258E+03 | 3.0094E+03 | 3.1777E+03 | 5.5915E+00 |
| 59.Pr | 6.9365E−03 | 3.4692E+03 | 3.5660E+03 | 3.8055E+03 | 6.7160E+00 |
| 61.Pm | 1.3120E−03 | 4.3930E+04 | 4.4027E+04 | 4.4143E+04 | 2.6506E−01 |
| | 7.0776E−03 | 3.2942E+03 | 3.3867E+03 | 3.6693E+03 | 8.3422E+00 |
| 62.Sm | 1.2497E−03 | 4.9310E+04 | 4.9409E+04 | 4.9579E+04 | 3.4327E−01 |
| 63.Eu | 8.3914E−03 | 1.9594E+03 | 2.0197E+03 | 2.1988E+03 | 8.8700E+00 |
| 64.Gd | 1.3739E−03 | 3.8588E+04 | 3.8681E+04 | 3.8848E+04 | 4.3322E−01 |
| 65.Tb | 7.6542E−03 | 2.5793E+03 | 2.6544E+03 | 2.8855E+03 | 8.7082E+00 |
| 67.Ho | 1.3879E−03 | 3.7382E+04 | 3.7474E+04 | 3.7738E+04 | 7.0407E−01 |

| Material | $E$, MeV | $\mu_{1en}$, cm$^{-1}$ | $\mu_1$, cm$^{-1}$ | $\mu_2$, cm$^{-1}$ | $R$, % |
|---|---|---|---|---|---|
| | 2.2651E−02 | 3.2657E+02 | 8.2189E+02 | 3.6153E+02 | 1.2734E+02 |
| 68.Er | 1.4404E−03 | 3.2849E+04 | 3.2939E+04 | 3.3193E+04 | 7.7002E−01 |
| | 2.4595E−02 | 2.9564E+02 | 7.0756E+02 | 3.2917E+02 | 1.1495E+02 |
| 69.Tm | 1.4870E−03 | 2.8830E+04 | 2.8917E+04 | 2.9148E+04 | 7.9849E−01 |
| | 2.6125E−02 | 2.7129E+02 | 6.1755E+02 | 3.0362E+02 | 1.0340E+02 |
| 70.Yb | 1.5750E−03 | 2.5627E+04 | 2.5714E+04 | 2.5952E+04 | 9.2477E−01 |
| | 9.4996E−03 | 1.4180E+03 | 1.4661E+03 | 1.6643E+03 | 1.3514E+01 |
| 71.Lu | 1.6185E−03 | 2.4417E+04 | 2.4504E+04 | 2.4734E+04 | 9.3670E−01 |
| | 2.8113E−02 | 2.3963E+02 | 5.0055E+02 | 2.7069E+02 | 8.4918E+01 |
| 72.Hf | 1.6712E−03 | 2.2952E+04 | 2.3039E+04 | 2.3226E+04 | 8.1073E−01 |
| | 3.0502E−03 | 2.2643E+04 | 2.3458E+04 | 2.2943E+04 | 2.2428E+00 |
| | 3.9707E−02 | 1.1759E+02 | 1.8633E+02 | 1.3516E+02 | 3.7857E+01 |
| 80.Hg | 1.3902E−03 | 3.7186E+04 | 3.7278E+04 | 3.7362E+04 | 2.2487E−01 |
| 81.Tl | 1.8719E−03 | 1.7374E+04 | 1.7461E+04 | 1.7515E+04 | 3.0794E−01 |
| | 2.2073E−03 | 1.1822E+04 | 1.1905E+04 | 1.1957E+04 | 4.4067E−01 |
| | 2.9858E−03 | 2.5310E+04 | 2.6246E+04 | 2.5946E+04 | 1.1550E+00 |
| | 3.7415E−03 | 1.6284E+04 | 1.6809E+04 | 1.6662E+04 | 8.8465E−01 |
| 82.Pb | 1.8155E−03 | 1.8942E+04 | 1.9029E+04 | 1.9071E+04 | 2.2161E−01 |
| | 2.3683E−03 | 1.0276E+04 | 1.0356E+04 | 1.0401E+04 | 4.3829E−01 |
| 83.Bi | 6.4981E−03 | 4.0127E+03 | 4.1229E+03 | 4.1309E+03 | 1.9483E−01 |
| | 1.2347E−02 | 8.0236E+02 | 8.3579E+02 | 8.4988E+02 | 1.6856E+00 |
| | 5.2246E−02 | 6.2392E+01 | 8.9709E+01 | 7.4782E+01 | 1.9960E+01 |
| 84.Po | 6.4178E−03 | 4.1122E+03 | 4.2248E+03 | 4.2347E+03 | 2.3503E−01 |
| | 1.3172E−02 | 6.7198E+02 | 7.0215E+02 | 7.1512E+02 | 1.8465E+00 |
| | 5.2989E−02 | 6.0546E+01 | 8.6846E+01 | 7.2832E+01 | 1.9242E+01 |
| 85.At | 1.6748E−03 | 2.2853E+04 | 2.2940E+04 | 2.2990E+04 | 2.1637E−01 |
| 87.Fr | 1.4799E−03 | 2.9444E+04 | 2.9532E+04 | 2.9575E+04 | 1.4463E−01 |
| 89.Ac | 1.4052E−03 | 3.5886E+04 | 3.5978E+04 | 3.6021E+04 | 1.2081E−01 |
| 91.Pa | 3.5081E−03 | 1.9077E+04 | 1.9718E+04 | 1.9769E+04 | 2.6004E−01 |
| 121. | 1.4464E−03 | 3.2334E+04 | 3.2424E+04 | 3.2550E+04 | 3.8931E−01 |
| 123. | 2.0157E−02 | 1.6762E+02 | 1.8274E+02 | 2.2371E+02 | 2.2417E+01 |
| 125. | 2.5252E−03 | 8.7687E+03 | 8.8462E+03 | 8.9887E+03 | 1.6106E+00 |
| | 1.4202E−02 | 5.0898E+02 | 5.3508E+02 | 6.3029E+02 | 1.7794E+01 |
| 130. | 2.3770E−03 | 1.0192E+04 | 1.0272E+04 | 1.0347E+04 | 7.3254E−01 |
| 45.RHODIUM | | | | | |
| 26.Fe | 2.0819E−02 | 1.6806E+02 | 1.8332E+02 | 1.9092E+02 | 4.1449E+00 |
| 27.Co | 2.9711E−03 | 5.7138E+03 | 5.7874E+03 | 5.7547E+03 | 5.6759E−01 |
| | 1.0202E−02 | 1.2254E+03 | 1.2716E+03 | 1.5946E+03 | 2.5399E+01 |
| 28.Ni | 9.3075E−03 | 1.6214E+03 | 1.6771E+03 | 2.3057E+03 | 3.7476E+01 |

| Material | $E$, MeV | $\mu_{1en}$, cm$^{-1}$ | $\mu_1$, cm$^{-1}$ | $\mu_2$, cm$^{-1}$ | $R$, % |
|---|---|---|---|---|---|
| 29.Cu | 9.6874E−03 | 1.4229E+03 | 1.4740E+03 | 2.1059E+03 | 4.2873E+01 |
| 30.Zn | 1.4469E−02 | 5.0222E+02 | 5.2897E+02 | 6.9404E+02 | 3.1206E+01 |
| 31.Ga | 2.0452E−02 | 1.7527E+02 | 1.9087E+02 | 2.2484E+02 | 1.7801E+01 |
| 32.Ge | 2.1714E−02 | 1.5044E+02 | 1.6489E+02 | 1.9885E+02 | 2.0595E+01 |
| 33.As | 1.9478E−02 | 2.0796E+02 | 2.2484E+02 | 2.9316E+02 | 3.0384E+01 |
| 39.Y | 2.3470E−03 | 1.1668E+04 | 1.1750E+04 | 1.1933E+04 | 1.5562E+00 |
| | 2.2141E−02 | 1.4205E+02 | 1.5611E+02 | 2.6306E+02 | 6.8506E+01 |
| 40.Zr | 1.8176E−02 | 2.6738E+02 | 2.8643E+02 | 6.0319E+02 | 1.1059E+02 |
| 43.Tc | 3.2251E−03 | 2.0780E+04 | 2.1596E+04 | 2.1435E+04 | 7.5176E−01 |
| | 2.4739E−02 | 2.8393E+02 | 7.1022E+02 | 6.4737E+02 | 9.7083E+00 |
| 44.Ru | 2.9387E−02 | 2.1936E+02 | 4.4787E+02 | 4.2562E+02 | 5.2256E+00 |
| 46.Pd | 3.3466E−03 | 1.8990E+04 | 1.9714E+04 | 1.9788E+04 | 3.7604E−01 |
| | 3.8501E−03 | 1.5746E+04 | 1.6294E+04 | 1.6365E+04 | 4.3460E−01 |
| 47.Ag | 2.1698E−02 | 1.5077E+02 | 1.6523E+02 | 1.6422E+02 | 6.1367E−01 |
| 57.La | 1.9332E−03 | 1.6990E+04 | 1.7076E+04 | 1.7062E+04 | 8.3461E−02 |
| | 2.0768E−02 | 1.6905E+02 | 1.8436E+02 | 1.8217E+02 | 1.2017E+00 |
| 58.Ce | 8.1350E−03 | 2.2340E+03 | 2.3043E+03 | 2.4102E+03 | 4.5976E+00 |
| 59.Pr | 1.3837E−03 | 4.0818E+04 | 4.0911E+04 | 4.0983E+04 | 1.7664E−01 |
| | 7.6188E−03 | 2.8078E+03 | 2.8935E+03 | 3.0644E+03 | 5.9062E+00 |
| 60.Nd | 1.3871E−03 | 4.0505E+04 | 4.0598E+04 | 4.0684E+04 | 2.1204E−01 |
| | 7.2665E−03 | 3.2731E+03 | 3.3714E+03 | 3.6089E+03 | 7.0441E+00 |
| 62.Sm | 1.3697E−03 | 4.2123E+04 | 4.2216E+04 | 4.2350E+04 | 3.1621E−01 |
| | 7.4174E−03 | 3.0739E+03 | 3.1668E+03 | 3.4521E+03 | 9.0094E+00 |
| 63.Eu | 1.1668E−02 | 9.7699E+02 | 1.0165E+03 | 1.0775E+03 | 6.0025E+00 |
| 64.Gd | 1.4051E−03 | 3.8829E+04 | 3.8921E+04 | 3.9090E+04 | 4.3452E−01 |
| 65.Tb | 1.3106E−03 | 4.7604E+04 | 4.7700E+04 | 4.7982E+04 | 5.8988E−01 |
| | 7.9858E−03 | 2.3233E+03 | 2.3958E+03 | 2.5908E+03 | 8.1379E+00 |
| | 8.0396E−03 | 2.2838E+03 | 2.3553E+03 | 2.5455E+03 | 8.0737E+00 |
| 67.Ho | 2.3756E−02 | 2.9759E+02 | 7.6573E+02 | 3.2968E+02 | 1.3226E+02 |
| 68.Er | 1.4452E−03 | 3.5106E+04 | 3.5195E+04 | 3.5477E+04 | 7.9894E−01 |
| | 2.5279E−02 | 2.7643E+02 | 6.7973E+02 | 3.0792E+02 | 1.2075E+02 |
| 69.Tm | 1.4906E−03 | 3.0890E+04 | 3.0978E+04 | 3.1237E+04 | 8.3615E−01 |
| | 2.6534E−02 | 2.5899E+02 | 6.0888E+02 | 2.8992E+02 | 1.1001E+02 |
| 71.Lu | 1.6229E−03 | 2.6322E+04 | 2.6409E+04 | 2.6667E+04 | 9.7837E−01 |
| | 2.8244E−02 | 2.3524E+02 | 5.1237E+02 | 2.6572E+02 | 9.2822E+01 |
| 72.Hf | 1.6766E−03 | 2.4709E+04 | 2.4796E+04 | 2.5016E+04 | 8.9060E−01 |
| | 3.2629E−03 | 2.0171E+04 | 2.0962E+04 | 2.0445E+04 | 2.5262E+00 |
| | 3.8887E−02 | 1.2846E+02 | 2.1628E+02 | 1.4733E+02 | 4.6798E+01 |
| 74.W | 1.3955E−03 | 3.9720E+04 | 3.9812E+04 | 3.9936E+04 | 3.1216E−01 |

| Material | $E$, MeV | $\mu_{1en}$, cm$^{-1}$ | $\mu_1$, cm$^{-1}$ | $\mu_2$, cm$^{-1}$ | $R$, % |
|---|---|---|---|---|---|
| 80.Hg | 1.7251E−03 | 2.3249E+04 | 2.3336E+04 | 2.3419E+04 | 3.5644E−01 |
| | 2.1995E−03 | 1.3075E+04 | 1.3159E+04 | 1.3231E+04 | 5.4742E−01 |
| 81.Tl | 4.5171E−03 | 1.0889E+04 | 1.1240E+04 | 1.1143E+04 | 8.7012E−01 |
| | 1.2042E−02 | 9.1362E+02 | 9.5145E+02 | 9.6863E+02 | 1.8053E+00 |
| 82.Pb | 4.5613E−03 | 1.0618E+04 | 1.0959E+04 | 1.0882E+04 | 7.1004E−01 |
| | 1.2497E−02 | 8.3650E+02 | 8.7226E+02 | 8.8862E+02 | 1.8761E+00 |
| 83.Bi | 9.8484E−03 | 1.3388E+03 | 1.3879E+03 | 1.4008E+03 | 9.3260E−01 |
| | 1.0200E−02 | 1.2257E+03 | 1.2719E+03 | 1.2850E+03 | 1.0288E+00 |
| | 4.6218E−02 | 8.8713E+01 | 1.3766E+02 | 1.0589E+02 | 2.9996E+01 |
| 84.Po | 9.7062E−03 | 1.4131E+03 | 1.4639E+03 | 1.4760E+03 | 8.2857E−01 |
| | 1.0558E−02 | 1.1651E+03 | 1.2097E+03 | 1.2218E+03 | 1.0030E+00 |
| | 4.6218E−02 | 8.8713E+01 | 1.3766E+02 | 1.0631E+02 | 2.9481E+01 |
| 85.At | 4.9232E−03 | 8.4068E+03 | 8.6642E+03 | 8.6445E+03 | 2.2724E−01 |
| 87.Fr | 1.8839E−03 | 1.8472E+04 | 1.8559E+04 | 1.8602E+04 | 2.3239E−01 |
| | 3.0480E−03 | 1.7437E+04 | 1.8067E+04 | 1.8019E+04 | 2.6223E−01 |
| | 4.8211E−03 | 9.0309E+03 | 9.3120E+03 | 9.3071E+03 | 5.2054E−02 |
| 89.Ac | 1.4780E−03 | 3.2060E+04 | 3.2148E+04 | 3.2192E+04 | 1.3658E−01 |
| 90.Th | 1.0276E−03 | 7.3878E+04 | 7.3989E+04 | 7.4042E+04 | 7.2667E−02 |
| | 1.3222E−03 | 4.6530E+04 | 4.6626E+04 | 4.6684E+04 | 1.2373E−01 |
| | 3.7251E−03 | 1.7163E+04 | 1.7774E+04 | 1.7823E+04 | 2.7833E−01 |
| | 4.0433E−03 | 1.3784E+04 | 1.4245E+04 | 1.4289E+04 | 3.0787E−01 |
| 121. | 1.4744E−03 | 3.2393E+04 | 3.2481E+04 | 3.2608E+04 | 3.9291E−01 |
| 123. | 2.1695E−02 | 1.5082E+02 | 1.6529E+02 | 2.0035E+02 | 2.1212E+01 |
| 125. | 2.5653E−03 | 9.5854E+03 | 9.6646E+03 | 9.8306E+03 | 1.7179E+00 |
| | 1.4705E−02 | 4.6227E+02 | 4.8794E+02 | 5.6852E+02 | 1.6514E+01 |
| 130. | 2.4603E−03 | 1.0587E+04 | 1.0668E+04 | 1.0769E+04 | 9.5318E−01 |

46.PALLADIUM

| Material | $E$, MeV | $\mu_{1en}$, cm$^{-1}$ | $\mu_1$, cm$^{-1}$ | $\mu_2$, cm$^{-1}$ | $R$, % |
|---|---|---|---|---|---|
| 26.Fe | 2.1698E−02 | 1.5743E+02 | 1.7194E+02 | 1.7881E+02 | 3.9938E+00 |
| 27.Co | 2.6171E−03 | 9.3764E+03 | 9.4546E+03 | 9.4284E+03 | 2.7820E−01 |
| | 3.1421E−03 | 4.9990E+03 | 5.0706E+03 | 5.0377E+03 | 6.5325E−01 |
| | 1.2120E−02 | 9.1980E+02 | 9.5789E+02 | 1.1778E+03 | 2.2960E+01 |
| 28.Ni | 9.5247E−03 | 1.5384E+03 | 1.5933E+03 | 2.1661E+03 | 3.5948E+01 |
| 29.Cu | 9.8127E−03 | 1.3856E+03 | 1.4363E+03 | 2.0372E+03 | 4.1833E+01 |
| 30.Zn | 1.2446E−03 | 5.5200E+04 | 5.5303E+04 | 5.5645E+04 | 6.1902E−01 |
| | 1.4719E−02 | 4.7065E+02 | 4.9650E+02 | 6.3997E+02 | 2.8897E+01 |
| 31.Ga | 2.1229E−02 | 1.6611E+02 | 1.8102E+02 | 2.1271E+02 | 1.7503E+01 |
| 32.Ge | 2.2597E−02 | 1.4079E+02 | 1.5451E+02 | 1.8551E+02 | 2.0063E+01 |
| 33.As | 1.9928E−02 | 1.9218E+02 | 2.0829E+02 | 2.6587E+02 | 2.7644E+01 |
| 34.Se | 2.4225E−02 | 1.1068E+02 | 1.2298E+02 | 1.5554E+02 | 2.6481E+01 |

| Material | $E$, MeV | $\mu_{1en}$, cm$^{-1}$ | $\mu_1$, cm$^{-1}$ | $\mu_2$, cm$^{-1}$ | $R$, % |
|---|---|---|---|---|---|
| 39.Y | 2.2292E−03 | 1.3192E+04 | 1.3274E+04 | 1.3505E+04 | 1.7409E+00 |
| | 2.2915E−02 | 1.3491E+02 | 1.4835E+02 | 2.4739E+02 | 6.6760E+01 |
| 40.Zr | 1.8419E−02 | 2.6257E+02 | 2.8126E+02 | 5.8555E+02 | 1.0819E+02 |
| 42.Mo | 2.4564E−02 | 2.6295E+02 | 6.9788E+02 | 5.7852E+02 | 2.0632E+01 |
| 43.Tc | 2.8923E−02 | 2.1297E+02 | 4.7225E+02 | 4.0627E+02 | 1.6241E+01 |
| 44.Ru | 3.9259E−02 | 1.2183E+02 | 2.1048E+02 | 1.9570E+02 | 7.5536E+00 |
| 45.Rh | 3.3466E−03 | 1.8990E+04 | 1.9788E+04 | 1.9714E+04 | 3.7604E−01 |
| 45.Rh | 3.8501E−03 | 1.5746E+04 | 1.6365E+04 | 1.6294E+04 | 4.3460E−01 |
| 57.La | 2.8870E−03 | 6.7225E+03 | 6.7981E+03 | 6.7721E+03 | 3.8289E−01 |
| | 2.1629E−02 | 1.5871E+02 | 1.7328E+02 | 1.7123E+02 | 1.1968E+00 |
| 58.Ce | 1.4422E−03 | 3.6399E+04 | 3.6496E+04 | 3.6531E+04 | 9.4263E−02 |
| | 9.6807E−03 | 1.4556E+03 | 1.5083E+03 | 1.5613E+03 | 3.5189E+00 |
| 59.Pr | 1.4151E−03 | 3.8980E+04 | 3.9078E+04 | 3.9138E+04 | 1.5412E−01 |
| | 7.7518E−03 | 2.6790E+03 | 2.7662E+03 | 2.9200E+03 | 5.5611E+00 |
| 60.Nd | 7.4047E−03 | 3.1424E+03 | 3.2440E+03 | 3.4612E+03 | 6.6928E+00 |
| 62.Sm | 1.4047E−03 | 3.9974E+04 | 4.0072E+04 | 4.0188E+04 | 2.8909E−01 |
| | 7.5498E−03 | 2.9487E+03 | 3.0443E+03 | 3.3222E+03 | 9.1293E+00 |
| 63.Eu | 1.3563E−02 | 6.7038E+02 | 7.0167E+02 | 7.3566E+02 | 4.8444E+00 |
| 64.Gd | 1.4158E−03 | 3.8912E+04 | 3.9010E+04 | 3.9173E+04 | 4.1661E−01 |
| 65.Tb | 1.3287E−03 | 4.7203E+04 | 4.7303E+04 | 4.7576E+04 | 5.7657E−01 |
| 66.Dy | 7.8159E−03 | 2.5934E+03 | 2.6779E+03 | 2.9210E+03 | 9.0761E+00 |
| 67.Ho | 2.5474E−02 | 2.5252E+02 | 6.5078E+02 | 2.8013E+02 | 1.3231E+02 |
| 68.Er | 1.4470E−03 | 3.5946E+04 | 3.6044E+04 | 3.6327E+04 | 7.8666E−01 |
| | 2.6586E−02 | 2.3976E+02 | 5.9322E+02 | 2.6735E+02 | 1.2188E+02 |
| 69.Tm | 1.4920E−03 | 3.1667E+04 | 3.1763E+04 | 3.2024E+04 | 8.2041E−01 |
| | 2.7540E−02 | 2.2883E+02 | 5.4384E+02 | 2.5633E+02 | 1.1217E+02 |
| 71.Lu | 1.6246E−03 | 2.7051E+04 | 2.7144E+04 | 2.7407E+04 | 9.6920E−01 |
| | 2.8899E−02 | 2.1324E+02 | 4.7350E+02 | 2.4087E+02 | 9.6577E+01 |
| 72.Hf | 1.6786E−03 | 2.5382E+04 | 2.5474E+04 | 2.5703E+04 | 8.9845E−01 |
| | 3.9615E−02 | 1.1880E+02 | 2.0256E+02 | 1.3652E+02 | 4.8374E+01 |
| 73.Ta | 1.7359E−03 | 2.3611E+04 | 2.3701E+04 | 2.3883E+04 | 7.6716E−01 |
| 74.W | 1.4639E−03 | 3.4341E+04 | 3.4438E+04 | 3.4555E+04 | 3.3876E−01 |
| | 1.7397E−03 | 2.3493E+04 | 2.3583E+04 | 2.3705E+04 | 5.1689E−01 |
| 80.Hg | 1.8943E−03 | 1.8714E+04 | 1.8801E+04 | 1.8880E+04 | 4.1904E−01 |
| | 2.1029E−03 | 1.4433E+04 | 1.4517E+04 | 1.4593E+04 | 5.2449E−01 |
| 81.Tl | 4.8698E−03 | 8.8422E+03 | 9.1469E+03 | 9.0547E+03 | 1.0178E+00 |
| | 1.1759E−02 | 9.8210E+02 | 1.0219E+03 | 1.0389E+03 | 1.6648E+00 |
| 82.Pb | 4.8819E−03 | 8.7673E+03 | 9.0687E+03 | 8.9877E+03 | 9.0059E−01 |
| | 1.2189E−02 | 9.0782E+02 | 9.4558E+02 | 9.6177E+02 | 1.7115E+00 |

| Material | $E$, MeV | $\mu_{1en}$, cm$^{-1}$ | $\mu_1$, cm$^{-1}$ | $\mu_2$, cm$^{-1}$ | $R$, % |
|---|---|---|---|---|---|
| 83.Bi | 4.7866E−02 | 7.9802E+01 | 1.2507E+02 | 9.5336E+01 | 3.1193E+01 |
| 84.Po | 4.7910E−02 | 7.9603E+01 | 1.2469E+02 | 9.5450E+01 | 3.0632E+01 |
| 85.At | 5.0987E−03 | 7.7409E+03 | 7.9993E+03 | 7.9597E+03 | 4.9824E−01 |
| 87.Fr | 1.9915E−03 | 1.5707E+04 | 1.5792E+04 | 1.5837E+04 | 2.8912E−01 |
| | 4.8855E−03 | 8.7455E+03 | 9.0459E+03 | 9.0126E+03 | 3.6876E−01 |
| 88.Ra | 2.5199E−02 | 2.5567E+02 | 6.6503E+02 | 3.4083E+02 | 9.5121E+01 |
| 89.Ac | 1.5000E−03 | 3.0907E+04 | 3.1003E+04 | 3.1037E+04 | 1.1209E−01 |
| | 4.7163E−03 | 9.7889E+03 | 1.0135E+04 | 1.0120E+04 | 1.4527E−01 |
| 90.Th | 1.3353E−03 | 4.6574E+04 | 4.6674E+04 | 4.6737E+04 | 1.3619E−01 |
| | 3.9251E−03 | 1.4977E+04 | 1.5557E+04 | 1.5541E+04 | 1.0281E−01 |
| 121. | 1.4841E−03 | 3.2413E+04 | 3.2509E+04 | 3.2629E+04 | 3.6672E−01 |
| 123. | 2.2575E−02 | 1.4121E+02 | 1.5495E+02 | 1.8699E+02 | 2.0673E+01 |
| 125. | 2.5761E−03 | 9.7801E+03 | 9.8587E+03 | 1.0030E+04 | 1.7427E+00 |
| | 1.4840E−02 | 4.4976E+02 | 4.7503E+02 | 5.5197E+02 | 1.6197E+01 |
| 130. | 2.5267E−03 | 1.0266E+04 | 1.0345E+04 | 1.0447E+04 | 9.7902E−01 |
| | | | 47.SILVER | | |
| 25.Mn | 2.4852E−02 | 1.0021E+02 | 1.1116E+02 | 1.1207E+02 | 8.1259E−01 |
| 26.Fe | 2.0006E−02 | 1.7788E+02 | 1.9268E+02 | 2.0213E+02 | 4.9001E+00 |
| 27.Co | 9.4356E−03 | 1.4859E+03 | 1.5404E+03 | 1.9919E+03 | 2.9311E+01 |
| 28.Ni | 8.6679E−03 | 1.8659E+03 | 1.9317E+03 | 2.7169E+03 | 4.0646E+01 |
| 29.Cu | 9.3737E−03 | 1.5165E+03 | 1.5719E+03 | 2.2779E+03 | 4.4914E+01 |
| 30.Zn | 1.3921E−02 | 5.7157E+02 | 5.9948E+02 | 8.1280E+02 | 3.5584E+01 |
| 31.Ga | 1.4797E−03 | 3.1020E+04 | 3.1105E+04 | 3.1288E+04 | 5.8906E−01 |
| | 2.4367E−03 | 1.0566E+04 | 1.0642E+04 | 1.0648E+04 | 5.9410E−02 |
| | 3.1490E−03 | 4.7714E+03 | 4.8363E+03 | 4.8133E+03 | 4.7593E−01 |
| | 1.9648E−02 | 1.9339E+02 | 2.0877E+02 | 2.5107E+02 | 2.0265E+01 |
| 32.Ge | 3.2501E−03 | 4.3946E+03 | 4.4585E+03 | 4.4358E+03 | 5.1074E−01 |
| | 2.1726E−02 | 1.5031E+02 | 1.6374E+02 | 1.9867E+02 | 2.1329E+01 |
| 33.As | 1.4931E−03 | 2.9828E+04 | 2.9913E+04 | 3.0194E+04 | 9.3910E−01 |
| | 1.5192E−03 | 2.8650E+04 | 2.8734E+04 | 2.8995E+04 | 9.0610E−01 |
| | 1.8657E−02 | 2.3676E+02 | 2.5373E+02 | 3.4294E+02 | 3.5156E+01 |
| 34.Se | 3.3283E−03 | 4.1033E+03 | 4.1665E+03 | 4.1492E+03 | 4.1768E−01 |
| | 2.4160E−02 | 1.1130E+02 | 1.2280E+02 | 1.5649E+02 | 2.7433E+01 |
| 39.Y | 2.2378E−02 | 1.3986E+02 | 1.5278E+02 | 2.5826E+02 | 6.9040E+01 |
| 42.Mo | 2.9496E−02 | 1.7868E+02 | 4.0723E+02 | 3.1422E+02 | 2.9602E+01 |
| 43.Tc | 4.2208E−02 | 9.4809E+01 | 1.6262E+02 | 1.4285E+02 | 1.3842E+01 |
| 44.Ru | 4.5881E−03 | 9.8128E+03 | 1.0204E+04 | 1.0097E+04 | 1.0660E+00 |
| 45.Rh | 2.1698E−02 | 1.5077E+02 | 1.6422E+02 | 1.6523E+02 | 6.1367E−01 |
| 57.La | 1.4987E−03 | 2.9328E+04 | 2.9412E+04 | 2.9433E+04 | 7.0303E−02 |

| Material | $E$, MeV | $\mu_{1en}$, cm$^{-1}$ | $\mu_1$, cm$^{-1}$ | $\mu_2$, cm$^{-1}$ | $R$, % |
|---|---|---|---|---|---|
| | 1.9813E−02 | 1.8614E+02 | 2.0125E+02 | 2.0024E+02 | 5.0596E−01 |
| 58.Ce | 1.4290E−03 | 3.5546E+04 | 3.5633E+04 | 3.5680E+04 | 1.3121E−01 |
| | 7.5679E−03 | 2.7331E+03 | 2.8271E+03 | 2.9635E+03 | 4.8246E+00 |
| 59.Pr | 1.3434E−03 | 4.3175E+04 | 4.3265E+04 | 4.3348E+04 | 1.9101E−01 |
| | 7.1124E−03 | 3.2986E+03 | 3.4120E+03 | 3.6144E+03 | 5.9335E+00 |
| 60.Nd | 1.3226E−03 | 4.5032E+04 | 4.5123E+04 | 4.5232E+04 | 2.4115E−01 |
| 61.Pm | 7.3121E−03 | 3.0507E+03 | 3.1556E+03 | 3.3995E+03 | 7.7318E+00 |
| 62.Sm | 1.3234E−03 | 4.4960E+04 | 4.5051E+04 | 4.5203E+04 | 3.3733E−01 |
| 63.Eu | 1.4975E−03 | 2.9431E+04 | 2.9515E+04 | 2.9611E+04 | 3.2353E−01 |
| | 1.5099E−03 | 2.8923E+04 | 2.9007E+04 | 2.9099E+04 | 3.1712E−01 |
| | 9.2252E−03 | 1.5900E+03 | 1.6476E+03 | 1.7736E+03 | 7.6435E+00 |
| 64.Gd | 1.3932E−03 | 3.8737E+04 | 3.8825E+04 | 3.8997E+04 | 4.4357E−01 |
| 65.Tb | 1.2882E−03 | 4.8102E+04 | 4.8195E+04 | 4.8485E+04 | 6.0274E−01 |
| 65.Tb | 7.7535E−03 | 2.5027E+03 | 2.5888E+03 | 2.7973E+03 | 8.0546E+00 |
| | 2.5853E−02 | 2.1031E+02 | 5.6676E+02 | 2.3185E+02 | 1.4445E+02 |
| 66.Dy | 2.6862E−02 | 2.0155E+02 | 5.2258E+02 | 2.2319E+02 | 1.3414E+02 |
| 67.Ho | 1.3907E−03 | 3.8963E+04 | 3.9051E+04 | 3.9336E+04 | 7.2850E−01 |
| | 2.7691E−02 | 1.9435E+02 | 4.8626E+02 | 2.1619E+02 | 1.2492E+02 |
| 68.Er | 1.4434E−03 | 3.4257E+04 | 3.4343E+04 | 3.4617E+04 | 7.9812E−01 |
| | 2.8435E−02 | 1.8789E+02 | 4.5370E+02 | 2.0997E+02 | 1.1608E+02 |
| 69.Tm | 1.4894E−03 | 3.0161E+04 | 3.0245E+04 | 3.0497E+04 | 8.3343E−01 |
| | 2.9095E−02 | 1.8216E+02 | 4.2477E+02 | 2.0435E+02 | 1.0786E+02 |
| | 5.9617E−02 | 4.2204E+01 | 6.2021E+01 | 1.1911E+02 | 9.2054E+01 |
| 70.Yb | 9.7400E−03 | 1.3352E+03 | 1.3852E+03 | 1.5477E+03 | 1.1730E+01 |
| | 2.5643E−02 | 2.1214E+02 | 5.7595E+02 | 2.3840E+02 | 1.4159E+02 |
| 71.Lu | 1.6214E−03 | 2.5669E+04 | 2.5753E+04 | 2.6005E+04 | 9.7609E−01 |
| | 3.0791E−02 | 1.6871E+02 | 3.6896E+02 | 1.9069E+02 | 9.3487E+01 |
| 72.Hf | 1.6747E−03 | 2.4114E+04 | 2.4198E+04 | 2.4410E+04 | 8.7692E−01 |
| | 4.8492E−02 | 6.9715E+01 | 1.1144E+02 | 8.1644E+01 | 3.6500E+01 |
| 74.W | 1.2818E−03 | 4.8667E+04 | 4.8761E+04 | 4.8888E+04 | 2.6159E−01 |
| 80.Hg | 1.4959E−03 | 2.9577E+04 | 2.9661E+04 | 2.9753E+04 | 3.1009E−01 |
| | 2.2635E−03 | 1.2176E+04 | 1.2256E+04 | 1.2331E+04 | 6.1057E−01 |
| 81.Tl | 1.2510E−02 | 8.0010E+02 | 8.3460E+02 | 8.5214E+02 | 2.1014E+00 |
| 82.Pb | 1.2987E−02 | 7.2284E+02 | 7.5511E+02 | 7.7204E+02 | 2.2421E+00 |
| 83.Bi | 7.3199E−03 | 3.0410E+03 | 3.1455E+03 | 3.1388E+03 | 2.1398E−01 |
| | 1.1664E−02 | 9.3699E+02 | 9.7543E+02 | 9.8826E+02 | 1.3155E+00 |
| 84.Po | 7.2349E−03 | 3.1466E+03 | 3.2547E+03 | 3.2482E+03 | 2.0045E−01 |
| | 1.2388E−02 | 8.1986E+02 | 8.5493E+02 | 8.6708E+02 | 1.4213E+00 |
| 85.At | 1.9567E−03 | 1.5889E+04 | 1.5973E+04 | 1.6020E+04 | 2.9339E−01 |

| Material | $E$, MeV | $\mu_{1en}$, cm$^{-1}$ | $\mu_1$, cm$^{-1}$ | $\mu_2$, cm$^{-1}$ | $R$, % |
|---|---|---|---|---|---|
| | 2.3885E−03 | 1.1013E+04 | 1.1090E+04 | 1.1135E+04 | 4.0160E−01 |
| 87.Fr | 1.7525E−03 | 2.1846E+04 | 2.1930E+04 | 2.1976E+04 | 2.0976E−01 |
| 88.Ra | 2.7987E−02 | 1.9178E+02 | 4.7330E+02 | 2.4929E+02 | 8.9858E+01 |
| 89.Ac | 1.4537E−03 | 3.3337E+04 | 3.3423E+04 | 3.3470E+04 | 1.4058E−01 |
| 90.Th | 1.1232E−03 | 6.2818E+04 | 6.2918E+04 | 6.2983E+04 | 1.0214E−01 |
| 121. | 1.4646E−03 | 3.2372E+04 | 3.2458E+04 | 3.2588E+04 | 4.0137E−01 |
| 123. | 3.2209E−03 | 4.5036E+03 | 4.5677E+03 | 4.5462E+03 | 4.7392E−01 |
| | 2.1693E−02 | 1.5085E+02 | 1.6431E+02 | 2.0038E+02 | 2.1957E+01 |
| 125. | 2.5574E−03 | 9.4427E+03 | 9.5168E+03 | 9.6841E+03 | 1.7579E+00 |
| | 1.4450E−02 | 4.8597E+02 | 5.1143E+02 | 5.9987E+02 | 1.7293E+01 |
| 130. | 2.4062E−03 | 1.0849E+04 | 1.0926E+04 | 1.1033E+04 | 9.8006E−01 |
| 48.CADMIUM | | | | | |
| 24.Cr | 2.5773E−02 | 7.9987E+01 | 8.8768E+01 | 8.8525E+01 | 2.7354E−01 |
| 25.Mn | 2.1476E−02 | 1.3480E+02 | 1.4632E+02 | 1.5073E+02 | 3.0147E+00 |
| 26.Fe | 2.2177E−03 | 1.0928E+04 | 1.0987E+04 | 1.0972E+04 | 1.4065E−01 |
| | 3.4580E−03 | 3.2768E+03 | 3.3277E+03 | 3.3055E+03 | 6.7345E−01 |
| 26.Fe | 9.1443E−03 | 1.3970E+03 | 1.4499E+03 | 1.7981E+03 | 2.4020E+01 |
| 30.Zn | 1.0610E−03 | 5.8826E+04 | 5.8912E+04 | 5.9336E+04 | 7.2068E−01 |
| | 9.8453E−03 | 1.1008E+03 | 1.1436E+03 | 1.7290E+03 | 5.1181E+01 |
| 31.Ga | 1.4554E−02 | 4.0376E+02 | 4.2520E+02 | 5.8140E+02 | 3.6737E+01 |
| 32.Ge | 1.6813E−02 | 2.7360E+02 | 2.9057E+02 | 3.9200E+02 | 3.4907E+01 |
| 33.As | 1.3971E−03 | 3.3137E+04 | 3.3216E+04 | 3.3560E+04 | 1.0353E+00 |
| | 1.4673E−02 | 3.8727E+02 | 4.0820E+02 | 6.1304E+02 | 5.0181E+01 |
| 34.Se | 2.0856E−02 | 1.4270E+02 | 1.5462E+02 | 2.0440E+02 | 3.2198E+01 |
| 39.Y | 1.9625E−02 | 1.6772E+02 | 1.8071E+02 | 3.2576E+02 | 8.0268E+01 |
| 41.Nb | 3.2193E−02 | 1.2626E+02 | 2.8798E+02 | 2.0136E+02 | 4.3020E+01 |
| 42.Mo | 4.8166E−02 | 5.8761E+01 | 9.7284E+01 | 8.2985E+01 | 1.7231E+01 |
| 43.Tc | 7.9919E−03 | 1.8891E+03 | 1.9586E+03 | 1.9444E+03 | 7.2709E−01 |
| 44.Ru | 2.7299E−03 | 6.8032E+03 | 6.8600E+03 | 6.8771E+03 | 2.4980E−01 |
| 50.Sn | 3.3232E−03 | 3.6743E+03 | 3.7265E+03 | 3.7200E+03 | 1.7572E−01 |
| | 2.3387E−02 | 1.1042E+02 | 1.2072E+02 | 1.2001E+02 | 5.9590E−01 |
| 51.Sb | 3.4250E−03 | 3.3741E+03 | 3.4254E+03 | 3.4158E+03 | 2.7972E−01 |
| | 2.4004E−02 | 1.0255E+02 | 1.1245E+02 | 1.1143E+02 | 9.1561E−01 |
| 52.Te | 2.5043E−02 | 8.9295E+01 | 9.8540E+01 | 9.7202E+01 | 1.3766E+00 |
| 57.La | 6.4737E−03 | 3.4945E+03 | 3.6258E+03 | 3.7911E+03 | 4.5607E+00 |
| 58.Ce | 1.0181E−03 | 6.2111E+04 | 6.2198E+04 | 6.2318E+04 | 1.9305E−01 |
| 59.Pr | 1.1079E−03 | 5.5245E+04 | 5.5330E+04 | 5.5456E+04 | 2.2932E−01 |
| | 6.7570E−03 | 3.1950E+03 | 3.3147E+03 | 3.4983E+03 | 5.5399E+00 |
| 60.Nd | 1.2961E−03 | 4.0861E+04 | 4.0943E+04 | 4.1034E+04 | 2.2356E−01 |

| Material | $E$, MeV | $\mu_{1en}$, cm$^{-1}$ | $\mu_1$, cm$^{-1}$ | $\mu_2$, cm$^{-1}$ | $R$, % |
|---|---|---|---|---|---|
| 61.Pm | 1.1507E−03 | 5.1975E+04 | 5.2059E+04 | 5.2237E+04 | 3.4238E−01 |
| | 5.8312E−02 | 3.7695E+01 | 5.7237E+01 | 8.6378E+01 | 5.0912E+01 |
| 62.Sm | 1.1752E−03 | 5.0099E+04 | 5.0182E+04 | 5.0375E+04 | 3.8458E−01 |
| | 5.8106E−02 | 3.8071E+01 | 5.7915E+01 | 9.2005E+01 | 5.8862E+01 |
| 64.Gd | 1.3302E−03 | 3.8250E+04 | 3.8330E+04 | 3.8510E+04 | 4.6938E−01 |
| | 2.7836E−02 | 1.5080E+02 | 3.9967E+02 | 1.6646E+02 | 1.4010E+02 |
| | 5.7615E−02 | 3.8970E+01 | 5.9531E+01 | 1.0612E+02 | 7.8267E+01 |
| 65.Tb | 2.8670E−02 | 1.4582E+02 | 3.7115E+02 | 1.6173E+02 | 1.2949E+02 |
| | 5.6777E−02 | 4.0502E+01 | 6.2288E+01 | 1.1900E+02 | 9.1041E+01 |
| 66.Dy | 1.3296E−03 | 3.8303E+04 | 3.8384E+04 | 3.8636E+04 | 6.5759E−01 |
| | 2.9279E−02 | 1.4218E+02 | 3.5031E+02 | 1.5828E+02 | 1.2132E+02 |
| | 5.6588E−02 | 4.0848E+01 | 6.2912E+01 | 1.2723E+02 | 1.0224E+02 |
| 67.Ho | 1.3825E−03 | 3.4258E+04 | 3.4337E+04 | 3.4581E+04 | 7.0863E−01 |
| | 2.9797E−02 | 1.3909E+02 | 3.3261E+02 | 1.5545E+02 | 1.1396E+02 |
| | 5.6579E−02 | 4.0865E+01 | 6.2941E+01 | 1.3456E+02 | 1.1378E+02 |
| 68.Er | 1.4349E−03 | 3.0248E+04 | 3.0327E+04 | 3.0560E+04 | 7.6817E−01 |
| | 3.2415E−02 | 1.2508E+02 | 2.8416E+02 | 1.4061E+02 | 1.0210E+02 |
| 69.Tm | 1.4831E−03 | 2.6567E+04 | 2.6645E+04 | 2.6855E+04 | 7.8667E−01 |
| | 3.5521E−02 | 1.0862E+02 | 2.3078E+02 | 1.2294E+02 | 8.7721E+01 |
| 70.Yb | 1.5671E−03 | 2.3584E+04 | 2.3660E+04 | 2.3879E+04 | 9.2516E−01 |
| | 2.8619E−02 | 1.4613E+02 | 3.7290E+02 | 1.6438E+02 | 1.2685E+02 |
| 71.Lu | 1.6138E−03 | 2.2408E+04 | 2.2482E+04 | 2.2694E+04 | 9.4327E−01 |
| | 3.9104E−02 | 8.9621E+01 | 1.6919E+02 | 1.0268E+02 | 6.4766E+01 |
| 72.Hf | 1.6656E−03 | 2.1104E+04 | 2.1176E+04 | 2.1342E+04 | 7.8262E−01 |
| 73.Ta | 1.4475E−03 | 2.9286E+04 | 2.9364E+04 | 2.9471E+04 | 3.6145E−01 |
| | 1.6571E−03 | 2.1319E+04 | 2.1392E+04 | 2.1491E+04 | 4.6566E−01 |
| 81.Tl | 1.4118E−03 | 3.2014E+04 | 3.2093E+04 | 3.2156E+04 | 1.9734E−01 |
| 82.Pb | 1.3861E−03 | 3.3981E+04 | 3.4061E+04 | 3.4120E+04 | 1.7311E−01 |
| 83.Bi | 1.8989E−03 | 1.5227E+04 | 1.5291E+04 | 1.5346E+04 | 3.5897E−01 |
| | 2.2114E−03 | 1.0978E+04 | 1.1038E+04 | 1.1092E+04 | 4.9529E−01 |
| 84.Po | 1.8529E−03 | 1.6385E+04 | 1.6451E+04 | 1.6500E+04 | 2.9752E−01 |
| | 2.4100E−03 | 9.3791E+03 | 9.4375E+03 | 9.4870E+03 | 5.2452E−01 |
| 85.At | 1.3725E−03 | 3.5021E+04 | 3.5101E+04 | 3.5161E+04 | 1.7078E−01 |
| 87.Fr | 1.3542E−03 | 3.6417E+04 | 3.6497E+04 | 3.6551E+04 | 1.4750E−01 |
| 88.Ra | 3.3666E−02 | 1.1845E+02 | 2.6267E+02 | 1.4812E+02 | 7.7336E+01 |
| 89.Ac | 1.0443E−03 | 6.0104E+04 | 6.0190E+04 | 6.0245E+04 | 9.1787E−02 |
| 121. | 1.4087E−03 | 3.2256E+04 | 3.2335E+04 | 3.2472E+04 | 4.2160E−01 |
| 123. | 1.4482E−03 | 2.9236E+04 | 2.9315E+04 | 2.9548E+04 | 7.9762E−01 |
| | 1.6896E−02 | 2.7045E+02 | 2.8731E+02 | 3.8964E+02 | 3.5616E+01 |

| Material | $E$, MeV | $\mu_{1en}$, cm$^{-1}$ | $\mu_1$, cm$^{-1}$ | $\mu_2$, cm$^{-1}$ | $R$, % |
|---|---|---|---|---|---|
| 125. | 2.5164E−03 | 8.5219E+03 | 8.5798E+03 | 8.7322E+03 | 1.7763E+00 |
| | 2.8775E−02 | 1.4519E+02 | 3.6756E+02 | 1.7585E+02 | 1.0901E+02 |
| 130. | 2.3656E−03 | 9.7367E+03 | 9.7953E+03 | 9.8777E+03 | 8.4108E−01 |
| 134. | 3.5095E−03 | 3.1248E+03 | 3.1752E+03 | 3.2193E+03 | 1.3876E+00 |
| | | | 49.INDIUM | | |
| 24.Cr | 2.3850E−02 | 9.7490E+01 | 1.0644E+02 | 1.0778E+02 | 1.2548E+00 |
| 25.Mn | 1.4077E−03 | 2.9132E+04 | 2.9202E+04 | 2.9219E+04 | 6.0710E−02 |
| | 9.6934E−03 | 1.0433E+03 | 1.0856E+03 | 1.2656E+03 | 1.6582E+01 |
| 26.Fe | 7.5981E−03 | 2.0595E+03 | 2.1416E+03 | 2.7698E+03 | 2.9331E+01 |
| 31.Ga | 1.2510E−03 | 3.9840E+04 | 3.9917E+04 | 4.0220E+04 | 7.5800E−01 |
| | 1.3231E−02 | 5.2693E+02 | 5.5167E+02 | 8.1075E+02 | 4.6964E+01 |
| 32.Ge | 1.3854E−03 | 3.0655E+04 | 3.0725E+04 | 3.0987E+04 | 8.4997E−01 |
| | 1.4503E−02 | 3.6905E+02 | 3.8856E+02 | 5.5945E+02 | 4.3980E+01 |
| 33.As | 1.3975E−02 | 4.3457E+02 | 4.5625E+02 | 7.1587E+02 | 5.6904E+01 |
| 34.Se | 1.4912E−03 | 2.3424E+04 | 2.3490E+04 | 2.3762E+04 | 1.1600E+00 |
| | 1.6450E−03 | 1.9531E+04 | 1.9594E+04 | 1.9796E+04 | 1.0309E+00 |
| | 1.8350E−02 | 1.9416E+02 | 2.0732E+02 | 2.9865E+02 | 4.4048E+01 |
| 39.Y | 2.1405E−03 | 1.0454E+04 | 1.0511E+04 | 1.0684E+04 | 1.6511E+00 |
| | 1.8696E−02 | 1.8248E+02 | 1.9520E+02 | 3.7395E+02 | 9.1576E+01 |
| 40.Zr | 2.8900E−02 | 1.1809E+02 | 3.1929E+02 | 1.9570E+02 | 6.3154E+01 |
| 41.Nb | 4.1111E−02 | 6.9486E+01 | 1.3007E+02 | 9.9493E+01 | 3.0733E+01 |
| 42.Mo | 4.5500E−03 | 7.3524E+03 | 7.7130E+03 | 7.5259E+03 | 2.4868E+00 |
| 43.Tc | 2.2465E−03 | 9.6827E+03 | 9.7385E+03 | 9.7582E+03 | 2.0226E−01 |
| 50.Sn | 4.5937E−02 | 5.6612E+01 | 1.0033E+02 | 1.0411E+02 | 3.7729E+00 |
| 51.Sb | 7.6021E−03 | 2.0558E+03 | 2.1377E+03 | 2.1515E+03 | 6.4442E−01 |
| 52.Te | 3.0041E−03 | 4.1882E+03 | 4.2357E+03 | 4.2293E+03 | 1.4956E−01 |
| | 2.1880E−02 | 1.1841E+02 | 1.2843E+02 | 1.2786E+02 | 4.4901E−01 |
| 57.La | 1.1560E−03 | 4.6330E+04 | 4.6411E+04 | 4.6468E+04 | 1.2223E−01 |
| | 5.9793E−03 | 3.6048E+03 | 3.7541E+03 | 3.9151E+03 | 4.2891E+00 |
| | 6.0459E−03 | 3.5176E+03 | 3.6627E+03 | 3.8182E+03 | 4.2462E+00 |
| 58.Ce | 1.1591E−03 | 4.6123E+04 | 4.6203E+04 | 4.6278E+04 | 1.6184E−01 |
| | 5.5007E−02 | 3.7990E+01 | 6.0674E+01 | 8.2011E+01 | 3.5165E+01 |
| 59.Pr | 5.3683E−02 | 4.0049E+01 | 6.4540E+01 | 9.2433E+01 | 4.3218E+01 |
| 60.Nd | 5.2831E−02 | 4.1374E+01 | 6.7029E+01 | 1.0180E+02 | 5.1874E+01 |
| 61.Pm | 1.0729E−03 | 5.2010E+04 | 5.2095E+04 | 5.2276E+04 | 3.4849E−01 |
| | 2.7945E−02 | 1.2206E+02 | 3.4584E+02 | 1.3422E+02 | 1.5766E+02 |
| | 4.9909E−02 | 4.6018E+01 | 7.5855E+01 | 1.2599E+02 | 6.6096E+01 |
| 62.Sm | 2.8467E−02 | 1.1989E+02 | 3.3133E+02 | 1.3226E+02 | 1.5052E+02 |
| | 5.0488E−02 | 4.5016E+01 | 7.3868E+01 | 1.2991E+02 | 7.5870E+01 |

| Material | $E$, MeV | $\mu_{1en}$, cm$^{-1}$ | $\mu_1$, cm$^{-1}$ | $\mu_2$, cm$^{-1}$ | $R$, % |
|---|---|---|---|---|---|
| 63.Eu | 1.4108E−03 | 2.8921E+04 | 2.8991E+04 | 2.9096E+04 | 3.6164E−01 |
| 64.Gd | 1.2800E−03 | 3.7861E+04 | 3.7936E+04 | 3.8121E+04 | 4.8834E−01 |
| | 2.9513E−02 | 1.1555E+02 | 3.0222E+02 | 1.2831E+02 | 1.3553E+02 |
| | 5.1736E−02 | 4.3076E+01 | 7.0224E+01 | 1.3891E+02 | 9.7806E+01 |
| 65.Tb | 1.2714E−03 | 3.8443E+04 | 3.8519E+04 | 3.8743E+04 | 5.8276E−01 |
| | 3.0840E−02 | 1.1007E+02 | 2.7593E+02 | 1.2285E+02 | 1.2460E+02 |
| 66.Dy | 1.3242E−03 | 3.4837E+04 | 3.4910E+04 | 3.5138E+04 | 6.5441E−01 |
| | 3.8125E−03 | 6.9942E+03 | 7.3350E+03 | 7.0826E+03 | 3.5628E+00 |
| | 3.4084E−02 | 9.6750E+01 | 2.2670E+02 | 1.0867E+02 | 1.0861E+02 |
| 67.Ho | 1.3772E−03 | 3.1216E+04 | 3.1287E+04 | 3.1507E+04 | 7.0240E−01 |
| | 3.6374E−02 | 8.7343E+01 | 1.9194E+02 | 9.8756E+01 | 9.4359E+01 |
| 68.Er | 1.4294E−03 | 2.7650E+04 | 2.7719E+04 | 2.7930E+04 | 7.6099E−01 |
| | 3.8198E−02 | 7.9853E+01 | 1.6427E+02 | 9.0883E+01 | 8.0748E+01 |
| 69.Tm | 1.4791E−03 | 2.4252E+04 | 2.4319E+04 | 2.4509E+04 | 7.8004E−01 |
| | 3.9658E−02 | 7.3855E+01 | 1.4211E+02 | 8.4591E+01 | 6.7996E+01 |
| 70.Yb | 1.5590E−03 | 2.1482E+04 | 2.1547E+04 | 2.1745E+04 | 9.2056E−01 |
| | 3.0916E−02 | 1.0976E+02 | 2.7476E+02 | 1.2368E+02 | 1.2215E+02 |
| 71.Lu | 1.6065E−03 | 2.0406E+04 | 2.0470E+04 | 2.0654E+04 | 9.0024E−01 |
| | 3.9474E−03 | 8.7326E+03 | 9.1847E+03 | 8.8652E+03 | 3.6044E+00 |
| | 4.2135E−03 | 7.5407E+03 | 7.9143E+03 | 7.6612E+03 | 3.3031E+00 |
| | 4.8364E−02 | 5.0138E+01 | 8.5373E+01 | 5.8694E+01 | 4.5454E+01 |
| 83.Bi | 1.3937E−03 | 3.0089E+04 | 3.0159E+04 | 3.0218E+04 | 1.9341E−01 |
| 84.Po | 1.3701E−03 | 3.1700E+04 | 3.1772E+04 | 3.1824E+04 | 1.6397E−01 |
| 88.Ra | 3.9698E−02 | 7.3689E+01 | 1.4149E+02 | 9.0387E+01 | 5.6543E+01 |
| 121. | 1.3633E−03 | 3.2162E+04 | 3.2234E+04 | 3.2378E+04 | 4.4666E−01 |
| 121. | 7.8640E−03 | 1.8098E+03 | 1.8811E+03 | 2.0048E+03 | 6.5753E+00 |
| 123. | 1.4572E−02 | 3.6057E+02 | 3.7980E+02 | 5.4495E+02 | 4.3484E+01 |
| 125. | 2.4938E−03 | 7.8827E+03 | 7.9358E+03 | 8.0678E+03 | 1.6630E+00 |
| | 3.2937E−02 | 1.0146E+02 | 2.4411E+02 | 1.2123E+02 | 1.0135E+02 |
| 130. | 2.3461E−03 | 8.9578E+03 | 9.0124E+03 | 9.0742E+03 | 6.8525E−01 |
| | 2.8603E−02 | 1.1932E+02 | 3.2754E+02 | 1.3925E+02 | 1.3522E+02 |
| 134. | 2.7802E−02 | 5.5525E+01 | 6.2333E+01 | 1.1305E+02 | 8.1361E+01 |

50.TIN

| Material | $E$, MeV | $\mu_{1en}$, cm$^{-1}$ | $\mu_1$, cm$^{-1}$ | $\mu_2$, cm$^{-1}$ | $R$, % |
|---|---|---|---|---|---|
| 25.Mn | 1.1045E−03 | 5.2109E+04 | 5.2198E+04 | 5.2264E+04 | 1.2704E−01 |
| | 1.4213E−02 | 4.2450E+02 | 4.4652E+02 | 4.9244E+02 | 1.0284E+01 |
| 26.Fe | 2.8845E−03 | 5.3286E+03 | 5.3780E+03 | 5.3626E+03 | 2.8748E−01 |
| | 7.8212E−03 | 1.9286E+03 | 2.0101E+03 | 2.5680E+03 | 2.7755E+01 |
| 31.Ga | 1.3911E−02 | 4.6355E+02 | 4.8697E+02 | 6.9273E+02 | 4.2252E+01 |
| 32.Ge | 1.4817E−02 | 3.4629E+02 | 3.6550E+02 | 5.1381E+02 | 4.0579E+01 |

| Material | $E$, MeV | $\mu_{1en}$, cm$^{-1}$ | $\mu_1$, cm$^{-1}$ | $\mu_2$, cm$^{-1}$ | $R$, % |
|---|---|---|---|---|---|
| 33.As | 1.4311E−02 | 4.1177E+02 | 4.3333E+02 | 6.6632E+02 | 5.3765E+01 |
| 34.Se | 1.9414E−02 | 1.6624E+02 | 1.7845E+02 | 2.4589E+02 | 3.7790E+01 |
| 39.Y | 1.9166E−02 | 1.7502E+02 | 1.8758E+02 | 3.4959E+02 | 8.6366E+01 |
| 40.Zr | 2.9542E−02 | 1.0992E+02 | 3.1125E+02 | 1.7584E+02 | 7.7009E+01 |
| 41.Nb | 4.1956E−02 | 6.6860E+01 | 1.2949E+02 | 9.5448E+01 | 3.5669E+01 |
| 43.Tc | 1.4875E−03 | 2.4915E+04 | 2.4982E+04 | 2.4996E+04 | 5.7112E−02 |
| | 2.0331E−02 | 1.4205E+02 | 1.5327E+02 | 1.5555E+02 | 1.4892E+00 |
| 48.Cd | 3.3232E−03 | 3.6743E+03 | 3.7200E+03 | 3.7265E+03 | 1.7572E−01 |
| | 2.3387E−02 | 1.1042E+02 | 1.2001E+02 | 1.2072E+02 | 5.9590E−01 |
| 49.In | 4.5937E−02 | 5.6612E+01 | 1.0411E+02 | 1.0033E+02 | 3.7729E+00 |
| 51.Sb | 3.8722E−03 | 2.3699E+03 | 2.4113E+03 | 2.4083E+03 | 1.2336E−01 |
| | 2.5901E−02 | 8.4405E+01 | 9.2639E+01 | 9.2334E+01 | 3.3010E−01 |
| 52.Te | 2.8534E−02 | 5.7161E+01 | 6.3981E+01 | 6.3372E+01 | 9.6224E−01 |
| 57.La | 1.2907E−03 | 3.8889E+04 | 3.8967E+04 | 3.9016E+04 | 1.2540E−01 |
| 58.Ce | 1.0851E−03 | 5.3493E+04 | 5.3583E+04 | 5.3674E+04 | 1.6997E−01 |
| | 5.6204E−02 | 3.6618E+01 | 5.9460E+01 | 7.7426E+01 | 3.0217E+01 |
| 59.Pr | 1.2277E−03 | 4.3362E+04 | 4.3444E+04 | 4.3529E+04 | 1.9485E−01 |
| | 5.4678E−02 | 3.8964E+01 | 6.4073E+01 | 8.8418E+01 | 3.7995E+01 |
| 60.Nd | 1.0238E−03 | 5.7841E+04 | 5.7935E+04 | 5.8097E+04 | 2.8112E−01 |
| | 5.3675E−02 | 4.0506E+01 | 6.7107E+01 | 9.8206E+01 | 4.6342E+01 |
| 61.Pm | 1.1061E−03 | 5.1995E+04 | 5.2084E+04 | 5.2260E+04 | 3.3708E−01 |
| | 5.0393E−02 | 4.5551E+01 | 7.7028E+01 | 1.2343E+02 | 6.0237E+01 |
| 62.Sm | 1.1254E−03 | 5.0627E+04 | 5.0714E+04 | 5.0908E+04 | 3.8217E−01 |
| | 5.1109E−02 | 4.4450E+01 | 7.4863E+01 | 1.2682E+02 | 6.9403E+01 |
| 63.Eu | 1.4554E−03 | 2.7195E+04 | 2.7263E+04 | 2.7358E+04 | 3.4889E−01 |
| | 7.7059E−03 | 2.0409E+03 | 2.1279E+03 | 2.2940E+03 | 7.8083E+00 |
| 64.Gd | 1.3027E−03 | 3.8037E+04 | 3.8114E+04 | 3.8297E+04 | 4.8112E−01 |
| | 2.9808E−02 | 1.0934E+02 | 3.0544E+02 | 1.2160E+02 | 1.5118E+02 |
| 64.Gd | 5.2226E−02 | 4.2734E+01 | 7.1488E+01 | 1.3618E+02 | 9.0491E+01 |
| 65.Tb | 1.2737E−03 | 4.0095E+04 | 4.0174E+04 | 4.0409E+04 | 5.8380E−01 |
| | 3.2478E−02 | 9.9744E+01 | 2.6177E+02 | 1.1161E+02 | 1.3455E+02 |
| 66.Dy | 1.3265E−03 | 3.6345E+04 | 3.6421E+04 | 3.6661E+04 | 6.5788E−01 |
| | 3.5039E−02 | 9.0261E+01 | 2.2098E+02 | 1.0159E+02 | 1.1752E+02 |
| 67.Ho | 1.3796E−03 | 3.2580E+04 | 3.2653E+04 | 3.2886E+04 | 7.1242E−01 |
| | 3.9682E−03 | 6.5061E+03 | 6.8310E+03 | 6.5955E+03 | 3.5710E+00 |
| | 3.6939E−02 | 8.3226E+01 | 1.9071E+02 | 9.4248E+01 | 1.0235E+02 |
| 68.Er | 1.4320E−03 | 2.8857E+04 | 2.8927E+04 | 2.9152E+04 | 7.7878E−01 |
| | 3.8510E−02 | 7.7412E+01 | 1.6570E+02 | 8.8199E+01 | 8.7869E+01 |
| 69.Tm | 1.4810E−03 | 2.5375E+04 | 2.5442E+04 | 2.5647E+04 | 8.0465E−01 |

| Material | $E$, MeV | $\mu_{1en}$, cm$^{-1}$ | $\mu_1$, cm$^{-1}$ | $\mu_2$, cm$^{-1}$ | $R$, % |
|---|---|---|---|---|---|
| | 3.9805E−02 | 7.2614E+01 | 1.4506E+02 | 8.3222E+01 | 7.4303E+01 |
| 70.Yb | 1.5631E−03 | 2.2525E+04 | 2.2590E+04 | 2.2804E+04 | 9.4667E−01 |
| | 3.2579E−02 | 9.9369E+01 | 2.6016E+02 | 1.1218E+02 | 1.3192E+02 |
| 71.Lu | 1.6102E−03 | 2.1402E+04 | 2.1467E+04 | 2.1670E+04 | 9.4602E−01 |
| | 4.8163E−02 | 5.0884E+01 | 8.9927E+01 | 5.9525E+01 | 5.1075E+01 |
| 72.Hf | 1.6627E−03 | 2.0151E+04 | 2.0214E+04 | 2.0370E+04 | 7.7171E−01 |
| 73.Ta | 1.2047E−03 | 4.4999E+04 | 4.5082E+04 | 4.5192E+04 | 2.4383E−01 |
| 81.Tl | 1.1503E−03 | 4.8862E+04 | 4.8948E+04 | 4.9011E+04 | 1.2789E−01 |
| 82.Pb | 1.0875E−03 | 5.3318E+04 | 5.3408E+04 | 5.3463E+04 | 1.0421E−01 |
| 83.Bi | 1.5491E−03 | 2.2857E+04 | 2.2922E+04 | 2.2983E+04 | 2.6473E−01 |
| | 2.4556E−03 | 8.6181E+03 | 8.6719E+03 | 8.7289E+03 | 6.5749E−01 |
| 84.Po | 1.4907E−03 | 2.4691E+04 | 2.4757E+04 | 2.4812E+04 | 2.2216E−01 |
| | 2.6791E−03 | 6.9034E+03 | 6.9549E+03 | 7.0087E+03 | 7.7389E−01 |
| 85.At | 1.1671E−03 | 4.7670E+04 | 4.7755E+04 | 4.7810E+04 | 1.1463E−01 |
| 87.Fr | 1.0558E−03 | 5.5572E+04 | 5.5663E+04 | 5.5712E+04 | 8.6654E−02 |
| | 1.2231E−03 | 4.3694E+04 | 4.3776E+04 | 4.3832E+04 | 1.2792E−01 |
| 88.Ra | 3.9881E−02 | 7.2336E+01 | 1.4386E+02 | 8.8643E+01 | 6.2294E+01 |
| 121. | 1.3848E−03 | 3.2206E+04 | 3.2279E+04 | 3.2422E+04 | 4.4374E−01 |
| 123. | 1.3973E−03 | 3.1320E+04 | 3.1392E+04 | 3.1663E+04 | 8.6437E−01 |
| | 1.4848E−02 | 3.4233E+02 | 3.6139E+02 | 5.0929E+02 | 4.0927E+01 |
| 125. | 2.5061E−03 | 8.2306E+03 | 8.2839E+03 | 8.4294E+03 | 1.7561E+00 |
| | 3.4270E−02 | 9.3110E+01 | 2.3323E+02 | 1.1118E+02 | 1.0978E+02 |
| 130. | 2.3566E−03 | 9.3774E+03 | 9.4323E+03 | 9.5071E+03 | 7.9370E−01 |
| 134. | 2.9139E−02 | 5.0897E+01 | 5.7392E+01 | 9.9049E+01 | 7.2583E+01 |

51.ANTIMONY

| Material | $E$, MeV | $\mu_{1en}$, cm$^{-1}$ | $\mu_1$, cm$^{-1}$ | $\mu_2$, cm$^{-1}$ | $R$, % |
|---|---|---|---|---|---|
| 25.Mn | 1.3502E−03 | 3.3491E+04 | 3.3566E+04 | 3.3591E+04 | 7.5888E−02 |
| | 9.8610E−03 | 9.8625E+02 | 1.0307E+03 | 1.1895E+03 | 1.5405E+01 |
| 26.Fe | 3.2575E−03 | 3.7501E+03 | 3.7931E+03 | 3.7804E+03 | 3.3537E−01 |
| | 7.5981E−03 | 2.0596E+03 | 2.1555E+03 | 2.7698E+03 | 2.8502E+01 |
| 31.Ga | 1.2865E−03 | 3.7825E+04 | 3.7903E+04 | 3.8180E+04 | 7.3191E−01 |
| | 1.3388E−02 | 5.1225E+02 | 5.3790E+02 | 7.8343E+02 | 4.5645E+01 |
| 32.Ge | 1.4079E−03 | 2.9561E+04 | 2.9633E+04 | 2.9879E+04 | 8.3078E−01 |
| | 1.4588E−02 | 3.6294E+02 | 3.8275E+02 | 5.4720E+02 | 4.2966E+01 |
| 33.As | 1.4057E−02 | 4.2905E+02 | 4.5144E+02 | 7.0387E+02 | 5.5917E+01 |
| 34.Se | 1.4961E−03 | 2.3560E+04 | 2.3627E+04 | 2.3900E+04 | 1.1571E+00 |
| | 1.5689E−03 | 2.1703E+04 | 2.1768E+04 | 2.2009E+04 | 1.1056E+00 |
| | 1.8733E−02 | 1.8411E+02 | 1.9676E+02 | 2.7966E+02 | 4.2129E+01 |
| 39.Y | 2.1071E−03 | 1.0972E+04 | 1.1025E+04 | 1.1219E+04 | 1.7565E+00 |
| | 1.8855E−02 | 1.7996E+02 | 1.9244E+02 | 3.6572E+02 | 9.0037E+01 |

| Material | $E$, MeV | $\mu_{1en}$, cm$^{-1}$ | $\mu_1$, cm$^{-1}$ | $\mu_2$, cm$^{-1}$ | $R$, % |
|---|---|---|---|---|---|
| 40.Zr | 3.4322E−02 | 8.1963E+01 | 2.1737E+02 | 1.2382E+02 | 7.5547E+01 |
| 41.Nb | 4.8850E−02 | 4.5429E+01 | 8.1916E+01 | 6.2442E+01 | 3.1186E+01 |
| 42.Mo | 4.8720E−03 | 5.9877E+03 | 6.3288E+03 | 6.1263E+03 | 3.3056E+00 |
| 43.Tc | 2.0941E−03 | 1.1069E+04 | 1.1122E+04 | 1.1148E+04 | 2.3262E−01 |
| | 2.0791E−02 | 1.3328E+02 | 1.4379E+02 | 1.4639E+02 | 1.8053E+00 |
| 48.Cd | 3.4250E−03 | 3.3741E+03 | 3.4158E+03 | 3.4254E+03 | 2.7972E−01 |
| | 2.4004E−02 | 1.0255E+02 | 1.1143E+02 | 1.1245E+02 | 9.1561E−01 |
| 49.In | 7.6021E−03 | 2.0558E+03 | 2.1515E+03 | 2.1377E+03 | 6.4442E−01 |
| 50.Sn | 3.8722E−03 | 2.3699E+03 | 2.4083E+03 | 2.4113E+03 | 1.2336E−01 |
| | 2.5901E−02 | 8.4405E+01 | 9.2334E+01 | 9.2639E+01 | 3.3010E−01 |
| 57.La | 1.1382E−03 | 4.7923E+04 | 4.8009E+04 | 4.8066E+04 | 1.1841E−01 |
| | 5.9654E−03 | 3.6207E+03 | 3.8021E+03 | 3.9327E+03 | 3.4347E+00 |
| | 6.0699E−03 | 3.4844E+03 | 3.6575E+03 | 3.7812E+03 | 3.3838E+00 |
| | 5.8527E−02 | 3.0903E+01 | 5.0285E+01 | 6.0144E+01 | 1.9606E+01 |
| 58.Ce | 1.1465E−03 | 4.7354E+04 | 4.7439E+04 | 4.7513E+04 | 1.5600E−01 |
| | 4.9161E−02 | 4.4725E+01 | 8.0032E+01 | 1.0770E+02 | 3.4576E+01 |
| 59.Pr | 4.8971E−02 | 4.5156E+01 | 8.1185E+01 | 1.1522E+02 | 4.1919E+01 |
| 60.Nd | 4.8897E−02 | 4.5323E+01 | 8.1632E+01 | 1.2232E+02 | 4.9846E+01 |
| 61.Pm | 1.0782E−03 | 5.2008E+04 | 5.2097E+04 | 5.2274E+04 | 3.3841E−01 |
| | 4.7800E−02 | 4.7811E+01 | 8.8290E+01 | 1.4275E+02 | 6.1680E+01 |
| 62.Sm | 4.8349E−02 | 4.6566E+01 | 8.4959E+01 | 1.4502E+02 | 7.0699E+01 |
| 63.Eu | 1.4259E−03 | 2.8336E+04 | 2.8407E+04 | 2.8507E+04 | 3.5180E−01 |
| 64.Gd | 1.2854E−03 | 3.7902E+04 | 3.7981E+04 | 3.8163E+04 | 4.7997E−01 |
| | 3.3774E−02 | 8.3553E+01 | 2.2527E+02 | 9.3625E+01 | 1.4061E+02 |
| 65.Tb | 1.2720E−03 | 3.8815E+04 | 3.8894E+04 | 3.9118E+04 | 5.7634E−01 |
| | 3.6129E−02 | 7.6725E+01 | 1.9136E+02 | 8.6549E+01 | 1.2110E+02 |
| 66.Dy | 1.3248E−03 | 3.5218E+04 | 3.5294E+04 | 3.5523E+04 | 6.4913E−01 |
| | 4.1554E−03 | 5.4722E+03 | 5.7665E+03 | 5.5508E+03 | 3.8855E+00 |
| | 3.7705E−02 | 7.2152E+01 | 1.6866E+02 | 8.1832E+01 | 1.0611E+02 |
| 67.Ho | 1.3779E−03 | 3.1605E+04 | 3.1679E+04 | 3.1900E+04 | 6.9965E−01 |
| | 3.8958E−02 | 6.8519E+01 | 1.5062E+02 | 7.8141E+01 | 9.2757E+01 |
| 68.Er | 1.4302E−03 | 2.8041E+04 | 2.8112E+04 | 2.8326E+04 | 7.6211E−01 |
| | 4.0342E−02 | 6.4722E+01 | 1.3355E+02 | 7.4242E+01 | 7.9885E+01 |
| 69.Tm | 1.4798E−03 | 2.4667E+04 | 2.4735E+04 | 2.4929E+04 | 7.8424E−01 |
| 69.Tm | 4.5557E−02 | 5.2897E+01 | 1.0190E+02 | 6.1384E+01 | 6.6009E+01 |
| 70.Yb | 1.5606E−03 | 2.1894E+04 | 2.1959E+04 | 2.2164E+04 | 9.2929E−01 |
| | 3.6268E−02 | 7.6321E+01 | 1.8936E+02 | 8.6661E+01 | 1.1851E+02 |
| 71.Lu | 1.6080E−03 | 2.0804E+04 | 2.0868E+04 | 2.1060E+04 | 9.2003E−01 |
| | 5.3687E−02 | 3.7669E+01 | 6.4280E+01 | 4.4755E+01 | 4.3626E+01 |

| Material | $E$, MeV | $\mu_{1en}$, cm$^{-1}$ | $\mu_1$, cm$^{-1}$ | $\mu_2$, cm$^{-1}$ | $R$, % |
|---|---|---|---|---|---|
| 83.Bi | 1.4371E−03 | 2.7572E+04 | 2.7642E+04 | 2.7700E+04 | 2.0859E−01 |
| | 2.5629E−03 | 7.5811E+03 | 7.6297E+03 | 7.6905E+03 | 7.9636E−01 |
| 84.Po | 1.4138E−03 | 2.9161E+04 | 2.9233E+04 | 2.9284E+04 | 1.7529E−01 |
| 85.At | 1.0341E−03 | 5.5006E+04 | 5.5098E+04 | 5.5152E+04 | 9.8809E−02 |
| 87.Fr | 1.1352E−03 | 4.8126E+04 | 4.8212E+04 | 4.8266E+04 | 1.1110E−01 |
| 88.Ra | 4.7141E−02 | 4.9304E+01 | 9.2287E+01 | 6.0184E+01 | 5.3342E+01 |
| 121. | 1.3695E−03 | 3.2175E+04 | 3.2249E+04 | 3.2390E+04 | 4.3991E−01 |
| | 7.8697E−03 | 1.8063E+03 | 1.8885E+03 | 2.0004E+03 | 5.9222E+00 |
| | 5.9389E−02 | 2.9699E+01 | 4.7793E+01 | 7.5693E+01 | 5.8377E+01 |
| 123. | 1.3590E−03 | 3.2889E+04 | 3.2964E+04 | 3.3256E+04 | 8.8487E−01 |
| | 1.4646E−02 | 3.5565E+02 | 3.7517E+02 | 5.3534E+02 | 4.2690E+01 |
| 125. | 2.4997E−03 | 8.0509E+03 | 8.1001E+03 | 8.2426E+03 | 1.7592E+00 |
| | 3.7537E−02 | 7.2639E+01 | 1.7108E+02 | 8.6549E+01 | 9.7668E+01 |
| 130. | 2.3511E−03 | 9.1571E+03 | 9.2076E+03 | 9.2798E+03 | 7.8484E−01 |
| | 4.2915E−02 | 5.8888E+01 | 1.1794E+02 | 1.0122E+02 | 1.6518E+01 |
| 134. | 2.9555E−02 | 4.9458E+01 | 5.5544E+01 | 9.4697E+01 | 7.0490E+01 |

52.TELLURIUM

| Material | $E$, MeV | $\mu_{1en}$, cm$^{-1}$ | $\mu_1$, cm$^{-1}$ | $\mu_2$, cm$^{-1}$ | $R$, % |
|---|---|---|---|---|---|
| 24.Cr | 3.1654E−02 | 3.7583E+01 | 4.2671E+01 | 4.1946E+01 | 1.7273E+00 |
| 25.Mn | 1.4730E−03 | 2.4181E+04 | 2.4246E+04 | 2.4254E+04 | 3.5227E−02 |
| | 7.9572E−03 | 1.6467E+03 | 1.7264E+03 | 2.0731E+03 | 2.0080E+01 |
| 26.Fe | 3.8662E−03 | 2.3129E+03 | 2.3492E+03 | 2.3384E+03 | 4.6428E−01 |
| | 4.1200E−03 | 1.8868E+03 | 1.9215E+03 | 1.9108E+03 | 5.6278E−01 |
| | 7.2850E−03 | 2.2433E+03 | 2.3595E+03 | 3.0529E+03 | 2.9390E+01 |
| 31.Ga | 1.1899E−03 | 4.2308E+04 | 4.2394E+04 | 4.2721E+04 | 7.6990E−01 |
| | 1.2577E−02 | 5.8781E+02 | 6.1725E+02 | 9.2413E+02 | 4.9716E+01 |
| 32.Ge | 1.3294E−03 | 3.3374E+04 | 3.3450E+04 | 3.3741E+04 | 8.7095E−01 |
| | 1.4280E−02 | 3.8529E+02 | 4.0614E+02 | 5.9201E+02 | 4.5766E+01 |
| 33.As | 1.3719E−02 | 4.5192E+02 | 4.7560E+02 | 7.5359E+02 | 5.8453E+01 |
| 34.Se | 1.4868E−03 | 2.3299E+04 | 2.3363E+04 | 2.3636E+04 | 1.1710E+00 |
| | 1.7682E−02 | 2.1171E+02 | 2.2525E+02 | 3.3180E+02 | 4.7300E+01 |
| 39.Y | 2.1524E−03 | 1.0287E+04 | 1.0336E+04 | 1.0512E+04 | 1.7061E+00 |
| | 1.8459E−02 | 1.8624E+02 | 1.9871E+02 | 3.8622E+02 | 9.4362E+01 |
| 40.Zr | 3.7770E−02 | 6.4305E+01 | 1.5692E+02 | 9.3628E+01 | 6.7600E+01 |
| 41.Nb | 4.7004E−03 | 5.3206E+03 | 5.6663E+03 | 5.4346E+03 | 4.2627E+00 |
| | 5.7427E−02 | 3.0120E+01 | 5.1016E+01 | 4.0315E+01 | 2.6544E+01 |
| 42.Mo | 5.9007E−03 | 3.5738E+03 | 3.7739E+03 | 3.6580E+03 | 3.1700E+00 |
| 43.Tc | 2.2840E−03 | 9.3414E+03 | 9.3889E+03 | 9.4161E+03 | 2.9046E−01 |
| 48.Cd | 2.5043E−02 | 8.9295E+01 | 9.7202E+01 | 9.8540E+01 | 1.3766E+00 |
| 49.In | 3.0041E−03 | 4.1882E+03 | 4.2293E+03 | 4.2357E+03 | 1.4956E−01 |

| Material | $E$, MeV | $\mu_{1en}$, cm$^{-1}$ | $\mu_1$, cm$^{-1}$ | $\mu_2$, cm$^{-1}$ | $R$, % |
|---|---|---|---|---|---|
| | 2.1880E−02 | 1.1841E+02 | 1.2786E+02 | 1.2843E+02 | 4.4901E−01 |
| 50.Sn | 2.8534E−02 | 5.7161E+01 | 6.3372E+01 | 6.3981E+01 | 9.6224E−01 |
| 57.La | 1.0266E−03 | 5.2772E+04 | 5.2870E+04 | 5.2924E+04 | 1.0126E−01 |
| | 4.8765E−02 | 4.1927E+01 | 7.8531E+01 | 9.7652E+01 | 2.4349E+01 |
| 58.Ce | 4.4572E−02 | 5.0169E+01 | 1.0258E+02 | 1.4335E+02 | 3.9745E+01 |
| 59.Pr | 4.4955E−02 | 4.9415E+01 | 1.0038E+02 | 1.4613E+02 | 4.5583E+01 |
| 60.Nd | 4.5325E−02 | 4.8688E+01 | 9.8256E+01 | 1.4976E+02 | 5.2420E+01 |
| 62.Sm | 3.3417E−02 | 7.4361E+01 | 2.1185E+02 | 8.3253E+01 | 1.5446E+02 |
| 63.Eu | 1.3810E−03 | 3.0072E+04 | 3.0143E+04 | 3.0254E+04 | 3.6653E−01 |
| 64.Gd | 1.2616E−03 | 3.7719E+04 | 3.7799E+04 | 3.7979E+04 | 4.7682E−01 |
| | 3.6673E−02 | 6.6839E+01 | 1.7076E+02 | 7.5484E+01 | 1.2623E+02 |
| 65.Tb | 1.2697E−03 | 3.7199E+04 | 3.7278E+04 | 3.7489E+04 | 5.6457E−01 |
| | 3.8288E−02 | 6.3110E+01 | 1.5040E+02 | 7.1728E+01 | 1.0968E+02 |
| 66.Dy | 1.3226E−03 | 3.3810E+04 | 3.3886E+04 | 3.4103E+04 | 6.3994E−01 |
| | 3.9423E−02 | 6.0489E+01 | 1.3608E+02 | 6.9106E+01 | 9.6913E+01 |
| 67.Ho | 1.3758E−03 | 3.0407E+04 | 3.0478E+04 | 3.0689E+04 | 6.9094E−01 |
| | 4.2119E−02 | 5.4989E+01 | 1.1664E+02 | 6.3280E+01 | 8.4322E+01 |
| 68.Er | 1.4281E−03 | 2.7059E+04 | 2.7127E+04 | 2.7331E+04 | 7.5337E−01 |
| | 4.6261E−02 | 4.6849E+01 | 9.2892E+01 | 5.4491E+01 | 7.0472E+01 |
| 69.Tm | 1.4783E−03 | 2.3838E+04 | 2.3902E+04 | 2.4089E+04 | 7.8110E−01 |
| | 4.9178E−02 | 4.1115E+01 | 7.6163E+01 | 4.8330E+01 | 5.7591E+01 |
| 70.Yb | 1.5579E−03 | 2.1171E+04 | 2.1232E+04 | 2.1429E+04 | 9.3116E−01 |
| | 3.8437E−02 | 6.2765E+01 | 1.4851E+02 | 7.1652E+01 | 1.0727E+02 |
| 71.Lu | 1.6054E−03 | 2.0118E+04 | 2.0178E+04 | 2.0361E+04 | 9.0862E−01 |
| | 5.9615E−02 | 2.7355E+01 | 4.4994E+01 | 3.3193E+01 | 3.5554E+01 |
| 83.Bi | 1.2580E−03 | 3.7947E+04 | 3.8028E+04 | 3.8078E+04 | 1.3329E−01 |
| 84.Po | 1.2126E−03 | 4.0855E+04 | 4.0939E+04 | 4.0982E+04 | 1.0342E−01 |
| 88.Ra | 5.3597E−02 | 3.4956E+01 | 6.1551E+01 | 4.2624E+01 | 4.4405E+01 |
| 112. | 4.6785E−03 | 5.3753E+03 | 5.7227E+03 | 5.6630E+03 | 1.0547E+00 |
| | 4.3982E−02 | 5.1329E+01 | 1.0596E+02 | 9.8356E+01 | 7.7319E+00 |
| 121. | 1.3488E−03 | 3.2132E+04 | 3.2206E+04 | 3.2347E+04 | 4.4063E−01 |
| | 7.5699E−03 | 1.9905E+03 | 2.0912E+03 | 2.2338E+03 | 6.8191E+00 |
| | 5.6474E−02 | 3.1323E+01 | 5.3637E+01 | 8.8438E+01 | 6.4882E+01 |
| 123. | 1.4382E−02 | 3.7311E+02 | 3.9345E+02 | 5.6948E+02 | 4.4738E+01 |
| 125. | 2.4924E−03 | 7.8440E+03 | 7.8896E+03 | 8.0275E+03 | 1.7478E+00 |
| | 3.9509E−02 | 6.0290E+01 | 1.3499E+02 | 7.1689E+01 | 8.8303E+01 |
| 130. | 2.3448E−03 | 8.9048E+03 | 8.9517E+03 | 9.0196E+03 | 7.5814E−01 |
| | 3.2689E−02 | 7.6042E+01 | 2.2103E+02 | 8.8573E+01 | 1.4954E+02 |
| 134. | 2.9259E−02 | 5.0480E+01 | 5.6338E+01 | 9.7788E+01 | 7.3575E+01 |

| Material | $E$, MeV | $\mu_{1en}$, cm$^{-1}$ | $\mu_1$, cm$^{-1}$ | $\mu_2$, cm$^{-1}$ | $R$, % |
|---|---|---|---|---|---|
| 53.IODINE | | | | | |
| 24.Cr | 1.5189E−03 | 1.8909E+04 | 1.8963E+04 | 1.8959E+04 | 2.1840E−02 |
| 25.Mn | 2.9458E−03 | 3.9591E+03 | 3.9937E+03 | 3.9868E+03 | 1.7121E−01 |
| 28.Ni | 3.5727E−02 | 5.4388E+01 | 1.5126E+02 | 6.2781E+01 | 1.4094E+02 |
| 29.Cu | 3.6645E−02 | 5.2889E+01 | 1.4217E+02 | 6.1773E+01 | 1.3015E+02 |
| 30.Zn | 1.0375E−03 | 4.1485E+04 | 4.1568E+04 | 4.1824E+04 | 6.1493E−01 |
| | 3.3745E−02 | 5.7628E+01 | 1.7089E+02 | 6.8235E+01 | 1.5045E+02 |
| 32.Ge | 1.2343E−02 | 5.2590E+02 | 5.5336E+02 | 8.7403E+02 | 5.7951E+01 |
| 34.Se | 1.4551E−02 | 3.0225E+02 | 3.1935E+02 | 5.1283E+02 | 6.0589E+01 |
| 38.Sr | 2.7503E−03 | 5.1662E+03 | 5.2028E+03 | 5.2621E+03 | 1.1391E+00 |
| | 2.9864E−02 | 3.8653E+01 | 4.3340E+01 | 5.6253E+01 | 2.9794E+01 |
| 39.Y | 3.3183E−02 | 5.8546E+01 | 1.7646E+02 | 8.6134E+01 | 1.0487E+02 |
| 40.Zr | 4.7007E−02 | 3.6895E+01 | 7.5167E+01 | 5.0320E+01 | 4.9380E+01 |
| 42.Mo | 1.9240E−03 | 1.1240E+04 | 1.1286E+04 | 1.1305E+04 | 1.6603E−01 |
| 59.Pr | 3.3503E−02 | 5.8023E+01 | 1.7329E+02 | 6.5027E+01 | 1.6649E+02 |
| 60.Nd | 3.5176E−02 | 5.5290E+01 | 1.5673E+02 | 6.2256E+01 | 1.5175E+02 |
| 61.Pm | 1.0502E−03 | 4.0452E+04 | 4.0534E+04 | 4.0655E+04 | 2.9818E−01 |
| | 3.7210E−02 | 5.1966E+01 | 1.3658E+02 | 5.8908E+01 | 1.3186E+02 |
| 62.Sm | 1.1032E−03 | 3.8801E+04 | 3.8883E+04 | 3.9016E+04 | 3.4345E−01 |
| | 3.8191E−02 | 5.0363E+01 | 1.2687E+02 | 5.7298E+01 | 1.2142E+02 |
| 63.Eu | 1.2075E−03 | 3.3668E+04 | 3.3743E+04 | 3.3882E+04 | 4.1258E−01 |
| | 5.2921E−02 | 2.9446E+01 | 5.3911E+01 | 8.6353E+01 | 6.0177E+01 |
| 64.Gd | 4.0360E−02 | 4.6867E+01 | 1.0722E+02 | 5.3797E+01 | 9.9298E+01 |
| 65.Tb | 1.2612E−03 | 3.1023E+04 | 3.1094E+04 | 3.1264E+04 | 5.4697E−01 |
| | 4.5360E−02 | 3.9365E+01 | 8.3107E+01 | 4.5752E+01 | 8.1649E+01 |
| 66.Dy | 1.3143E−03 | 2.8408E+04 | 2.8475E+04 | 2.8652E+04 | 6.2081E−01 |
| | 4.8270E−02 | 3.5000E+01 | 6.9077E+01 | 4.1102E+01 | 6.8061E+01 |
| 67.Ho | 1.3670E−03 | 2.5812E+04 | 2.5875E+04 | 2.6044E+04 | 6.5352E−01 |
| | 5.1007E−02 | 3.1385E+01 | 5.8385E+01 | 3.7241E+01 | 5.6775E+01 |
| 68.Er | 1.4196E−03 | 2.3227E+04 | 2.3286E+04 | 2.3449E+04 | 7.0034E−01 |
| | 4.9853E−03 | 3.9193E+03 | 4.1811E+03 | 3.9949E+03 | 4.6623E+00 |
| | 5.0479E−03 | 3.8076E+03 | 4.0599E+03 | 3.8823E+03 | 4.5756E+00 |
| | 5.6174E−02 | 2.6150E+01 | 4.6306E+01 | 3.1528E+01 | 4.6875E+01 |
| 69.Tm | 1.4727E−03 | 2.0609E+04 | 2.0665E+04 | 2.0816E+04 | 7.3007E−01 |
| 70.Yb | 1.5473E−03 | 1.8371E+04 | 1.8424E+04 | 1.8589E+04 | 8.9211E−01 |
| | 4.6052E−02 | 3.8327E+01 | 7.9772E+01 | 4.4539E+01 | 7.9108E+01 |
| 71.Lu | 1.5955E−03 | 1.7458E+04 | 1.7510E+04 | 1.7651E+04 | 8.0414E−01 |
| | 9.0937E−03 | 1.0377E+03 | 1.0912E+03 | 1.0874E+03 | 3.4353E−01 |
| 72.Hf | 1.0133E−03 | 4.3590E+04 | 4.3677E+04 | 4.3736E+04 | 1.3627E−01 |

| Material | $E$, MeV | $\mu_{1en}$, cm$^{-1}$ | $\mu_1$, cm$^{-1}$ | $\mu_2$, cm$^{-1}$ | $R$, % |
|---|---|---|---|---|---|
| | 1.5880E−03 | 1.7600E+04 | 1.7653E+04 | 1.7747E+04 | 5.3201E−01 |
| 88.Ra | 1.1258E−02 | 6.3572E+02 | 6.6827E+02 | 6.6704E+02 | 1.8517E−01 |
| 112. | 3.2812E−03 | 3.0969E+03 | 3.1295E+03 | 3.1352E+03 | 1.8379E−01 |
| | 2.2922E−02 | 9.3436E+01 | 1.0107E+02 | 1.0160E+02 | 5.2374E−01 |
| 113. | 4.4109E−03 | 1.3815E+03 | 1.4092E+03 | 1.5592E+03 | 1.0646E+01 |
| 121. | 1.2431E−03 | 3.1912E+04 | 3.1984E+04 | 3.2128E+04 | 4.4952E−01 |
| | 3.6756E−02 | 5.2708E+01 | 1.4108E+02 | 5.9692E+01 | 1.3635E+02 |
| 123. | 1.2852E−02 | 4.7435E+02 | 4.9943E+02 | 7.6739E+02 | 5.3655E+01 |
| 125. | 4.9450E−02 | 3.3230E+01 | 6.3391E+01 | 3.9795E+01 | 5.9293E+01 |
| 130. | 2.1568E−03 | 8.8323E+03 | 8.8750E+03 | 8.8959E+03 | 2.3498E−01 |
| | 2.3016E−03 | 7.9378E+03 | 7.9791E+03 | 8.0135E+03 | 4.3191E−01 |
| | 1.1900E−02 | 5.7069E+02 | 6.0022E+02 | 6.0219E+02 | 3.2735E−01 |
| 134. | 2.7666E−02 | 5.5994E+01 | 6.1614E+01 | 1.1446E+02 | 8.5778E+01 |
| | | | 54.XENON | | |
| 3.Li | 2.8893E−03 | 5.0222E+00 | 5.0629E+00 | 5.1854E+00 | 2.4186E+00 |
| 4.Be | 8.7688E−03 | 1.3078E+00 | 1.3801E+00 | 1.7380E+00 | 2.5934E+01 |
| | 3.3760E−02 | 3.1879E−02 | 3.6318E−02 | 3.2060E−01 | 7.8275E+02 |
| | 5.8180E−02 | 2.6903E−02 | 4.7807E−02 | 2.7796E−01 | 4.8141E+02 |
| 5.B | 3.9041E−02 | 5.2624E−02 | 1.3463E−01 | 4.3108E−01 | 2.2020E+02 |
| | 4.2480E−02 | 4.7352E−02 | 1.1094E−01 | 4.1742E−01 | 2.7627E+02 |
| 17.Cl | 4.6722E−03 | 1.3977E+00 | 1.4272E+00 | 1.4763E+00 | 3.4383E+00 |
| 35.Br | 3.8001E−02 | 5.4236E−02 | 1.4560E−01 | 6.9484E−02 | 1.0954E+02 |
| 36.Kr | 2.7776E−02 | 6.4059E−02 | 7.0439E−02 | 9.3057E−02 | 3.2109E+01 |
| 102. | 3.7543E−02 | 5.4945E−02 | 1.5042E−01 | 2.4319E−01 | 6.1666E+01 |
| 106. | 3.9646E−02 | 5.1686E−02 | 1.2824E−01 | 2.8271E−01 | 1.2044E+02 |
| | 5.2499E−02 | 3.3132E−02 | 6.3059E−02 | 2.4581E−01 | 2.8981E+02 |
| 142. | 3.7286E−02 | 5.5344E−02 | 1.5314E−01 | 2.6664E−01 | 7.4113E+01 |
| | 5.8457E−02 | 2.6599E−02 | 4.7062E−02 | 2.1134E−01 | 3.4906E+02 |
| | | | 55.CESIUM | | |
| 22.Ti | 2.8644E−03 | 1.8978E+03 | 1.9122E+03 | 1.9110E+03 | 6.0396E−02 |
| 23.V | 3.6818E−02 | 1.8666E+01 | 5.5908E+01 | 2.1116E+01 | 1.6476E+02 |
| 24.Cr | 4.1609E−02 | 1.6430E+01 | 4.1459E+01 | 1.8997E+01 | 1.1824E+02 |
| 25.Mn | 4.6485E−02 | 1.4086E+01 | 3.1952E+01 | 1.6557E+01 | 9.2977E+01 |
| 26.Fe | 5.2965E−02 | 1.1304E+01 | 2.2237E+01 | 1.3659E+01 | 6.2798E+01 |
| 28.Ni | 5.4989E−03 | 1.2581E+03 | 1.3590E+03 | 1.2839E+03 | 5.8492E+00 |
| 34.Se | 5.8846E−02 | 9.1399E+00 | 1.6562E+01 | 1.1326E+01 | 4.6238E+01 |
| 37.Rb | 1.8709E−02 | 6.4270E+01 | 6.8732E+01 | 1.1675E+02 | 6.9867E+01 |
| 38.Sr | 4.4244E−02 | 1.5163E+01 | 3.6321E+01 | 2.0074E+01 | 8.0937E+01 |
| 39.Y | 1.0197E−03 | 1.6819E+04 | 1.6859E+04 | 1.6850E+04 | 5.3076E−02 |

| Material | $E$, MeV | $\mu_{1en}$, cm$^{-1}$ | $\mu_1$, cm$^{-1}$ | $\mu_2$, cm$^{-1}$ | $R$, % |
|---|---|---|---|---|---|
| | 1.1173E−03 | 1.4753E+04 | 1.4790E+04 | 1.4783E+04 | 4.7187E−02 |
| | 7.0404E−03 | 8.5707E+02 | 9.1626E+02 | 8.7677E+02 | 4.5037E+00 |
| 56.Ba | 3.6292E−02 | 1.8907E+01 | 5.7776E+01 | 2.1624E+01 | 1.6719E+02 |
| 63.Eu | 1.1346E−03 | 1.4264E+04 | 1.4300E+04 | 1.4352E+04 | 3.6325E−01 |
| | 5.8301E−03 | 1.2560E+03 | 1.3501E+03 | 1.2878E+03 | 4.8369E+00 |
| 64.Gd | 1.1257E−03 | 1.4515E+04 | 1.4552E+04 | 1.4599E+04 | 3.2506E−01 |
| 118. | 7.5738E−03 | 6.9601E+02 | 7.4156E+02 | 7.5421E+02 | 1.7056E+00 |
| 123. | 1.1164E−03 | 1.4777E+04 | 1.4814E+04 | 1.4885E+04 | 4.7621E−01 |
| 133. | 2.9173E−02 | 1.8672E+01 | 2.0707E+01 | 3.6361E+01 | 7.5602E+01 |
| 134. | 1.1217E−03 | 1.4628E+04 | 1.4665E+04 | 1.4658E+04 | 4.9382E−02 |

56.BARIUM

| Material | $E$, MeV | $\mu_{1en}$, cm$^{-1}$ | $\mu_1$, cm$^{-1}$ | $\mu_2$, cm$^{-1}$ | $R$, % |
|---|---|---|---|---|---|
| 20.Ca | 4.9100E−03 | 8.8380E+02 | 9.0263E+02 | 9.9502E+02 | 1.0236E+01 |
| 23.V | 1.4324E−03 | 1.7697E+04 | 1.7751E+04 | 1.7739E+04 | 6.7384E−02 |
| | 2.8908E−02 | 3.8107E+01 | 4.2110E+01 | 4.2082E+01 | 6.5512E−02 |
| | 3.2401E−02 | 2.6424E+01 | 2.9688E+01 | 2.9460E+01 | 7.7311E−01 |
| 24.Cr | 3.5651E−03 | 2.1399E+03 | 2.1634E+03 | 2.1615E+03 | 9.0439E−02 |
| 26.Fe | 3.7593E−02 | 3.2606E+01 | 1.0120E+02 | 3.7193E+01 | 1.7210E+02 |
| 27.Co | 3.9925E−02 | 3.0998E+01 | 8.6466E+01 | 3.5761E+01 | 1.4179E+02 |
| 28.Ni | 4.4998E−02 | 2.6910E+01 | 6.7137E+01 | 3.1490E+01 | 1.1320E+02 |
| 29.Cu | 4.6631E−02 | 2.5591E+01 | 6.0978E+01 | 3.0202E+01 | 1.0190E+02 |
| 30.Zn | 1.0216E−03 | 2.8460E+04 | 2.8535E+04 | 2.8668E+04 | 4.6795E−01 |
| | 4.2272E−02 | 2.9111E+01 | 7.7422E+01 | 3.4365E+01 | 1.2529E+02 |
| 31.Ga | 1.1235E−03 | 2.6517E+04 | 2.6589E+04 | 2.6759E+04 | 6.3891E−01 |
| | 3.9068E−02 | 3.1589E+01 | 9.1882E+01 | 3.7704E+01 | 1.4370E+02 |
| 32.Ge | 1.2209E−03 | 2.3614E+04 | 2.3683E+04 | 2.3865E+04 | 7.6771E−01 |
| | 3.8625E−02 | 3.1895E+01 | 9.4682E+01 | 3.8634E+01 | 1.4508E+02 |
| 33.As | 4.1190E−02 | 2.9986E+01 | 8.1506E+01 | 3.6605E+01 | 1.2267E+02 |
| 34.Se | 1.2981E−02 | 3.7247E+02 | 3.9528E+02 | 6.8047E+02 | 7.2152E+01 |
| | 3.7869E−02 | 3.2416E+01 | 9.9461E+01 | 4.0745E+01 | 1.4410E+02 |
| 38.Sr | 2.3718E−02 | 7.1576E+01 | 7.7489E+01 | 1.2227E+02 | 5.7792E+01 |
| 39.Y | 4.5426E−02 | 2.6564E+01 | 6.5522E+01 | 3.5746E+01 | 8.3296E+01 |
| 40.Zr | 5.7644E−03 | 2.1437E+03 | 2.3160E+03 | 2.1885E+03 | 5.8285E+00 |
| 41.Nb | 1.4762E−03 | 1.6402E+04 | 1.6453E+04 | 1.6454E+04 | 9.8887E−03 |
| | 1.6703E−02 | 1.7038E+02 | 1.8152E+02 | 1.8275E+02 | 6.8098E−01 |
| 55.Cs | 3.6292E−02 | 1.8907E+01 | 2.1624E+01 | 5.7776E+01 | 1.6719E+02 |
| 57.La | 3.7559E−02 | 3.2629E+01 | 1.0142E+02 | 3.7380E+01 | 1.7131E+02 |
| 58.Ce | 3.9662E−02 | 3.1180E+01 | 8.8131E+01 | 3.6061E+01 | 1.4439E+02 |
| 59.Pr | 4.1023E−02 | 3.0120E+01 | 8.2134E+01 | 3.4993E+01 | 1.3471E+02 |
| 60.Nd | 4.2994E−02 | 2.8529E+01 | 7.4699E+01 | 3.3327E+01 | 1.2414E+02 |

| Material | $E$, MeV | $\mu_{1en}$, cm$^{-1}$ | $\mu_1$, cm$^{-1}$ | $\mu_2$, cm$^{-1}$ | $R$, % |
|---|---|---|---|---|---|
| 61.Pm | 1.0384E−03 | 2.7443E+04 | 2.7515E+04 | 2.7584E+04 | 2.5079E−01 |
| 62.Sm | 1.0925E−03 | 2.8127E+04 | 2.8204E+04 | 2.8282E+04 | 2.7430E−01 |
| 63.Eu | 1.1577E−03 | 2.6405E+04 | 2.6480E+04 | 2.6571E+04 | 3.4383E−01 |
| | 3.9906E−02 | 3.1012E+01 | 8.6590E+01 | 3.5592E+01 | 1.4329E+02 |
| 64.Gd | 1.2073E−03 | 2.4166E+04 | 2.4237E+04 | 2.4331E+04 | 3.8921E−01 |
| 65.Tb | 1.2473E−03 | 2.2612E+04 | 2.2678E+04 | 2.2777E+04 | 4.3800E−01 |
| 66.Dy | 1.3011E−03 | 2.1584E+04 | 2.1646E+04 | 2.1760E+04 | 5.2743E−01 |
| 67.Ho | 1.3548E−03 | 1.9995E+04 | 2.0054E+04 | 2.0163E+04 | 5.4176E−01 |
| | 7.1007E−03 | 1.6069E+03 | 1.7278E+03 | 1.6577E+03 | 4.2310E+00 |
| 70.Yb | 1.5354E−03 | 1.5157E+04 | 1.5206E+04 | 1.5329E+04 | 8.0909E−01 |
| 71.Lu | 1.0968E−03 | 2.7884E+04 | 2.7961E+04 | 2.8000E+04 | 1.3943E−01 |
| | 1.2310E−03 | 2.3230E+04 | 2.3298E+04 | 2.3344E+04 | 1.9738E−01 |
| 88.Ra | 2.1276E−03 | 7.4323E+03 | 7.4692E+03 | 7.4916E+03 | 2.9998E−01 |
| 121. | 1.2117E−03 | 2.3968E+04 | 2.4038E+04 | 2.4119E+04 | 3.3595E−01 |
| | 4.7301E−02 | 2.5049E+01 | 5.8449E+01 | 2.9540E+01 | 9.7866E+01 |
| 123. | 3.8674E−02 | 3.1861E+01 | 9.4372E+01 | 3.8678E+01 | 1.4399E+02 |
| 125. | 7.1315E−03 | 1.5893E+03 | 1.7086E+03 | 1.6397E+03 | 4.2033E+00 |

57.LANTHANUM

| Material | $E$, MeV | $\mu_{1en}$, cm$^{-1}$ | $\mu_1$, cm$^{-1}$ | $\mu_2$, cm$^{-1}$ | $R$, % |
|---|---|---|---|---|---|
| 21.Sc | 4.7813E−03 | 1.8150E+03 | 1.8494E+03 | 2.1221E+03 | 1.4747E+01 |
| 24.Cr | 1.0604E−03 | 4.8965E+04 | 4.9107E+04 | 4.9079E+04 | 5.7171E−02 |
| 26.Fe | 1.4337E−03 | 3.2587E+04 | 3.2698E+04 | 3.2697E+04 | 2.8254E−03 |
| | 3.6979E−02 | 3.4587E+01 | 3.9481E+01 | 3.9392E+01 | 2.2578E−01 |
| 27.Co | 2.7345E−03 | 8.1617E+03 | 8.2145E+03 | 8.2101E+03 | 5.4287E−02 |
| | 7.8945E−03 | 2.1262E+03 | 2.2836E+03 | 2.9897E+03 | 3.0918E+01 |
| 30.Zn | 3.9007E−03 | 3.0382E+03 | 3.0778E+03 | 3.0719E+03 | 1.9431E−01 |
| | 1.2996E−02 | 6.8867E+02 | 7.3339E+02 | 1.0134E+03 | 3.8176E+01 |
| 31.Ga | 1.7951E−03 | 2.0902E+04 | 2.0985E+04 | 2.1072E+04 | 4.1660E−01 |
| | 1.9601E−02 | 1.9509E+02 | 2.0968E+02 | 2.5362E+02 | 2.0957E+01 |
| 32.Ge | 2.8337E−02 | 7.8103E+01 | 8.5895E+01 | 9.8839E+01 | 1.5069E+01 |
| 33.As | 1.4791E−03 | 3.0309E+04 | 3.0416E+04 | 3.0683E+04 | 8.7851E−01 |
| | 1.5159E−03 | 2.8810E+04 | 2.8914E+04 | 2.9158E+04 | 8.4305E−01 |
| | 4.5915E−03 | 2.0419E+03 | 2.0774E+03 | 2.0697E+03 | 3.7122E−01 |
| | 5.2966E−03 | 1.3506E+03 | 1.3827E+03 | 1.3733E+03 | 6.8380E−01 |
| | 1.8389E−02 | 2.4619E+02 | 2.6358E+02 | 3.5924E+02 | 3.6293E+01 |
| 34.Se | 3.5794E−02 | 3.8581E+01 | 4.3768E+01 | 4.8938E+01 | 1.1811E+01 |
| 39.Y | 2.2962E−03 | 1.2299E+04 | 1.2361E+04 | 1.2585E+04 | 1.8100E+00 |
| | 2.5892E−02 | 1.0749E+02 | 1.1700E+02 | 1.8721E+02 | 6.0007E+01 |
| 40.Zr | 3.9979E−02 | 5.2995E+01 | 1.5894E+02 | 7.4287E+01 | 1.1396E+02 |
| 41.Nb | 5.3160E−02 | 3.6862E+01 | 7.8337E+01 | 4.9865E+01 | 5.7097E+01 |

| Material | $E$, MeV | $\mu_{1en}$, cm$^{-1}$ | $\mu_1$, cm$^{-1}$ | $\mu_2$, cm$^{-1}$ | $R$, % |
|---|---|---|---|---|---|
| 43.Tc | 1.3427E−03 | 3.5784E+04 | 3.5899E+04 | 3.5868E+04 | 8.6155E−02 |
| | 6.8594E−03 | 3.1231E+03 | 3.3820E+03 | 3.2052E+03 | 5.5141E+00 |
| 44.Ru | 1.4570E−03 | 3.1418E+04 | 3.1527E+04 | 3.1507E+04 | 6.1661E−02 |
| | 1.4285E−02 | 4.9587E+02 | 5.2806E+02 | 5.2165E+02 | 1.2273E+00 |
| 45.Rh | 1.9332E−03 | 1.6990E+04 | 1.7062E+04 | 1.7076E+04 | 8.3461E−02 |
| | 2.0768E−02 | 1.6905E+02 | 1.8217E+02 | 1.8436E+02 | 1.2017E+00 |
| 46.Pd | 2.8870E−03 | 6.7225E+03 | 6.7721E+03 | 6.7981E+03 | 3.8289E−01 |
| | 2.1629E−02 | 1.5871E+02 | 1.7123E+02 | 1.7328E+02 | 1.1968E+00 |
| 47.Ag | 1.4987E−03 | 2.9328E+04 | 2.9433E+04 | 2.9412E+04 | 7.0303E−02 |
| | 1.9813E−02 | 1.8614E+02 | 2.0024E+02 | 2.0125E+02 | 5.0596E−01 |
| 48.Cd | 6.4737E−03 | 3.4945E+03 | 3.7911E+03 | 3.6258E+03 | 4.5607E+00 |
| 49.In | 1.1560E−03 | 4.6330E+04 | 4.6468E+04 | 4.6411E+04 | 1.2223E−01 |
| | 5.9793E−03 | 3.6048E+03 | 3.9151E+03 | 3.7541E+03 | 4.2891E+00 |
| | 6.0459E−03 | 3.5176E+03 | 3.8182E+03 | 3.6627E+03 | 4.2462E+00 |
| 50.Sn | 1.2907E−03 | 3.8889E+04 | 3.9016E+04 | 3.8967E+04 | 1.2540E−01 |
| 51.Sb | 1.1382E−03 | 4.7923E+04 | 4.8066E+04 | 4.8009E+04 | 1.1841E−01 |
| | 5.9654E−03 | 3.6207E+03 | 3.9327E+03 | 3.8021E+03 | 3.4347E+00 |
| | 6.0699E−03 | 3.4844E+03 | 3.7812E+03 | 3.6575E+03 | 3.3838E+00 |
| | 5.8527E−02 | 3.0903E+01 | 6.0144E+01 | 5.0285E+01 | 1.9606E+01 |
| 52.Te | 1.0266E−03 | 5.2772E+04 | 5.2924E+04 | 5.2870E+04 | 1.0126E−01 |
| | 4.8765E−02 | 4.1927E+01 | 9.7652E+01 | 7.8531E+01 | 2.4349E+01 |
| 56.Ba | 3.7559E−02 | 3.2629E+01 | 3.7380E+01 | 1.0142E+02 | 1.7131E+02 |
| 58.Ce | 1.1646E−03 | 4.5578E+04 | 4.5714E+04 | 4.5732E+04 | 4.0316E−02 |
| 59.Pr | 1.2320E−03 | 4.2947E+04 | 4.3084E+04 | 4.3112E+04 | 6.4327E−02 |
| 59.Pr | 6.6324E−03 | 3.3417E+03 | 3.6227E+03 | 3.6634E+03 | 1.1233E+00 |
| 63.Eu | 1.5043E−03 | 2.9140E+04 | 2.9245E+04 | 2.9317E+04 | 2.4952E−01 |
| | 1.6913E−03 | 2.3843E+04 | 2.3933E+04 | 2.3986E+04 | 2.2291E−01 |
| 64.Gd | 1.3047E−03 | 3.8052E+04 | 3.8176E+04 | 3.8313E+04 | 3.5889E−01 |
| | 7.4929E−03 | 2.5130E+03 | 2.7098E+03 | 2.7915E+03 | 3.0168E+00 |
| 65.Tb | 1.2736E−03 | 3.9991E+04 | 4.0121E+04 | 4.0303E+04 | 4.5455E−01 |
| | 3.9875E−02 | 5.3100E+01 | 1.6009E+02 | 6.0831E+01 | 1.6317E+02 |
| 66.Dy | 1.3271E−03 | 3.6715E+04 | 3.6833E+04 | 3.7034E+04 | 5.4386E−01 |
| | 4.2667E−02 | 4.9613E+01 | 1.4013E+02 | 5.7177E+01 | 1.4509E+02 |
| 67.Ho | 1.3839E−03 | 3.5087E+04 | 3.5202E+04 | 3.5419E+04 | 6.1661E−01 |
| | 4.5156E−02 | 4.6475E+01 | 1.2279E+02 | 5.3893E+01 | 1.2785E+02 |
| 68.Er | 1.4393E−03 | 3.2308E+04 | 3.2418E+04 | 3.2645E+04 | 6.9991E−01 |
| | 4.7264E−02 | 4.3818E+01 | 1.0811E+02 | 5.1141E+01 | 1.1139E+02 |
| 69.Tm | 1.4888E−03 | 2.9826E+04 | 2.9931E+04 | 3.0158E+04 | 7.5622E−01 |
| | 4.9032E−02 | 4.1591E+01 | 9.5794E+01 | 4.8856E+01 | 9.6072E+01 |

| Material | $E$, MeV | $\mu_{1en}$, cm$^{-1}$ | $\mu_1$, cm$^{-1}$ | $\mu_2$, cm$^{-1}$ | $R$, % |
|---|---|---|---|---|---|
| 70.Yb | 4.0022E−02 | 5.2946E+01 | 1.5856E+02 | 6.0781E+01 | 1.6087E+02 |
| 71.Lu | 1.6217E−03 | 2.5813E+04 | 2.5908E+04 | 2.6150E+04 | 9.3372E−01 |
| | 5.5898E−02 | 3.3822E+01 | 6.9056E+01 | 4.0443E+01 | 7.0752E+01 |
| 72.Hf | 1.6753E−03 | 2.4296E+04 | 2.4387E+04 | 2.4595E+04 | 8.5298E−01 |
| | 7.9106E−03 | 2.1108E+03 | 2.2666E+03 | 2.1905E+03 | 3.4722E+00 |
| 80.Hg | 2.1699E−03 | 1.3492E+04 | 1.3556E+04 | 1.3649E+04 | 6.8523E−01 |
| 83.Bi | 1.0524E−03 | 4.9860E+04 | 5.0004E+04 | 4.9996E+04 | 1.6830E−02 |
| | 1.2697E−02 | 7.3340E+02 | 7.8103E+02 | 7.7900E+02 | 2.6121E−01 |
| 84.Po | 1.0467E−03 | 5.0500E+04 | 5.0646E+04 | 5.0630E+04 | 3.1594E−02 |
| | 1.3416E−02 | 6.2581E+02 | 6.6644E+02 | 6.6768E+02 | 1.8535E−01 |
| 87.Fr | 1.2161E−03 | 4.4079E+04 | 4.4219E+04 | 4.4217E+04 | 3.3217E−03 |
| | 1.8514E−03 | 1.9306E+04 | 1.9385E+04 | 1.9436E+04 | 2.6481E−01 |
| 88.Ra | 5.0168E−02 | 4.0183E+01 | 8.8478E+01 | 4.8940E+01 | 8.0789E+01 |
| 112. | 2.8462E−02 | 7.6596E+01 | 8.4301E+01 | 1.5734E+02 | 8.6647E+01 |
| | 4.7944E−02 | 4.2961E+01 | 1.0337E+02 | 7.7155E+01 | 3.3979E+01 |
| 121. | 1.4391E−03 | 3.2319E+04 | 3.2429E+04 | 3.2535E+04 | 3.2605E−01 |
| | 5.9838E−02 | 2.9449E+01 | 5.5703E+01 | 7.3734E+01 | 3.2370E+01 |
| 123. | 2.8180E−02 | 7.9993E+01 | 8.7896E+01 | 1.0184E+02 | 1.5860E+01 |
| 125. | 2.5716E−03 | 9.6995E+03 | 9.7556E+03 | 9.9478E+03 | 1.9697E+00 |
| | 1.4190E−02 | 5.1015E+02 | 5.4326E+02 | 6.3184E+02 | 1.6306E+01 |
| | 4.3318E−02 | 4.8792E+01 | 1.3560E+02 | 5.8088E+01 | 1.3344E+02 |
| 130. | 2.4958E−03 | 1.0416E+04 | 1.0473E+04 | 1.0597E+04 | 1.1804E+00 |
| | 5.2383E−02 | 3.7725E+01 | 8.0972E+01 | 5.8915E+01 | 3.7439E+01 |
| 134. | 3.8663E−02 | 2.8909E+01 | 3.3386E+01 | 4.7397E+01 | 4.1966E+01 |
| | | | 58.CERIUM | | |
| 25.Mn | 1.0833E−03 | 5.3720E+04 | 5.3902E+04 | 5.3880E+04 | 4.0491E−02 |
| 26.Fe | 1.3449E−03 | 4.0510E+04 | 4.0651E+04 | 4.0650E+04 | 3.1711E−03 |
| 27.Co | 1.4890E−03 | 3.3960E+04 | 3.4082E+04 | 3.4099E+04 | 5.1175E−02 |
| | 1.3531E−02 | 6.9498E+02 | 7.4307E+02 | 8.7121E+02 | 1.7244E+01 |
| 28.Ni | 2.7856E−03 | 8.8160E+03 | 8.8755E+03 | 8.8714E+03 | 4.5507E−02 |
| | 9.4899E−03 | 1.5517E+03 | 1.6662E+03 | 2.1885E+03 | 3.1349E+01 |
| 29.Cu | 3.6410E−03 | 4.3611E+03 | 4.4086E+03 | 4.4033E+03 | 1.2075E−01 |
| | 9.8301E−03 | 1.3804E+03 | 1.4793E+03 | 2.0277E+03 | 3.7068E+01 |
| 30.Zn | 1.0457E−03 | 5.8556E+04 | 5.8752E+04 | 5.9069E+04 | 5.3976E−01 |
| | 1.8189E−03 | 2.3109E+04 | 2.3204E+04 | 2.3270E+04 | 2.8563E−01 |
| | 1.7752E−02 | 3.1282E+02 | 3.3513E+02 | 4.0631E+02 | 2.1238E+01 |
| 33.As | 2.8953E−02 | 8.1311E+01 | 8.9771E+01 | 1.0463E+02 | 1.6555E+01 |
| 39.Y | 2.5600E−03 | 1.1246E+04 | 1.1311E+04 | 1.1491E+04 | 1.5891E+00 |
| | 2.9401E−02 | 7.5142E+01 | 8.3229E+01 | 1.1623E+02 | 3.9651E+01 |

| Material | $E$, MeV | $\mu_{1en}$, cm$^{-1}$ | $\mu_1$, cm$^{-1}$ | $\mu_2$, cm$^{-1}$ | $R$, % |
|---|---|---|---|---|---|
| 40.Zr | 2.2473E−03 | 1.4613E+04 | 1.4686E+04 | 1.4968E+04 | 1.9191E+00 |
| | 1.9058E−02 | 2.4992E+02 | 2.6852E+02 | 5.3917E+02 | 1.0079E+02 |
| 41.Nb | 4.9025E−02 | 4.4886E+01 | 1.0876E+02 | 6.1606E+01 | 7.6538E+01 |
| 43.Tc | 1.0547E−03 | 5.7396E+04 | 5.7589E+04 | 5.7487E+04 | 1.7702E−01 |
| 44.Ru | 1.3683E−03 | 3.9073E+04 | 3.9212E+04 | 3.9167E+04 | 1.1518E−01 |
| | 7.3747E−03 | 2.9258E+03 | 3.1777E+03 | 3.0094E+03 | 5.5915E+00 |
| 45.Rh | 8.1350E−03 | 2.2340E+03 | 2.4102E+03 | 2.3043E+03 | 4.5976E+00 |
| 46.Pd | 1.4422E−03 | 3.6399E+04 | 3.6531E+04 | 3.6496E+04 | 9.4263E−02 |
| | 9.6807E−03 | 1.4556E+03 | 1.5613E+03 | 1.5083E+03 | 3.5189E+00 |
| 47.Ag | 1.4290E−03 | 3.5546E+04 | 3.5680E+04 | 3.5633E+04 | 1.3121E−01 |
| | 7.5679E−03 | 2.7331E+03 | 2.9635E+03 | 2.8271E+03 | 4.8246E+00 |
| 48.Cd | 1.0181E−03 | 6.2111E+04 | 6.2318E+04 | 6.2198E+04 | 1.9305E−01 |
| 49.In | 1.1591E−03 | 4.6123E+04 | 4.6278E+04 | 4.6203E+04 | 1.6184E−01 |
| | 5.5007E−02 | 3.7990E+01 | 8.2011E+01 | 6.0674E+01 | 3.5165E+01 |
| 50.Sn | 1.0851E−03 | 5.3493E+04 | 5.3674E+04 | 5.3583E+04 | 1.6997E−01 |
| | 5.6204E−02 | 3.6618E+01 | 7.7426E+01 | 5.9460E+01 | 3.0217E+01 |
| 51.Sb | 1.1465E−03 | 4.7354E+04 | 4.7513E+04 | 4.7439E+04 | 1.5600E−01 |
| | 4.9161E−02 | 4.4725E+01 | 1.0770E+02 | 8.0032E+01 | 3.4576E+01 |
| 52.Te | 4.4572E−02 | 5.0169E+01 | 1.4335E+02 | 1.0258E+02 | 3.9745E+01 |
| 56.Ba | 3.9662E−02 | 3.1180E+01 | 3.6061E+01 | 8.8131E+01 | 1.4439E+02 |
| 57.La | 1.1646E−03 | 4.5578E+04 | 4.5732E+04 | 4.5714E+04 | 4.0316E−02 |
| 59.Pr | 4.7335E−02 | 4.6891E+01 | 1.2188E+02 | 1.2781E+02 | 4.8625E+00 |
| 60.Nd | 1.0680E−03 | 5.5681E+04 | 5.5868E+04 | 5.5924E+04 | 9.9571E−02 |
| | 4.7730E−02 | 4.6423E+01 | 1.1882E+02 | 1.3129E+02 | 1.0497E+01 |
| 61.Pm | 1.0991E−03 | 5.1998E+04 | 5.2175E+04 | 5.2263E+04 | 1.6976E−01 |
| 62.Sm | 1.1117E−03 | 5.0773E+04 | 5.0944E+04 | 5.1055E+04 | 2.1800E−01 |
| | 1.1862E−03 | 4.9982E+04 | 5.0155E+04 | 5.0258E+04 | 2.0441E−01 |
| 63.Eu | 2.9077E−03 | 7.5019E+03 | 7.5582E+03 | 7.5639E+03 | 7.5553E−02 |
| | 2.2630E−02 | 1.6836E+02 | 1.8208E+02 | 1.8378E+02 | 9.3354E−01 |
| 64.Gd | 1.3763E−03 | 3.8606E+04 | 3.8744E+04 | 3.8867E+04 | 3.1696E−01 |
| 65.Tb | 7.9541E−03 | 2.3478E+03 | 2.5353E+03 | 2.6190E+03 | 3.2999E+00 |
| | 8.0480E−03 | 2.2778E+03 | 2.4580E+03 | 2.5386E+03 | 3.2774E+00 |
| 66.Dy | 4.0686E−02 | 5.4779E+01 | 1.7353E+02 | 6.2859E+01 | 1.7606E+02 |
| 67.Ho | 1.3888E−03 | 3.7883E+04 | 3.8020E+04 | 3.8244E+04 | 5.9103E−01 |
| | 4.3301E−02 | 5.1677E+01 | 1.5322E+02 | 5.9628E+01 | 1.5695E+02 |
| 68.Er | 1.4474E−03 | 3.6130E+04 | 3.6261E+04 | 3.6513E+04 | 6.9597E−01 |
| | 4.5543E−02 | 4.9017E+01 | 1.3580E+02 | 5.6886E+01 | 1.3873E+02 |
| 69.Tm | 1.4954E−03 | 3.3626E+04 | 3.3746E+04 | 3.4009E+04 | 7.7833E−01 |
| | 4.7442E−02 | 4.6765E+01 | 1.2106E+02 | 5.4589E+01 | 1.2176E+02 |

| Material | $E$, MeV | $\mu_{1en}$, cm$^{-1}$ | $\mu_1$, cm$^{-1}$ | $\mu_2$, cm$^{-1}$ | $R$, % |
|---|---|---|---|---|---|
| 70.Yb | 1.6155E−03 | 2.9662E+04 | 2.9773E+04 | 3.0046E+04 | 9.1954E−01 |
| 71.Lu | 1.6296E−03 | 2.9208E+04 | 2.9318E+04 | 2.9597E+04 | 9.5321E−01 |
| | 5.9527E−03 | 3.0854E+03 | 3.3294E+03 | 3.1629E+03 | 5.2631E+00 |
| | 6.0514E−03 | 2.9619E+03 | 3.1935E+03 | 3.0381E+03 | 5.1162E+00 |
| | 5.0596E−02 | 4.3047E+01 | 9.8906E+01 | 5.0784E+01 | 9.4758E+01 |
| 72.Hf | 1.6848E−03 | 2.7430E+04 | 2.7535E+04 | 2.7790E+04 | 9.2743E−01 |
| 73.Ta | 1.1043E−03 | 5.1494E+04 | 5.1668E+04 | 5.1690E+04 | 4.2466E−02 |
| | 1.7414E−03 | 2.5606E+04 | 2.5707E+04 | 2.5920E+04 | 8.3022E−01 |
| 80.Hg | 1.3251E−03 | 4.1868E+04 | 4.2015E+04 | 4.2044E+04 | 7.0307E−02 |
| | 2.3013E−03 | 1.4031E+04 | 1.4103E+04 | 1.4258E+04 | 1.0993E+00 |
| 81.Tl | 1.0945E−03 | 5.2456E+04 | 5.2633E+04 | 5.2606E+04 | 5.2513E−02 |
| | 2.3894E−03 | 1.3082E+04 | 1.3152E+04 | 1.3328E+04 | 1.3446E+00 |
| | 1.1569E−02 | 1.0282E+03 | 1.1003E+03 | 1.0862E+03 | 1.2919E+00 |
| 82.Pb | 1.0853E−03 | 5.3462E+04 | 5.3643E+04 | 5.3608E+04 | 6.6076E−02 |
| | 1.1946E−02 | 9.6423E+02 | 1.0317E+03 | 1.0196E+03 | 1.1817E+00 |
| 83.Bi | 7.6476E−03 | 2.6536E+03 | 2.8751E+03 | 2.7433E+03 | 4.8069E+00 |
| 84.Po | 7.6762E−03 | 2.6251E+03 | 2.8434E+03 | 2.7154E+03 | 4.7151E+00 |
| 85.At | 1.1032E−03 | 5.1603E+04 | 5.1778E+04 | 5.1743E+04 | 6.7204E−02 |
| | 1.4050E−02 | 6.0671E+02 | 6.4846E+02 | 6.5006E+02 | 2.4692E−01 |
| 88.Ra | 4.8282E−02 | 4.5768E+01 | 1.1453E+02 | 5.5822E+01 | 1.0517E+02 |
| 89.Ac | 2.4436E−03 | 1.2498E+04 | 1.2567E+04 | 1.2621E+04 | 4.3016E−01 |
| 112. | 3.6717E−03 | 4.2584E+03 | 4.3056E+03 | 4.4052E+03 | 2.3133E+00 |
| | 2.9727E−02 | 7.0659E+01 | 7.8475E+01 | 1.3920E+02 | 7.7380E+01 |
| | 4.4479E−02 | 5.0280E+01 | 1.4407E+02 | 9.5697E+01 | 5.0547E+01 |
| 125. | 4.1198E−02 | 5.4171E+01 | 1.6955E+02 | 6.4410E+01 | 1.6323E+02 |
| 130. | 2.7567E−03 | 9.1279E+03 | 9.1881E+03 | 9.2980E+03 | 1.1960E+00 |
| | 1.4254E−02 | 5.7207E+02 | 6.1133E+02 | 6.8815E+02 | 1.2565E+01 |
| | 4.8013E−02 | 4.6086E+01 | 1.1661E+02 | 7.5017E+01 | 5.5452E+01 |

59.PRASEODYMIUM

| Material | $E$, MeV | $\mu_{1en}$, cm$^{-1}$ | $\mu_1$, cm$^{-1}$ | $\mu_2$, cm$^{-1}$ | $R$, % |
|---|---|---|---|---|---|
| 27.Co | 1.4749E−03 | 3.5483E+04 | 3.5629E+04 | 3.5630E+04 | 3.5632E−03 |
| 28.Ni | 1.9328E−03 | 2.0754E+04 | 2.0849E+04 | 2.0855E+04 | 3.0605E−02 |
| | 1.1850E−02 | 1.0435E+03 | 1.1224E+03 | 1.4053E+03 | 2.5207E+01 |
| 29.Cu | 2.6965E−03 | 1.0461E+04 | 1.0530E+04 | 1.0530E+04 | 2.7730E−03 |
| 29.Cu | 1.2629E−02 | 9.0323E+02 | 9.7093E+02 | 1.2662E+03 | 3.0412E+01 |
| 30.Zn | 1.0805E−03 | 5.9170E+04 | 5.9396E+04 | 5.9676E+04 | 4.7182E−01 |
| | 2.9012E−02 | 8.6490E+01 | 9.5464E+01 | 1.0381E+02 | 8.7395E+00 |
| 33.As | 4.0841E−02 | 3.0497E+01 | 3.5403E+01 | 3.7230E+01 | 5.1589E+00 |
| 39.Y | 2.8823E−03 | 8.3215E+03 | 8.3851E+03 | 8.4886E+03 | 1.2343E+00 |
| | 3.4712E−02 | 5.3221E+01 | 5.9863E+01 | 7.7487E+01 | 2.9440E+01 |

| Material | $E$, MeV | $\mu_{1en}$, cm$^{-1}$ | $\mu_1$, cm$^{-1}$ | $\mu_2$, cm$^{-1}$ | $R$, % |
|---|---|---|---|---|---|
| 40.Zr | 1.9618E−02 | 2.3885E+02 | 2.5749E+02 | 4.9858E+02 | 9.3635E+01 |
| 41.Nb | 4.8921E−02 | 4.5209E+01 | 1.1560E+02 | 6.2103E+01 | 8.6139E+01 |
| 42.Mo | 5.9196E−02 | 3.4038E+01 | 7.0191E+01 | 4.5952E+01 | 5.2750E+01 |
| 43.Tc | 1.1789E−03 | 4.8074E+04 | 4.8258E+04 | 4.8162E+04 | 2.0024E−01 |
| 44.Ru | 6.9365E−03 | 3.4692E+03 | 3.8055E+03 | 3.5660E+03 | 6.7160E+00 |
| 45.Rh | 1.3837E−03 | 4.0818E+04 | 4.0983E+04 | 4.0911E+04 | 1.7664E−01 |
|  | 7.6188E−03 | 2.8078E+03 | 3.0644E+03 | 2.8935E+03 | 5.9062E+00 |
| 46.Pd | 1.4151E−03 | 3.8980E+04 | 3.9138E+04 | 3.9078E+04 | 1.5412E−01 |
|  | 7.7518E−03 | 2.6790E+03 | 2.9200E+03 | 2.7662E+03 | 5.5611E+00 |
| 47.Ag | 1.3434E−03 | 4.3175E+04 | 4.3348E+04 | 4.3265E+04 | 1.9101E−01 |
|  | 7.1124E−03 | 3.2986E+03 | 3.6144E+03 | 3.4120E+03 | 5.9335E+00 |
| 48.Cd | 1.1079E−03 | 5.5245E+04 | 5.5456E+04 | 5.5330E+04 | 2.2932E−01 |
|  | 6.7570E−03 | 3.1950E+03 | 3.4983E+03 | 3.3147E+03 | 5.5399E+00 |
| 49.In | 5.3683E−02 | 4.0049E+01 | 9.2433E+01 | 6.4540E+01 | 4.3218E+01 |
| 50.Sn | 1.2277E−03 | 4.3362E+04 | 4.3529E+04 | 4.3444E+04 | 1.9485E−01 |
|  | 5.4678E−02 | 3.8964E+01 | 8.8418E+01 | 6.4073E+01 | 3.7995E+01 |
| 51.Sb | 4.8971E−02 | 4.5156E+01 | 1.1522E+02 | 8.1185E+01 | 4.1919E+01 |
| 52.Te | 4.4955E−02 | 4.9415E+01 | 1.4613E+02 | 1.0038E+02 | 4.5583E+01 |
| 53.I | 3.3503E−02 | 5.8023E+01 | 6.5027E+01 | 1.7329E+02 | 1.6649E+02 |
| 56.Ba | 4.1023E−02 | 3.0120E+01 | 3.4993E+01 | 8.2134E+01 | 1.3471E+02 |
| 57.La | 1.2320E−03 | 4.2947E+04 | 4.3112E+04 | 4.3084E+04 | 6.4327E−02 |
|  | 6.6324E−03 | 3.3417E+03 | 3.6634E+03 | 3.6227E+03 | 1.1233E+00 |
| 58.Ce | 4.7335E−02 | 4.6891E+01 | 1.2781E+02 | 1.2188E+02 | 4.8625E+00 |
| 60.Nd | 1.1330E−03 | 5.2508E+04 | 5.2709E+04 | 5.2731E+04 | 4.2242E−02 |
|  | 1.3724E−03 | 4.1482E+04 | 4.1649E+04 | 4.1666E+04 | 4.0771E−02 |
|  | 1.5575E−03 | 3.3418E+04 | 3.3553E+04 | 3.3566E+04 | 3.6823E−02 |
|  | 4.8148E−02 | 4.6029E+01 | 1.2155E+02 | 1.2808E+02 | 5.3686E+00 |
| 61.Pm | 1.1385E−03 | 5.1981E+04 | 5.2180E+04 | 5.2243E+04 | 1.2177E−01 |
| 62.Sm | 1.1558E−03 | 5.0304E+04 | 5.0497E+04 | 5.0583E+04 | 1.6952E−01 |
| 64.Gd | 1.4162E−03 | 3.8915E+04 | 3.9073E+04 | 3.9176E+04 | 2.6234E−01 |
| 66.Dy | 7.8779E−03 | 2.5567E+03 | 2.7830E+03 | 2.8785E+03 | 3.4313E+00 |
|  | 8.2315E−03 | 2.3156E+03 | 2.5152E+03 | 2.5993E+03 | 3.3432E+00 |
| 67.Ho | 4.3592E−02 | 5.0861E+01 | 1.5663E+02 | 5.8729E+01 | 1.6670E+02 |
| 68.Er | 1.4492E−03 | 3.6985E+04 | 3.7137E+04 | 3.7379E+04 | 6.5216E−01 |
|  | 4.5658E−02 | 4.8670E+01 | 1.4072E+02 | 5.6503E+01 | 1.4906E+02 |
| 69.Tm | 1.4964E−03 | 3.4222E+04 | 3.4364E+04 | 3.4614E+04 | 7.2734E−01 |
| 69.Tm | 4.7436E−02 | 4.6784E+01 | 1.2704E+02 | 5.4611E+01 | 1.3262E+02 |
| 70.Yb | 1.7013E−03 | 2.8566E+04 | 2.8686E+04 | 2.8937E+04 | 8.7602E−01 |
| 71.Lu | 1.6335E−03 | 3.0854E+04 | 3.0982E+04 | 3.1268E+04 | 9.2442E−01 |

| Material | $E$, MeV | $\mu_{1en}$, cm$^{-1}$ | $\mu_1$, cm$^{-1}$ | $\mu_2$, cm$^{-1}$ | $R$, % |
|---|---|---|---|---|---|
| | 5.0029E−02 | 4.4033E+01 | 1.0718E+02 | 5.1889E+01 | 1.0655E+02 |
| 72.Hf | 1.6893E−03 | 2.8971E+04 | 2.9092E+04 | 2.9361E+04 | 9.2332E−01 |
| 73.Ta | 1.2232E−03 | 4.3803E+04 | 4.3971E+04 | 4.3995E+04 | 5.5319E−02 |
| | 1.7455E−03 | 2.7073E+04 | 2.7188E+04 | 2.7418E+04 | 8.4378E−01 |
| 74.W | 1.3754E−03 | 4.1304E+04 | 4.1470E+04 | 4.1521E+04 | 1.2175E−01 |
| 75.Re | 1.6747E−03 | 2.9463E+04 | 2.9586E+04 | 2.9715E+04 | 4.3703E−01 |
| | 1.8300E−03 | 2.4224E+04 | 2.4330E+04 | 2.4468E+04 | 5.6756E−01 |
| 80.Hg | 1.0763E−03 | 5.9780E+04 | 6.0008E+04 | 5.9956E+04 | 8.6789E−02 |
| | 2.3087E−03 | 1.4929E+04 | 1.5008E+04 | 1.5189E+04 | 1.2013E+00 |
| | 1.1895E−02 | 1.0355E+03 | 1.1137E+03 | 1.0987E+03 | 1.3682E+00 |
| 81.Tl | 1.2118E−03 | 4.4897E+04 | 4.5069E+04 | 4.5044E+04 | 5.5093E−02 |
| | 2.3972E−03 | 1.3910E+04 | 1.3986E+04 | 1.4185E+04 | 1.4218E+00 |
| | 1.0511E−02 | 1.2848E+03 | 1.3829E+03 | 1.3496E+03 | 2.4674E+00 |
| 82.Pb | 1.2002E−03 | 4.6022E+04 | 4.6198E+04 | 4.6165E+04 | 7.2549E−02 |
| | 1.0744E−02 | 1.2428E+03 | 1.3375E+03 | 1.3053E+03 | 2.4630E+00 |
| 83.Bi | 7.0547E−03 | 3.3546E+03 | 3.6772E+03 | 3.4590E+03 | 6.3067E+00 |
| 84.Po | 7.0779E−03 | 3.3321E+03 | 3.6519E+03 | 3.4377E+03 | 6.2302E+00 |
| 85.At | 1.2114E−03 | 4.4942E+04 | 4.5115E+04 | 4.5082E+04 | 7.1839E−02 |
| | 1.2158E−02 | 9.8806E+02 | 1.0625E+03 | 1.0425E+03 | 1.9229E+00 |
| 87.Fr | 1.2260E−03 | 4.3533E+04 | 4.3700E+04 | 4.3671E+04 | 6.6675E−02 |
| 88.Ra | 4.8224E−02 | 4.5949E+01 | 1.2097E+02 | 5.6045E+01 | 1.1584E+02 |
| 89.Ac | 1.1231E−03 | 5.3462E+04 | 5.3667E+04 | 5.3603E+04 | 1.1916E−01 |
| 112. | 6.1572E−03 | 2.9990E+03 | 3.2523E+03 | 3.1412E+03 | 3.5382E+00 |
| | 4.4820E−02 | 4.9559E+01 | 1.4717E+02 | 9.3870E+01 | 5.6785E+01 |
| 116. | 3.6140E−02 | 4.7552E+01 | 5.3766E+01 | 1.3524E+02 | 1.5153E+02 |
| 121. | 1.6016E−03 | 3.1928E+04 | 3.2059E+04 | 3.2141E+04 | 2.5404E−01 |
| | 2.4543E−03 | 1.3253E+04 | 1.3328E+04 | 1.3351E+04 | 1.7738E−01 |
| 130. | 1.4677E−02 | 5.3417E+02 | 5.7254E+02 | 6.4085E+02 | 1.1932E+01 |
| | 4.7955E−02 | 4.6234E+01 | 1.2304E+02 | 7.5319E+01 | 6.3358E+01 |
| 60.NEODYMIUM | | | | | |
| 25.Mn | 1.0382E−03 | 5.7140E+04 | 5.7392E+04 | 5.7310E+04 | 1.4330E−01 |
| 27.Co | 1.4310E−03 | 4.0221E+04 | 4.0399E+04 | 4.0393E+04 | 1.6634E−02 |
| 28.Ni | 1.6888E−03 | 3.0204E+04 | 3.0341E+04 | 3.0348E+04 | 2.4320E−02 |
| | 1.4933E−02 | 5.2184E+02 | 5.6084E+02 | 6.4693E+02 | 1.5349E+01 |
| 29.Cu | 1.9161E−03 | 2.2575E+04 | 2.2683E+04 | 2.2702E+04 | 8.6210E−02 |
| | 1.4670E−02 | 5.7218E+02 | 6.1554E+02 | 7.4745E+02 | 2.1430E+01 |
| 30.Zn | 1.4160E−03 | 4.1091E+04 | 4.1273E+04 | 4.1400E+04 | 3.0638E−01 |
| 39.Y | 3.9890E−02 | 3.5196E+01 | 4.0587E+01 | 4.8216E+01 | 1.8796E+01 |
| 40.Zr | 2.1242E−02 | 2.1549E+02 | 2.3330E+02 | 4.3243E+02 | 8.5349E+01 |

| Material | $E$, MeV | $\mu_{1en}$, cm$^{-1}$ | $\mu_1$, cm$^{-1}$ | $\mu_2$, cm$^{-1}$ | $R$, % |
|---|---|---|---|---|---|
| 41.Nb | 4.8879E−02 | 4.5340E+01 | 1.2246E+02 | 6.2305E+01 | 9.6550E+01 |
| 42.Mo | 5.8325E−02 | 3.5726E+01 | 7.8410E+01 | 4.8411E+01 | 6.1966E+01 |
| 43.Tc | 1.0953E−03 | 5.4349E+04 | 5.4584E+04 | 5.4439E+04 | 2.6649E−01 |
| 45.Rh | 1.3871E−03 | 4.0505E+04 | 4.0684E+04 | 4.0598E+04 | 2.1204E−01 |
| | 7.2665E−03 | 3.2731E+03 | 3.6089E+03 | 3.3714E+03 | 7.0441E+00 |
| 46.Pd | 7.4047E−03 | 3.1424E+03 | 3.4612E+03 | 3.2440E+03 | 6.6928E+00 |
| 47.Ag | 1.3226E−03 | 4.5032E+04 | 4.5232E+04 | 4.5123E+04 | 2.4115E−01 |
| 48.Cd | 1.2961E−03 | 4.0861E+04 | 4.1034E+04 | 4.0943E+04 | 2.2356E−01 |
| 49.In | 5.2831E−02 | 4.1374E+01 | 1.0180E+02 | 6.7029E+01 | 5.1874E+01 |
| 50.Sn | 1.0238E−03 | 5.7841E+04 | 5.8097E+04 | 5.7935E+04 | 2.8112E−01 |
| | 5.3675E−02 | 4.0506E+01 | 9.8206E+01 | 6.7107E+01 | 4.6342E+01 |
| 51.Sb | 4.8897E−02 | 4.5323E+01 | 1.2232E+02 | 8.1632E+01 | 4.9846E+01 |
| 52.Te | 4.5325E−02 | 4.8688E+01 | 1.4976E+02 | 9.8256E+01 | 5.2420E+01 |
| 53.I | 3.5176E−02 | 5.5290E+01 | 6.2256E+01 | 1.5673E+02 | 1.5175E+02 |
| 56.Ba | 4.2994E−02 | 2.8529E+01 | 3.3327E+01 | 7.4699E+01 | 1.2414E+02 |
| 58.Ce | 1.0680E−03 | 5.5681E+04 | 5.5924E+04 | 5.5868E+04 | 9.9571E−02 |
| | 4.7730E−02 | 4.6423E+01 | 1.3129E+02 | 1.1882E+02 | 1.0497E+01 |
| 59.Pr | 1.1330E−03 | 5.2508E+04 | 5.2731E+04 | 5.2709E+04 | 4.2242E−02 |
| | 1.3724E−03 | 4.1482E+04 | 4.1666E+04 | 4.1649E+04 | 4.0771E−02 |
| | 1.5575E−03 | 3.3418E+04 | 3.3566E+04 | 3.3553E+04 | 3.6823E−02 |
| | 4.8148E−02 | 4.6029E+01 | 1.2808E+02 | 1.2155E+02 | 5.3686E+00 |
| 61.Pm | 1.1432E−03 | 5.1978E+04 | 5.2199E+04 | 5.2241E+04 | 8.0701E−02 |
| 62.Sm | 1.1680E−03 | 5.0175E+04 | 5.0388E+04 | 5.0453E+04 | 1.2801E−01 |
| | 1.3242E−03 | 4.4913E+04 | 4.5113E+04 | 4.5156E+04 | 9.5914E−02 |
| 64.Gd | 1.4492E−03 | 3.9170E+04 | 3.9343E+04 | 3.9431E+04 | 2.2258E−01 |
| 67.Ho | 8.1182E−03 | 2.5141E+03 | 2.7517E+03 | 2.8479E+03 | 3.4944E+00 |
| | 4.3882E−02 | 5.0048E+01 | 1.6085E+02 | 5.7832E+01 | 1.7813E+02 |
| 68.Er | 4.5800E−02 | 4.8241E+01 | 1.4612E+02 | 5.6029E+01 | 1.6079E+02 |
| 69.Tm | 1.4999E−03 | 3.6230E+04 | 3.6389E+04 | 3.6649E+04 | 7.1467E−01 |
| | 4.7472E−02 | 4.6666E+01 | 1.3327E+02 | 5.4479E+01 | 1.4462E+02 |
| 70.Yb | 1.7675E−03 | 2.7562E+04 | 2.7688E+04 | 2.7919E+04 | 8.3318E−01 |
| 71.Lu | 1.6360E−03 | 3.1972E+04 | 3.2116E+04 | 3.2403E+04 | 8.9327E−01 |
| | 4.9927E−02 | 4.4353E+01 | 1.1441E+02 | 5.2246E+01 | 1.1898E+02 |
| 72.Hf | 1.6915E−03 | 3.0112E+04 | 3.0249E+04 | 3.0523E+04 | 9.0456E−01 |
| 73.Ta | 1.7486E−03 | 2.8195E+04 | 2.8324E+04 | 2.8563E+04 | 8.4288E−01 |
| | 9.4529E−03 | 1.7709E+03 | 1.9256E+03 | 1.8556E+03 | 3.7723E+00 |
| 74.W | 1.3774E−03 | 4.1151E+04 | 4.1333E+04 | 4.1368E+04 | 8.4026E−02 |
| | 1.8114E−03 | 2.6089E+04 | 2.6210E+04 | 2.6414E+04 | 7.7907E−01 |
| 75.Re | 1.4958E−03 | 3.6466E+04 | 3.6626E+04 | 3.6718E+04 | 2.5217E−01 |

| Material | $E$, MeV | $\mu_{1en}$, cm$^{-1}$ | $\mu_1$, cm$^{-1}$ | $\mu_2$, cm$^{-1}$ | $R$, % |
|---|---|---|---|---|---|
| | 1.5123E−03 | 3.5626E+04 | 3.5782E+04 | 3.5878E+04 | 2.6771E−01 |
| | 1.8490E−03 | 2.4828E+04 | 2.4945E+04 | 2.5104E+04 | 6.4106E−01 |
| 80.Hg | 2.3165E−03 | 1.5875E+04 | 1.5960E+04 | 1.6168E+04 | 1.2990E+00 |
| 80.Hg | 1.1175E−02 | 1.2413E+03 | 1.3426E+03 | 1.3098E+03 | 2.5007E+00 |
| 81.Tl | 2.4054E−03 | 1.4782E+04 | 1.4865E+04 | 1.5088E+04 | 1.5014E+00 |
| | 7.7852E−03 | 2.7829E+03 | 3.0545E+03 | 2.8786E+03 | 6.1113E+00 |
| 82.Pb | 7.8040E−03 | 2.7652E+03 | 3.0344E+03 | 2.8611E+03 | 6.0582E+00 |
| 85.At | 7.8101E−03 | 2.7593E+03 | 3.0278E+03 | 2.8571E+03 | 5.9743E+00 |
| 87.Fr | 1.0458E−03 | 5.6769E+04 | 5.7019E+04 | 5.6909E+04 | 1.9306E−01 |
| 88.Ra | 4.8219E−02 | 4.5962E+01 | 1.2753E+02 | 5.6061E+01 | 1.2748E+02 |
| 89.Ac | 1.1350E−03 | 5.2410E+04 | 5.2633E+04 | 5.2551E+04 | 1.5585E−01 |
| 112. | 4.5157E−02 | 4.8846E+01 | 1.5105E+02 | 9.2065E+01 | 6.4070E+01 |
| 116. | 3.7382E−02 | 4.5885E+01 | 5.2114E+01 | 1.2506E+02 | 1.3997E+02 |
| 121. | 2.2832E−03 | 1.6284E+04 | 1.6371E+04 | 1.6401E+04 | 1.8768E−01 |
| | 8.8558E−03 | 2.1034E+03 | 2.2952E+03 | 2.3682E+03 | 3.1822E+00 |
| 125. | 2.6351E−03 | 1.1962E+04 | 1.2036E+04 | 1.2288E+04 | 2.0898E+00 |
| 130. | 1.0004E−03 | 4.5736E+04 | 4.5937E+04 | 4.5837E+04 | 2.1731E−01 |
| | 6.2196E−03 | 3.0810E+03 | 3.3625E+03 | 3.2288E+03 | 4.1414E+00 |
| | 4.7969E−02 | 4.6197E+01 | 1.2945E+02 | 7.5244E+01 | 7.2040E+01 |
| | | | 61.PROMETHIUM | | |
| 22.Ti | 1.0354E−03 | 2.5394E+04 | 2.5525E+04 | 2.5434E+04 | 3.5974E−01 |
| 23.V | 1.0473E−03 | 3.7212E+04 | 3.7399E+04 | 3.7282E+04 | 3.1578E−01 |
| 25.Mn | 1.1060E−03 | 5.1995E+04 | 5.2260E+04 | 5.2150E+04 | 2.0996E−01 |
| 26.Fe | 1.2888E−03 | 4.5514E+04 | 4.5736E+04 | 4.5673E+04 | 1.3662E−01 |
| 27.Co | 1.3891E−03 | 4.4751E+04 | 4.4966E+04 | 4.4946E+04 | 4.6341E−02 |
| 29.Cu | 1.4886E−03 | 4.0603E+04 | 4.0804E+04 | 4.0837E+04 | 8.1947E−02 |
| | 1.5576E−03 | 3.7036E+04 | 3.7220E+04 | 3.7246E+04 | 7.1219E−02 |
| | 4.3672E−02 | 3.0816E+01 | 3.5985E+01 | 3.6165E+01 | 5.0045E−01 |
| 40.Zr | 1.0364E−03 | 2.6123E+04 | 2.6258E+04 | 2.6168E+04 | 3.4318E−01 |
| | 2.6227E−02 | 1.5209E+02 | 1.6634E+02 | 2.7833E+02 | 6.7325E+01 |
| 41.Nb | 1.0472E−03 | 3.7077E+04 | 3.7264E+04 | 3.7144E+04 | 3.2297E−01 |
| | 1.9016E−02 | 3.2038E+02 | 3.4658E+02 | 7.5001E+02 | 1.1640E+02 |
| | 4.8191E−02 | 4.7478E+01 | 1.3964E+02 | 6.5598E+01 | 1.1287E+02 |
| 42.Mo | 5.6255E−02 | 3.9736E+01 | 9.6002E+01 | 5.4255E+01 | 7.6946E+01 |
| 43.Tc | 1.1268E−03 | 5.1986E+04 | 5.2249E+04 | 5.2075E+04 | 3.3462E−01 |
| 44.Ru | 1.3120E−03 | 4.3930E+04 | 4.4143E+04 | 4.4027E+04 | 2.6506E−01 |
| | 7.0776E−03 | 3.2942E+03 | 3.6693E+03 | 3.3867E+03 | 8.3422E+00 |
| 47.Ag | 7.3121E−03 | 3.0507E+03 | 3.3995E+03 | 3.1556E+03 | 7.7318E+00 |
| 48.Cd | 1.1507E−03 | 5.1975E+04 | 5.2237E+04 | 5.2059E+04 | 3.4238E−01 |

| Material | $E$, MeV | $\mu_{1en}$, cm$^{-1}$ | $\mu_1$, cm$^{-1}$ | $\mu_2$, cm$^{-1}$ | $R$, % |
|---|---|---|---|---|---|
| | 5.8312E−02 | 3.7695E+01 | 8.6378E+01 | 5.7237E+01 | 5.0912E+01 |
| 49.In | 1.0729E−03 | 5.2010E+04 | 5.2276E+04 | 5.2095E+04 | 3.4849E−01 |
| | 2.7945E−02 | 1.2206E+02 | 1.3422E+02 | 3.4584E+02 | 1.5766E+02 |
| | 4.9909E−02 | 4.6018E+01 | 1.2599E+02 | 7.5855E+01 | 6.6096E+01 |
| 50.Sn | 1.1061E−03 | 5.1995E+04 | 5.2260E+04 | 5.2084E+04 | 3.3708E−01 |
| | 5.0393E−02 | 4.5551E+01 | 1.2343E+02 | 7.7028E+01 | 6.0237E+01 |
| 51.Sb | 1.0782E−03 | 5.2008E+04 | 5.2274E+04 | 5.2097E+04 | 3.3841E−01 |
| | 4.7800E−02 | 4.7811E+01 | 1.4275E+02 | 8.8290E+01 | 6.1680E+01 |
| 53.I | 1.0502E−03 | 4.0452E+04 | 4.0655E+04 | 4.0534E+04 | 2.9818E−01 |
| | 3.7210E−02 | 5.1966E+01 | 5.8908E+01 | 1.3658E+02 | 1.3186E+02 |
| 56.Ba | 1.0384E−03 | 2.7442E+04 | 2.7584E+04 | 2.7515E+04 | 2.5079E−01 |
| 58.Ce | 1.0991E−03 | 5.1998E+04 | 5.2263E+04 | 5.2175E+04 | 1.6976E−01 |
| 59.Pr | 1.1385E−03 | 5.1981E+04 | 5.2243E+04 | 5.2180E+04 | 1.2177E−01 |
| 60.Nd | 1.1432E−03 | 5.1978E+04 | 5.2241E+04 | 5.2199E+04 | 8.0701E−02 |
| 62.Sm | 1.2302E−03 | 4.9516E+04 | 4.9762E+04 | 4.9787E+04 | 5.0742E−02 |
| | 1.6913E−03 | 3.2451E+04 | 3.2613E+04 | 3.2636E+04 | 6.9866E−02 |
| | 5.5964E−02 | 4.0024E+01 | 9.7363E+01 | 1.0266E+02 | 5.4440E+00 |
| 64.Gd | 1.4704E−03 | 3.9334E+04 | 3.9529E+04 | 3.9595E+04 | 1.6572E−01 |
| | 8.1025E−03 | 2.7599E+03 | 3.0454E+03 | 3.1195E+03 | 2.4348E+00 |
| | 5.5629E−02 | 4.0357E+01 | 9.8933E+01 | 1.1720E+02 | 1.8466E+01 |
| 65.Tb | 1.3672E−03 | 4.6347E+04 | 4.6568E+04 | 4.6710E+04 | 3.0491E−01 |
| | 5.3177E−02 | 4.2789E+01 | 1.1040E+02 | 1.3950E+02 | 2.6356E+01 |
| 66.Dy | 1.0279E−03 | 2.0295E+04 | 2.0400E+04 | 2.0388E+04 | 6.0507E−02 |
| | 1.3577E−03 | 4.7043E+04 | 4.7267E+04 | 4.7460E+04 | 4.0781E−01 |
| 67.Ho | 1.0302E−03 | 2.1843E+04 | 2.1956E+04 | 2.1938E+04 | 7.9930E−02 |
| 68.Er | 1.0327E−03 | 2.3593E+04 | 2.3714E+04 | 2.3692E+04 | 9.3088E−02 |
| | 4.5214E−02 | 5.0009E+01 | 1.6329E+02 | 5.7982E+01 | 1.8162E+02 |
| 69.Tm | 1.0355E−03 | 2.5504E+04 | 2.5635E+04 | 2.5606E+04 | 1.1360E−01 |
| | 9.3775E−03 | 1.9921E+03 | 2.1828E+03 | 2.2699E+03 | 3.9904E+00 |
| | 4.6880E−02 | 4.8593E+01 | 1.5006E+02 | 5.6615E+01 | 1.6505E+02 |
| 70.Yb | 1.0269E−03 | 1.9626E+04 | 1.9728E+04 | 1.9700E+04 | 1.3966E−01 |
| | 1.0194E−02 | 1.5764E+03 | 1.7169E+03 | 1.8622E+03 | 8.4627E+00 |
| 71.Lu | 1.0408E−03 | 2.9828E+04 | 2.9981E+04 | 2.9945E+04 | 1.1964E−01 |
| | 1.6385E−03 | 3.3023E+04 | 3.3192E+04 | 3.3469E+04 | 8.3713E−01 |
| | 4.9349E−02 | 4.6495E+01 | 1.3044E+02 | 5.4633E+01 | 1.3876E+02 |
| 72.Hf | 1.0514E−03 | 4.1719E+04 | 4.1928E+04 | 4.1865E+04 | 1.4859E−01 |
| | 1.6957E−03 | 3.2298E+04 | 3.2459E+04 | 3.2747E+04 | 8.8897E−01 |
| 73.Ta | 1.0965E−03 | 5.2000E+04 | 5.2265E+04 | 5.2196E+04 | 1.3082E−01 |
| | 1.7544E−03 | 3.0289E+04 | 3.0442E+04 | 3.0700E+04 | 8.4846E−01 |

| Material | $E$, MeV | $\mu_{1en}$, cm$^{-1}$ | $\mu_1$, cm$^{-1}$ | $\mu_2$, cm$^{-1}$ | $R$, % |
|---|---|---|---|---|---|
| | 7.5916E−03 | 3.2138E+03 | 3.5631E+03 | 3.3215E+03 | 7.2735E+00 |
| 74.W | 1.8172E−03 | 2.8142E+04 | 2.8288E+04 | 2.8510E+04 | 7.8763E−01 |
| 75.Re | 1.4484E−03 | 4.0738E+04 | 4.0938E+04 | 4.0990E+04 | 1.2610E−01 |
| | 1.8827E−03 | 2.5899E+04 | 2.6037E+04 | 2.6232E+04 | 7.5169E−01 |
| 76.Os | 1.8563E−03 | 2.6802E+04 | 2.6943E+04 | 2.7050E+04 | 3.9933E−01 |
| 78.Pt | 2.1123E−03 | 2.0360E+04 | 2.0477E+04 | 2.0603E+04 | 6.1762E−01 |
| 79.Au | 1.9409E−03 | 2.3906E+04 | 2.4036E+04 | 2.4140E+04 | 4.3273E−01 |
| | 2.2062E−03 | 1.9087E+04 | 1.9199E+04 | 1.9350E+04 | 7.8790E−01 |
| 80.Hg | 1.1849E−03 | 5.1959E+04 | 5.2220E+04 | 5.2136E+04 | 1.6161E−01 |
| 80.Hg | 2.3292E−03 | 1.7418E+04 | 1.7524E+04 | 1.7766E+04 | 1.3812E+00 |
| | 7.9561E−03 | 2.8638E+03 | 3.1630E+03 | 2.9666E+03 | 6.6191E+00 |
| 81.Tl | 1.1016E−03 | 5.1997E+04 | 5.2262E+04 | 5.2147E+04 | 2.1982E−01 |
| | 2.4187E−03 | 1.6203E+04 | 1.6305E+04 | 1.6558E+04 | 1.5557E+00 |
| 82.Pb | 1.1080E−03 | 5.1994E+04 | 5.2259E+04 | 5.2140E+04 | 2.2860E−01 |
| 83.Bi | 7.3093E−03 | 3.0536E+03 | 3.4033E+03 | 3.1517E+03 | 7.9853E+00 |
| 84.Po | 7.3404E−03 | 3.0219E+03 | 3.3617E+03 | 3.1208E+03 | 7.7186E+00 |
| 85.At | 1.0967E−03 | 5.2000E+04 | 5.2264E+04 | 5.2140E+04 | 2.3946E−01 |
| 87.Fr | 1.0902E−03 | 5.2003E+04 | 5.2268E+04 | 5.2143E+04 | 2.4009E−01 |
| 88.Ra | 1.0399E−03 | 2.8828E+04 | 2.8977E+04 | 2.8898E+04 | 2.7151E−01 |
| | 3.1469E−03 | 7.6931E+03 | 7.7628E+03 | 7.9565E+03 | 2.4954E+00 |
| | 4.7556E−02 | 4.8018E+01 | 1.4468E+02 | 5.8597E+01 | 1.4691E+02 |
| 89.Ac | 1.1399E−03 | 5.1980E+04 | 5.2243E+04 | 5.2121E+04 | 2.3349E−01 |
| | 7.9397E−03 | 2.8795E+03 | 3.1809E+03 | 2.9877E+03 | 6.4655E+00 |
| 112. | 3.8072E−03 | 4.8865E+03 | 4.9447E+03 | 5.0829E+03 | 2.7948E+00 |
| 116. | 1.0478E−03 | 3.7739E+04 | 3.7929E+04 | 3.7825E+04 | 2.7548E−01 |
| | 3.8932E−02 | 4.3805E+01 | 5.0095E+01 | 1.1235E+02 | 1.2428E+02 |
| 118. | 1.0274E−03 | 1.9919E+04 | 2.0022E+04 | 1.9973E+04 | 2.4404E−01 |
| 121. | 2.8593E−03 | 1.0226E+04 | 1.0305E+04 | 1.0360E+04 | 5.3942E−01 |
| | 4.2244E−02 | 3.3898E+01 | 3.9345E+01 | 3.9246E+01 | 2.5126E−01 |
| 125. | 1.0391E−03 | 2.7944E+04 | 2.8088E+04 | 2.8019E+04 | 2.4851E−01 |
| | 2.8142E−03 | 1.0838E+04 | 1.0919E+04 | 1.1129E+04 | 1.9203E+00 |
| 130. | 1.0511E−03 | 4.1407E+04 | 4.1614E+04 | 4.1500E+04 | 2.7575E−01 |
| | 2.9833E−03 | 8.5446E+03 | 8.6177E+03 | 8.7064E+03 | 1.0297E+00 |
| | 3.0612E−03 | 8.0574E+03 | 8.1286E+03 | 8.2109E+03 | 1.0121E+00 |
| | 1.7686E−02 | 4.0079E+02 | 4.3296E+02 | 4.8012E+02 | 1.0893E+01 |
| | 4.7084E−02 | 4.8419E+01 | 1.4843E+02 | 7.9791E+01 | 8.6027E+01 |

62.SAMARIUM

| Material | $E$, MeV | $\mu_{1en}$, cm$^{-1}$ | $\mu_1$, cm$^{-1}$ | $\mu_2$, cm$^{-1}$ | $R$, % |
|---|---|---|---|---|---|
| 21.Sc | 1.0011E−03 | 1.5612E+04 | 1.5687E+04 | 1.5633E+04 | 3.4343E−01 |
| 22.Ti | 1.0861E−03 | 2.3658E+04 | 2.3790E+04 | 2.3695E+04 | 4.0003E−01 |

| Material | $E$, MeV | $\mu_{1en}$, cm$^{-1}$ | $\mu_1$, cm$^{-1}$ | $\mu_2$, cm$^{-1}$ | $R$, % |
|---|---|---|---|---|---|
| 23.V | 1.0991E−03 | 3.4591E+04 | 3.4783E+04 | 3.4658E+04 | 3.6157E−01 |
| 25.Mn | 1.1239E−03 | 5.0643E+04 | 5.0925E+04 | 5.0794E+04 | 2.5743E−01 |
| 26.Fe | 1.2458E−03 | 4.9351E+04 | 4.9620E+04 | 4.9526E+04 | 1.9105E−01 |
| 28.Ni | 1.4596E−03 | 4.2421E+04 | 4.2653E+04 | 4.2629E+04 | 5.6529E−02 |
| 29.Cu | 1.4907E−03 | 4.0366E+04 | 4.0586E+04 | 4.0599E+04 | 3.0635E−02 |
| | 1.5236E−03 | 3.8410E+04 | 3.8622E+04 | 3.8628E+04 | 1.6789E−02 |
| 40.Zr | 1.0872E−03 | 2.4419E+04 | 2.4556E+04 | 2.4464E+04 | 3.7568E−01 |
| | 2.7824E−02 | 1.3177E+02 | 1.4500E+02 | 2.2893E+02 | 5.7886E+01 |
| 41.Nb | 1.0990E−03 | 3.4580E+04 | 3.4771E+04 | 3.4645E+04 | 3.6385E−01 |
| | 2.4075E−03 | 1.7308E+04 | 1.7418E+04 | 1.7767E+04 | 2.0070E+00 |
| | 1.9459E−02 | 3.1092E+02 | 3.3748E+02 | 7.0994E+02 | 1.1037E+02 |
| | 4.8522E−02 | 4.6450E+01 | 1.4370E+02 | 6.4015E+01 | 1.2447E+02 |
| 42.Mo | 5.6232E−02 | 3.9780E+01 | 1.0133E+02 | 5.4319E+01 | 8.6544E+01 |
| 43.Tc | 1.1481E−03 | 5.0386E+04 | 5.0665E+04 | 5.0475E+04 | 3.7765E−01 |
| 44.Ru | 1.2497E−03 | 4.9310E+04 | 4.9579E+04 | 4.9409E+04 | 3.4327E−01 |
| 45.Rh | 1.3697E−03 | 4.2123E+04 | 4.2350E+04 | 4.2216E+04 | 3.1621E−01 |
| | 7.4174E−03 | 3.0739E+03 | 3.4521E+03 | 3.1668E+03 | 9.0094E+00 |
| 46.Pd | 1.4047E−03 | 3.9974E+04 | 4.0188E+04 | 4.0072E+04 | 2.8909E−01 |
| | 7.5498E−03 | 2.9487E+03 | 3.3222E+03 | 3.0443E+03 | 9.1293E+00 |
| 47.Ag | 1.3234E−03 | 4.4960E+04 | 4.5203E+04 | 4.5051E+04 | 3.3733E−01 |
| 48.Cd | 1.1752E−03 | 5.0099E+04 | 5.0375E+04 | 5.0182E+04 | 3.8458E−01 |
| | 5.8106E−02 | 3.8071E+01 | 9.2005E+01 | 5.7915E+01 | 5.8862E+01 |
| 49.In | 2.8467E−02 | 1.1989E+02 | 1.3226E+02 | 3.3133E+02 | 1.5052E+02 |
| | 5.0488E−02 | 4.5016E+01 | 1.2991E+02 | 7.3868E+01 | 7.5870E+01 |
| 50.Sn | 1.1254E−03 | 5.0627E+04 | 5.0908E+04 | 5.0714E+04 | 3.8217E−01 |
| | 5.1109E−02 | 4.4450E+01 | 1.2682E+02 | 7.4863E+01 | 6.9403E+01 |
| 51.Sb | 4.8349E−02 | 4.6566E+01 | 1.4502E+02 | 8.4959E+01 | 7.0699E+01 |
| 52.Te | 3.3417E−02 | 7.4361E+01 | 8.3253E+01 | 2.1185E+02 | 1.5446E+02 |
| 53.I | 1.1032E−03 | 3.8801E+04 | 3.9016E+04 | 3.8883E+04 | 3.4345E−01 |
| | 3.8191E−02 | 5.0363E+01 | 5.7298E+01 | 1.2687E+02 | 1.2142E+02 |
| 56.Ba | 1.0925E−03 | 2.8127E+04 | 2.8282E+04 | 2.8204E+04 | 2.7430E−01 |
| 58.Ce | 1.1117E−03 | 5.0773E+04 | 5.1055E+04 | 5.0944E+04 | 2.1800E−01 |
| | 1.1862E−03 | 4.9982E+04 | 5.0258E+04 | 5.0155E+04 | 2.0441E−01 |
| 59.Pr | 1.1558E−03 | 5.0304E+04 | 5.0583E+04 | 5.0497E+04 | 1.6952E−01 |
| 60.Nd | 1.1680E−03 | 5.0175E+04 | 5.0453E+04 | 5.0388E+04 | 1.2801E−01 |
| | 1.3242E−03 | 4.4913E+04 | 4.5156E+04 | 4.5113E+04 | 9.5914E−02 |
| 61.Pm | 1.2302E−03 | 4.9516E+04 | 4.9787E+04 | 4.9762E+04 | 5.0742E−02 |
| | 1.6913E−03 | 3.2451E+04 | 3.2636E+04 | 3.2613E+04 | 6.9866E−02 |
| | 5.5964E−02 | 4.0024E+01 | 1.0266E+02 | 9.7363E+01 | 5.4440E+00 |

| Material | $E$, MeV | $\mu_{1en}$, $cm^{-1}$ | $\mu_1$, $cm^{-1}$ | $\mu_2$, $cm^{-1}$ | $R$, % |
|---|---|---|---|---|---|
| 64.Gd | 5.5502E−02 | 4.0445E+01 | 1.0496E+02 | 1.1791E+02 | 1.2332E+01 |
| 65.Tb | 8.6183E−03 | 2.5616E+03 | 2.8445E+03 | 2.9092E+03 | 2.2734E+00 |
| | 5.2366E−02 | 4.3304E+01 | 1.2057E+02 | 1.4412E+02 | 1.9535E+01 |
| 67.Ho | 1.0809E−03 | 2.0047E+04 | 2.0161E+04 | 2.0139E+04 | 1.0970E−01 |
| 68.Er | 1.0833E−03 | 2.1706E+04 | 2.1829E+04 | 2.1806E+04 | 1.0563E−01 |
| 69.Tm | 1.0859E−03 | 2.3497E+04 | 2.3629E+04 | 2.3600E+04 | 1.2357E−01 |
| | 4.7283E−02 | 4.7279E+01 | 1.5321E+02 | 5.5159E+01 | 1.7776E+02 |
| 71.Lu | 1.0924E−03 | 2.8038E+04 | 2.8192E+04 | 2.8154E+04 | 1.3570E−01 |
| | 4.9546E−02 | 4.5765E+01 | 1.3583E+02 | 5.3820E+01 | 1.5238E+02 |
| 72.Hf | 1.1035E−03 | 3.9154E+04 | 3.9371E+04 | 3.9300E+04 | 1.8014E−01 |
| | 1.6957E−03 | 3.2259E+04 | 3.2442E+04 | 3.2707E+04 | 8.1757E−01 |
| 73.Ta | 1.1162E−03 | 5.0725E+04 | 5.1007E+04 | 5.0920E+04 | 1.6989E−01 |
| | 1.7573E−03 | 3.1307E+04 | 3.1480E+04 | 3.1739E+04 | 8.2408E−01 |
| 74.W | 1.3485E−03 | 4.3418E+04 | 4.3652E+04 | 4.3636E+04 | 3.7222E−02 |
| | 1.8201E−03 | 2.9193E+04 | 2.9356E+04 | 2.9583E+04 | 7.7360E−01 |
| 75.Re | 1.8867E−03 | 2.6951E+04 | 2.7103E+04 | 2.7309E+04 | 7.5845E−01 |
| 76.Os | 1.6065E−03 | 3.6335E+04 | 3.6537E+04 | 3.6584E+04 | 1.2771E−01 |
| 77.Ir | 1.9514E−03 | 2.4776E+04 | 2.4918E+04 | 2.5024E+04 | 4.2810E−01 |
| 78.Pt | 1.9593E−03 | 2.4509E+04 | 2.4650E+04 | 2.4767E+04 | 4.7283E−01 |
| 79.Au | 1.6161E−03 | 3.5843E+04 | 3.6042E+04 | 3.6090E+04 | 1.3397E−01 |
| | 2.2121E−03 | 2.0104E+04 | 2.0226E+04 | 2.0402E+04 | 8.6899E−01 |
| 80.Hg | 1.2169E−03 | 4.9657E+04 | 4.9929E+04 | 4.9833E+04 | 1.9281E−01 |
| | 2.3366E−03 | 1.8322E+04 | 1.8436E+04 | 1.8703E+04 | 1.4441E+00 |
| | 7.7398E−03 | 3.1871E+03 | 3.5604E+03 | 3.2958E+03 | 8.0295E+00 |
| 81.Tl | 1.1224E−03 | 5.0659E+04 | 5.0941E+04 | 5.0808E+04 | 2.6045E−01 |
| | 2.4265E−03 | 1.7035E+04 | 1.7143E+04 | 1.7419E+04 | 1.6062E+00 |
| 82.Pb | 1.1298E−03 | 5.0580E+04 | 5.0861E+04 | 5.0725E+04 | 2.6903E 01 |
| | 2.4923E−03 | 1.6094E+04 | 1.6199E+04 | 1.6470E+04 | 1.6743E+00 |
| 85.At | 1.1177E−03 | 5.0708E+04 | 5.0991E+04 | 5.0848E+04 | 2.7984E−01 |
| 88.Ra | 1.0907E−03 | 2.6838E+04 | 2.6987E+04 | 2.6908E+04 | 2.9163E−01 |
| | 4.7935E−02 | 4.6843E+01 | 1.4820E+02 | 5.7148E+01 | 1.5933E+02 |
| 89.Ac | 1.1592E−03 | 5.0269E+04 | 5.0547E+04 | 5.0410E+04 | 2.7198E−01 |
| 116. | 1.1003E−03 | 3.5854E+04 | 3.6052E+04 | 3.5936E+04 | 3.2403E−01 |
| | 3.9701E−02 | 4.2773E+01 | 4.9088E+01 | 1.0605E+02 | 1.1604E+02 |
| 121. | 2.9953E−03 | 8.8918E+03 | 8.9667E+03 | 9.0114E+03 | 4.9835E−01 |
| | 5.4593E−03 | 2.0330E+03 | 2.0784E+03 | 2.0799E+03 | 7.1573E−02 |
| | 6.0289E−03 | 1.5203E+03 | 1.5619E+03 | 1.5617E+03 | 9.7235E−03 |
| 125. | 1.0887E−03 | 2.5484E+04 | 2.5626E+04 | 2.5559E+04 | 2.6219E−01 |
| | 2.8947E−03 | 1.0333E+04 | 1.0414E+04 | 1.0608E+04 | 1.8695E+00 |

| Material | $E$, MeV | $\mu_{1en}$, cm$^{-1}$ | $\mu_1$, cm$^{-1}$ | $\mu_2$, cm$^{-1}$ | $R$, % |
|---|---|---|---|---|---|
| 130. | 1.1037E−03 | 3.9352E+04 | 3.9570E+04 | 3.9446E+04 | 3.1528E−01 |
| | 3.8534E−03 | 4.9832E+03 | 5.0438E+03 | 5.0844E+03 | 8.0411E−01 |
| | 4.5039E−03 | 3.3819E+03 | 3.4352E+03 | 3.4569E+03 | 6.3235E−01 |
| | 2.6467E−02 | 1.5686E+02 | 1.7193E+02 | 1.8371E+02 | 6.8545E+00 |
| | 3.1668E−02 | 8.3151E+01 | 9.2762E+01 | 9.6769E+01 | 4.3196E+00 |
| | 4.7631E−02 | 4.7047E+01 | 1.5054E+02 | 7.6982E+01 | 9.5550E+01 |
| | | | 63.EUROPIUM | | |
| 21.Sc | 1.1315E−03 | 1.2980E+04 | 1.3060E+04 | 1.2999E+04 | 4.6782E−01 |
| | 6.9541E−03 | 7.7987E+02 | 8.0671E+02 | 8.7543E+02 | 8.5189E+00 |
| 22.Ti | 1.1498E−03 | 2.1476E+04 | 2.1609E+04 | 2.1512E+04 | 4.5362E−01 |
| 24.Cr | 1.2986E−03 | 3.2890E+04 | 3.3090E+04 | 3.2969E+04 | 3.6933E−01 |
| 25.Mn | 1.4101E−03 | 2.8945E+04 | 2.9120E+04 | 2.9032E+04 | 3.0202E−01 |
| 27.Co | 1.8811E−03 | 1.9805E+04 | 1.9929E+04 | 1.9891E+04 | 1.8876E−01 |
| | 9.7200E−03 | 1.3708E+03 | 1.5212E+03 | 1.8138E+03 | 1.9235E+01 |
| 28.Ni | 2.8052E−03 | 8.5835E+03 | 8.6504E+03 | 8.6382E+03 | 1.4182E−01 |
| 29.Cu | 3.5016E−03 | 4.8605E+03 | 4.9108E+03 | 4.9048E+03 | 1.2195E−01 |
| | 9.4271E−03 | 1.5006E+03 | 1.6706E+03 | 2.2486E+03 | 3.4603E+01 |
| 30.Zn | 1.9784E−03 | 1.7577E+04 | 1.7686E+04 | 1.7697E+04 | 6.4583E−02 |
| 30.Zn | 1.6227E−02 | 3.8056E+02 | 4.1410E+02 | 5.0201E+02 | 2.1229E+01 |
| 31.Ga | 1.6279E−03 | 2.5930E+04 | 2.6085E+04 | 2.6148E+04 | 2.4061E−01 |
| 32.Ge | 1.5460E−03 | 2.7513E+04 | 2.7680E+04 | 2.7790E+04 | 3.9530E−01 |
| 33.As | 1.1217E−03 | 9.3445E+03 | 9.3969E+03 | 9.3778E+03 | 2.0408E−01 |
| | 1.4815E−03 | 3.0226E+04 | 3.0415E+04 | 3.0598E+04 | 6.0488E−01 |
| | 1.9526E−03 | 1.8168E+04 | 1.8281E+04 | 1.8357E+04 | 4.1701E−01 |
| | 2.9511E−02 | 7.4566E+01 | 8.2736E+01 | 9.4866E+01 | 1.4661E+01 |
| 39.Y | 1.1349E−03 | 1.4380E+04 | 1.4468E+04 | 1.4410E+04 | 4.0573E−01 |
| | 2.5100E−03 | 1.1699E+04 | 1.1780E+04 | 1.1957E+04 | 1.4974E+00 |
| | 2.9608E−02 | 7.3237E+01 | 8.1304E+01 | 1.1205E+02 | 3.7815E+01 |
| 40.Zr | 1.1511E−03 | 2.2275E+04 | 2.2414E+04 | 2.2319E+04 | 4.2453E−01 |
| | 2.2584E−03 | 1.4354E+04 | 1.4447E+04 | 1.4703E+04 | 1.7699E+00 |
| | 1.8995E−02 | 2.5117E+02 | 2.7345E+02 | 5.4373E+02 | 9.8841E+01 |
| | 4.9467E−02 | 3.1281E+01 | 9.9845E+01 | 4.1971E+01 | 1.3789E+02 |
| 41.Nb | 7.0437E−03 | 1.9106E+03 | 2.1156E+03 | 1.9568E+03 | 8.1148E+00 |
| 42.Mo | 1.2823E−03 | 3.3029E+04 | 3.3232E+04 | 3.3101E+04 | 3.9785E−01 |
| 43.Tc | 1.4590E−03 | 2.7057E+04 | 2.7219E+04 | 2.7138E+04 | 2.9918E−01 |
| 44.Ru | 8.3914E−03 | 1.9594E+03 | 2.1988E+03 | 2.0197E+03 | 8.8700E+00 |
| 45.Rh | 1.1668E−02 | 9.7699E+02 | 1.0775E+03 | 1.0165E+03 | 6.0025E+00 |
| 46.Pd | 1.3563E−02 | 6.7038E+02 | 7.3566E+02 | 7.0167E+02 | 4.8444E+00 |
| 47.Ag | 1.4975E−03 | 2.9431E+04 | 2.9611E+04 | 2.9515E+04 | 3.2353E−01 |

| Material | $E$, MeV | $\mu_{1en}$, cm$^{-1}$ | $\mu_1$, cm$^{-1}$ | $\mu_2$, cm$^{-1}$ | $R$, % |
|---|---|---|---|---|---|
| | 1.5099E−03 | 2.8923E+04 | 2.9099E+04 | 2.9007E+04 | 3.1712E−01 |
| | 9.2252E−03 | 1.5900E+03 | 1.7736E+03 | 1.6476E+03 | 7.6435E+00 |
| 49.In | 1.4108E−03 | 2.8921E+04 | 2.9096E+04 | 2.8991E+04 | 3.6164E−01 |
| 50.Sn | 1.4554E−03 | 2.7195E+04 | 2.7358E+04 | 2.7263E+04 | 3.4889E−01 |
| | 7.7059E−03 | 2.0409E+03 | 2.2940E+03 | 2.1279E+03 | 7.8083E+00 |
| 51.Sb | 1.4259E−03 | 2.8336E+04 | 2.8507E+04 | 2.8407E+04 | 3.5180E−01 |
| 52.Te | 1.3810E−03 | 3.0072E+04 | 3.0254E+04 | 3.0143E+04 | 3.6653E−01 |
| 53.I | 1.2075E−03 | 3.3668E+04 | 3.3882E+04 | 3.3743E+04 | 4.1258E−01 |
| | 5.2921E−02 | 2.9446E+01 | 8.6353E+01 | 5.3911E+01 | 6.0177E+01 |
| 55.Cs | 1.1346E−03 | 1.4264E+04 | 1.4352E+04 | 1.4300E+04 | 3.6325E−01 |
| | 5.8301E−03 | 1.2560E+03 | 1.2878E+03 | 1.3501E+03 | 4.8369E+00 |
| 56.Ba | 1.1577E−03 | 2.6405E+04 | 2.6571E+04 | 2.6480E+04 | 3.4383E−01 |
| | 3.9906E−02 | 3.1012E+01 | 3.5592E+01 | 8.6590E+01 | 1.4329E+02 |
| 57.La | 1.5043E−03 | 2.9140E+04 | 2.9317E+04 | 2.9245E+04 | 2.4952E−01 |
| | 1.6913E−03 | 2.3843E+04 | 2.3986E+04 | 2.3933E+04 | 2.2291E−01 |
| 58.Ce | 2.9077E−03 | 7.5019E+03 | 7.5639E+03 | 7.5582E+03 | 7.5553E−02 |
| | 2.2630E−02 | 1.6836E+02 | 1.8378E+02 | 1.8208E+02 | 9.3354E−01 |
| 64.Gd | 1.1347E−03 | 1.4301E+04 | 1.4389E+04 | 1.4384E+04 | 3.4197E−02 |
| 65.Tb | 1.1375E−03 | 1.5461E+04 | 1.5556E+04 | 1.5543E+04 | 8.2017E−02 |
| | 1.2642E−03 | 3.3184E+04 | 3.3389E+04 | 3.3442E+04 | 1.5680E−01 |
| | 4.8563E−02 | 3.1630E+01 | 1.0468E+02 | 3.7254E+01 | 1.8098E+02 |
| 66.Dy | 1.1401E−03 | 1.6561E+04 | 1.6663E+04 | 1.6646E+04 | 9.6856E−02 |
| | 1.3205E−03 | 3.2413E+04 | 3.2610E+04 | 3.2693E+04 | 2.5494E−01 |
| | 4.9736E−02 | 3.1177E+01 | 9.8405E+01 | 3.6897E+01 | 1.6670E+02 |
| 67.Ho | 1.1432E−03 | 1.7841E+04 | 1.7951E+04 | 1.7930E+04 | 1.1333E−01 |
| | 1.3756E−03 | 3.0282E+04 | 3.0466E+04 | 3.0563E+04 | 3.2107E−01 |
| | 5.1933E−02 | 2.9997E+01 | 8.9951E+01 | 3.5698E+01 | 1.5198E+02 |
| 68.Er | 1.1465E−03 | 1.9351E+04 | 1.9469E+04 | 1.9450E+04 | 9.7564E−02 |
| | 1.4305E−03 | 2.8158E+04 | 2.8328E+04 | 2.8445E+04 | 4.1194E−01 |
| | 5.4640E−02 | 2.8487E+01 | 8.0086E+01 | 3.4132E+01 | 1.3463E+02 |
| 69.Tm | 1.1491E−03 | 2.0981E+04 | 2.1110E+04 | 2.1083E+04 | 1.2857E−01 |
| | 1.4888E−03 | 2.9863E+04 | 3.0048E+04 | 3.0196E+04 | 4.9309E−01 |
| | 7.0248E−03 | 1.9226E+03 | 2.1292E+03 | 1.9816E+03 | 7.4487E+00 |
| | 5.7418E−02 | 2.6937E+01 | 6.9964E+01 | 3.2515E+01 | 1.1518E+02 |
| 70.Yb | 1.1413E−03 | 1.7061E+04 | 1.7166E+04 | 1.7133E+04 | 1.8958E−01 |
| | 4.8863E−02 | 3.1514E+01 | 1.0307E+02 | 3.6969E+01 | 1.7882E+02 |
| 71.Lu | 1.1568E−03 | 2.5806E+04 | 2.5968E+04 | 2.5921E+04 | 1.8148E−01 |
| | 1.6224E−03 | 2.6112E+04 | 2.6267E+04 | 2.6454E+04 | 7.0903E−01 |
| 72.Hf | 1.2168E−03 | 3.3589E+04 | 3.3801E+04 | 3.3735E+04 | 1.9549E−01 |

| Material | $E$, MeV | $\mu_{1en}$, cm$^{-1}$ | $\mu_1$, cm$^{-1}$ | $\mu_2$, cm$^{-1}$ | $R$, % |
|---|---|---|---|---|---|
| | 1.6755E−03 | 2.4363E+04 | 2.4509E+04 | 2.4664E+04 | 6.3001E−01 |
| 80.Hg | 1.4988E−03 | 2.9368E+04 | 2.9547E+04 | 2.9544E+04 | 9.3543E−03 |
| | 1.5022E−03 | 2.9223E+04 | 2.9401E+04 | 2.9399E+04 | 5.6669E−03 |
| | 1.6406E−03 | 2.5513E+04 | 2.5666E+04 | 2.5686E+04 | 7.6722E−02 |
| | 2.3003E−03 | 1.3912E+04 | 1.4002E+04 | 1.4135E+04 | 9.4401E−01 |
| 81.Tl | 1.2006E−02 | 9.2226E+02 | 1.0165E+03 | 9.7749E+02 | 3.9924E+00 |
| 82.Pb | 1.2406E−02 | 8.5760E+02 | 9.4443E+02 | 9.1027E+02 | 3.7530E+00 |
| 83.Bi | 1.4200E−03 | 2.8564E+04 | 2.8736E+04 | 2.8692E+04 | 1.5334E−01 |
| | 1.0519E−02 | 1.1628E+03 | 1.2848E+03 | 1.2204E+03 | 5.2740E+00 |
| 84.Po | 1.4321E−03 | 2.8096E+04 | 2.8266E+04 | 2.8219E+04 | 1.6604E−01 |
| | 1.0875E−02 | 1.1052E+03 | 1.2205E+03 | 1.1603E+03 | 5.1898E+00 |
| 87.Fr | 1.5733E−03 | 2.6449E+04 | 2.6610E+04 | 2.6579E+04 | 1.1814E−01 |
| 88.Ra | 1.1541E−03 | 2.4126E+04 | 2.4277E+04 | 2.4195E+04 | 3.4029E−01 |
| | 5.9688E−02 | 2.5671E+01 | 6.1694E+01 | 3.1405E+01 | 9.6447E+01 |
| 89.Ac | 1.9732E−03 | 1.7695E+04 | 1.7804E+04 | 1.7826E+04 | 1.2266E−01 |
| | 2.2553E−03 | 1.4387E+04 | 1.4480E+04 | 1.4513E+04 | 2.2936E−01 |
| 112. | 1.2864E−03 | 3.2993E+04 | 3.3196E+04 | 3.3063E+04 | 4.0106E−01 |
| | 2.9834E−02 | 7.0156E+01 | 7.7985E+01 | 1.3766E+02 | 7.6522E+01 |
| 113. | 1.1334E−03 | 1.3748E+04 | 1.3833E+04 | 1.3801E+04 | 2.3320E−01 |
| 118. | 1.1428E−03 | 1.7678E+04 | 1.7786E+04 | 1.7727E+04 | 3.3054E−01 |
| 121. | 1.1349E−03 | 1.4372E+04 | 1.4461E+04 | 1.4443E+04 | 1.2214E−01 |
| | 1.3288E−03 | 3.2090E+04 | 3.2285E+04 | 3.2306E+04 | 6.4937E−02 |
| 123. | 1.1520E−03 | 2.2844E+04 | 2.2986E+04 | 2.3049E+04 | 2.7340E−01 |
| | 1.5760E−03 | 2.6342E+04 | 2.6502E+04 | 2.6612E+04 | 4.1458E−01 |
| 125. | 1.1513E−03 | 2.2401E+04 | 2.2540E+04 | 2.2475E+04 | 2.8728E−01 |
| | 5.1141E−02 | 3.0439E+01 | 9.2838E+01 | 3.6528E+01 | 1.5416E+02 |
| 130. | 1.2224E−03 | 3.3540E+04 | 3.3752E+04 | 3.3629E+04 | 3.6537E−01 |
| | 2.7509E−03 | 9.1569E+03 | 9.2263E+03 | 9.3273E+03 | 1.0947E+00 |
| 134. | 1.1348E−03 | 1.4366E+04 | 1.4454E+04 | 1.4395E+04 | 4.1028E−01 |
| | 6.6531E−03 | 8.9358E+02 | 9.2171E+02 | 9.2167E+02 | 4.2382E−03 |
| 64.GADILINIUM | | | | | |
| 22.Ti | 1.2008E−03 | 1.9734E+04 | 1.9867E+04 | 1.9767E+04 | 5.0557E−01 |
| | 6.8200E−03 | 1.3224E+03 | 1.3643E+03 | 1.5345E+03 | 1.2473E+01 |
| 23.V | 1.2139E−03 | 2.8772E+04 | 2.8969E+04 | 2.8829E+04 | 4.8380E−01 |
| 24.Cr | 1.2306E−03 | 3.7479E+04 | 3.7739E+04 | 3.7568E+04 | 4.5720E−01 |
| 25.Mn | 1.2914E−03 | 3.7949E+04 | 3.8209E+04 | 3.8062E+04 | 3.8665E−01 |
| 26.Fe | 1.3671E−03 | 3.8535E+04 | 3.8795E+04 | 3.8667E+04 | 3.3111E−01 |
| 27.Co | 1.4413E−03 | 3.9109E+04 | 3.9370E+04 | 3.9275E+04 | 2.4141E−01 |
| 28.Ni | 1.4841E−03 | 3.9440E+04 | 3.9701E+04 | 3.9630E+04 | 1.7961E−01 |

| Material | $E$, MeV | $\mu_{1en}$, cm$^{-1}$ | $\mu_1$, cm$^{-1}$ | $\mu_2$, cm$^{-1}$ | $R$, % |
|---|---|---|---|---|---|
| 29.Cu | 1.4983E−03 | 3.9550E+04 | 3.9810E+04 | 3.9775E+04 | 8.8417E−02 |
| | 1.5099E−03 | 3.8961E+04 | 3.9218E+04 | 3.9183E+04 | 9.0482E−02 |
| 30.Zn | 1.4402E−03 | 3.9100E+04 | 3.9361E+04 | 3.9390E+04 | 7.4094E−02 |
| 31.Ga | 1.2852E−03 | 3.7901E+04 | 3.8162E+04 | 3.8257E+04 | 2.5141E−01 |
| | 1.3580E−03 | 3.8464E+04 | 3.8725E+04 | 3.8817E+04 | 2.3926E−01 |
| 39.Y | 1.1033E−03 | 1.5049E+04 | 1.5135E+04 | 1.5079E+04 | 3.6701E−01 |
| 40.Zr | 1.2021E−03 | 2.0564E+04 | 2.0703E+04 | 2.0607E+04 | 4.6866E−01 |
| | 2.6960E−03 | 1.5052E+04 | 1.5173E+04 | 1.5409E+04 | 1.5540E+00 |
| | 3.1881E−02 | 9.4463E+01 | 1.0547E+02 | 1.4520E+02 | 3.7675E+01 |
| 41.Nb | 1.2143E−03 | 2.9027E+04 | 2.9225E+04 | 2.9088E+04 | 4.7320E−01 |
| | 2.3105E−02 | 2.5026E+02 | 2.7406E+02 | 5.2666E+02 | 9.2167E+01 |
| 42.Mo | 5.6107E−02 | 4.0023E+01 | 1.1454E+02 | 5.4674E+01 | 1.0949E+02 |
| 43.Tc | 1.3117E−03 | 3.8106E+04 | 3.8367E+04 | 3.8191E+04 | 4.6051E−01 |
| 44.Ru | 1.3739E−03 | 3.8588E+04 | 3.8848E+04 | 3.8681E+04 | 4.3322E−01 |
| 45.Rh | 1.4051E−03 | 3.8829E+04 | 3.9090E+04 | 3.8921E+04 | 4.3452E−01 |
| 46.Pd | 1.4158E−03 | 3.8912E+04 | 3.9173E+04 | 3.9010E+04 | 4.1661E−01 |
| 47.Ag | 1.3932E−03 | 3.8737E+04 | 3.8997E+04 | 3.8825E+04 | 4.4357E−01 |
| 48.Cd | 1.3302E−03 | 3.8250E+04 | 3.8510E+04 | 3.8330E+04 | 4.6938E−01 |
| | 2.7836E−02 | 1.5080E+02 | 1.6646E+02 | 3.9967E+02 | 1.4010E+02 |
| | 5.7615E−02 | 3.8970E+01 | 1.0612E+02 | 5.9531E+01 | 7.8267E+01 |
| 49.In | 1.2800E−03 | 3.7861E+04 | 3.8121E+04 | 3.7936E+04 | 4.8834E−01 |
| | 2.9513E−02 | 1.1555E+02 | 1.2831E+02 | 3.0222E+02 | 1.3553E+02 |
| | 5.1736E−02 | 4.3076E+01 | 1.3891E+02 | 7.0224E+01 | 9.7806E+01 |
| 50.Sn | 1.3027E−03 | 3.8037E+04 | 3.8297E+04 | 3.8114E+04 | 4.8112E−01 |
| | 2.9808E−02 | 1.0934E+02 | 1.2160E+02 | 3.0544E+02 | 1.5118E+02 |
| | 5.2226E−02 | 4.2734E+01 | 1.3618E+02 | 7.1488E+01 | 9.0491E+01 |
| 51.Sb | 1.2854E−03 | 3.7902E+04 | 3.8163E+04 | 3.7981E+04 | 4.7997E−01 |
| 51.Sb | 3.3774E−02 | 8.3553E+01 | 9.3625E+01 | 2.2527E+02 | 1.4061E+02 |
| 52.Te | 1.2616E−03 | 3.7719E+04 | 3.7979E+04 | 3.7799E+04 | 4.7682E−01 |
| | 3.6673E−02 | 6.6839E+01 | 7.5484E+01 | 1.7076E+02 | 1.2623E+02 |
| 53.I | 4.0360E−02 | 4.6867E+01 | 5.3797E+01 | 1.0722E+02 | 9.9298E+01 |
| 55.Cs | 1.1257E−03 | 1.4515E+04 | 1.4599E+04 | 1.4552E+04 | 3.2506E−01 |
| 56.Ba | 1.2073E−03 | 2.4166E+04 | 2.4331E+04 | 2.4237E+04 | 3.8921E−01 |
| 57.La | 1.3047E−03 | 3.8052E+04 | 3.8313E+04 | 3.8176E+04 | 3.5889E−01 |
| | 7.4929E−03 | 2.5130E+03 | 2.7915E+03 | 2.7098E+03 | 3.0168E+00 |
| 58.Ce | 1.3763E−03 | 3.8606E+04 | 3.8867E+04 | 3.8744E+04 | 3.1696E−01 |
| 59.Pr | 1.4162E−03 | 3.8915E+04 | 3.9176E+04 | 3.9073E+04 | 2.6234E−01 |
| 60.Nd | 1.4492E−03 | 3.9170E+04 | 3.9431E+04 | 3.9343E+04 | 2.2258E−01 |
| 61.Pm | 1.4704E−03 | 3.9334E+04 | 3.9595E+04 | 3.9529E+04 | 1.6572E−01 |

| Material | $E$, MeV | $\mu_{1en}$, cm$^{-1}$ | $\mu_1$, cm$^{-1}$ | $\mu_2$, cm$^{-1}$ | $R$, % |
|---|---|---|---|---|---|
| | 8.1025E−03 | 2.7599E+03 | 3.1195E+03 | 3.0454E+03 | 2.4348E+00 |
| | 5.5629E−02 | 4.0357E+01 | 1.1720E+02 | 9.8933E+01 | 1.8466E+01 |
| 62.Sm | 5.5502E−02 | 4.0445E+01 | 1.1791E+02 | 1.0496E+02 | 1.2332E+01 |
| 63.Eu | 1.1347E−03 | 1.4301E+04 | 1.4384E+04 | 1.4389E+04 | 3.4197E−02 |
| 65.Tb | 1.2705E−03 | 3.7788E+04 | 3.8048E+04 | 3.8083E+04 | 9.0202E−02 |
| 66.Dy | 1.1863E−03 | 1.5475E+04 | 1.5573E+04 | 1.5561E+04 | 7.6835E−02 |
| | 1.3295E−03 | 3.8244E+04 | 3.8504E+04 | 3.8576E+04 | 1.8697E−01 |
| 67.Ho | 1.1898E−03 | 1.6524E+04 | 1.6630E+04 | 1.6612E+04 | 1.1058E−01 |
| | 1.3902E−03 | 3.8714E+04 | 3.8974E+04 | 3.9084E+04 | 2.8157E−01 |
| 68.Er | 1.1938E−03 | 1.7679E+04 | 1.7795E+04 | 1.7778E+04 | 9.2052E−02 |
| 69.Tm | 1.1983E−03 | 1.9017E+04 | 1.9145E+04 | 1.9120E+04 | 1.3034E−01 |
| 70.Yb | 1.1881E−03 | 1.6012E+04 | 1.6114E+04 | 1.6084E+04 | 1.8961E−01 |
| | 2.7898E−03 | 1.3528E+04 | 1.3641E+04 | 1.3691E+04 | 3.6462E−01 |
| | 1.3939E−02 | 9.3646E+02 | 1.0325E+03 | 1.0846E+03 | 5.0419E+00 |
| 71.Lu | 1.2071E−03 | 2.4059E+04 | 2.4223E+04 | 2.4173E+04 | 2.0688E−01 |
| 72.Hf | 1.7033E−03 | 3.6166E+04 | 3.6414E+04 | 3.6685E+04 | 7.4300E−01 |
| | 7.6815E−03 | 2.3626E+03 | 2.6201E+03 | 2.4456E+03 | 7.1328E+00 |
| 73.Ta | 1.3113E−03 | 3.8103E+04 | 3.8363E+04 | 3.8292E+04 | 1.8611E−01 |
| | 1.7634E−03 | 3.3500E+04 | 3.3727E+04 | 3.3978E+04 | 7.4486E−01 |
| 74.W | 1.4067E−03 | 3.8841E+04 | 3.9102E+04 | 3.9057E+04 | 1.1471E−01 |
| | 1.8253E−03 | 3.1046E+04 | 3.1257E+04 | 3.1475E+04 | 6.9898E−01 |
| 75.Re | 1.4645E−03 | 3.9289E+04 | 3.9549E+04 | 3.9541E+04 | 2.1378E−02 |
| | 1.8930E−03 | 2.9850E+04 | 3.0046E+04 | 3.0272E+04 | 7.5263E−01 |
| | 1.0476E−02 | 1.7911E+03 | 1.9950E+03 | 1.8909E+03 | 5.5062E+00 |
| 77.Ir | 1.6644E−03 | 3.5908E+04 | 3.6153E+04 | 3.6170E+04 | 4.6979E−02 |
| | 2.0484E−03 | 2.5576E+04 | 2.5754E+04 | 2.5930E+04 | 6.8299E−01 |
| 78.Pt | 1.6601E−03 | 3.6126E+04 | 3.6372E+04 | 3.6384E+04 | 3.1188E−02 |
| | 2.1327E−03 | 2.4205E+04 | 2.4376E+04 | 2.4562E+04 | 7.6597E−01 |
| 79.Au | 2.2270E−03 | 2.2673E+04 | 2.2835E+04 | 2.3056E+04 | 9.6660E−01 |
| | 1.1577E−02 | 1.5193E+03 | 1.6890E+03 | 1.6102E+03 | 4.8942E+00 |
| 80.Hg | 1.3710E−03 | 3.8565E+04 | 3.8826E+04 | 3.8741E+04 | 2.1823E−01 |
| | 2.3488E−03 | 2.0693E+04 | 2.0845E+04 | 2.1145E+04 | 1.4406E+00 |
| | 7.9402E−03 | 2.8875E+03 | 3.2686E+03 | 2.9907E+03 | 9.2914E+00 |
| | 8.2440E−03 | 2.6491E+03 | 2.9894E+03 | 2.7478E+03 | 8.7947E+00 |
| 81.Tl | 1.3167E−03 | 3.8145E+04 | 3.8405E+04 | 3.8289E+04 | 3.0233E−01 |
| | 2.4458E−03 | 1.9117E+04 | 1.9260E+04 | 1.9570E+04 | 1.6085E+00 |
| 82.Pb | 1.3213E−03 | 3.8180E+04 | 3.8441E+04 | 3.8320E+04 | 3.1430E−01 |
| | 2.5182E−03 | 1.7942E+04 | 1.8078E+04 | 1.8394E+04 | 1.7450E+00 |
| 83.Bi | 1.2619E−03 | 3.7721E+04 | 3.7982E+04 | 3.7852E+04 | 3.4172E−01 |

| Material | $E$, MeV | $\mu_{1en}$, cm$^{-1}$ | $\mu_1$, cm$^{-1}$ | $\mu_2$, cm$^{-1}$ | $R$, % |
|---|---|---|---|---|---|
| | 2.5821E−03 | 1.6903E+04 | 1.7034E+04 | 1.7354E+04 | 1.8758E+00 |
| 84.Po | 1.2660E−03 | 3.7753E+04 | 3.8013E+04 | 3.7878E+04 | 3.5688E−01 |
| 85.At | 1.3212E−03 | 3.8180E+04 | 3.8440E+04 | 3.8320E+04 | 3.1498E−01 |
| 87.Fr | 1.3223E−03 | 3.8188E+04 | 3.8449E+04 | 3.8323E+04 | 3.2768E−01 |
| 88.Ra | 1.2045E−03 | 2.2204E+04 | 2.2355E+04 | 2.2269E+04 | 3.8484E−01 |
| 89.Ac | 1.3564E−03 | 3.8452E+04 | 3.8713E+04 | 3.8589E+04 | 3.2013E−01 |
| | 8.2621E−03 | 2.6350E+03 | 2.9728E+03 | 2.7365E+03 | 8.6361E+00 |
| 90.Th | 1.4599E−03 | 3.9253E+04 | 3.9513E+04 | 3.9408E+04 | 2.6794E−01 |
| | 9.8168E−03 | 2.0232E+03 | 2.2609E+03 | 2.1137E+03 | 6.9614E+00 |
| 112. | 3.5732E−02 | 7.2261E+01 | 8.1369E+01 | 1.7015E+02 | 1.0910E+02 |
| 116. | 1.2142E−03 | 2.9015E+04 | 2.9214E+04 | 2.9083E+04 | 4.4971E−01 |
| | 4.5612E−02 | 3.5288E+01 | 4.1098E+01 | 7.8033E+01 | 8.9871E+01 |
| 118. | 1.1888E−03 | 1.6218E+04 | 1.6322E+04 | 1.6264E+04 | 3.5748E−01 |
| 121. | 1.1697E−03 | 1.3468E+04 | 1.3549E+04 | 1.3537E+04 | 8.9485E−02 |
| 123. | 1.1162E−03 | 1.4741E+04 | 1.4826E+04 | 1.4849E+04 | 1.5395E−01 |
| | 1.2041E−03 | 2.1965E+04 | 2.2114E+04 | 2.2159E+04 | 2.0211E−01 |
| 125. | 1.2024E−03 | 2.0722E+04 | 2.0862E+04 | 2.0794E+04 | 3.2614E−01 |
| | 1.9281E−02 | 3.6715E+02 | 4.0117E+02 | 4.6485E+02 | 1.5874E+01 |
| 134. | 1.0306E−03 | 1.7114E+04 | 1.7196E+04 | 1.7145E+04 | 2.9867E−01 |
| | 1.1171E−03 | 1.4719E+04 | 1.4804E+04 | 1.4749E+04 | 3.7192E−01 |
| | | | 65.TERBIUM | | |
| 23.V | 1.2545E−03 | 2.6713E+04 | 2.6917E+04 | 2.6768E+04 | 5.5574E−01 |
| 24.Cr | 1.2667E−03 | 3.5039E+04 | 3.5312E+04 | 3.5123E+04 | 5.3892E−01 |
| 25.Mn | 1.2727E−03 | 3.9362E+04 | 3.9669E+04 | 3.9479E+04 | 4.8134E−01 |
| 27.Co | 1.3761E−03 | 4.6150E+04 | 4.6511E+04 | 4.6352E+04 | 3.4306E−01 |
| 28.Ni | 1.4407E−03 | 4.4715E+04 | 4.5060E+04 | 4.4936E+04 | 2.7461E−01 |
| 29.Cu | 1.4532E−03 | 4.4439E+04 | 4.4780E+04 | 4.4705E+04 | 1.6911E−01 |
| 30.Zn | 1.3466E−03 | 4.6805E+04 | 4.7174E+04 | 4.7169E+04 | 9.5236E−03 |
| 31.Ga | 1.2718E−03 | 3.8662E+04 | 3.8965E+04 | 3.9028E+04 | 1.6286E−01 |
| 32.Ge | 1.2665E−03 | 3.4827E+04 | 3.5098E+04 | 3.5223E+04 | 3.5518E−01 |
| 40.Zr | 1.2415E−03 | 1.9245E+04 | 1.9378E+04 | 1.9288E+04 | 4.6987E−01 |
| | 2.9542E−03 | 1.1850E+04 | 1.1954E+04 | 1.2113E+04 | 1.3364E+00 |
| | 3.9663E−03 | 5.6256E+03 | 5.7005E+03 | 5.7364E+03 | 6.2991E−01 |
| 40.Zr | 7.1970E−03 | 1.2645E+03 | 1.3075E+03 | 1.2947E+03 | 9.9077E−01 |
| | 3.9514E−02 | 5.5374E+01 | 6.3307E+01 | 7.8356E+01 | 2.3772E+01 |
| 41.Nb | 1.2551E−03 | 2.7058E+04 | 2.7264E+04 | 2.7117E+04 | 5.4161E−01 |
| | 2.6348E−02 | 1.9898E+02 | 2.1953E+02 | 3.8641E+02 | 7.6016E+01 |
| 42.Mo | 1.2654E−03 | 3.4069E+04 | 3.4334E+04 | 3.4140E+04 | 5.6738E−01 |
| | 2.5474E−03 | 1.9009E+04 | 1.9160E+04 | 1.9555E+04 | 2.0622E+00 |

| Material | $E$, MeV | $\mu_{1en}$, cm$^{-1}$ | $\mu_1$, cm$^{-1}$ | $\mu_2$, cm$^{-1}$ | $R$, % |
|---|---|---|---|---|---|
| | 2.0579E−02 | 3.3104E+02 | 3.6313E+02 | 7.9208E+02 | 1.1813E+02 |
| | 5.5412E−02 | 4.1369E+01 | 1.2677E+02 | 5.6635E+01 | 1.2384E+02 |
| 43.Tc | 1.2748E−03 | 4.0878E+04 | 4.1197E+04 | 4.0963E+04 | 5.7165E−01 |
| 44.Ru | 7.6542E−03 | 2.5793E+03 | 2.8855E+03 | 2.6544E+03 | 8.7082E+00 |
| 45.Rh | 1.3106E−03 | 4.7604E+04 | 4.7982E+04 | 4.7700E+04 | 5.8988E−01 |
| | 7.9858E−03 | 2.3233E+03 | 2.5908E+03 | 2.3958E+03 | 8.1379E+00 |
| | 8.0396E−03 | 2.2838E+03 | 2.5455E+03 | 2.3553E+03 | 8.0737E+00 |
| 46.Pd | 1.3287E−03 | 4.7203E+04 | 4.7576E+04 | 4.7303E+04 | 5.7657E−01 |
| 47.Ag | 1.2882E−03 | 4.8102E+04 | 4.8485E+04 | 4.8195E+04 | 6.0274E−01 |
| | 7.7535E−03 | 2.5027E+03 | 2.7973E+03 | 2.5888E+03 | 8.0546E+00 |
| | 2.5853E−02 | 2.1031E+02 | 2.3185E+02 | 5.6676E+02 | 1.4445E+02 |
| 48.Cd | 2.8670E−02 | 1.4582E+02 | 1.6173E+02 | 3.7115E+02 | 1.2949E+02 |
| | 5.6777E−02 | 4.0502E+01 | 1.1900E+02 | 6.2288E+01 | 9.1041E+01 |
| 49.In | 1.2714E−03 | 3.8443E+04 | 3.8743E+04 | 3.8519E+04 | 5.8276E−01 |
| | 3.0840E−02 | 1.1007E+02 | 1.2285E+02 | 2.7593E+02 | 1.2460E+02 |
| 50.Sn | 1.2737E−03 | 4.0095E+04 | 4.0409E+04 | 4.0174E+04 | 5.8380E−01 |
| | 3.2478E−02 | 9.9744E+01 | 1.1161E+02 | 2.6177E+02 | 1.3455E+02 |
| 51.Sb | 1.2720E−03 | 3.8815E+04 | 3.9118E+04 | 3.8894E+04 | 5.7634E−01 |
| | 3.6129E−02 | 7.6725E+01 | 8.6549E+01 | 1.9136E+02 | 1.2110E+02 |
| 52.Te | 1.2697E−03 | 3.7199E+04 | 3.7489E+04 | 3.7278E+04 | 5.6457E−01 |
| | 3.8288E−02 | 6.3110E+01 | 7.1728E+01 | 1.5040E+02 | 1.0968E+02 |
| 53.I | 1.2612E−03 | 3.1023E+04 | 3.1264E+04 | 3.1094E+04 | 5.4697E−01 |
| | 4.5360E−02 | 3.9365E+01 | 4.5752E+01 | 8.3107E+01 | 8.1649E+01 |
| 56.Ba | 1.2473E−03 | 2.2612E+04 | 2.2777E+04 | 2.2678E+04 | 4.3800E−01 |
| 57.La | 1.2736E−03 | 3.9991E+04 | 4.0303E+04 | 4.0121E+04 | 4.5455E−01 |
| | 3.9875E−02 | 5.3100E+01 | 6.0831E+01 | 1.6009E+02 | 1.6317E+02 |
| 58.Ce | 7.9541E−03 | 2.3478E+03 | 2.6190E+03 | 2.5353E+03 | 3.2999E+00 |
| | 8.0480E−03 | 2.2778E+03 | 2.5386E+03 | 2.4580E+03 | 3.2774E+00 |
| 61.Pm | 1.3672E−03 | 4.6347E+04 | 4.6710E+04 | 4.6568E+04 | 3.0491E−01 |
| | 5.3177E−02 | 4.2789E+01 | 1.3950E+02 | 1.1040E+02 | 2.6356E+01 |
| 62.Sm | 8.6183E−03 | 2.5616E+03 | 2.9092E+03 | 2.8445E+03 | 2.2734E+00 |
| | 5.2366E−02 | 4.3304E+01 | 1.4412E+02 | 1.2057E+02 | 1.9535E+01 |
| 63.Eu | 1.1375E−03 | 1.5461E+04 | 1.5543E+04 | 1.5556E+04 | 8.2017E−02 |
| | 1.2642E−03 | 3.3184E+04 | 3.3442E+04 | 3.3389E+04 | 1.5680E−01 |
| | 4.8563E−02 | 3.1630E+01 | 3.7254E+01 | 1.0468E+02 | 1.8098E+02 |
| 64.Gd | 1.2705E−03 | 3.7788E+04 | 3.8083E+04 | 3.8048E+04 | 9.0202E−02 |
| 66.Dy | 1.3359E−03 | 4.7042E+04 | 4.7413E+04 | 4.7461E+04 | 1.0005E−01 |
| 67.Ho | 1.3942E−03 | 4.5749E+04 | 4.6106E+04 | 4.6208E+04 | 2.2158E−01 |
| | 1.7349E−03 | 3.5597E+04 | 3.5862E+04 | 3.5927E+04 | 1.8060E−01 |

| Material | $E$, MeV | $\mu_{1en}$, cm$^{-1}$ | $\mu_1$, cm$^{-1}$ | $\mu_2$, cm$^{-1}$ | $R$, % |
|---|---|---|---|---|---|
| 68.Er | 1.4534E−03 | 4.4434E+04 | 4.4775E+04 | 4.4923E+04 | 3.3232E−01 |
| 70.Yb | 4.2276E−03 | 4.9045E+03 | 4.9754E+03 | 4.9814E+03 | 1.1981E−01 |
| | 2.9837E−02 | 1.1911E+02 | 1.3269E+02 | 1.3409E+02 | 1.0561E+00 |
| 71.Lu | 1.2474E−03 | 2.2662E+04 | 2.2827E+04 | 2.2775E+04 | 2.2859E−01 |
| | 1.6962E−03 | 3.7452E+04 | 3.7730E+04 | 3.7971E+04 | 6.4089E−01 |
| 72.Hf | 1.2617E−03 | 3.1383E+04 | 3.1626E+04 | 3.1529E+04 | 3.0863E−01 |
| | 1.7049E−03 | 3.7035E+04 | 3.7309E+04 | 3.7568E+04 | 6.9508E−01 |
| | 5.9489E−02 | 3.8779E+01 | 1.0355E+02 | 4.6919E+01 | 1.2070E+02 |
| 73.Ta | 1.2743E−03 | 4.0495E+04 | 4.0812E+04 | 4.0686E+04 | 3.0995E−01 |
| | 1.7647E−03 | 3.4169E+04 | 3.4425E+04 | 3.4661E+04 | 6.8457E−01 |
| | 1.7681E−03 | 3.6116E+04 | 3.6388E+04 | 3.6644E+04 | 7.0585E−01 |
| 74.W | 1.2894E−03 | 4.8076E+04 | 4.8459E+04 | 4.8296E+04 | 3.3679E−01 |
| | 1.8320E−03 | 3.3454E+04 | 3.3709E+04 | 3.3934E+04 | 6.6630E−01 |
| 75.Re | 1.3924E−03 | 4.5790E+04 | 4.6146E+04 | 4.6042E+04 | 2.2693E−01 |
| | 1.8955E−03 | 3.0997E+04 | 3.1234E+04 | 3.1444E+04 | 6.7310E−01 |
| | 9.7666E−03 | 2.2047E+03 | 2.4881E+03 | 2.3132E+03 | 7.5607E+00 |
| 76.Os | 1.4618E−03 | 4.4249E+04 | 4.4588E+04 | 4.4501E+04 | 1.9603E−01 |
| | 1.0771E−02 | 1.8544E+03 | 2.0835E+03 | 1.9603E+03 | 6.2843E+00 |
| 77.Ir | 1.4865E−03 | 4.3698E+04 | 4.4031E+04 | 4.3968E+04 | 1.4320E−01 |
| | 1.5474E−03 | 4.0446E+04 | 4.0751E+04 | 4.0713E+04 | 9.2646E−02 |
| | 2.0568E−03 | 2.7646E+04 | 2.7854E+04 | 2.8065E+04 | 7.5805E−01 |
| | 1.1165E−02 | 1.7500E+03 | 1.9645E+03 | 1.8537E+03 | 5.9817E+00 |
| 78.Pt | 1.4872E−03 | 4.3683E+04 | 4.4016E+04 | 4.3941E+04 | 1.7076E−01 |
| | 1.5450E−03 | 4.0596E+04 | 4.0901E+04 | 4.0853E+04 | 1.1864E−01 |
| | 2.1421E−03 | 2.6144E+04 | 2.6342E+04 | 2.6567E+04 | 8.5389E−01 |
| | 1.1266E−02 | 1.7234E+03 | 1.9343E+03 | 1.8247E+03 | 6.0077E+00 |
| 79.Au | 1.4572E−03 | 4.4351E+04 | 4.4691E+04 | 4.4602E+04 | 1.9947E−01 |
| | 2.2375E−03 | 2.4465E+04 | 2.4652E+04 | 2.4908E+04 | 1.0370E+00 |
| | 1.0772E−02 | 1.8542E+03 | 2.0832E+03 | 1.9529E+03 | 6.6749E+00 |
| 80.Hg | 2.3566E−03 | 2.2368E+04 | 2.2541E+04 | 2.2868E+04 | 1.4527E+00 |
| 81.Tl | 1.2748E−03 | 4.0843E+04 | 4.1163E+04 | 4.0989E+04 | 4.2369E−01 |
| | 2.4590E−03 | 2.0566E+04 | 2.0727E+04 | 2.1063E+04 | 1.6234E+00 |
| 82.Pb | 2.5366E−03 | 1.9200E+04 | 1.9352E+04 | 1.9702E+04 | 1.8077E+00 |
| 83.Bi | 1.2698E−03 | 3.7265E+04 | 3.7555E+04 | 3.7396E+04 | 4.2689E−01 |
| | 2.6320E−03 | 1.7521E+04 | 1.7663E+04 | 1.8018E+04 | 2.0097E+00 |
| | 7.8162E−03 | 2.4543E+03 | 2.7416E+03 | 2.5398E+03 | 7.9458E+00 |
| 84.Po | 1.2702E−03 | 3.7511E+04 | 3.7803E+04 | 3.7636E+04 | 4.4484E−01 |
| | 7.8292E−03 | 2.4442E+03 | 2.7299E+03 | 2.5306E+03 | 7.8778E+00 |
| 87.Fr | 1.2747E−03 | 4.0826E+04 | 4.1146E+04 | 4.0963E+04 | 4.4652E−01 |

| Material | $E$, MeV | $\mu_{1en}$, cm$^{-1}$ | $\mu_1$, cm$^{-1}$ | $\mu_2$, cm$^{-1}$ | $R$, % |
|---|---|---|---|---|---|
| 88.Ra | 1.2454E−03 | 2.1516E+04 | 2.1671E+04 | 2.1586E+04 | 3.9410E−01 |
| | 3.3554E−03 | 9.0509E+03 | 9.1409E+03 | 9.3922E+03 | 2.7498E+00 |
| 90.Th | 1.3064E−03 | 4.7698E+04 | 4.8076E+04 | 4.7853E+04 | 4.6624E−01 |
| 91.Pa | 2.6225E−03 | 1.7689E+04 | 1.7831E+04 | 1.7873E+04 | 2.3700E−01 |
| | 3.2916E−03 | 9.4087E+03 | 9.5002E+03 | 9.5778E+03 | 8.1663E−01 |
| 112. | 1.2656E−03 | 3.4226E+04 | 3.4493E+04 | 3.4297E+04 | 5.7044E−01 |
| | 3.7797E−02 | 6.6201E+01 | 7.5093E+01 | 1.4572E+02 | 9.4049E+01 |
| 116. | 1.2568E−03 | 2.8015E+04 | 2.8230E+04 | 2.8084E+04 | 5.2000E−01 |
| | 4.8622E−02 | 3.1487E+01 | 3.7098E+01 | 6.4319E+01 | 7.3378E+01 |
| 121. | 1.2625E−03 | 3.1952E+04 | 3.2200E+04 | 3.2168E+04 | 1.0107E−01 |
| 123. | 1.1228E−03 | 1.5807E+04 | 1.5889E+04 | 1.5925E+04 | 2.2493E−01 |
| | 1.2444E−03 | 2.0907E+04 | 2.1056E+04 | 2.1090E+04 | 1.5952E−01 |
| 125. | 1.2418E−03 | 1.9426E+04 | 1.9560E+04 | 1.9497E+04 | 3.2515E−01 |
| | 3.8008E−03 | 6.5539E+03 | 6.6329E+03 | 6.7156E+03 | 1.2466E+00 |
| | 2.7970E−02 | 1.6184E+02 | 1.7914E+02 | 1.9719E+02 | 1.0074E+01 |
| 130. | 1.2620E−03 | 3.1604E+04 | 3.1849E+04 | 3.1691E+04 | 5.0032E−01 |
| | 3.3602E−02 | 9.2659E+01 | 1.0390E+02 | 1.8411E+02 | 7.7210E+01 |

66.DYSPROSIUM

| Material | $E$, MeV | $\mu_{1en}$, cm$^{-1}$ | $\mu_1$, cm$^{-1}$ | $\mu_2$, cm$^{-1}$ | $R$, % |
|---|---|---|---|---|---|
| 23.V | 1.3061E−03 | 2.4101E+04 | 2.4303E+04 | 2.4152E+04 | 6.2387E−01 |
| 24.Cr | 1.3191E−03 | 3.1506E+04 | 3.1777E+04 | 3.1582E+04 | 6.1934E−01 |
| 25.Mn | 1.3251E−03 | 3.5393E+04 | 3.5700E+04 | 3.5499E+04 | 5.6603E−01 |
| 27.Co | 1.3678E−03 | 4.7044E+04 | 4.7459E+04 | 4.7250E+04 | 4.4216E−01 |
| 28.Ni | 1.4216E−03 | 4.7047E+04 | 4.7457E+04 | 4.7281E+04 | 3.7021E−01 |
| 29.Cu | 1.4291E−03 | 4.7047E+04 | 4.7456E+04 | 4.7334E+04 | 2.5818E−01 |
| 30.Zn | 1.3437E−03 | 4.7043E+04 | 4.7460E+04 | 4.7409E+04 | 1.0879E−01 |
| 31.Ga | 1.3322E−03 | 4.0038E+04 | 4.0387E+04 | 4.0409E+04 | 5.5614E−02 |
| 32.Ge | 1.3223E−03 | 3.3563E+04 | 3.3854E+04 | 3.3933E+04 | 2.3539E−01 |
| 40.Zr | 5.1281E−02 | 2.8596E+01 | 3.4039E+01 | 3.8137E+01 | 1.2039E+01 |
| 41.Nb | 1.3070E−03 | 2.4559E+04 | 2.4765E+04 | 2.4617E+04 | 6.0143E−01 |
| | 2.8085E−02 | 1.7151E+02 | 1.9035E+02 | 3.1129E+02 | 6.3535E+01 |
| 42.Mo | 1.3180E−03 | 3.0823E+04 | 3.1089E+04 | 3.0895E+04 | 6.2834E−01 |
| | 2.3897E−02 | 2.7434E+02 | 3.0277E+02 | 6.1424E+02 | 1.0287E+02 |
| | 5.5312E−02 | 4.1563E+01 | 1.3455E+02 | 5.6918E+01 | 1.3640E+02 |
| 43.Tc | 1.3274E−03 | 3.6928E+04 | 3.7249E+04 | 3.7013E+04 | 6.3851E−01 |
| | 5.9744E−02 | 3.9080E+01 | 1.0911E+02 | 5.3435E+01 | 1.0420E+02 |
| 46.Pd | 7.8159E−03 | 2.5934E+03 | 2.9210E+03 | 2.6779E+03 | 9.0761E+00 |
| 47.Ag | 2.6862E−02 | 2.0155E+02 | 2.2319E+02 | 5.2258E+02 | 1.3414E+02 |
| 48.Cd | 1.3296E−03 | 3.8303E+04 | 3.8636E+04 | 3.8384E+04 | 6.5759E−01 |
| | 2.9279E−02 | 1.4218E+02 | 1.5828E+02 | 3.5031E+02 | 1.2132E+02 |

| Material | $E$, MeV | $\mu_{1en}$, cm$^{-1}$ | $\mu_1$, cm$^{-1}$ | $\mu_2$, cm$^{-1}$ | $R$, % |
|---|---|---|---|---|---|
| | 5.6588E−02 | 4.0848E+01 | 1.2723E+02 | 6.2912E+01 | 1.0224E+02 |
| 49.In | 1.3242E−03 | 3.4837E+04 | 3.5138E+04 | 3.4910E+04 | 6.5441E−01 |
| | 3.8125E−03 | 6.9942E+03 | 7.0826E+03 | 7.3350E+03 | 3.5628E+00 |
| 49.In | 3.4084E−02 | 9.6750E+01 | 1.0867E+02 | 2.2670E+02 | 1.0861E+02 |
| 50.Sn | 1.3265E−03 | 3.6345E+04 | 3.6661E+04 | 3.6421E+04 | 6.5788E−01 |
| | 3.5039E−02 | 9.0261E+01 | 1.0159E+02 | 2.2098E+02 | 1.1752E+02 |
| 51.Sb | 1.3248E−03 | 3.5218E+04 | 3.5523E+04 | 3.5294E+04 | 6.4913E−01 |
| | 4.1554E−03 | 5.4722E+03 | 5.5508E+03 | 5.7665E+03 | 3.8855E+00 |
| | 3.7705E−02 | 7.2152E+01 | 8.1832E+01 | 1.6866E+02 | 1.0611E+02 |
| 52.Te | 1.3226E−03 | 3.3810E+04 | 3.4103E+04 | 3.3886E+04 | 6.3994E−01 |
| | 3.9423E−02 | 6.0489E+01 | 6.9106E+01 | 1.3608E+02 | 9.6913E+01 |
| 53.I | 1.3143E−03 | 2.8408E+04 | 2.8652E+04 | 2.8475E+04 | 6.2081E−01 |
| | 4.8270E−02 | 3.5000E+01 | 4.1102E+01 | 6.9077E+01 | 6.8061E+01 |
| 56.Ba | 1.3011E−03 | 2.1584E+04 | 2.1760E+04 | 2.1646E+04 | 5.2743E−01 |
| 57.La | 1.3271E−03 | 3.6715E+04 | 3.7034E+04 | 3.6833E+04 | 5.4386E−01 |
| | 4.2667E−02 | 4.9613E+01 | 5.7177E+01 | 1.4013E+02 | 1.4509E+02 |
| 58.Ce | 4.0686E−02 | 5.4779E+01 | 6.2859E+01 | 1.7353E+02 | 1.7606E+02 |
| 59.Pr | 7.8779E−03 | 2.5567E+03 | 2.8785E+03 | 2.7830E+03 | 3.4313E+00 |
| | 8.2315E−03 | 2.3156E+03 | 2.5993E+03 | 2.5152E+03 | 3.3432E+00 |
| 61.Pm | 1.0279E−03 | 2.0295E+04 | 2.0388E+04 | 2.0400E+04 | 6.0507E−02 |
| | 1.3577E−03 | 4.7043E+04 | 4.7460E+04 | 4.7267E+04 | 4.0781E−01 |
| 63.Eu | 1.1401E−03 | 1.6561E+04 | 1.6646E+04 | 1.6663E+04 | 9.6856E−02 |
| | 1.3205E−03 | 3.2413E+04 | 3.2693E+04 | 3.2610E+04 | 2.5494E−01 |
| | 4.9736E−02 | 3.1177E+01 | 3.6897E+01 | 9.8405E+01 | 1.6670E+02 |
| 64.Gd | 1.1863E−03 | 1.5475E+04 | 1.5561E+04 | 1.5573E+04 | 7.6835E−02 |
| | 1.3295E−03 | 3.8244E+04 | 3.8576E+04 | 3.8504E+04 | 1.8697E−01 |
| 65.Tb | 1.3359E−03 | 4.7042E+04 | 4.7461E+04 | 4.7413E+04 | 1.0005E−01 |
| 67.Ho | 1.4207E−03 | 4.7047E+04 | 4.7457E+04 | 4.7516E+04 | 1.2481E−01 |
| | 1.9179E−03 | 3.2479E+04 | 3.2754E+04 | 3.2780E+04 | 8.1736E−02 |
| | 2.1002E−03 | 2.8140E+04 | 2.8381E+04 | 2.8394E+04 | 4.6507E−02 |
| | 5.6463E−02 | 4.0918E+01 | 1.2795E+02 | 1.3522E+02 | 5.6811E+00 |
| 68.Er | 1.4656E−03 | 4.7049E+04 | 4.7454E+04 | 4.7567E+04 | 2.3793E−01 |
| | 1.8024E−03 | 3.5071E+04 | 3.5364E+04 | 3.5432E+04 | 1.9102E−01 |
| | 5.7815E−02 | 4.0161E+01 | 1.2018E+02 | 1.3545E+02 | 1.2703E+01 |
| 69.Tm | 1.5520E−03 | 4.3735E+04 | 4.4107E+04 | 4.4254E+04 | 3.3526E−01 |
| | 1.6835E−03 | 4.1086E+04 | 4.1433E+04 | 4.1563E+04 | 3.1390E−01 |
| 70.Yb | 1.0905E−03 | 1.8202E+04 | 1.8290E+04 | 1.8275E+04 | 8.5543E−02 |
| 71.Lu | 1.2997E−03 | 2.0851E+04 | 2.1020E+04 | 2.0963E+04 | 2.7245E−01 |
| | 1.7715E−03 | 3.6476E+04 | 3.6785E+04 | 3.6979E+04 | 5.2629E−01 |

| Material | $E$, MeV | $\mu_{1en}$, cm$^{-1}$ | $\mu_1$, cm$^{-1}$ | $\mu_2$, cm$^{-1}$ | $R$, % |
|---|---|---|---|---|---|
| 72.Hf | 1.3149E−03 | 2.8769E+04 | 2.9016E+04 | 2.8916E+04 | 3.4832E−01 |
| | 1.7100E−03 | 3.9659E+04 | 3.9995E+04 | 4.0240E+04 | 6.1160E−01 |
| | 5.9253E−02 | 3.9355E+01 | 1.1193E+02 | 4.7567E+01 | 1.3532E+02 |
| 73.Ta | 1.3276E−03 | 3.7045E+04 | 3.7366E+04 | 3.7233E+04 | 3.5719E−01 |
| | 1.7690E−03 | 3.6594E+04 | 3.6904E+04 | 3.7131E+04 | 6.1543E−01 |
| 74.W | 1.8327E−03 | 3.3691E+04 | 3.3969E+04 | 3.4175E+04 | 6.0820E−01 |
| 75.Re | 1.3784E−03 | 4.7044E+04 | 4.7459E+04 | 4.7297E+04 | 3.4255E−01 |
| | 1.9002E−03 | 3.3143E+04 | 3.3423E+04 | 3.3638E+04 | 6.4104E−01 |
| | 9.0499E−03 | 2.7719E+03 | 3.1819E+03 | 2.8910E+03 | 1.0060E+01 |
| 76.Os | 1.4339E−03 | 4.7047E+04 | 4.7456E+04 | 4.7302E+04 | 3.2631E−01 |
| | 1.0266E−02 | 2.1093E+03 | 2.3954E+03 | 2.2212E+03 | 7.8425E+00 |
| 77.Ir | 1.4547E−03 | 4.7048E+04 | 4.7455E+04 | 4.7319E+04 | 2.8615E−01 |
| | 2.0616E−03 | 2.8837E+04 | 2.9083E+04 | 2.9293E+04 | 7.2242E−01 |
| | 1.0666E−02 | 1.9976E+03 | 2.2666E+03 | 2.1068E+03 | 7.5846E+00 |
| 78.Pt | 1.4552E−03 | 4.7048E+04 | 4.7455E+04 | 4.7306E+04 | 3.1501E−01 |
| | 2.1476E−03 | 2.7284E+04 | 2.7519E+04 | 2.7745E+04 | 8.2396E−01 |
| | 1.0693E−02 | 1.9899E+03 | 2.2578E+03 | 2.0978E+03 | 7.6267E+00 |
| 79.Au | 1.4299E−03 | 4.7047E+04 | 4.7456E+04 | 4.7298E+04 | 3.3370E−01 |
| | 2.2438E−03 | 2.5548E+04 | 2.5769E+04 | 2.6026E+04 | 9.9623E−01 |
| | 9.9632E−03 | 2.2064E+03 | 2.5083E+03 | 2.3133E+03 | 8.4289E+00 |
| 80.Hg | 2.3615E−03 | 2.3422E+04 | 2.3628E+04 | 2.3953E+04 | 1.3769E+00 |
| 81.Tl | 1.3282E−03 | 3.7403E+04 | 3.7728E+04 | 3.7548E+04 | 4.8065E−01 |
| | 2.4676E−03 | 2.1506E+04 | 2.1698E+04 | 2.2033E+04 | 1.5452E+00 |
| 82.Pb | 1.3286E−03 | 3.7703E+04 | 3.8031E+04 | 3.7843E+04 | 4.9604E−01 |
| | 2.5529E−03 | 1.9966E+04 | 2.0146E+04 | 2.0486E+04 | 1.6881E+00 |
| 83.Bi | 1.3232E−03 | 3.4173E+04 | 3.4468E+04 | 3.4303E+04 | 4.8335E−01 |
| | 2.6860E−03 | 1.7563E+04 | 1.7725E+04 | 1.8051E+04 | 1.8374E+00 |
| | 1.3679E−02 | 1.1550E+03 | 1.2948E+03 | 1.4564E+03 | 1.2480E+01 |
| 84.Po | 1.3236E−03 | 3.4406E+04 | 3.4705E+04 | 3.4531E+04 | 5.0271E−01 |
| | 1.3896E−02 | 1.0942E+03 | 1.2247E+03 | 1.3911E+03 | 1.3589E+01 |
| 85.At | 1.3287E−03 | 3.7720E+04 | 3.8048E+04 | 3.7860E+04 | 4.9640E−01 |
| 87.Fr | 1.3288E−03 | 3.7826E+04 | 3.8155E+04 | 3.7961E+04 | 5.1103E−01 |
| 88.Ra | 1.2982E−03 | 2.0101E+04 | 2.0263E+04 | 2.0169E+04 | 4.6309E−01 |
| | 1.9877E−02 | 3.8023E+02 | 4.1871E+02 | 5.1993E+02 | 2.4173E+01 |
| 89.Ac | 1.3318E−03 | 3.9749E+04 | 4.0095E+04 | 3.9887E+04 | 5.2159E−01 |
| 112. | 1.3185E−03 | 3.1097E+04 | 3.1365E+04 | 3.1165E+04 | 6.3947E−01 |
| | 3.9178E−02 | 6.2149E+01 | 7.0917E+01 | 1.2938E+02 | 8.2442E+01 |
| 116. | 1.3097E−03 | 2.5962E+04 | 2.6182E+04 | 2.6028E+04 | 5.9072E−01 |
| | 5.1297E−02 | 2.8572E+01 | 3.4013E+01 | 5.5149E+01 | 6.2141E+01 |

| Material | $E$, MeV | $\mu_{1en}$, cm$^{-1}$ | $\mu_1$, cm$^{-1}$ | $\mu_2$, cm$^{-1}$ | $R$, % |
|---|---|---|---|---|---|
| 121. | 1.1885E−03 | 1.5422E+04 | 1.5508E+04 | 1.5510E+04 | 1.6600E−02 |
| | 1.3200E−03 | 3.2072E+04 | 3.2349E+04 | 3.2287E+04 | 1.8943E−01 |
| 123. | 1.1297E−03 | 1.6888E+04 | 1.6974E+04 | 1.7017E+04 | 2.5285E−01 |
| | 1.2966E−03 | 1.9289E+04 | 1.9443E+04 | 1.9454E+04 | 5.7240E−02 |
| | 1.3005E−03 | 2.1293E+04 | 2.1467E+04 | 2.1478E+04 | 5.1078E−02 |
| 125. | 3.9215E−03 | 6.3370E+03 | 6.4212E+03 | 6.4916E+03 | 1.0963E+00 |
| | 3.8777E−02 | 6.4871E+01 | 7.3887E+01 | 7.7202E+01 | 4.4857E+00 |
| 130. | 1.3152E−03 | 2.8998E+04 | 2.9247E+04 | 2.9082E+04 | 5.6616E−01 |
| | 3.6373E−02 | 8.1202E+01 | 9.1707E+01 | 1.5470E+02 | 6.8687E+01 |

67.HOLMIUM

| Material | $E$, MeV | $\mu_{1en}$, cm$^{-1}$ | $\mu_1$, cm$^{-1}$ | $\mu_2$, cm$^{-1}$ | $R$, % |
|---|---|---|---|---|---|
| 23.V | 1.3579E−03 | 2.1474E+04 | 2.1658E+04 | 2.1521E+04 | 6.3617E−01 |
| | 5.7433E−03 | 2.6037E+03 | 2.6647E+03 | 3.2107E+03 | 2.0488E+01 |
| 24.Cr | 1.3715E−03 | 2.7965E+04 | 2.8221E+04 | 2.8033E+04 | 6.7000E−01 |
| 25.Mn | 1.3775E−03 | 3.1416E+04 | 3.1709E+04 | 3.1511E+04 | 6.3099E−01 |
| 26.Fe | 1.3868E−03 | 3.6770E+04 | 3.7120E+04 | 3.6896E+04 | 6.0715E−01 |
| 28.Ni | 1.4213E−03 | 4.7077E+04 | 4.7546E+04 | 4.7312E+04 | 4.9550E−01 |
| 29.Cu | 1.4265E−03 | 4.7331E+04 | 4.7803E+04 | 4.7620E+04 | 3.8286E−01 |
| 31.Ga | 1.3867E−03 | 3.6705E+04 | 3.7054E+04 | 3.7038E+04 | 4.3051E−02 |
| 32.Ge | 1.3769E−03 | 3.1066E+04 | 3.1356E+04 | 3.1403E+04 | 1.5248E−01 |
| 33.As | 1.3815E−03 | 3.3677E+04 | 3.3994E+04 | 3.4110E+04 | 3.4126E−01 |
| 41.Nb | 1.3591E−03 | 2.2045E+04 | 2.2236E+04 | 2.2102E+04 | 6.0704E−01 |
| | 2.4835E−03 | 2.2060E+04 | 2.2270E+04 | 2.2689E+04 | 1.8793E+00 |
| | 2.9284E−02 | 1.5255E+02 | 1.7025E+02 | 2.5943E+02 | 5.2386E+01 |
| 42.Mo | 1.3708E−03 | 2.7572E+04 | 2.7824E+04 | 2.7643E+04 | 6.5362E−01 |
| | 2.6033E−02 | 2.3785E+02 | 2.6401E+02 | 4.9979E+02 | 8.9309E+01 |
| 43.Tc | 1.3802E−03 | 3.2966E+04 | 3.3275E+04 | 3.3049E+04 | 6.8454E−01 |
| | 2.3430E−02 | 3.0614E+02 | 3.3907E+02 | 7.2281E+02 | 1.1317E+02 |
| | 5.9567E−02 | 3.9479E+01 | 1.1758E+02 | 5.4034E+01 | 1.1761E+02 |
| 44.Ru | 1.3879E−03 | 3.7382E+04 | 3.7738E+04 | 3.7474E+04 | 7.0407E−01 |
| | 2.2651E−02 | 3.2657E+02 | 3.6153E+02 | 8.2189E+02 | 1.2734E+02 |
| 45.Rh | 2.3756E−02 | 2.9759E+02 | 3.2968E+02 | 7.6573E+02 | 1.3226E+02 |
| 46.Pd | 2.5474E−02 | 2.5252E+02 | 2.8013E+02 | 6.5078E+02 | 1.3231E+02 |
| 47.Ag | 1.3907E−03 | 3.8963E+04 | 3.9336E+04 | 3.9051E+04 | 7.2850E−01 |
| | 2.7691E−02 | 1.9435E+02 | 2.1619E+02 | 4.8626E+02 | 1.2492E+02 |
| 48.Cd | 1.3825E−03 | 3.4258E+04 | 3.4581E+04 | 3.4337E+04 | 7.0863E−01 |
| | 2.9797E−02 | 1.3909E+02 | 1.5545E+02 | 3.3261E+02 | 1.1396E+02 |
| | 5.6579E−02 | 4.0865E+01 | 1.3456E+02 | 6.2941E+01 | 1.1378E+02 |
| 49.In | 1.3772E−03 | 3.1216E+04 | 3.1507E+04 | 3.1287E+04 | 7.0240E−01 |
| | 3.6374E−02 | 8.7343E+01 | 9.8756E+01 | 1.9194E+02 | 9.4359E+01 |

| Material | $E$, MeV | $\mu_{1en}$, cm$^{-1}$ | $\mu_1$, cm$^{-1}$ | $\mu_2$, cm$^{-1}$ | $R$, % |
|---|---|---|---|---|---|
| 50.Sn | 1.3796E−03 | 3.2580E+04 | 3.2886E+04 | 3.2653E+04 | 7.1242E−01 |
| | 3.9682E−03 | 6.5061E+03 | 6.5955E+03 | 6.8310E+03 | 3.5710E+00 |
| | 3.6939E−02 | 8.3226E+01 | 9.4248E+01 | 1.9071E+02 | 1.0235E+02 |
| 51.Sb | 1.3779E−03 | 3.1605E+04 | 3.1900E+04 | 3.1679E+04 | 6.9965E−01 |
| | 3.8958E−02 | 6.8519E+01 | 7.8141E+01 | 1.5062E+02 | 9.2757E+01 |
| 52.Te | 1.3758E−03 | 3.0407E+04 | 3.0689E+04 | 3.0478E+04 | 6.9094E−01 |
| | 4.2119E−02 | 5.4989E+01 | 6.3280E+01 | 1.1664E+02 | 8.4322E+01 |
| 53.I | 1.3670E−03 | 2.5812E+04 | 2.6044E+04 | 2.5875E+04 | 6.5352E−01 |
| | 5.1007E−02 | 3.1385E+01 | 3.7241E+01 | 5.8385E+01 | 5.6775E+01 |
| 56.Ba | 1.3548E−03 | 1.9995E+04 | 2.0163E+04 | 2.0054E+04 | 5.4176E−01 |
| | 7.1007E−03 | 1.6069E+03 | 1.6577E+03 | 1.7278E+03 | 4.2310E+00 |
| 57.La | 1.3839E−03 | 3.5087E+04 | 3.5419E+04 | 3.5202E+04 | 6.1661E−01 |
| | 4.5156E−02 | 4.6475E+01 | 5.3893E+01 | 1.2279E+02 | 1.2785E+02 |
| 58.Ce | 1.3888E−03 | 3.7883E+04 | 3.8244E+04 | 3.8020E+04 | 5.9103E−01 |
| | 4.3301E−02 | 5.1677E+01 | 5.9628E+01 | 1.5322E+02 | 1.5695E+02 |
| 59.Pr | 4.3592E−02 | 5.0861E+01 | 5.8729E+01 | 1.5663E+02 | 1.6670E+02 |
| 60.Nd | 8.1182E−03 | 2.5141E+03 | 2.8479E+03 | 2.7517E+03 | 3.4944E+00 |
| | 4.3882E−02 | 5.0048E+01 | 5.7832E+01 | 1.6085E+02 | 1.7813E+02 |
| 61.Pm | 1.0302E−03 | 2.1843E+04 | 2.1938E+04 | 2.1956E+04 | 7.9930E−02 |
| 62.Sm | 1.0809E−03 | 2.0047E+04 | 2.0139E+04 | 2.0161E+04 | 1.0970E−01 |
| 63.Eu | 1.1432E−03 | 1.7841E+04 | 1.7930E+04 | 1.7951E+04 | 1.1333E−01 |
| | 1.3756E−03 | 3.0282E+04 | 3.0563E+04 | 3.0466E+04 | 3.2107E−01 |
| | 5.1933E−02 | 2.9997E+01 | 3.5698E+01 | 8.9951E+01 | 1.5198E+02 |
| 64.Gd | 1.1898E−03 | 1.6524E+04 | 1.6612E+04 | 1.6630E+04 | 1.1058E−01 |
| | 1.3902E−03 | 3.8714E+04 | 3.9084E+04 | 3.8974E+04 | 2.8157E−01 |
| 65.Tb | 1.3942E−03 | 4.5749E+04 | 4.6208E+04 | 4.6106E+04 | 2.2158E−01 |
| | 1.7349E−03 | 3.5597E+04 | 3.5927E+04 | 3.5862E+04 | 1.8060E−01 |
| 66.Dy | 1.4207E−03 | 4.7047E+04 | 4.7516E+04 | 4.7457E+04 | 1.2481E−01 |
| | 1.9179E−03 | 3.2479E+04 | 3.2780E+04 | 3.2754E+04 | 8.1736E−02 |
| | 2.1002E−03 | 2.8140E+04 | 2.8394E+04 | 2.8381E+04 | 4.6507E−02 |
| | 5.6463E−02 | 4.0918E+01 | 1.3522E+02 | 1.2795E+02 | 5.6811E+00 |
| 68.Er | 1.4789E−03 | 4.9890E+04 | 5.0383E+04 | 5.0439E+04 | 1.1190E−01 |
| | 2.1921E−03 | 2.7310E+04 | 2.7564E+04 | 2.7586E+04 | 7.8332E−02 |
| | 5.8834E−02 | 3.9819E+01 | 1.2175E+02 | 1.2987E+02 | 6.6696E+00 |
| 69.Tm | 1.6362E−03 | 4.2039E+04 | 4.2441E+04 | 4.2532E+04 | 2.1302E−01 |
| | 5.9986E−02 | 3.9285E+01 | 1.1520E+02 | 1.3089E+02 | 1.3619E+01 |
| 71.Lu | 1.3527E−03 | 1.9011E+04 | 1.9168E+04 | 1.9123E+04 | 2.3691E−01 |
| | 1.7090E−03 | 3.7286E+04 | 3.7635E+04 | 3.7802E+04 | 4.4452E−01 |
| | 1.8475E−03 | 3.5491E+04 | 3.5826E+04 | 3.5977E+04 | 4.2241E−01 |

| Material | $E$, MeV | $\mu_{1en}$, cm$^{-1}$ | $\mu_1$, cm$^{-1}$ | $\mu_2$, cm$^{-1}$ | $R$, % |
|---|---|---|---|---|---|
| | 1.0759E−02 | 2.0839E+03 | 2.3885E+03 | 2.5046E+03 | 4.8641E+00 |
| 72.Hf | 1.3678E−03 | 2.6168E+04 | 2.6405E+04 | 2.6315E+04 | 3.4234E−01 |
| | 1.7058E−03 | 3.7495E+04 | 3.7847E+04 | 3.8037E+04 | 5.0419E−01 |
| | 5.9116E−02 | 3.9688E+01 | 1.2015E+02 | 4.7941E+01 | 1.5061E+02 |
| 73.Ta | 1.3813E−03 | 3.3572E+04 | 3.3888E+04 | 3.3759E+04 | 3.8166E−01 |
| | 1.7733E−03 | 3.9116E+04 | 3.9487E+04 | 3.9701E+04 | 5.4116E−01 |
| 74.W | 1.8388E−03 | 3.5865E+04 | 3.6204E+04 | 3.6396E+04 | 5.2949E−01 |
| 75.Re | 1.3933E−03 | 4.5706E+04 | 4.6164E+04 | 4.5959E+04 | 4.4781E−01 |
| | 1.9004E−03 | 3.3228E+04 | 3.3538E+04 | 3.3725E+04 | 5.5711E−01 |
| 76.Os | 1.4296E−03 | 4.7483E+04 | 4.7955E+04 | 4.7737E+04 | 4.5700E−01 |
| | 9.7600E−03 | 2.4536E+03 | 2.8260E+03 | 2.5728E+03 | 9.8441E+00 |
| 77.Ir | 1.4439E−03 | 4.8181E+04 | 4.8659E+04 | 4.8452E+04 | 4.2727E−01 |
| | 2.0634E−03 | 2.9297E+04 | 2.9561E+04 | 2.9767E+04 | 6.9856E−01 |
| | 1.0101E−02 | 2.2773E+03 | 2.6145E+03 | 2.3928E+03 | 9.2644E+00 |
| 78.Pt | 1.4442E−03 | 4.8197E+04 | 4.8676E+04 | 4.8454E+04 | 4.5672E−01 |
| | 2.1513E−03 | 2.8046E+04 | 2.8307E+04 | 2.8533E+04 | 8.0035E−01 |
| | 1.0031E−02 | 2.2977E+03 | 2.6383E+03 | 2.4132E+03 | 9.3282E+00 |
| 79.Au | 1.4269E−03 | 4.7349E+04 | 4.7821E+04 | 4.7600E+04 | 4.6328E−01 |
| | 2.2481E−03 | 2.6303E+04 | 2.6548E+04 | 2.6806E+04 | 9.6947E−01 |
| 79.Au | 9.4335E−03 | 2.6532E+03 | 3.0669E+03 | 2.7693E+03 | 1.0745E+01 |
| 80.Hg | 1.3879E−03 | 3.7353E+04 | 3.7709E+04 | 3.7529E+04 | 4.7915E−01 |
| | 2.3651E−03 | 2.4194E+04 | 2.4422E+04 | 2.4747E+04 | 1.3321E+00 |
| 81.Tl | 1.3819E−03 | 3.3940E+04 | 3.4260E+04 | 3.4084E+04 | 5.1767E−01 |
| | 2.4742E−03 | 2.2228E+04 | 2.2440E+04 | 2.2777E+04 | 1.5036E+00 |
| | 8.7574E−03 | 2.0852E+03 | 2.3474E+03 | 2.1670E+03 | 8.3239E+00 |
| 82.Pb | 1.3824E−03 | 3.4220E+04 | 3.4542E+04 | 3.4359E+04 | 5.3532E−01 |
| | 2.5658E−03 | 2.0577E+04 | 2.0774E+04 | 2.1111E+04 | 1.6205E+00 |
| | 8.6451E−03 | 2.1535E+03 | 2.4269E+03 | 2.2366E+03 | 8.5055E+00 |
| 83.Bi | 1.3769E−03 | 3.1060E+04 | 3.1349E+04 | 3.1189E+04 | 5.1361E−01 |
| | 1.4321E−02 | 1.0369E+03 | 1.1654E+03 | 1.2980E+03 | 1.1383E+01 |
| 84.Po | 1.3773E−03 | 3.1281E+04 | 3.1573E+04 | 3.1405E+04 | 5.3562E−01 |
| | 2.7562E−03 | 1.7147E+04 | 1.7315E+04 | 1.7657E+04 | 1.9725E+00 |
| | 1.4442E−02 | 1.0015E+03 | 1.1240E+03 | 1.2651E+03 | 1.2552E+01 |
| 85.At | 1.3827E−03 | 3.4392E+04 | 3.4716E+04 | 3.4532E+04 | 5.3458E−01 |
| | 8.5649E−03 | 2.2023E+03 | 2.4836E+03 | 2.2872E+03 | 8.5856E+00 |
| 87.Fr | 1.3834E−03 | 3.4797E+04 | 3.5126E+04 | 3.4931E+04 | 5.5985E−01 |
| 88.Ra | 1.3520E−03 | 1.8657E+04 | 1.8810E+04 | 1.8725E+04 | 4.5360E−01 |
| | 3.8479E−03 | 7.2821E+03 | 7.3768E+03 | 7.5327E+03 | 2.1138E+00 |
| | 4.4608E−03 | 5.0553E+03 | 5.1348E+03 | 5.2206E+03 | 1.6707E+00 |

| Material | $E$, MeV | $\mu_{1en}$, cm$^{-1}$ | $\mu_1$, cm$^{-1}$ | $\mu_2$, cm$^{-1}$ | $R$, % |
|---|---|---|---|---|---|
| | 2.6423E−02 | 2.2762E+02 | 2.5277E+02 | 3.0064E+02 | 1.8940E+01 |
| 89.Ac | 1.3870E−03 | 3.6847E+04 | 3.7197E+04 | 3.6982E+04 | 5.8077E−01 |
| 90.Th | 9.2919E−03 | 2.3969E+03 | 2.7609E+03 | 2.4982E+03 | 1.0516E+01 |
| 91.Pa | 1.5000E−03 | 5.0922E+04 | 5.1423E+04 | 5.1137E+04 | 5.5954E−01 |
| | 1.5001E−03 | 5.0916E+04 | 5.1417E+04 | 5.1131E+04 | 5.5947E−01 |
| 112. | 1.3715E−03 | 2.7953E+04 | 2.8210E+04 | 2.8020E+04 | 6.7642E−01 |
| | 4.1726E−02 | 5.6092E+01 | 6.4496E+01 | 1.1042E+02 | 7.1211E+01 |
| 116. | 1.3630E−03 | 2.3895E+04 | 2.4106E+04 | 2.3958E+04 | 6.1879E−01 |
| | 5.5315E−02 | 2.4930E+01 | 3.0064E+01 | 4.6180E+01 | 5.3607E+01 |
| 121. | 1.1931E−03 | 1.6448E+04 | 1.6536E+04 | 1.6544E+04 | 5.2656E−02 |
| | 1.3789E−03 | 3.2194E+04 | 3.2495E+04 | 3.2410E+04 | 2.6400E−01 |
| 123. | 1.1380E−03 | 1.8025E+04 | 1.8114E+04 | 1.8167E+04 | 2.9107E−01 |
| | 1.3787E−03 | 3.2083E+04 | 3.2383E+04 | 3.2437E+04 | 1.6723E−01 |
| 125. | 7.0737E−03 | 1.6229E+03 | 1.6739E+03 | 1.6740E+03 | 4.6964E−03 |
| | 5.3846E−02 | 2.7130E+01 | 3.2511E+01 | 3.2672E+01 | 4.9748E−01 |
| 130. | 1.3683E−03 | 2.6400E+04 | 2.6639E+04 | 2.6482E+04 | 5.9256E−01 |
| | 3.8325E−02 | 7.3132E+01 | 8.3193E+01 | 1.3398E+02 | 6.1042E+01 |
| | | | 68.ERBIUM | | |
| 22.Ti | 1.4031E−03 | 1.2810E+04 | 1.2909E+04 | 1.2836E+04 | 5.7265E−01 |
| 23.V | 1.4098E−03 | 1.8842E+04 | 1.9008E+04 | 1.8885E+04 | 6.5200E−01 |
| | 7.8529E−03 | 1.2527E+03 | 1.3009E+03 | 1.4656E+03 | 1.2657E+01 |
| 24.Cr | 1.4224E−03 | 2.4528E+04 | 2.4768E+04 | 2.4590E+04 | 7.2467E−01 |
| 25.Mn | 1.4291E−03 | 2.7512E+04 | 2.7790E+04 | 2.7594E+04 | 7.0751E−01 |
| 26.Fe | 1.4389E−03 | 3.2126E+04 | 3.2460E+04 | 3.2234E+04 | 7.0398E−01 |
| 27.Co | 1.4514E−03 | 3.8020E+04 | 3.8426E+04 | 3.8180E+04 | 6.4373E−01 |
| 29.Cu | 1.4534E−03 | 4.4419E+04 | 4.4909E+04 | 4.4685E+04 | 5.0202E−01 |
| 30.Zn | 1.4517E−03 | 3.8153E+04 | 3.8561E+04 | 3.8434E+04 | 3.3044E−01 |
| 31.Ga | 1.4415E−03 | 3.3355E+04 | 3.3705E+04 | 3.3650E+04 | 1.6270E−01 |
| 32.Ge | 1.4385E−03 | 3.1912E+04 | 3.2244E+04 | 3.2247E+04 | 8.4317E−03 |
| 33.As | 1.4381E−03 | 3.1725E+04 | 3.2055E+04 | 3.2124E+04 | 2.1475E−01 |
| 41.Nb | 1.4114E−03 | 1.9527E+04 | 1.9702E+04 | 1.9581E+04 | 6.1669E−01 |
| | 3.2757E−02 | 1.2240E+02 | 1.3767E+02 | 1.9438E+02 | 4.1197E+01 |
| 42.Mo | 1.4222E−03 | 2.4402E+04 | 2.4640E+04 | 2.4473E+04 | 6.8002E−01 |
| | 2.7622E−02 | 2.1070E+02 | 2.3520E+02 | 4.1464E+02 | 7.6293E+01 |
| 43.Tc | 1.4324E−03 | 2.9051E+04 | 2.9348E+04 | 2.9133E+04 | 7.3931E−01 |
| | 2.5429E−02 | 2.7223E+02 | 3.0328E+02 | 6.0763E+02 | 1.0036E+02 |
| | 5.9519E−02 | 3.9589E+01 | 1.2612E+02 | 5.4200E+01 | 1.3269E+02 |
| 44.Ru | 1.4404E−03 | 3.2849E+04 | 3.3193E+04 | 3.2939E+04 | 7.7002E−01 |
| | 2.4595E−02 | 2.9564E+02 | 3.2917E+02 | 7.0756E+02 | 1.1495E+02 |

| Material | $E$, MeV | $\mu_{1en}$, cm$^{-1}$ | $\mu_1$, cm$^{-1}$ | $\mu_2$, cm$^{-1}$ | $R$, % |
|---|---|---|---|---|---|
| 45.Rh | 1.4452E−03 | 3.5106E+04 | 3.5477E+04 | 3.5195E+04 | 7.9894E−01 |
| | 2.5279E−02 | 2.7643E+02 | 3.0792E+02 | 6.7973E+02 | 1.2075E+02 |
| 46.Pd | 1.4470E−03 | 3.5946E+04 | 3.6327E+04 | 3.6044E+04 | 7.8666E−01 |
| | 2.6586E−02 | 2.3976E+02 | 2.6735E+02 | 5.9322E+02 | 1.2188E+02 |
| 47.Ag | 1.4434E−03 | 3.4257E+04 | 3.4617E+04 | 3.4343E+04 | 7.9812E−01 |
| | 2.8435E−02 | 1.8789E+02 | 2.0997E+02 | 4.5370E+02 | 1.1608E+02 |
| 48.Cd | 1.4349E−03 | 3.0248E+04 | 3.0560E+04 | 3.0327E+04 | 7.6817E−01 |
| | 3.2415E−02 | 1.2508E+02 | 1.4061E+02 | 2.8416E+02 | 1.0210E+02 |
| 49.In | 1.4294E−03 | 2.7650E+04 | 2.7930E+04 | 2.7719E+04 | 7.6099E−01 |
| | 3.8198E−02 | 7.9853E+01 | 9.0883E+01 | 1.6427E+02 | 8.0748E+01 |
| 50.Sn | 1.4320E−03 | 2.8857E+04 | 2.9152E+04 | 2.8927E+04 | 7.7878E−01 |
| | 3.8510E−02 | 7.7412E+01 | 8.8199E+01 | 1.6570E+02 | 8.7869E+01 |
| 51.Sb | 1.4302E−03 | 2.8041E+04 | 2.8326E+04 | 2.8112E+04 | 7.6211E−01 |
| | 4.0342E−02 | 6.4722E+01 | 7.4242E+01 | 1.3355E+02 | 7.9885E+01 |
| 52.Te | 1.4281E−03 | 2.7059E+04 | 2.7331E+04 | 2.7127E+04 | 7.5337E−01 |
| | 4.6261E−02 | 4.6849E+01 | 5.4491E+01 | 9.2892E+01 | 7.0472E+01 |
| 53.I | 1.4196E−03 | 2.3227E+04 | 2.3449E+04 | 2.3286E+04 | 7.0034E−01 |
| | 4.9853E−03 | 3.9193E+03 | 3.9949E+03 | 4.1811E+03 | 4.6623E+00 |
| | 5.0479E−03 | 3.8076E+03 | 3.8823E+03 | 4.0599E+03 | 4.5756E+00 |
| | 5.6174E−02 | 2.6150E+01 | 3.1528E+01 | 4.6306E+01 | 4.6875E+01 |
| 57.La | 1.4393E−03 | 3.2308E+04 | 3.2645E+04 | 3.2418E+04 | 6.9991E−01 |
| | 4.7264E−02 | 4.3818E+01 | 5.1141E+01 | 1.0811E+02 | 1.1139E+02 |
| 58.Ce | 1.4474E−03 | 3.6130E+04 | 3.6513E+04 | 3.6261E+04 | 6.9597E−01 |
| | 4.5543E−02 | 4.9017E+01 | 5.6886E+01 | 1.3580E+02 | 1.3873E+02 |
| 59.Pr | 1.4492E−03 | 3.6985E+04 | 3.7379E+04 | 3.7137E+04 | 6.5216E−01 |
| 59.Pr | 4.5658E−02 | 4.8670E+01 | 5.6503E+01 | 1.4072E+02 | 1.4906E+02 |
| 60.Nd | 4.5800E−02 | 4.8241E+01 | 5.6029E+01 | 1.4612E+02 | 1.6079E+02 |
| 61.Pm | 1.0327E−03 | 2.3593E+04 | 2.3692E+04 | 2.3714E+04 | 9.3088E−02 |
| | 4.5214E−02 | 5.0009E+01 | 5.7982E+01 | 1.6329E+02 | 1.8162E+02 |
| 62.Sm | 1.0833E−03 | 2.1706E+04 | 2.1806E+04 | 2.1829E+04 | 1.0563E−01 |
| 63.Eu | 1.1465E−03 | 1.9351E+04 | 1.9450E+04 | 1.9469E+04 | 9.7564E−02 |
| | 1.4305E−03 | 2.8158E+04 | 2.8445E+04 | 2.8328E+04 | 4.1194E−01 |
| | 5.4640E−02 | 2.8487E+01 | 3.4132E+01 | 8.0086E+01 | 1.3463E+02 |
| 64.Gd | 1.1938E−03 | 1.7679E+04 | 1.7778E+04 | 1.7795E+04 | 9.2052E−02 |
| 65.Tb | 1.4534E−03 | 4.4434E+04 | 4.4923E+04 | 4.4775E+04 | 3.3232E−01 |
| 66.Dy | 1.4656E−03 | 4.7049E+04 | 4.7567E+04 | 4.7454E+04 | 2.3793E−01 |
| | 1.8024E−03 | 3.5071E+04 | 3.5432E+04 | 3.5364E+04 | 1.9102E−01 |
| | 5.7815E−02 | 4.0161E+01 | 1.3545E+02 | 1.2018E+02 | 1.2703E+01 |
| 67.Ho | 1.4789E−03 | 4.9890E+04 | 5.0439E+04 | 5.0383E+04 | 1.1190E−01 |

| Material | $E$, MeV | $\mu_{1en}$, cm$^{-1}$ | $\mu_1$, cm$^{-1}$ | $\mu_2$, cm$^{-1}$ | $R$, % |
|---|---|---|---|---|---|
| | 2.1921E−03 | 2.7310E+04 | 2.7586E+04 | 2.7564E+04 | 7.8332E−02 |
| | 5.8834E−02 | 3.9819E+01 | 1.2987E+02 | 1.2175E+02 | 6.6696E+00 |
| 69.Tm | 1.7383E−03 | 3.9174E+04 | 3.9585E+04 | 3.9626E+04 | 1.0294E−01 |
| | 2.2829E−03 | 2.6684E+04 | 2.6951E+04 | 2.6973E+04 | 8.0469E−02 |
| | 5.9967E−02 | 3.9439E+01 | 1.2366E+02 | 1.3027E+02 | 5.3457E+00 |
| 71.Lu | 1.7827E−03 | 3.6332E+04 | 3.6708E+04 | 3.6832E+04 | 3.3685E−01 |
| | 1.9394E−03 | 3.4300E+04 | 3.4649E+04 | 3.4766E+04 | 3.3612E−01 |
| 72.Hf | 1.4204E−03 | 2.3586E+04 | 2.3813E+04 | 2.3732E+04 | 3.4148E−01 |
| | 1.7123E−03 | 4.0834E+04 | 4.1266E+04 | 4.1436E+04 | 4.1182E−01 |
| | 1.0631E−02 | 2.2468E+03 | 2.6052E+03 | 2.6001E+03 | 1.9607E−01 |
| | 5.9099E−02 | 3.9730E+01 | 1.2842E+02 | 4.7988E+01 | 1.6760E+02 |
| 73.Ta | 1.4347E−03 | 3.0118E+04 | 3.0428E+04 | 3.0303E+04 | 4.1248E−01 |
| | 1.7699E−03 | 3.7149E+04 | 3.7536E+04 | 3.7697E+04 | 4.2962E−01 |
| 74.W | 1.4465E−03 | 3.5708E+04 | 3.6086E+04 | 3.5923E+04 | 4.5574E−01 |
| | 1.8438E−03 | 3.8529E+04 | 3.8929E+04 | 3.9114E+04 | 4.7627E−01 |
| 75.Re | 1.9059E−03 | 3.5781E+04 | 3.6149E+04 | 3.6334E+04 | 5.1337E−01 |
| | 9.5507E−03 | 2.3756E+03 | 2.7595E+03 | 2.4873E+03 | 1.0944E+01 |
| 76.Os | 1.4555E−03 | 4.4878E+04 | 4.5372E+04 | 4.5130E+04 | 5.3713E−01 |
| 77.Ir | 1.4620E−03 | 4.6276E+04 | 4.6786E+04 | 4.6547E+04 | 5.1373E−01 |
| | 2.0708E−03 | 3.1103E+04 | 3.1414E+04 | 3.1630E+04 | 6.8741E−01 |
| 78.Pt | 1.4622E−03 | 4.6312E+04 | 4.6822E+04 | 4.6569E+04 | 5.4297E−01 |
| | 2.1533E−03 | 2.8471E+04 | 2.8757E+04 | 2.8972E+04 | 7.4846E−01 |
| 79.Au | 1.4543E−03 | 4.4630E+04 | 4.5122E+04 | 4.4881E+04 | 5.3658E−01 |
| | 2.2506E−03 | 2.7269E+04 | 2.7543E+04 | 2.7800E+04 | 9.3305E−01 |
| 80.Hg | 1.4418E−03 | 3.3473E+04 | 3.3824E+04 | 3.3649E+04 | 5.1974E−01 |
| | 2.3694E−03 | 2.5117E+04 | 2.5370E+04 | 2.5697E+04 | 1.2889E+00 |
| 81.Tl | 1.4355E−03 | 3.0492E+04 | 3.0807E+04 | 3.0634E+04 | 5.6388E−01 |
| | 2.4819E−03 | 2.3078E+04 | 2.3312E+04 | 2.3653E+04 | 1.4642E+00 |
| 81.Tl | 1.3509E−02 | 1.3558E+03 | 1.5497E+03 | 1.7607E+03 | 1.3615E+01 |
| 82.Pb | 1.4360E−03 | 3.0749E+04 | 3.1067E+04 | 3.0887E+04 | 5.8380E−01 |
| | 2.5809E−03 | 2.1285E+04 | 2.1502E+04 | 2.1836E+04 | 1.5534E+00 |
| | 1.3449E−02 | 1.3741E+03 | 1.5715E+03 | 1.7190E+03 | 9.3876E+00 |
| 83.Bi | 1.4301E−03 | 2.7979E+04 | 2.8263E+04 | 2.8107E+04 | 5.5487E−01 |
| | 1.4855E−02 | 9.3872E+02 | 1.0558E+03 | 1.1663E+03 | 1.0471E+01 |
| | 1.5406E−02 | 8.5578E+02 | 9.5957E+02 | 1.0566E+03 | 1.0112E+01 |
| 84.Po | 1.4305E−03 | 2.8186E+04 | 2.8473E+04 | 2.8308E+04 | 5.8024E−01 |
| | 2.7049E−03 | 1.9036E+04 | 1.9232E+04 | 1.9608E+04 | 1.9535E+00 |
| | 1.4909E−02 | 9.2213E+02 | 1.0361E+03 | 1.1572E+03 | 1.1681E+01 |
| | 1.5334E−02 | 8.6258E+02 | 9.6727E+02 | 1.0776E+03 | 1.1406E+01 |

| Material | $E$, MeV | $\mu_{1en}$, cm$^{-1}$ | $\mu_1$, cm$^{-1}$ | $\mu_2$, cm$^{-1}$ | $R$, % |
|---|---|---|---|---|---|
| 85.At | 1.4367E−03 | 3.1069E+04 | 3.1391E+04 | 3.1209E+04 | 5.8282E−01 |
| 87.Fr | 1.4381E−03 | 3.1762E+04 | 3.2092E+04 | 3.1893E+04 | 6.2237E−01 |
| 88.Ra | 4.7686E−03 | 4.5486E+03 | 4.6289E+03 | 4.7010E+03 | 1.5575E+00 |
| | 2.9673E−02 | 1.5314E+02 | 1.7152E+02 | 1.9393E+02 | 1.3065E+01 |
| 89.Ac | 1.4427E−03 | 3.3917E+04 | 3.4273E+04 | 3.4050E+04 | 6.5494E−01 |
| 91.Pa | 1.4880E−03 | 5.1844E+04 | 5.2414E+04 | 5.2059E+04 | 6.8224E−01 |
| | 1.6932E−03 | 4.2062E+04 | 4.2509E+04 | 4.2271E+04 | 5.6180E−01 |
| | 1.5760E−02 | 8.2253E+02 | 9.2196E+02 | 8.8635E+02 | 4.0174E+00 |
| 92.U | 3.4696E−03 | 1.0445E+04 | 1.0568E+04 | 1.0648E+04 | 7.6303E−01 |
| 112. | 1.4232E−03 | 2.4889E+04 | 2.5133E+04 | 2.4954E+04 | 7.1877E−01 |
| | 4.6627E−02 | 4.5742E+01 | 5.3267E+01 | 8.4200E+01 | 5.8071E+01 |
| 116. | 1.4164E−03 | 2.1822E+04 | 2.2027E+04 | 2.1881E+04 | 6.6418E−01 |
| | 5.6671E−03 | 2.9162E+03 | 2.9830E+03 | 3.1155E+03 | 4.4445E+00 |
| 121. | 1.1982E−03 | 1.7576E+04 | 1.7676E+04 | 1.7682E+04 | 3.6176E−02 |
| | 1.4393E−03 | 3.2320E+04 | 3.2657E+04 | 3.2535E+04 | 3.7279E−01 |
| | 5.0649E−02 | 3.4569E+01 | 4.0911E+01 | 1.1390E+02 | 1.7842E+02 |
| 123. | 1.4340E−03 | 2.9816E+04 | 3.0123E+04 | 3.0137E+04 | 4.7812E−02 |
| 130. | 1.4209E−03 | 2.3825E+04 | 2.4055E+04 | 2.3905E+04 | 6.3045E−01 |
| | 3.9877E−02 | 6.6714E+01 | 7.6438E+01 | 1.1750E+02 | 5.3718E+01 |

## 69.THULIUM

| Material | $E$, MeV | $\mu_{1en}$, cm$^{-1}$ | $\mu_1$, cm$^{-1}$ | $\mu_2$, cm$^{-1}$ | $R$, % |
|---|---|---|---|---|---|
| 22.Ti | 1.0560E−03 | 2.4688E+04 | 2.4791E+04 | 2.4727E+04 | 2.5763E−01 |
| | 1.2893E−03 | 1.6704E+04 | 1.6804E+04 | 1.6734E+04 | 4.1442E−01 |
| 24.Cr | 1.4735E−03 | 2.1078E+04 | 2.1292E+04 | 2.1132E+04 | 7.5362E−01 |
| 25.Mn | 1.4783E−03 | 2.3782E+04 | 2.4032E+04 | 2.3854E+04 | 7.4689E−01 |
| 26.Fe | 1.4855E−03 | 2.7967E+04 | 2.8274E+04 | 2.8059E+04 | 7.6678E−01 |
| 27.Co | 1.4949E−03 | 3.3325E+04 | 3.3704E+04 | 3.3461E+04 | 7.2633E−01 |
| 28.Ni | 1.5073E−03 | 3.7232E+04 | 3.7661E+04 | 3.7409E+04 | 6.7356E−01 |
| 30.Zn | 1.4968E−03 | 3.4438E+04 | 3.4832E+04 | 3.4683E+04 | 4.3082E−01 |
| 31.Ga | 1.4898E−03 | 3.0405E+04 | 3.0745E+04 | 3.0666E+04 | 2.5694E−01 |
| 32.Ge | 1.4881E−03 | 2.9442E+04 | 2.9769E+04 | 2.9743E+04 | 8.6935E−02 |
| 33.As | 1.4890E−03 | 2.9968E+04 | 3.0302E+04 | 3.0336E+04 | 1.1158E−01 |
| 34.Se | 1.4769E−03 | 2.3025E+04 | 2.3264E+04 | 2.3358E+04 | 4.0204E−01 |
| 40.Zr | 1.3780E−03 | 1.4664E+04 | 1.4760E+04 | 1.4704E+04 | 3.7982E−01 |
| 41.Nb | 7.0794E−03 | 1.8850E+03 | 1.9436E+03 | 1.9307E+03 | 6.6500E−01 |
| | 8.3554E−03 | 1.1251E+03 | 1.1738E+03 | 1.1576E+03 | 1.3991E+00 |
| | 3.8754E−02 | 8.1446E+01 | 9.2965E+01 | 1.2021E+02 | 2.9311E+01 |
| 42.Mo | 1.4738E−03 | 2.1218E+04 | 2.1434E+04 | 2.1290E+04 | 6.7498E−01 |
| | 2.8835E−02 | 1.8997E+02 | 2.1306E+02 | 3.4964E+02 | 6.4105E+01 |
| 43.Tc | 1.4811E−03 | 2.5399E+04 | 2.5670E+04 | 2.5479E+04 | 7.4956E−01 |

| Material | $E$, MeV | $\mu_{1en}$, cm$^{-1}$ | $\mu_1$, cm$^{-1}$ | $\mu_2$, cm$^{-1}$ | $R$, % |
|---|---|---|---|---|---|
| | 2.6957E−02 | 2.4631E+02 | 2.7580E+02 | 5.1956E+02 | 8.8382E+01 |
| 44.Ru | 1.4870E−03 | 2.8830E+04 | 2.9148E+04 | 2.8917E+04 | 7.9849E−01 |
| | 2.6125E−02 | 2.7129E+02 | 3.0362E+02 | 6.1755E+02 | 1.0340E+02 |
| 45.Rh | 1.4906E−03 | 3.0890E+04 | 3.1237E+04 | 3.0978E+04 | 8.3615E−01 |
| | 2.6534E−02 | 2.5899E+02 | 2.8992E+02 | 6.0888E+02 | 1.1001E+02 |
| 46.Pd | 1.4920E−03 | 3.1667E+04 | 3.2024E+04 | 3.1763E+04 | 8.2041E−01 |
| | 2.7540E−02 | 2.2883E+02 | 2.5633E+02 | 5.4384E+02 | 1.1217E+02 |
| 47.Ag | 1.4894E−03 | 3.0161E+04 | 3.0497E+04 | 3.0245E+04 | 8.3343E−01 |
| | 2.9095E−02 | 1.8216E+02 | 2.0435E+02 | 4.2477E+02 | 1.0786E+02 |
| | 5.9617E−02 | 4.2204E+01 | 1.1911E+02 | 6.2021E+01 | 9.2054E+01 |
| 48.Cd | 1.4831E−03 | 2.6567E+04 | 2.6855E+04 | 2.6645E+04 | 7.8667E−01 |
| | 3.5521E−02 | 1.0862E+02 | 1.2294E+02 | 2.3078E+02 | 8.7721E+01 |
| 49.In | 1.4791E−03 | 2.4252E+04 | 2.4509E+04 | 2.4319E+04 | 7.8004E−01 |
| | 3.9658E−02 | 7.3855E+01 | 8.4591E+01 | 1.4211E+02 | 6.7996E+01 |
| 50.Sn | 1.4810E−03 | 2.5375E+04 | 2.5647E+04 | 2.5442E+04 | 8.0465E−01 |
| | 3.9805E−02 | 7.2614E+01 | 8.3222E+01 | 1.4506E+02 | 7.4303E+01 |
| 51.Sb | 1.4798E−03 | 2.4667E+04 | 2.4929E+04 | 2.4735E+04 | 7.8424E−01 |
| | 4.5557E−02 | 5.2897E+01 | 6.1384E+01 | 1.0190E+02 | 6.6009E+01 |
| 52.Te | 1.4783E−03 | 2.3838E+04 | 2.4089E+04 | 2.3902E+04 | 7.8110E−01 |
| | 4.9178E−02 | 4.1115E+01 | 4.8330E+01 | 7.6163E+01 | 5.7591E+01 |
| 53.I | 1.4727E−03 | 2.0609E+04 | 2.0816E+04 | 2.0665E+04 | 7.3007E−01 |
| 57.La | 1.4888E−03 | 2.9826E+04 | 3.0158E+04 | 2.9931E+04 | 7.5622E−01 |
| | 4.9032E−02 | 4.1591E+01 | 4.8856E+01 | 9.5794E+01 | 9.6072E+01 |
| 58.Ce | 1.4954E−03 | 3.3626E+04 | 3.4009E+04 | 3.3746E+04 | 7.7833E−01 |
| | 4.7442E−02 | 4.6765E+01 | 5.4589E+01 | 1.2106E+02 | 1.2176E+02 |
| 59.Pr | 1.4964E−03 | 3.4222E+04 | 3.4614E+04 | 3.4364E+04 | 7.2734E−01 |
| | 4.7436E−02 | 4.6784E+01 | 5.4611E+01 | 1.2704E+02 | 1.3262E+02 |
| 60.Nd | 1.4999E−03 | 3.6230E+04 | 3.6649E+04 | 3.6389E+04 | 7.1467E−01 |
| | 4.7472E−02 | 4.6666E+01 | 5.4479E+01 | 1.3327E+02 | 1.4462E+02 |
| 61.Pm | 1.0355E−03 | 2.5504E+04 | 2.5606E+04 | 2.5635E+04 | 1.1360E−01 |
| | 9.3775E−03 | 1.9921E+03 | 2.2699E+03 | 2.1828E+03 | 3.9904E+00 |
| | 4.6880E−02 | 4.8593E+01 | 5.6615E+01 | 1.5006E+02 | 1.6505E+02 |
| 62.Sm | 1.0859E−03 | 2.3497E+04 | 2.3600E+04 | 2.3629E+04 | 1.2357E−01 |
| | 4.7283E−02 | 4.7279E+01 | 5.5159E+01 | 1.5321E+02 | 1.7776E+02 |
| 63.Eu | 1.1491E−03 | 2.0981E+04 | 2.1083E+04 | 2.1110E+04 | 1.2857E−01 |
| | 1.4888E−03 | 2.9863E+04 | 3.0196E+04 | 3.0048E+04 | 4.9309E−01 |
| | 7.0248E−03 | 1.9226E+03 | 1.9816E+03 | 2.1292E+03 | 7.4487E+00 |
| | 5.7418E−02 | 2.6937E+01 | 3.2515E+01 | 6.9964E+01 | 1.1518E+02 |
| 64.Gd | 1.1983E−03 | 1.9017E+04 | 1.9120E+04 | 1.9145E+04 | 1.3034E−01 |

| Material | $E$, MeV | $\mu_{1en}$, cm$^{-1}$ | $\mu_1$, cm$^{-1}$ | $\mu_2$, cm$^{-1}$ | $R$, % |
|---|---|---|---|---|---|
| 66.Dy | 1.5520E−03 | 4.3735E+04 | 4.4254E+04 | 4.4107E+04 | 3.3526E−01 |
| | 1.6835E−03 | 4.1086E+04 | 4.1563E+04 | 4.1433E+04 | 3.1390E−01 |
| 67.Ho | 1.6362E−03 | 4.2039E+04 | 4.2532E+04 | 4.2441E+04 | 2.1302E−01 |
| | 5.9986E−02 | 3.9285E+01 | 1.3089E+02 | 1.1520E+02 | 1.3619E+01 |
| 68.Er | 1.7383E−03 | 3.9174E+04 | 3.9626E+04 | 3.9585E+04 | 1.0294E−01 |
| | 2.2829E−03 | 2.6684E+04 | 2.6973E+04 | 2.6951E+04 | 8.0469E−02 |
| | 5.9967E−02 | 3.9439E+01 | 1.3027E+02 | 1.2366E+02 | 5.3457E+00 |
| 71.Lu | 1.8338E−03 | 3.5670E+04 | 3.6076E+04 | 3.6159E+04 | 2.2874E−01 |
| 72.Hf | 1.4734E−03 | 2.0980E+04 | 2.1192E+04 | 2.1127E+04 | 3.1049E−01 |
| | 1.7110E−03 | 4.0173E+04 | 4.0638E+04 | 4.0763E+04 | 3.0689E−01 |
| | 1.0273E−02 | 2.4636E+03 | 2.8916E+03 | 2.8627E+03 | 1.0124E+00 |
| 73.Ta | 1.4838E−03 | 2.6942E+04 | 2.7235E+04 | 2.7126E+04 | 4.0230E−01 |
| | 1.7713E−03 | 3.7961E+04 | 3.8397E+04 | 3.8524E+04 | 3.3023E−01 |
| 74.W | 1.4927E−03 | 3.2073E+04 | 3.2436E+04 | 3.2286E+04 | 4.6423E−01 |
| | 1.8378E−03 | 3.5520E+04 | 3.5924E+04 | 3.6043E+04 | 3.3036E−01 |
| 75.Re | 1.4997E−03 | 3.6117E+04 | 3.6534E+04 | 3.6369E+04 | 4.5370E−01 |
| | 1.9108E−03 | 3.8015E+04 | 3.8446E+04 | 3.8617E+04 | 4.4605E−01 |
| 76.Os | 9.9641E−03 | 2.2749E+03 | 2.6615E+03 | 2.3906E+03 | 1.1332E+01 |
| 77.Ir | 2.0717E−03 | 3.1335E+04 | 3.1678E+04 | 3.1870E+04 | 6.0479E−01 |
| 78.Pt | 2.1616E−03 | 3.0237E+04 | 3.0575E+04 | 3.0797E+04 | 7.2613E−01 |
| 79.Au | 2.2514E−03 | 2.7567E+04 | 2.7869E+04 | 2.8105E+04 | 8.4686E−01 |
| | 9.7395E−03 | 2.3951E+03 | 2.8096E+03 | 2.5059E+03 | 1.2119E+01 |
| 80.Hg | 1.4892E−03 | 3.0060E+04 | 3.0396E+04 | 3.0237E+04 | 5.2585E−01 |
| | 2.3733E−03 | 2.5965E+04 | 2.6242E+04 | 2.6570E+04 | 1.2477E+00 |
| 81.Tl | 1.4844E−03 | 2.7337E+04 | 2.7635E+04 | 2.7478E+04 | 5.7197E−01 |
| | 1.4270E−02 | 1.1868E+03 | 1.3585E+03 | 1.4932E+03 | 9.9176E+00 |
| 82.Pb | 1.4849E−03 | 2.7584E+04 | 2.7886E+04 | 2.7721E+04 | 5.9514E−01 |
| | 1.4202E−02 | 1.2085E+03 | 1.3846E+03 | 1.4995E+03 | 8.2986E+00 |
| 83.Bi | 1.4805E−03 | 2.5060E+04 | 2.5327E+04 | 2.5187E+04 | 5.5673E−01 |
| | 5.9446E−02 | 4.3555E+01 | 1.1366E+02 | 5.2704E+01 | 1.1567E+02 |
| 84.Po | 1.4808E−03 | 2.5263E+04 | 2.5533E+04 | 2.5384E+04 | 5.8519E−01 |
| | 5.9422E−02 | 4.3747E+01 | 1.1289E+02 | 5.3030E+01 | 1.1288E+02 |
| 85.At | 1.4857E−03 | 2.8052E+04 | 2.8359E+04 | 2.8192E+04 | 5.9552E−01 |
| | 1.4641E−02 | 1.0683E+03 | 1.2162E+03 | 1.3621E+03 | 1.1996E+01 |
| | 1.6341E−02 | 8.1982E+02 | 9.2550E+02 | 1.0255E+03 | 1.0807E+01 |
| 87.Fr | 1.4874E−03 | 2.9030E+04 | 2.9351E+04 | 2.9160E+04 | 6.5438E−01 |
| | 1.6292E−02 | 8.2475E+02 | 9.3113E+02 | 1.0537E+03 | 1.3161E+01 |
| 88.Ra | 4.9416E−03 | 4.3601E+03 | 4.4427E+03 | 4.4987E+03 | 1.2602E+00 |
| | 3.9521E−02 | 7.5003E+01 | 8.5857E+01 | 9.2082E+01 | 7.2502E+00 |

| Material | $E$, MeV | $\mu_{1en}$, cm$^{-1}$ | $\mu_1$, cm$^{-1}$ | $\mu_2$, cm$^{-1}$ | $R$, % |
|---|---|---|---|---|---|
| 89.Ac | 1.4914E−03 | 3.1355E+04 | 3.1708E+04 | 3.1487E+04 | 7.0311E−01 |
| 90.Th | 1.5037E−03 | 3.6770E+04 | 3.7194E+04 | 3.6922E+04 | 7.3634E−01 |
| 91.Pa | 1.8276E−03 | 3.5895E+04 | 3.6305E+04 | 3.6100E+04 | 5.6577E−01 |
| | 1.2992E−02 | 1.5950E+03 | 1.8487E+03 | 1.6844E+03 | 9.7505E+00 |
| 92.U | 2.8799E−03 | 1.6851E+04 | 1.7040E+04 | 1.7071E+04 | 1.8132E−01 |
| 112. | 1.4749E−03 | 2.1832E+04 | 2.2055E+04 | 2.1895E+04 | 7.3361E−01 |
| | 4.9842E−02 | 3.8953E+01 | 4.5933E+01 | 6.6997E+01 | 4.5857E+01 |
| 116. | 1.4711E−03 | 1.9700E+04 | 1.9895E+04 | 1.9756E+04 | 7.0195E−01 |
| | 5.7324E−03 | 3.0430E+03 | 3.1139E+03 | 3.2544E+03 | 4.5128E+00 |
| 121. | 1.2023E−03 | 1.8861E+04 | 1.8963E+04 | 1.8977E+04 | 7.0521E−02 |
| | 1.4933E−03 | 3.2432E+04 | 3.2799E+04 | 3.2648E+04 | 4.6418E−01 |
| | 5.3533E−02 | 3.2962E+01 | 3.9245E+01 | 1.0129E+02 | 1.5810E+02 |
| 123. | 1.4851E−03 | 2.7723E+04 | 2.8026E+04 | 2.8013E+04 | 4.6504E−02 |
| 130. | 1.4738E−03 | 2.1233E+04 | 2.1449E+04 | 2.1311E+04 | 6.4722E−01 |
| | 4.6422E−02 | 5.0082E+01 | 5.8265E+01 | 8.3195E+01 | 4.2787E+01 |

70.YTTERBIUM

| Material | $E$, MeV | $\mu_{1en}$, cm$^{-1}$ | $\mu_1$, cm$^{-1}$ | $\mu_2$, cm$^{-1}$ | $R$, % |
|---|---|---|---|---|---|
| 23.V | 1.5305E−03 | 1.3813E+04 | 1.3965E+04 | 1.3849E+04 | 8.3727E−01 |
| 24.Cr | 1.5472E−03 | 1.8334E+04 | 1.8552E+04 | 1.8383E+04 | 9.1497E−01 |
| 25.Mn | 1.5565E−03 | 2.0822E+04 | 2.1076E+04 | 2.0887E+04 | 9.0511E−01 |
| 26.Fe | 1.5714E−03 | 2.4690E+04 | 2.5001E+04 | 2.4771E+04 | 9.2767E−01 |
| 27.Co | 1.5768E−03 | 3.0158E+04 | 3.0548E+04 | 3.0281E+04 | 8.7953E−01 |
| 28.Ni | 1.7457E−03 | 2.7997E+04 | 2.8362E+04 | 2.8131E+04 | 8.1850E−01 |
| 29.Cu | 1.8282E−03 | 2.6122E+04 | 2.6455E+04 | 2.6270E+04 | 7.0442E−01 |
| 30.Zn | 1.6385E−03 | 2.9368E+04 | 2.9749E+04 | 2.9575E+04 | 5.8806E−01 |
| 33.As | 1.5875E−03 | 3.0020E+04 | 3.0409E+04 | 3.0381E+04 | 9.1501E−02 |
| 34.Se | 1.5608E−03 | 2.1935E+04 | 2.2205E+04 | 2.2245E+04 | 1.8025E−01 |
| 40.Zr | 3.9899E−03 | 5.4875E+03 | 5.5695E+03 | 5.5950E+03 | 4.5785E−01 |
| | 4.0786E−02 | 5.1094E+01 | 5.8722E+01 | 7.1436E+01 | 2.1650E+01 |
| 41.Nb | 1.5339E−03 | 1.4734E+04 | 1.4899E+04 | 1.4785E+04 | 7.6881E−01 |
| | 2.3813E−03 | 1.7947E+04 | 1.8159E+04 | 1.8421E+04 | 1.4395E+00 |
| | 2.5958E−02 | 2.0514E+02 | 2.3055E+02 | 4.0325E+02 | 7.4905E+01 |
| 42.Mo | 1.5483E−03 | 1.8649E+04 | 1.8871E+04 | 1.8720E+04 | 8.0623E−01 |
| | 2.0000E−02 | 3.3734E+02 | 3.7880E+02 | 8.2320E+02 | 1.1732E+02 |
| 43.Tc | 1.5628E−03 | 2.2463E+04 | 2.2741E+04 | 2.2544E+04 | 8.7514E−01 |
| 44.Ru | 1.5750E−03 | 2.5627E+04 | 2.5952E+04 | 2.5714E+04 | 9.2477E−01 |
| | 9.4996E−03 | 1.4180E+03 | 1.6643E+03 | 1.4661E+03 | 1.3514E+01 |
| 47.Ag | 9.7400E−03 | 1.3352E+03 | 1.5477E+03 | 1.3852E+03 | 1.1730E+01 |
| | 2.5643E−02 | 2.1214E+02 | 2.3840E+02 | 5.7595E+02 | 1.4159E+02 |
| 48.Cd | 1.5671E−03 | 2.3584E+04 | 2.3879E+04 | 2.3660E+04 | 9.2516E−01 |

| Material | $E$, MeV | $\mu_{1en}$, cm$^{-1}$ | $\mu_1$, cm$^{-1}$ | $\mu_2$, cm$^{-1}$ | $R$, % |
|---|---|---|---|---|---|
| | 2.8619E−02 | 1.4613E+02 | 1.6438E+02 | 3.7290E+02 | 1.2685E+02 |
| 49.In | 1.5590E−03 | 2.1482E+04 | 2.1745E+04 | 2.1547E+04 | 9.2056E−01 |
| | 3.0916E−02 | 1.0976E+02 | 1.2368E+02 | 2.7476E+02 | 1.2215E+02 |
| 50.Sn | 1.5631E−03 | 2.2525E+04 | 2.2804E+04 | 2.2590E+04 | 9.4667E−01 |
| | 3.2579E−02 | 9.9369E+01 | 1.1218E+02 | 2.6016E+02 | 1.3192E+02 |
| 51.Sb | 1.5606E−03 | 2.1894E+04 | 2.2164E+04 | 2.1959E+04 | 9.2929E−01 |
| | 3.6268E−02 | 7.6321E+01 | 8.6661E+01 | 1.8936E+02 | 1.1851E+02 |
| 52.Te | 1.5579E−03 | 2.1171E+04 | 2.1429E+04 | 2.1232E+04 | 9.3116E−01 |
| | 3.8437E−02 | 6.2765E+01 | 7.1652E+01 | 1.4851E+02 | 1.0727E+02 |
| 53.I | 1.5473E−03 | 1.8371E+04 | 1.8589E+04 | 1.8424E+04 | 8.9211E−01 |
| | 4.6052E−02 | 3.8327E+01 | 4.4539E+01 | 7.9772E+01 | 7.9108E+01 |
| 56.Ba | 1.5354E−03 | 1.5157E+04 | 1.5329E+04 | 1.5206E+04 | 8.0909E−01 |
| 57.La | 4.0022E−02 | 5.2946E+01 | 6.0781E+01 | 1.5856E+02 | 1.6087E+02 |
| 58.Ce | 1.6155E−03 | 2.9662E+04 | 3.0046E+04 | 2.9773E+04 | 9.1954E−01 |
| 59.Pr | 1.7013E−03 | 2.8566E+04 | 2.8937E+04 | 2.8686E+04 | 8.7602E−01 |
| 60.Nd | 1.7675E−03 | 2.7562E+04 | 2.7919E+04 | 2.7688E+04 | 8.3318E−01 |
| 61.Pm | 1.0269E−03 | 1.9626E+04 | 1.9700E+04 | 1.9728E+04 | 1.3966E−01 |
| | 1.0194E−02 | 1.5764E+03 | 1.8622E+03 | 1.7169E+03 | 8.4627E+00 |
| 63.Eu | 1.1413E−03 | 1.7061E+04 | 1.7133E+04 | 1.7166E+04 | 1.8958E−01 |
| | 4.8863E−02 | 3.1514E+01 | 3.6969E+01 | 1.0307E+02 | 1.7882E+02 |
| 64.Gd | 1.1881E−03 | 1.6012E+04 | 1.6084E+04 | 1.6114E+04 | 1.8961E−01 |
| | 2.7898E−03 | 1.3528E+04 | 1.3691E+04 | 1.3641E+04 | 3.6462E−01 |
| | 1.3939E−02 | 9.3646E+02 | 1.0846E+03 | 1.0325E+03 | 5.0419E+00 |
| 65.Tb | 4.2276E−03 | 4.9045E+03 | 4.9814E+03 | 4.9754E+03 | 1.1981E−01 |
| | 2.9837E−02 | 1.1911E+02 | 1.3409E+02 | 1.3269E+02 | 1.0561E+00 |
| 66.Dy | 1.0905E−03 | 1.8202E+04 | 1.8275E+04 | 1.8290E+04 | 8.5543E−02 |
| 71.Lu | 1.5289E−03 | 1.3389E+04 | 1.3535E+04 | 1.3498E+04 | 2.7789E−01 |
| | 1.6302E−03 | 2.9474E+04 | 2.9856E+04 | 2.9867E+04 | 3.6222E−02 |
| 72.Hf | 1.5479E−03 | 1.8544E+04 | 1.8764E+04 | 1.8690E+04 | 3.9446E−01 |
| | 1.6888E−03 | 2.8726E+04 | 2.9099E+04 | 2.9111E+04 | 4.2292E−02 |
| 73.Ta | 1.5683E−03 | 2.3901E+04 | 2.4200E+04 | 2.4080E+04 | 5.0163E−01 |
| | 1.7480E−03 | 2.7968E+04 | 2.8332E+04 | 2.8332E+04 | 3.3987E−03 |
| 74.W | 1.8125E−03 | 2.6494E+04 | 2.6833E+04 | 2.6828E+04 | 1.9504E−02 |
| 75.Re | 1.6968E−03 | 2.8623E+04 | 2.8995E+04 | 2.8875E+04 | 4.1473E−01 |
| | 1.8634E−03 | 2.5287E+04 | 2.5605E+04 | 2.5588E+04 | 6.8713E−02 |
| 76.Os | 1.9495E−03 | 2.3246E+04 | 2.3529E+04 | 2.3495E+04 | 1.4696E−01 |
| 77.Ir | 2.0426E−03 | 2.4151E+04 | 2.4445E+04 | 2.4459E+04 | 5.6696E−02 |
| 78.Pt | 2.1226E−03 | 2.2098E+04 | 2.2364E+04 | 2.2383E+04 | 8.4319E−02 |
| 79.Au | 2.2181E−03 | 2.1136E+04 | 2.1388E+04 | 2.1468E+04 | 3.7530E−01 |

| Material | $E$, MeV | $\mu_{1en}$, cm$^{-1}$ | $\mu_1$, cm$^{-1}$ | $\mu_2$, cm$^{-1}$ | $R$, % |
|---|---|---|---|---|---|
| | 1.1917E−02 | 1.3781E+03 | 1.6212E+03 | 1.4657E+03 | 1.0612E+01 |
| 80.Hg | 2.3396E−03 | 1.8710E+04 | 1.8933E+04 | 1.9105E+04 | 9.0751E−01 |
| 81.Tl | 1.5711E−03 | 2.4621E+04 | 2.4931E+04 | 2.4762E+04 | 6.8309E−01 |
| | 2.4352E−03 | 1.7957E+04 | 1.8167E+04 | 1.8373E+04 | 1.1333E+00 |
| 82.Pb | 1.5720E−03 | 2.4855E+04 | 2.5169E+04 | 2.4990E+04 | 7.1493E−01 |
| | 2.5060E−03 | 1.7073E+04 | 1.7273E+04 | 1.7489E+04 | 1.2475E+00 |
| 83.Bi | 1.5632E−03 | 2.2551E+04 | 2.2830E+04 | 2.2677E+04 | 6.7752E−01 |
| 84.Po | 1.5639E−03 | 2.2743E+04 | 2.3025E+04 | 2.2863E+04 | 7.0851E−01 |
| 85.At | 1.5739E−03 | 2.5345E+04 | 2.5665E+04 | 2.5483E+04 | 7.1408E−01 |
| 88.Ra | 1.5321E−03 | 1.4258E+04 | 1.4416E+04 | 1.4323E+04 | 6.5347E−01 |
| | 3.4076E−03 | 8.6727E+03 | 8.7856E+03 | 9.0000E+03 | 2.4403E+00 |
| 89.Ac | 1.0366E−02 | 1.5158E+03 | 1.7872E+03 | 1.5871E+03 | 1.2608E+01 |
| 90.Th | 1.8131E−03 | 2.6480E+04 | 2.6819E+04 | 2.6633E+04 | 7.0002E−01 |
| | 1.3678E−02 | 9.9336E+02 | 1.1537E+03 | 1.0528E+03 | 9.5884E+00 |
| 91.Pa | 3.3588E−03 | 8.9398E+03 | 9.0553E+03 | 9.1075E+03 | 5.7650E−01 |
| 112. | 1.5508E−03 | 1.9319E+04 | 1.9550E+04 | 1.9380E+04 | 8.8021E−01 |
| | 3.7967E−02 | 6.5704E+01 | 7.4906E+01 | 1.4371E+02 | 9.1858E+01 |
| 116. | 1.5450E−03 | 1.7762E+04 | 1.7971E+04 | 1.7815E+04 | 8.7311E−01 |
| | 4.9147E−02 | 3.0824E+01 | 3.6202E+01 | 6.1928E+01 | 7.1060E+01 |
| 118. | 1.0412E−03 | 1.9306E+04 | 1.9379E+04 | 1.9358E+04 | 1.0848E−01 |
| | 1.2129E−03 | 1.5455E+04 | 1.5526E+04 | 1.5499E+04 | 1.7854E−01 |
| 121. | 1.1909E−03 | 1.5950E+04 | 1.6021E+04 | 1.6042E+04 | 1.3122E−01 |
| | 1.6706E−03 | 2.8957E+04 | 2.9333E+04 | 2.9154E+04 | 6.1389E−01 |
| | 1.7380E−03 | 2.8096E+04 | 2.8461E+04 | 2.8281E+04 | 6.3875E−01 |
| 123. | 1.1324E−03 | 1.7260E+04 | 1.7333E+04 | 1.7394E+04 | 3.5173E−01 |
| 125. | 3.7760E−03 | 6.6579E+03 | 6.7513E+03 | 6.8226E+03 | 1.0572E+00 |
| | 2.7086E−02 | 1.8012E+02 | 2.0251E+02 | 2.2064E+02 | 8.9536E+00 |
| 130. | 1.5496E−03 | 1.8999E+04 | 1.9226E+04 | 1.9074E+04 | 7.9515E−01 |
| | 3.3754E−02 | 9.2030E+01 | 1.0405E+02 | 1.8250E+02 | 7.5389E+01 |
| **71.LUTETIUM** | | | | | |
| 24.Cr | 1.5952E−03 | 1.7359E+04 | 1.7550E+04 | 1.7406E+04 | 8.2599E−01 |
| | 7.2551E−03 | 2.0173E+03 | 2.0811E+03 | 2.5122E+03 | 2.0718E+01 |
| 25.Mn | 1.6039E−03 | 1.9721E+04 | 1.9957E+04 | 1.9784E+04 | 8.7625E−01 |
| | 6.7882E−03 | 2.3837E+03 | 2.4523E+03 | 3.1362E+03 | 2.7891E+01 |
| 26.Fe | 1.6162E−03 | 2.3441E+04 | 2.3742E+04 | 2.3518E+04 | 9.5312E−01 |
| 27.Co | 1.6278E−03 | 2.8422E+04 | 2.8799E+04 | 2.8540E+04 | 9.0918E−01 |
| 28.Ni | 1.6366E−03 | 3.2222E+04 | 3.2657E+04 | 3.2376E+04 | 8.6744E−01 |
| 30.Zn | 1.0241E−03 | 3.0408E+04 | 3.0525E+04 | 3.0635E+04 | 3.6102E−01 |
| | 1.6306E−03 | 2.9642E+04 | 3.0037E+04 | 2.9851E+04 | 6.2478E−01 |

| Material | $E$, MeV | $\mu_{1en}$, cm$^{-1}$ | $\mu_1$, cm$^{-1}$ | $\mu_2$, cm$^{-1}$ | $R$, % |
|---|---|---|---|---|---|
| 31.Ga | 1.1245E−03 | 2.6924E+04 | 2.7040E+04 | 2.7171E+04 | 4.8564E−01 |
| | 1.6224E−03 | 2.6097E+04 | 2.6439E+04 | 2.6316E+04 | 4.6600E−01 |
| 32.Ge | 1.2207E−03 | 2.3589E+04 | 2.3702E+04 | 2.3839E+04 | 5.7649E−01 |
| | 1.6207E−03 | 2.5341E+04 | 2.5672E+04 | 2.5593E+04 | 3.0762E−01 |
| 33.As | 1.6284E−03 | 2.8692E+04 | 2.9074E+04 | 2.9034E+04 | 1.3646E−01 |
| 34.Se | 1.6072E−03 | 2.0610E+04 | 2.0862E+04 | 2.0895E+04 | 1.5918E−01 |
| 42.Mo | 1.5964E−03 | 1.7700E+04 | 1.7897E+04 | 1.7770E+04 | 7.1873E−01 |
| 42.Mo | 3.4238E−02 | 1.3592E+02 | 1.5421E+02 | 2.2153E+02 | 4.3658E+01 |
| 43.Tc | 1.6099E−03 | 2.1328E+04 | 2.1594E+04 | 2.1409E+04 | 8.6576E−01 |
| | 2.8891E−02 | 2.1351E+02 | 2.4118E+02 | 4.0812E+02 | 6.9222E+01 |
| 44.Ru | 1.6185E−03 | 2.4417E+04 | 2.4734E+04 | 2.4504E+04 | 9.3670E−01 |
| | 2.8113E−02 | 2.3963E+02 | 2.7069E+02 | 5.0055E+02 | 8.4918E+01 |
| 45.Rh | 1.6229E−03 | 2.6322E+04 | 2.6667E+04 | 2.6409E+04 | 9.7837E−01 |
| | 2.8244E−02 | 2.3524E+02 | 2.6572E+02 | 5.1237E+02 | 9.2822E+01 |
| 46.Pd | 1.6246E−03 | 2.7051E+04 | 2.7407E+04 | 2.7144E+04 | 9.6920E−01 |
| | 2.8899E−02 | 2.1324E+02 | 2.4087E+02 | 4.7350E+02 | 9.6577E+01 |
| 47.Ag | 1.6214E−03 | 2.5669E+04 | 2.6005E+04 | 2.5753E+04 | 9.7609E−01 |
| | 3.0791E−02 | 1.6871E+02 | 1.9069E+02 | 3.6896E+02 | 9.3487E+01 |
| 48.Cd | 1.6138E−03 | 2.2408E+04 | 2.2694E+04 | 2.2482E+04 | 9.4327E−01 |
| | 3.9104E−02 | 8.9621E+01 | 1.0268E+02 | 1.6919E+02 | 6.4766E+01 |
| 49.In | 1.6065E−03 | 2.0406E+04 | 2.0654E+04 | 2.0470E+04 | 9.0024E−01 |
| | 3.9474E−03 | 8.7326E+03 | 8.8652E+03 | 9.1847E+03 | 3.6044E+00 |
| | 4.2135E−03 | 7.5407E+03 | 7.6612E+03 | 7.9143E+03 | 3.3031E+00 |
| | 4.8364E−02 | 5.0138E+01 | 5.8694E+01 | 8.5373E+01 | 4.5454E+01 |
| 50.Sn | 1.6102E−03 | 2.1402E+04 | 2.1670E+04 | 2.1467E+04 | 9.4602E−01 |
| | 4.8163E−02 | 5.0884E+01 | 5.9525E+01 | 8.9927E+01 | 5.1075E+01 |
| 51.Sb | 1.6080E−03 | 2.0804E+04 | 2.1060E+04 | 2.0868E+04 | 9.2003E−01 |
| | 5.3687E−02 | 3.7669E+01 | 4.4755E+01 | 6.4280E+01 | 4.3626E+01 |
| 52.Te | 1.6054E−03 | 2.0118E+04 | 2.0361E+04 | 2.0178E+04 | 9.0862E−01 |
| | 5.9615E−02 | 2.7355E+01 | 3.3193E+01 | 4.4994E+01 | 3.5554E+01 |
| 53.I | 1.5955E−03 | 1.7458E+04 | 1.7651E+04 | 1.7510E+04 | 8.0414E−01 |
| | 9.0937E−03 | 1.0377E+03 | 1.0874E+03 | 1.0912E+03 | 3.4353E−01 |
| 56.Ba | 1.0968E−03 | 2.7884E+04 | 2.8000E+04 | 2.7961E+04 | 1.3943E−01 |
| | 1.2310E−03 | 2.3230E+04 | 2.3344E+04 | 2.3298E+04 | 1.9738E−01 |
| 57.La | 1.6217E−03 | 2.5813E+04 | 2.6150E+04 | 2.5908E+04 | 9.3372E−01 |
| | 5.5898E−02 | 3.3822E+01 | 4.0443E+01 | 6.9056E+01 | 7.0752E+01 |
| 58.Ce | 1.6296E−03 | 2.9208E+04 | 2.9597E+04 | 2.9318E+04 | 9.5321E−01 |
| | 5.9527E−03 | 3.0854E+03 | 3.1629E+03 | 3.3294E+03 | 5.2631E+00 |
| | 6.0514E−03 | 2.9619E+03 | 3.0381E+03 | 3.1935E+03 | 5.1162E+00 |

| Material | $E$, MeV | $\mu_{1en}$, cm$^{-1}$ | $\mu_1$, cm$^{-1}$ | $\mu_2$, cm$^{-1}$ | $R$, % |
|---|---|---|---|---|---|
| | 5.0596E−02 | 4.3047E+01 | 5.0784E+01 | 9.8906E+01 | 9.4758E+01 |
| 59.Pr | 1.6335E−03 | 3.0854E+04 | 3.1268E+04 | 3.0982E+04 | 9.2442E−01 |
| | 5.0029E−02 | 4.4033E+01 | 5.1889E+01 | 1.0718E+02 | 1.0655E+02 |
| 60.Nd | 1.6360E−03 | 3.1972E+04 | 3.2403E+04 | 3.2116E+04 | 8.9327E−01 |
| | 4.9927E−02 | 4.4353E+01 | 5.2246E+01 | 1.1441E+02 | 1.1898E+02 |
| 61.Pm | 1.0408E−03 | 2.9828E+04 | 2.9945E+04 | 2.9981E+04 | 1.1964E−01 |
| | 1.6385E−03 | 3.3023E+04 | 3.3469E+04 | 3.3192E+04 | 8.3713E−01 |
| | 4.9349E−02 | 4.6495E+01 | 5.4633E+01 | 1.3044E+02 | 1.3876E+02 |
| 62.Sm | 1.0924E−03 | 2.8038E+04 | 2.8154E+04 | 2.8192E+04 | 1.3570E−01 |
| | 4.9546E−02 | 4.5765E+01 | 5.3820E+01 | 1.3583E+02 | 1.5238E+02 |
| 63.Eu | 1.1568E−03 | 2.5806E+04 | 2.5921E+04 | 2.5968E+04 | 1.8148E−01 |
| | 1.6224E−03 | 2.6112E+04 | 2.6454E+04 | 2.6267E+04 | 7.0903E−01 |
| 64.Gd | 1.2071E−03 | 2.4059E+04 | 2.4173E+04 | 2.4223E+04 | 2.0688E−01 |
| 65.Tb | 1.2474E−03 | 2.2662E+04 | 2.2775E+04 | 2.2827E+04 | 2.2859E−01 |
| | 1.6962E−03 | 3.7452E+04 | 3.7971E+04 | 3.7730E+04 | 6.4089E−01 |
| 66.Dy | 1.2997E−03 | 2.0851E+04 | 2.0963E+04 | 2.1020E+04 | 2.7245E−01 |
| | 1.7715E−03 | 3.6476E+04 | 3.6979E+04 | 3.6785E+04 | 5.2629E−01 |
| 67.Ho | 1.3527E−03 | 1.9011E+04 | 1.9123E+04 | 1.9168E+04 | 2.3691E−01 |
| | 1.7090E−03 | 3.7286E+04 | 3.7802E+04 | 3.7635E+04 | 4.4452E−01 |
| | 1.8475E−03 | 3.5491E+04 | 3.5977E+04 | 3.5826E+04 | 4.2241E−01 |
| | 1.0759E−02 | 2.0839E+03 | 2.5046E+03 | 2.3885E+03 | 4.8641E+00 |
| 68.Er | 1.7827E−03 | 3.6332E+04 | 3.6832E+04 | 3.6708E+04 | 3.3685E−01 |
| | 1.9394E−03 | 3.4300E+04 | 3.4766E+04 | 3.4649E+04 | 3.3612E−01 |
| 69.Tm | 1.8338E−03 | 3.5670E+04 | 3.6159E+04 | 3.6076E+04 | 2.2874E−01 |
| 70.Yb | 1.5289E−03 | 1.3389E+04 | 1.3498E+04 | 1.3535E+04 | 2.7789E−01 |
| | 1.6302E−03 | 2.9474E+04 | 2.9867E+04 | 2.9856E+04 | 3.6222E−02 |
| 72.Hf | 1.5954E−03 | 1.7426E+04 | 1.7618E+04 | 1.7572E+04 | 2.6247E−01 |
| | 1.7055E−03 | 3.7332E+04 | 3.7849E+04 | 3.7871E+04 | 5.8549E−02 |
| 73.Ta | 1.6142E−03 | 2.2566E+04 | 2.2855E+04 | 2.2741E+04 | 4.9835E−01 |
| | 1.7688E−03 | 3.6512E+04 | 3.7015E+04 | 3.7047E+04 | 8.8193E−02 |
| 74.W | 1.6252E−03 | 2.7315E+04 | 2.7676E+04 | 2.7528E+04 | 5.3753E−01 |
| | 1.8381E−03 | 3.5614E+04 | 3.6102E+04 | 3.6139E+04 | 1.0290E−01 |
| | 9.3443E−03 | 2.2336E+03 | 2.5956E+03 | 2.3360E+03 | 1.1112E+01 |
| 75.Re | 1.6338E−03 | 3.1013E+04 | 3.1430E+04 | 3.1266E+04 | 5.2460E−01 |
| | 1.9037E−03 | 3.4763E+04 | 3.5236E+04 | 3.5293E+04 | 1.6063E−01 |
| 77.Ir | 2.0823E−03 | 3.5358E+04 | 3.5835E+04 | 3.6000E+04 | 4.6143E−01 |
| 78.Pt | 2.1656E−03 | 3.2129E+04 | 3.2558E+04 | 3.2739E+04 | 5.5520E−01 |
| 79.Au | 2.2555E−03 | 2.9111E+04 | 2.9490E+04 | 2.9694E+04 | 6.9236E−01 |
| 80.Hg | 1.6222E−03 | 2.6006E+04 | 2.6347E+04 | 2.6179E+04 | 6.4030E−01 |

| Material | $E$, MeV | $\mu_{1en}$, cm$^{-1}$ | $\mu_1$, cm$^{-1}$ | $\mu_2$, cm$^{-1}$ | $R$, % |
|---|---|---|---|---|---|
| | 2.3796E−03 | 2.7331E+04 | 2.7683E+04 | 2.7975E+04 | 1.0544E+00 |
| 81.Tl | 1.6164E−03 | 2.3529E+04 | 2.3832E+04 | 2.3670E+04 | 6.8579E−01 |
| 82.Pb | 1.6170E−03 | 2.3763E+04 | 2.4069E+04 | 2.3896E+04 | 7.2371E−01 |
| 83.Bi | 1.6106E−03 | 2.1516E+04 | 2.1786E+04 | 2.1641E+04 | 6.6927E−01 |
| 84.Po | 1.6113E−03 | 2.1700E+04 | 2.1973E+04 | 2.1820E+04 | 7.0475E−01 |
| 85.At | 1.6181E−03 | 2.4252E+04 | 2.4566E+04 | 2.4390E+04 | 7.2261E−01 |
| | 2.8369E−03 | 1.9509E+04 | 1.9760E+04 | 2.0128E+04 | 1.8596E+00 |
| 87.Fr | 1.6204E−03 | 2.5238E+04 | 2.5567E+04 | 2.5368E+04 | 7.8375E−01 |
| | 3.0888E−03 | 1.5872E+04 | 1.6081E+04 | 1.6389E+04 | 1.9155E+00 |
| 88.Ra | 1.4004E−03 | 1.7358E+04 | 1.7468E+04 | 1.7425E+04 | 2.4960E−01 |
| 89.Ac | 1.6254E−03 | 2.7403E+04 | 2.7765E+04 | 2.7534E+04 | 8.3785E−01 |
| | 3.2377E−03 | 1.4633E+04 | 1.4829E+04 | 1.5142E+04 | 2.1112E+00 |
| 90.Th | 1.6369E−03 | 3.2341E+04 | 3.2777E+04 | 3.2493E+04 | 8.7396E−01 |
| 91.Pa | 1.8320E−03 | 3.5692E+04 | 3.6181E+04 | 3.5897E+04 | 7.9209E−01 |
| 92.U | 2.2020E−03 | 3.0907E+04 | 3.1315E+04 | 3.1147E+04 | 5.3951E−01 |
| | 2.4075E−03 | 2.6645E+04 | 2.6988E+04 | 2.6879E+04 | 4.0602E−01 |
| | 1.6884E−02 | 8.5779E+02 | 9.8278E+02 | 9.2974E+02 | 5.7053E+00 |
| 112. | 1.5989E−03 | 1.8350E+04 | 1.8560E+04 | 1.8410E+04 | 8.1675E−01 |
| 116. | 1.5934E−03 | 1.6883E+04 | 1.7065E+04 | 1.6935E+04 | 7.6703E−01 |
| 121. | 1.2116E−03 | 2.3905E+04 | 2.4019E+04 | 2.4055E+04 | 1.5170E−01 |
| | 1.6327E−03 | 3.0541E+04 | 3.0950E+04 | 3.0745E+04 | 6.6499E−01 |
| | 5.7740E−02 | 3.0617E+01 | 3.6850E+01 | 8.2902E+01 | 1.2497E+02 |
| 123. | 1.6201E−03 | 2.5097E+04 | 2.5423E+04 | 2.5353E+04 | 2.7773E−01 |
| 130. | 1.5978E−03 | 1.8074E+04 | 1.8278E+04 | 1.8147E+04 | 7.2128E−01 |
| | 5.9213E−02 | 2.8055E+01 | 3.3977E+01 | 4.2020E+01 | 2.3673E+01 |

72.HAFNIUM

| Material | $E$, MeV | $\mu_{1en}$, cm$^{-1}$ | $\mu_1$, cm$^{-1}$ | $\mu_2$, cm$^{-1}$ | $R$, % |
|---|---|---|---|---|---|
| 24.Cr | 1.4793E−03 | 2.0688E+04 | 2.0834E+04 | 2.0741E+04 | 4.4928E−01 |
| | 1.6178E−03 | 1.6899E+04 | 1.7046E+04 | 1.6946E+04 | 5.8735E−01 |
| 26.Fe | 1.6683E−03 | 2.1991E+04 | 2.2246E+04 | 2.2065E+04 | 8.2351E−01 |
| 27.Co | 1.6822E−03 | 2.6572E+04 | 2.6915E+04 | 2.6682E+04 | 8.7328E−01 |
| | 7.8986E−03 | 2.1239E+03 | 2.2039E+03 | 2.9859E+03 | 3.5483E+01 |
| 28.Ni | 1.6915E−03 | 3.0099E+04 | 3.0509E+04 | 3.0243E+04 | 8.7999E−01 |
| 29.Cu | 1.6942E−03 | 3.1526E+04 | 3.1962E+04 | 3.1705E+04 | 8.0980E−01 |
| 30.Zn | 1.0385E−03 | 4.2353E+04 | 4.2499E+04 | 4.2700E+04 | 4.7382E−01 |
| | 1.6857E−03 | 2.7730E+04 | 2.8096E+04 | 2.7925E+04 | 6.1385E−01 |
| 31.Ga | 1.6759E−03 | 2.4488E+04 | 2.4791E+04 | 2.4692E+04 | 4.0260E−01 |
| 32.Ge | 1.6738E−03 | 2.3796E+04 | 2.4086E+04 | 2.4030E+04 | 2.3504E−01 |
| 33.As | 1.6832E−03 | 2.6913E+04 | 2.7263E+04 | 2.7228E+04 | 1.2760E−01 |
| 34.Se | 1.6669E−03 | 2.1519E+04 | 2.1765E+04 | 2.1811E+04 | 2.1142E−01 |

| Material | $E$, MeV | $\mu_{1en}$, cm$^{-1}$ | $\mu_1$, cm$^{-1}$ | $\mu_2$, cm$^{-1}$ | $R$, % |
|---|---|---|---|---|---|
| 42.Mo | 1.4944E−03 | 1.9948E+04 | 2.0094E+04 | 2.0019E+04 | 3.7401E−01 |
| | 1.5184E−03 | 1.9239E+04 | 1.9386E+04 | 1.9311E+04 | 3.8928E−01 |
| 43.Tc | 1.6624E−03 | 2.0062E+04 | 2.0280E+04 | 2.0143E+04 | 6.8102E−01 |
| | 3.9873E−03 | 1.1753E+04 | 1.1940E+04 | 1.2070E+04 | 1.0853E+00 |
| | 5.4577E−02 | 5.0750E+01 | 6.0375E+01 | 7.0964E+01 | 1.7539E+01 |
| 44.Ru | 1.6712E−03 | 2.2952E+04 | 2.3226E+04 | 2.3039E+04 | 8.1073E−01 |
| | 3.0502E−03 | 2.2643E+04 | 2.2943E+04 | 2.3458E+04 | 2.2428E+00 |
| | 3.9707E−02 | 1.1759E+02 | 1.3516E+02 | 1.8633E+02 | 3.7857E+01 |
| 45.Rh | 1.6766E−03 | 2.4709E+04 | 2.5016E+04 | 2.4796E+04 | 8.9060E−01 |
| | 3.2629E−03 | 2.0171E+04 | 2.0445E+04 | 2.0962E+04 | 2.5262E+00 |
| | 3.8887E−02 | 1.2846E+02 | 1.4733E+02 | 2.1628E+02 | 4.6798E+01 |
| 46.Pd | 1.6786E−03 | 2.5382E+04 | 2.5703E+04 | 2.5474E+04 | 8.9845E−01 |
| | 3.9615E−02 | 1.1880E+02 | 1.3652E+02 | 2.0256E+02 | 4.8374E+01 |
| 47.Ag | 1.6747E−03 | 2.4114E+04 | 2.4410E+04 | 2.4198E+04 | 8.7692E−01 |
| | 4.8492E−02 | 6.9715E+01 | 8.1644E+01 | 1.1144E+02 | 3.6500E+01 |
| 48.Cd | 1.6656E−03 | 2.1104E+04 | 2.1342E+04 | 2.1176E+04 | 7.8262E−01 |
| 50.Sn | 1.6627E−03 | 2.0151E+04 | 2.0370E+04 | 2.0214E+04 | 7.7171E−01 |
| 53.I | 1.0133E−03 | 4.3590E+04 | 4.3736E+04 | 4.3677E+04 | 1.3627E−01 |
| | 1.5880E−03 | 1.7600E+04 | 1.7747E+04 | 1.7653E+04 | 5.3201E−01 |
| 57.La | 1.6753E−03 | 2.4295E+04 | 2.4595E+04 | 2.4387E+04 | 8.5298E−01 |
| | 7.9106E−03 | 2.1108E+03 | 2.1905E+03 | 2.2666E+03 | 3.4722E+00 |
| 58.Ce | 1.6848E−03 | 2.7430E+04 | 2.7790E+04 | 2.7535E+04 | 9.2743E−01 |
| 59.Pr | 1.6893E−03 | 2.8971E+04 | 2.9361E+04 | 2.9092E+04 | 9.2332E−01 |
| 60.Nd | 1.6915E−03 | 3.0112E+04 | 3.0523E+04 | 3.0249E+04 | 9.0456E−01 |
| 61.Pm | 1.0514E−03 | 4.1719E+04 | 4.1865E+04 | 4.1928E+04 | 1.4859E−01 |
| | 1.6957E−03 | 3.2298E+04 | 3.2747E+04 | 3.2459E+04 | 8.8897E−01 |
| 62.Sm | 1.1035E−03 | 3.9154E+04 | 3.9300E+04 | 3.9371E+04 | 1.8014E−01 |
| | 1.6957E−03 | 3.2259E+04 | 3.2707E+04 | 3.2442E+04 | 8.1757E−01 |
| 63.Eu | 1.2168E−03 | 3.3589E+04 | 3.3735E+04 | 3.3801E+04 | 1.9549E−01 |
| | 1.6755E−03 | 2.4363E+04 | 2.4664E+04 | 2.4509E+04 | 6.3001E−01 |
| 64.Gd | 1.7033E−03 | 3.6166E+04 | 3.6685E+04 | 3.6414E+04 | 7.4300E−01 |
| | 7.6815E−03 | 2.3626E+03 | 2.4456E+03 | 2.6201E+03 | 7.1328E+00 |
| 65.Tb | 1.2617E−03 | 3.1383E+04 | 3.1529E+04 | 3.1626E+04 | 3.0863E−01 |
| | 1.7049E−03 | 3.7035E+04 | 3.7568E+04 | 3.7309E+04 | 6.9508E−01 |
| | 5.9489E−02 | 3.8779E+01 | 4.6919E+01 | 1.0355E+02 | 1.2070E+02 |
| 66.Dy | 1.3149E−03 | 2.8769E+04 | 2.8916E+04 | 2.9016E+04 | 3.4832E−01 |
| | 1.7100E−03 | 3.9659E+04 | 4.0240E+04 | 3.9995E+04 | 6.1160E−01 |
| | 5.9253E−02 | 3.9355E+01 | 4.7567E+01 | 1.1193E+02 | 1.3532E+02 |
| 67.Ho | 1.3678E−03 | 2.6168E+04 | 2.6315E+04 | 2.6405E+04 | 3.4234E−01 |

| Material | $E$, MeV | $\mu_{1en}$, cm$^{-1}$ | $\mu_1$, cm$^{-1}$ | $\mu_2$, cm$^{-1}$ | $R$, % |
|---|---|---|---|---|---|
| | 1.7058E−03 | 3.7495E+04 | 3.8037E+04 | 3.7847E+04 | 5.0419E−01 |
| | 5.9116E−02 | 3.9688E+01 | 4.7941E+01 | 1.2015E+02 | 1.5061E+02 |
| 68.Er | 1.4204E−03 | 2.3586E+04 | 2.3732E+04 | 2.3813E+04 | 3.4148E−01 |
| | 1.7123E−03 | 4.0834E+04 | 4.1436E+04 | 4.1266E+04 | 4.1182E−01 |
| | 1.0631E−02 | 2.2468E+03 | 2.6001E+03 | 2.6052E+03 | 1.9607E−01 |
| | 5.9099E−02 | 3.9730E+01 | 4.7988E+01 | 1.2842E+02 | 1.6760E+02 |
| 69.Tm | 1.4734E−03 | 2.0980E+04 | 2.1127E+04 | 2.1192E+04 | 3.1049E−01 |
| | 1.7110E−03 | 4.0173E+04 | 4.0763E+04 | 4.0638E+04 | 3.0689E−01 |
| | 1.0273E−02 | 2.4636E+03 | 2.8627E+03 | 2.8916E+03 | 1.0124E+00 |
| 70.Yb | 1.5479E−03 | 1.8544E+04 | 1.8690E+04 | 1.8764E+04 | 3.9446E−01 |
| | 1.6888E−03 | 2.8726E+04 | 2.9111E+04 | 2.9099E+04 | 4.2292E−02 |
| 71.Lu | 1.5954E−03 | 1.7426E+04 | 1.7572E+04 | 1.7618E+04 | 2.6247E−01 |
| | 1.7055E−03 | 3.7332E+04 | 3.7871E+04 | 3.7849E+04 | 5.8549E−02 |
| 73.Ta | 1.6655E−03 | 2.1073E+04 | 2.1310E+04 | 2.1245E+04 | 3.1001E−01 |
| | 1.7888E−03 | 4.8010E+04 | 4.8722E+04 | 4.8762E+04 | 8.2339E−02 |
| 74.W | 1.6790E−03 | 2.5519E+04 | 2.5843E+04 | 2.5732E+04 | 4.3189E−01 |
| | 1.8593E−03 | 4.7739E+04 | 4.8444E+04 | 4.8514E+04 | 1.4458E−01 |
| | 1.1365E−02 | 2.9070E+03 | 3.4929E+03 | 3.4068E+03 | 2.5255E+00 |
| 75.Re | 1.6891E−03 | 2.8914E+04 | 2.9303E+04 | 2.9166E+04 | 4.6866E−01 |
| 75.Re | 1.9313E−03 | 4.7461E+04 | 4.8160E+04 | 4.8272E+04 | 2.3154E−01 |
| 76.Os | 1.6969E−03 | 3.2887E+04 | 3.3346E+04 | 3.3135E+04 | 6.3830E−01 |
| | 1.9838E−03 | 4.7259E+04 | 4.7953E+04 | 4.8094E+04 | 2.9374E−01 |
| 77.Ir | 1.7001E−03 | 3.4524E+04 | 3.5013E+04 | 3.4784E+04 | 6.5818E−01 |
| | 2.0942E−03 | 4.2092E+04 | 4.2691E+04 | 4.2896E+04 | 4.7855E−01 |
| 78.Pt | 1.7002E−03 | 3.4571E+04 | 3.5061E+04 | 3.4829E+04 | 6.6742E−01 |
| | 2.1906E−03 | 4.3861E+04 | 4.4491E+04 | 4.4775E+04 | 6.3660E−01 |
| 79.Au | 1.6969E−03 | 3.2875E+04 | 3.3334E+04 | 3.3118E+04 | 6.5226E−01 |
| | 2.2833E−03 | 3.9695E+04 | 4.0258E+04 | 4.0577E+04 | 7.9157E−01 |
| 80.Hg | 1.6761E−03 | 2.4562E+04 | 2.4866E+04 | 2.4733E+04 | 5.3969E−01 |
| | 2.7884E−03 | 2.8073E+04 | 2.8450E+04 | 2.8767E+04 | 1.1152E+00 |
| | 1.4497E−02 | 1.6766E+03 | 1.9630E+03 | 2.2671E+03 | 1.5495E+01 |
| 81.Tl | 1.6691E−03 | 2.2260E+04 | 2.2520E+04 | 2.2400E+04 | 5.3397E−01 |
| | 3.3751E−03 | 1.8868E+04 | 1.9128E+04 | 1.9330E+04 | 1.0552E+00 |
| 82.Pb | 1.6698E−03 | 2.2480E+04 | 2.2745E+04 | 2.2613E+04 | 5.8459E−01 |
| | 3.3863E−03 | 1.8737E+04 | 1.8996E+04 | 1.9240E+04 | 1.2817E+00 |
| | 1.6260E−02 | 1.2857E+03 | 1.4885E+03 | 1.6821E+03 | 1.3005E+01 |
| 83.Bi | 1.6634E−03 | 2.0365E+04 | 2.0589E+04 | 2.0489E+04 | 4.8831E−01 |
| | 3.9543E−03 | 1.2137E+04 | 1.2328E+04 | 1.2464E+04 | 1.0991E+00 |
| | 2.7365E−02 | 3.6919E+02 | 4.1915E+02 | 4.5619E+02 | 8.8378E+00 |

| Material | $E$, MeV | $\mu_{1en}$, cm$^{-1}$ | $\mu_1$, cm$^{-1}$ | $\mu_2$, cm$^{-1}$ | $R$, % |
|---|---|---|---|---|---|
| 84.Po | 1.6639E−03 | 2.0543E+04 | 2.0770E+04 | 2.0661E+04 | 5.2704E−01 |
| | 3.9580E−03 | 1.2094E+04 | 1.2285E+04 | 1.2429E+04 | 1.1734E+00 |
| | 4.1038E−03 | 1.1094E+04 | 1.1274E+04 | 1.1401E+04 | 1.1279E+00 |
| | 2.8254E−02 | 3.2775E+02 | 3.7194E+02 | 4.0627E+02 | 9.2293E+00 |
| 85.At | 1.6712E−03 | 2.2942E+04 | 2.3215E+04 | 2.3078E+04 | 5.9323E−01 |
| | 2.9535E−03 | 2.4292E+04 | 2.4613E+04 | 2.5114E+04 | 2.0324E+00 |
| | 3.5253E−03 | 1.7122E+04 | 1.7365E+04 | 1.7638E+04 | 1.5716E+00 |
| | 1.9322E−02 | 8.1635E+02 | 9.3309E+02 | 1.0757E+03 | 1.5286E+01 |
| 87.Fr | 1.6740E−03 | 2.3862E+04 | 2.4153E+04 | 2.3992E+04 | 6.7223E−01 |
| | 3.1511E−03 | 2.1470E+04 | 2.1758E+04 | 2.2259E+04 | 2.3025E+00 |
| | 1.9549E−02 | 7.8164E+02 | 8.9203E+02 | 1.0575E+03 | 1.8554E+01 |
| 89.Ac | 1.6801E−03 | 2.5877E+04 | 2.6208E+04 | 2.6008E+04 | 7.6675E−01 |
| 90.Th | 1.6922E−03 | 3.0501E+04 | 3.0918E+04 | 3.0653E+04 | 8.6405E−01 |
| 91.Pa | 1.7130E−03 | 4.1154E+04 | 4.1761E+04 | 4.1362E+04 | 9.6387E−01 |
| | 9.9086E−03 | 2.6866E+03 | 3.1335E+03 | 2.8106E+03 | 1.1489E+01 |
| | 1.0116E−02 | 2.5588E+03 | 2.9779E+03 | 2.6790E+03 | 1.1159E+01 |
| 92.U | 1.7743E−03 | 4.8066E+04 | 4.8779E+04 | 4.8321E+04 | 9.4867E−01 |
| 121. | 1.2506E−03 | 3.1928E+04 | 3.2074E+04 | 3.2143E+04 | 2.1622E−01 |
| | 1.6873E−03 | 2.8260E+04 | 2.8636E+04 | 2.8454E+04 | 6.4269E−01 |
| | 1.6909E−03 | 2.9807E+04 | 3.0212E+04 | 3.0007E+04 | 6.8249E−01 |
| 123. | 1.6732E−03 | 2.3598E+04 | 2.3884E+04 | 2.3837E+04 | 1.9782E−01 |
| 130. | 1.0407E−03 | 4.2241E+04 | 4.2387E+04 | 4.2335E+04 | 1.2267E−01 |
| 73.TANTALUM | | | | | |
| 25.Mn | 1.1615E−03 | 4.7795E+04 | 4.7990E+04 | 4.7938E+04 | 1.0826E−01 |
| 27.Co | 1.7388E−03 | 2.4648E+04 | 2.4942E+04 | 2.4752E+04 | 7.6847E−01 |
| 28.Ni | 1.7478E−03 | 2.7916E+04 | 2.8278E+04 | 2.8049E+04 | 8.1370E−01 |
| 29.Cu | 1.7515E−03 | 2.9218E+04 | 2.9607E+04 | 2.9383E+04 | 7.6196E−01 |
| 30.Zn | 1.7419E−03 | 2.5781E+04 | 2.6099E+04 | 2.5961E+04 | 5.2857E−01 |
| 33.As | 1.3776E−03 | 3.3811E+04 | 3.3998E+04 | 3.4247E+04 | 7.2996E−01 |
| | 1.7399E−03 | 2.5072E+04 | 2.5375E+04 | 2.5361E+04 | 5.4918E−02 |
| 43.Tc | 1.3151E−03 | 3.7855E+04 | 3.8044E+04 | 3.7939E+04 | 2.7557E−01 |
| 46.Pd | 1.7359E−03 | 2.3611E+04 | 2.3883E+04 | 2.3701E+04 | 7.6716E−01 |
| 48.Cd | 1.4475E−03 | 2.9286E+04 | 2.9471E+04 | 2.9364E+04 | 3.6145E−01 |
| | 1.6571E−03 | 2.1319E+04 | 2.1491E+04 | 2.1392E+04 | 4.6566E−01 |
| 50.Sn | 1.2047E−03 | 4.4999E+04 | 4.5192E+04 | 4.5082E+04 | 2.4383E−01 |
| 58.Ce | 1.1043E−03 | 5.1494E+04 | 5.1690E+04 | 5.1668E+04 | 4.2466E−02 |
| | 1.7414E−03 | 2.5606E+04 | 2.5920E+04 | 2.5707E+04 | 8.3022E−01 |
| 59.Pr | 1.2232E−03 | 4.3803E+04 | 4.3995E+04 | 4.3971E+04 | 5.5319E−02 |
| | 1.7455E−03 | 2.7073E+04 | 2.7418E+04 | 2.7188E+04 | 8.4378E−01 |

| Material | $E$, MeV | $\mu_{1en}$, cm$^{-1}$ | $\mu_1$, cm$^{-1}$ | $\mu_2$, cm$^{-1}$ | $R$, % |
|---|---|---|---|---|---|
| 60.Nd | 1.7486E−03 | 2.8195E+04 | 2.8563E+04 | 2.8324E+04 | 8.4288E−01 |
| | 9.4529E−03 | 1.7709E+03 | 1.8556E+03 | 1.9256E+03 | 3.7723E+00 |
| 61.Pm | 1.0965E−03 | 5.2000E+04 | 5.2196E+04 | 5.2265E+04 | 1.3082E−01 |
| | 1.7544E−03 | 3.0289E+04 | 3.0700E+04 | 3.0442E+04 | 8.4846E−01 |
| | 7.5916E−03 | 3.2138E+03 | 3.3215E+03 | 3.5631E+03 | 7.2735E+00 |
| 62.Sm | 1.1162E−03 | 5.0725E+04 | 5.0920E+04 | 5.1007E+04 | 1.6989E−01 |
| | 1.7573E−03 | 3.1307E+04 | 3.1739E+04 | 3.1480E+04 | 8.2408E−01 |
| 64.Gd | 1.3113E−03 | 3.8103E+04 | 3.8292E+04 | 3.8363E+04 | 1.8611E−01 |
| | 1.7634E−03 | 3.3500E+04 | 3.3978E+04 | 3.3727E+04 | 7.4486E−01 |
| 65.Tb | 1.2743E−03 | 4.0495E+04 | 4.0686E+04 | 4.0812E+04 | 3.0995E−01 |
| | 1.7647E−03 | 3.4169E+04 | 3.4661E+04 | 3.4425E+04 | 6.8457E−01 |
| | 1.7681E−03 | 3.6116E+04 | 3.6644E+04 | 3.6388E+04 | 7.0585E−01 |
| 66.Dy | 1.3276E−03 | 3.7045E+04 | 3.7233E+04 | 3.7366E+04 | 3.5719E−01 |
| | 1.7690E−03 | 3.6594E+04 | 3.7131E+04 | 3.6904E+04 | 6.1543E−01 |
| 67.Ho | 1.3813E−03 | 3.3572E+04 | 3.3759E+04 | 3.3888E+04 | 3.8166E−01 |
| | 1.7733E−03 | 3.9116E+04 | 3.9701E+04 | 3.9487E+04 | 5.4116E−01 |
| 68.Er | 1.4347E−03 | 3.0118E+04 | 3.0303E+04 | 3.0428E+04 | 4.1248E−01 |
| | 1.7699E−03 | 3.7149E+04 | 3.7697E+04 | 3.7536E+04 | 4.2962E−01 |
| 69.Tm | 1.4838E−03 | 2.6942E+04 | 2.7126E+04 | 2.7235E+04 | 4.0230E−01 |
| | 1.7713E−03 | 3.7961E+04 | 3.8524E+04 | 3.8397E+04 | 3.3023E−01 |
| 70.Yb | 1.5683E−03 | 2.3901E+04 | 2.4080E+04 | 2.4200E+04 | 5.0163E−01 |
| | 1.7480E−03 | 2.7968E+04 | 2.8332E+04 | 2.8332E+04 | 3.3987E−03 |
| 71.Lu | 1.6142E−03 | 2.2566E+04 | 2.2741E+04 | 2.2855E+04 | 4.9835E−01 |
| | 1.7688E−03 | 3.6512E+04 | 3.7047E+04 | 3.7015E+04 | 8.8193E−02 |
| 72.Hf | 1.6655E−03 | 2.1073E+04 | 2.1245E+04 | 2.1310E+04 | 3.1001E−01 |
| | 1.7888E−03 | 4.8010E+04 | 4.8762E+04 | 4.8722E+04 | 8.2339E−02 |
| 74.W | 1.7359E−03 | 2.3619E+04 | 2.3892E+04 | 2.3832E+04 | 2.5271E−01 |
| 75.Re | 1.7448E−03 | 2.6804E+04 | 2.7143E+04 | 2.7056E+04 | 3.2049E−01 |
| 76.Os | 1.7554E−03 | 3.0651E+04 | 3.1071E+04 | 3.0900E+04 | 5.5330E−01 |
| 77.Ir | 1.7598E−03 | 3.2209E+04 | 3.2660E+04 | 3.2466E+04 | 5.9857E−01 |
| | 2.1155E−03 | 5.4134E+04 | 5.4994E+04 | 5.5225E+04 | 4.1944E−01 |
| 78.Pt | 1.7599E−03 | 3.2252E+04 | 3.2705E+04 | 3.2510E+04 | 6.0054E−01 |
| | 2.2720E−03 | 5.2373E+04 | 5.3187E+04 | 5.3524E+04 | 6.3318E−01 |
| 79.Au | 1.7556E−03 | 3.0715E+04 | 3.1136E+04 | 3.0956E+04 | 5.7922E−01 |
| | 2.4191E−03 | 4.5005E+04 | 4.5685E+04 | 4.6052E+04 | 8.0445E−01 |
| | 2.4803E−03 | 4.4945E+04 | 4.5621E+04 | 4.6003E+04 | 8.3688E−01 |
| 80.Hg | 3.8667E−03 | 1.7115E+04 | 1.7388E+04 | 1.7500E+04 | 6.4725E−01 |
| | 2.7620E−02 | 4.6321E+02 | 5.2849E+02 | 5.5531E+02 | 5.0761E+00 |
| 85.At | 1.0075E−03 | 5.7756E+04 | 5.7955E+04 | 5.7896E+04 | 1.0287E−01 |

| Material | $E$, MeV | $\mu_{1en}$, cm$^{-1}$ | $\mu_1$, cm$^{-1}$ | $\mu_2$, cm$^{-1}$ | $R$, % |
|---|---|---|---|---|---|
| | 1.0913E−03 | 5.2336E+04 | 5.2533E+04 | 5.2476E+04 | 1.0817E−01 |
| 87.Fr | 1.0729E−03 | 5.3525E+04 | 5.3722E+04 | 5.3665E+04 | 1.0691E−01 |
| | 1.2356E−03 | 4.2996E+04 | 4.3188E+04 | 4.3134E+04 | 1.2596E−01 |
| | 9.2767E−03 | 1.8750E+03 | 1.9615E+03 | 1.9531E+03 | 4.3211E−01 |
| 89.Ac | 1.7377E−03 | 2.4269E+04 | 2.4555E+04 | 2.4400E+04 | 6.3581E−01 |
| | 3.9593E−02 | 1.5517E+02 | 1.7854E+02 | 1.9172E+02 | 7.3862E+00 |
| 90.Th | 1.7497E−03 | 2.8589E+04 | 2.8965E+04 | 2.8741E+04 | 7.7880E−01 |
| | 2.5655E−02 | 5.8127E+02 | 6.6414E+02 | 7.9221E+02 | 1.9283E+01 |
| 91.Pa | 1.7722E−03 | 3.8438E+04 | 3.9010E+04 | 3.8645E+04 | 9.4488E−01 |
| 92.U | 1.7876E−03 | 4.7299E+04 | 4.8038E+04 | 4.7554E+04 | 1.0184E+00 |
| | 1.0427E−02 | 3.0638E+03 | 3.5929E+03 | 3.2097E+03 | 1.1940E+01 |
| 121. | 1.4018E−03 | 3.2242E+04 | 3.2428E+04 | 3.2458E+04 | 9.0488E−02 |
| | 1.7474E−03 | 2.7756E+04 | 2.8114E+04 | 2.7938E+04 | 6.3262E−01 |
| | 9.0871E−03 | 1.9869E+03 | 2.0755E+03 | 2.2331E+03 | 7.5958E+00 |
| 123. | 1.4485E−03 | 2.9223E+04 | 2.9408E+04 | 2.9535E+04 | 4.3359E−01 |
| | | | 74.TUNGSTEN | | |
| 26.Fe | 1.0405E−03 | 6.7661E+04 | 6.7891E+04 | 6.7907E+04 | 2.3222E−02 |
| 28.Ni | 1.8098E−03 | 2.5516E+04 | 2.5830E+04 | 2.5639E+04 | 7.4266E−01 |
| 29.Cu | 1.8132E−03 | 2.6728E+04 | 2.7066E+04 | 2.6879E+04 | 6.9825E−01 |
| 45.Rh | 1.3955E−03 | 3.9720E+04 | 3.9936E+04 | 3.9812E+04 | 3.1216E−01 |
| 46.Pd | 1.4639E−03 | 3.4341E+04 | 3.4555E+04 | 3.4438E+04 | 3.3876E−01 |
| | 1.7397E−03 | 2.3493E+04 | 2.3705E+04 | 2.3583E+04 | 5.1689E−01 |
| 47.Ag | 1.2818E−03 | 4.8667E+04 | 4.8888E+04 | 4.8761E+04 | 2.6159E−01 |
| 59.Pr | 1.3754E−03 | 4.1304E+04 | 4.1521E+04 | 4.1470E+04 | 1.2175E−01 |
| 60.Nd | 1.3774E−03 | 4.1151E+04 | 4.1368E+04 | 4.1333E+04 | 8.4026E−02 |
| | 1.8114E−03 | 2.6089E+04 | 2.6414E+04 | 2.6210E+04 | 7.7907E−01 |
| 61.Pm | 1.8172E−03 | 2.8142E+04 | 2.8510E+04 | 2.8288E+04 | 7.8763E−01 |
| 62.Sm | 1.3485E−03 | 4.3418E+04 | 4.3636E+04 | 4.3652E+04 | 3.7222E−02 |
| | 1.8201E−03 | 2.9193E+04 | 2.9583E+04 | 2.9356E+04 | 7.7360E−01 |
| 64.Gd | 1.4067E−03 | 3.8841E+04 | 3.9057E+04 | 3.9102E+04 | 1.1471E−01 |
| | 1.8253E−03 | 3.1046E+04 | 3.1475E+04 | 3.1257E+04 | 6.9898E−01 |
| 65.Tb | 1.2894E−03 | 4.8076E+04 | 4.8296E+04 | 4.8459E+04 | 3.3679E−01 |
| 65.Tb | 1.8320E−03 | 3.3454E+04 | 3.3934E+04 | 3.3709E+04 | 6.6630E−01 |
| 66.Dy | 1.8327E−03 | 3.3691E+04 | 3.4175E+04 | 3.3969E+04 | 6.0820E−01 |
| 67.Ho | 1.8388E−03 | 3.5865E+04 | 3.6396E+04 | 3.6204E+04 | 5.2949E−01 |
| 68.Er | 1.4465E−03 | 3.5708E+04 | 3.5923E+04 | 3.6086E+04 | 4.5574E−01 |
| | 1.8438E−03 | 3.8529E+04 | 3.9114E+04 | 3.8929E+04 | 4.7627E−01 |
| 69.Tm | 1.4927E−03 | 3.2073E+04 | 3.2286E+04 | 3.2436E+04 | 4.6423E−01 |
| | 1.8378E−03 | 3.5520E+04 | 3.6043E+04 | 3.5924E+04 | 3.3036E−01 |

| Material | $E$, MeV | $\mu_{1en}$, cm$^{-1}$ | $\mu_1$, cm$^{-1}$ | $\mu_2$, cm$^{-1}$ | $R$, % |
|---|---|---|---|---|---|
| 70.Yb | 1.8125E−03 | 2.6494E+04 | 2.6828E+04 | 2.6833E+04 | 1.9504E−02 |
| 71.Lu | 1.6252E−03 | 2.7315E+04 | 2.7528E+04 | 2.7676E+04 | 5.3753E−01 |
| | 1.8381E−03 | 3.5614E+04 | 3.6139E+04 | 3.6102E+04 | 1.0290E−01 |
| | 9.3443E−03 | 2.2336E+03 | 2.3360E+03 | 2.5956E+03 | 1.1112E+01 |
| 72.Hf | 1.6790E−03 | 2.5519E+04 | 2.5732E+04 | 2.5843E+04 | 4.3189E−01 |
| | 1.8593E−03 | 4.7739E+04 | 4.8514E+04 | 4.8444E+04 | 1.4458E−01 |
| | 1.1365E−02 | 2.9070E+03 | 3.4068E+03 | 3.4929E+03 | 2.5255E+00 |
| 73.Ta | 1.7359E−03 | 2.3619E+04 | 2.3832E+04 | 2.3892E+04 | 2.5271E−01 |
| 76.Os | 1.8175E−03 | 2.8281E+04 | 2.8653E+04 | 2.8529E+04 | 4.3124E−01 |
| | 2.1510E−03 | 6.3248E+04 | 6.4352E+04 | 6.4480E+04 | 1.9976E−01 |
| | 2.3000E−03 | 6.1130E+04 | 6.2137E+04 | 6.2324E+04 | 3.0110E−01 |
| 77.Ir | 1.8218E−03 | 2.9802E+04 | 3.0205E+04 | 3.0057E+04 | 4.9433E−01 |
| | 2.2300E−03 | 5.7429E+04 | 5.8413E+04 | 5.8632E+04 | 3.7433E−01 |
| | 2.3774E−03 | 5.6515E+04 | 5.7460E+04 | 5.7711E+04 | 4.3714E−01 |
| 78.Pt | 1.8219E−03 | 2.9844E+04 | 3.0248E+04 | 3.0101E+04 | 4.8730E−01 |
| | 2.4653E−03 | 5.1748E+04 | 5.2607E+04 | 5.2899E+04 | 5.5481E−01 |
| | 1.3816E−02 | 2.8733E+03 | 3.4630E+03 | 3.6545E+03 | 5.5301E+00 |
| 79.Au | 1.8180E−03 | 2.8425E+04 | 2.8799E+04 | 2.8664E+04 | 4.7251E−01 |
| 89.Ac | 1.6082E−03 | 2.7885E+04 | 2.8098E+04 | 2.8016E+04 | 2.9050E−01 |
| 90.Th | 1.8126E−03 | 2.6499E+04 | 2.6833E+04 | 2.6651E+04 | 6.8118E−01 |
| | 5.6450E−03 | 7.9828E+03 | 8.1659E+03 | 8.2558E+03 | 1.1003E+00 |
| | 4.4348E−02 | 1.4317E+02 | 1.6632E+02 | 1.7715E+02 | 6.5145E+00 |
| 91.Pa | 1.8376E−03 | 3.5437E+04 | 3.5958E+04 | 3.5642E+04 | 8.8826E−01 |
| | 3.6459E−03 | 2.4524E+04 | 2.4921E+04 | 2.5531E+04 | 2.4480E+00 |
| 92.U | 1.8523E−03 | 4.3581E+04 | 4.4271E+04 | 4.3833E+04 | 9.9861E−01 |
| 121. | 1.4883E−03 | 3.2421E+04 | 3.2634E+04 | 3.2637E+04 | 9.2048E−03 |
| | 1.8101E−03 | 2.5636E+04 | 2.5952E+04 | 2.5803E+04 | 5.7710E−01 |
| | | | 75.RHENIUM | | |
| 27.Co | 1.3146E−03 | 5.2791E+04 | 5.3044E+04 | 5.3027E+04 | 3.1035E−02 |
| 28.Ni | 1.8372E−03 | 2.4455E+04 | 2.4711E+04 | 2.4573E+04 | 5.6269E−01 |
| 29.Cu | 1.8553E−03 | 2.5029E+04 | 2.5316E+04 | 2.5170E+04 | 5.7843E−01 |
| 59.Pr | 1.6747E−03 | 2.9463E+04 | 2.9715E+04 | 2.9586E+04 | 4.3703E−01 |
| | 1.8300E−03 | 2.4224E+04 | 2.4468E+04 | 2.4330E+04 | 5.6756E−01 |
| 60.Nd | 1.4958E−03 | 3.6466E+04 | 3.6718E+04 | 3.6626E+04 | 2.5217E−01 |
| | 1.5123E−03 | 3.5626E+04 | 3.5878E+04 | 3.5782E+04 | 2.6771E−01 |
| 60.Nd | 1.8490E−03 | 2.4828E+04 | 2.5104E+04 | 2.4945E+04 | 6.4106E−01 |
| 61.Pm | 1.4484E−03 | 4.0738E+04 | 4.0990E+04 | 4.0938E+04 | 1.2610E−01 |
| | 1.8827E−03 | 2.5899E+04 | 2.6232E+04 | 2.6037E+04 | 7.5169E−01 |
| 62.Sm | 1.8867E−03 | 2.6951E+04 | 2.7309E+04 | 2.7103E+04 | 7.5845E−01 |

| Material | $E$, MeV | $\mu_{1en}$, $cm^{-1}$ | $\mu_1$, $cm^{-1}$ | $\mu_2$, $cm^{-1}$ | $R$, % |
|---|---|---|---|---|---|
| 64.Gd | 1.4645E−03 | 3.9289E+04 | 3.9541E+04 | 3.9549E+04 | 2.1378E−02 |
| | 1.8930E−03 | 2.9850E+04 | 3.0272E+04 | 3.0046E+04 | 7.5263E−01 |
| | 1.0476E−02 | 1.7911E+03 | 1.8909E+03 | 1.9950E+03 | 5.5062E+00 |
| 65.Tb | 1.3924E−03 | 4.5790E+04 | 4.6042E+04 | 4.6146E+04 | 2.2693E−01 |
| | 1.8955E−03 | 3.0997E+04 | 3.1444E+04 | 3.1234E+04 | 6.7310E−01 |
| | 9.7666E−03 | 2.2047E+03 | 2.3132E+03 | 2.4881E+03 | 7.5607E+00 |
| 66.Dy | 1.3784E−03 | 4.7044E+04 | 4.7297E+04 | 4.7459E+04 | 3.4255E−01 |
| | 1.9002E−03 | 3.3143E+04 | 3.3638E+04 | 3.3423E+04 | 6.4104E−01 |
| | 9.0499E−03 | 2.7719E+03 | 2.8910E+03 | 3.1819E+03 | 1.0060E+01 |
| 67.Ho | 1.3933E−03 | 4.5706E+04 | 4.5959E+04 | 4.6164E+04 | 4.4781E−01 |
| | 1.9004E−03 | 3.3228E+04 | 3.3725E+04 | 3.3538E+04 | 5.5711E−01 |
| 68.Er | 1.9059E−03 | 3.5781E+04 | 3.6334E+04 | 3.6149E+04 | 5.1337E−01 |
| | 9.5507E−03 | 2.3756E+03 | 2.4873E+03 | 2.7595E+03 | 1.0944E+01 |
| 69.Tm | 1.4997E−03 | 3.6117E+04 | 3.6369E+04 | 3.6534E+04 | 4.5370E−01 |
| | 1.9108E−03 | 3.8015E+04 | 3.8617E+04 | 3.8446E+04 | 4.4605E−01 |
| 70.Yb | 1.6968E−03 | 2.8623E+04 | 2.8875E+04 | 2.8995E+04 | 4.1473E−01 |
| | 1.8634E−03 | 2.5287E+04 | 2.5588E+04 | 2.5605E+04 | 6.8713E−02 |
| 71.Lu | 1.6338E−03 | 3.1013E+04 | 3.1266E+04 | 3.1430E+04 | 5.2460E−01 |
| | 1.9037E−03 | 3.4763E+04 | 3.5293E+04 | 3.5236E+04 | 1.6063E−01 |
| 72.Hf | 1.6891E−03 | 2.8914E+04 | 2.9166E+04 | 2.9303E+04 | 4.6866E−01 |
| | 1.9313E−03 | 4.7461E+04 | 4.8272E+04 | 4.8160E+04 | 2.3154E−01 |
| 73.Ta | 1.7448E−03 | 2.6804E+04 | 2.7056E+04 | 2.7143E+04 | 3.2049E−01 |
| 76.Os | 1.8812E−03 | 2.5852E+04 | 2.6183E+04 | 2.6100E+04 | 3.1541E−01 |
| | 2.2532E−03 | 6.2544E+04 | 6.3703E+04 | 6.3772E+04 | 1.0755E−01 |
| 77.Ir | 1.8874E−03 | 2.7258E+04 | 2.7623E+04 | 2.7509E+04 | 4.1171E−01 |
| | 2.3422E−03 | 5.7175E+04 | 5.8217E+04 | 5.8395E+04 | 3.0581E−01 |
| 78.Pt | 1.8875E−03 | 2.7298E+04 | 2.7664E+04 | 2.7555E+04 | 3.9339E−01 |
| 79.Au | 1.8846E−03 | 2.5975E+04 | 2.6311E+04 | 2.6211E+04 | 3.8293E−01 |
| | 2.7831E−03 | 4.6547E+04 | 4.7325E+04 | 4.7609E+04 | 5.9993E−01 |
| | 3.6848E−03 | 2.6911E+04 | 2.7378E+04 | 2.7481E+04 | 3.7747E−01 |
| | 1.7479E−02 | 1.8853E+03 | 2.2386E+03 | 2.3498E+03 | 4.9698E+00 |
| 90.Th | 1.4744E−03 | 3.8402E+04 | 3.8654E+04 | 3.8556E+04 | 2.5448E−01 |
| | 1.8560E−03 | 2.5052E+04 | 2.5340E+04 | 2.5205E+04 | 5.3838E−01 |
| 91.Pa | 1.8991E−03 | 3.2618E+04 | 3.3101E+04 | 3.2821E+04 | 8.5352E−01 |
| | 2.6376E−02 | 7.2427E+02 | 8.3793E+02 | 9.8885E+02 | 1.8011E+01 |
| 92.U | 1.9151E−03 | 3.9975E+04 | 4.0620E+04 | 4.0225E+04 | 9.8326E−01 |
| | 2.1414E−02 | 1.1218E+03 | 1.3039E+03 | 1.7577E+03 | 3.4806E+01 |
| 121. | 1.5729E−03 | 3.3326E+04 | 3.3579E+04 | 3.3548E+04 | 9.1625E−02 |
| 121. | 1.8428E−03 | 2.4632E+04 | 2.4898E+04 | 2.4794E+04 | 4.1847E−01 |

| Material | $E$, MeV | $\mu_{1en}$, cm$^{-1}$ | $\mu_1$, cm$^{-1}$ | $\mu_2$, cm$^{-1}$ | $R$, % |
|---|---|---|---|---|---|
| | | | 76.OSMIUM | | |
| 28.Ni | 1.3620E−03 | 5.4285E+04 | 5.4545E+04 | 5.4563E+04 | 3.1532E−02 |
| 29.Cu | 1.0238E−03 | 8.8312E+04 | 8.8603E+04 | 8.8965E+04 | 4.0843E−01 |
| | 1.3675E−03 | 5.3736E+04 | 5.3997E+04 | 5.4078E+04 | 1.5070E−01 |
| 61.Pm | 1.8563E−03 | 2.6802E+04 | 2.7050E+04 | 2.6943E+04 | 3.9933E−01 |
| 62.Sm | 1.6065E−03 | 3.6335E+04 | 3.6584E+04 | 3.6537E+04 | 1.2771E−01 |
| 65.Tb | 1.4618E−03 | 4.4249E+04 | 4.4501E+04 | 4.4588E+04 | 1.9603E−01 |
| | 1.0771E−02 | 1.8544E+03 | 1.9603E+03 | 2.0835E+03 | 6.2843E+00 |
| 66.Dy | 1.4339E−03 | 4.7047E+04 | 4.7302E+04 | 4.7456E+04 | 3.2631E−01 |
| | 1.0266E−02 | 2.1093E+03 | 2.2212E+03 | 2.3954E+03 | 7.8425E+00 |
| 67.Ho | 1.4296E−03 | 4.7483E+04 | 4.7737E+04 | 4.7955E+04 | 4.5700E−01 |
| | 9.7600E−03 | 2.4536E+03 | 2.5728E+03 | 2.8260E+03 | 9.8441E+00 |
| 68.Er | 1.4555E−03 | 4.4878E+04 | 4.5130E+04 | 4.5372E+04 | 5.3713E−01 |
| 69.Tm | 9.9641E−03 | 2.2749E+03 | 2.3906E+03 | 2.6615E+03 | 1.1332E+01 |
| 70.Yb | 1.9495E−03 | 2.3246E+04 | 2.3495E+04 | 2.3529E+04 | 1.4696E−01 |
| 72.Hf | 1.6969E−03 | 3.2887E+04 | 3.3135E+04 | 3.3346E+04 | 6.3830E−01 |
| | 1.9838E−03 | 4.7259E+04 | 4.8094E+04 | 4.7953E+04 | 2.9374E−01 |
| 73.Ta | 1.7554E−03 | 3.0651E+04 | 3.0900E+04 | 3.1071E+04 | 5.5330E−01 |
| 74.W | 1.8175E−03 | 2.8281E+04 | 2.8529E+04 | 2.8653E+04 | 4.3124E−01 |
| | 2.1510E−03 | 6.3248E+04 | 6.4480E+04 | 6.4352E+04 | 1.9976E−01 |
| | 2.3000E−03 | 6.1130E+04 | 6.2324E+04 | 6.2137E+04 | 3.0110E−01 |
| 75.Re | 1.8812E−03 | 2.5852E+04 | 2.6100E+04 | 2.6183E+04 | 3.1541E−01 |
| | 2.2532E−03 | 6.2544E+04 | 6.3772E+04 | 6.3703E+04 | 1.0755E−01 |
| 78.Pt | 3.8107E−03 | 2.6752E+04 | 2.7248E+04 | 2.7299E+04 | 1.8606E−01 |
| | 1.9444E−02 | 1.5091E+03 | 1.7830E+03 | 1.8204E+03 | 2.0960E+00 |
| 79.Au | 1.7059E−03 | 3.2541E+04 | 3.2789E+04 | 3.2784E+04 | 1.5454E−02 |
| | 1.0770E−02 | 1.8552E+03 | 1.9611E+03 | 1.9539E+03 | 3.6789E−01 |
| 91.Pa | 2.9761E−02 | 4.9943E+02 | 5.7621E+02 | 6.5055E+02 | 1.2902E+01 |
| | | | 77.IRIDIUM | | |
| 28.Ni | 1.2097E−03 | 7.2795E+04 | 7.3077E+04 | 7.3183E+04 | 1.4521E−01 |
| 62.Sm | 1.9514E−03 | 2.4776E+04 | 2.5024E+04 | 2.4918E+04 | 4.2810E−01 |
| 64.Gd | 1.6644E−03 | 3.5908E+04 | 3.6170E+04 | 3.6153E+04 | 4.6979E−02 |
| | 2.0484E−03 | 2.5576E+04 | 2.5930E+04 | 2.5754E+04 | 6.8299E−01 |
| 65.Tb | 1.4865E−03 | 4.3698E+04 | 4.3968E+04 | 4.4031E+04 | 1.4320E−01 |
| | 1.5474E−03 | 4.0446E+04 | 4.0713E+04 | 4.0751E+04 | 9.2646E−02 |
| | 2.0568E−03 | 2.7646E+04 | 2.8065E+04 | 2.7854E+04 | 7.5805E−01 |
| | 1.1165E−02 | 1.7500E+03 | 1.8537E+03 | 1.9645E+03 | 5.9817E+00 |
| 66.Dy | 1.4547E−03 | 4.7048E+04 | 4.7319E+04 | 4.7455E+04 | 2.8615E−01 |
| | 2.0616E−03 | 2.8837E+04 | 2.9293E+04 | 2.9083E+04 | 7.2242E−01 |

| Material | $E$, MeV | $\mu_{1en}$, cm$^{-1}$ | $\mu_1$, cm$^{-1}$ | $\mu_2$, cm$^{-1}$ | $R$, % |
|---|---|---|---|---|---|
| | 1.0666E−02 | 1.9976E+03 | 2.1068E+03 | 2.2666E+03 | 7.5846E+00 |
| 67.Ho | 1.4439E−03 | 4.8181E+04 | 4.8452E+04 | 4.8659E+04 | 4.2727E−01 |
| 67.Ho | 2.0634E−03 | 2.9297E+04 | 2.9767E+04 | 2.9561E+04 | 6.9856E−01 |
| | 1.0101E−02 | 2.2773E+03 | 2.3928E+03 | 2.6145E+03 | 9.2644E+00 |
| 68.Er | 1.4620E−03 | 4.6276E+04 | 4.6547E+04 | 4.6786E+04 | 5.1373E−01 |
| | 2.0708E−03 | 3.1103E+04 | 3.1630E+04 | 3.1414E+04 | 6.8741E−01 |
| 69.Tm | 2.0717E−03 | 3.1335E+04 | 3.1870E+04 | 3.1678E+04 | 6.0479E−01 |
| 70.Yb | 2.0426E−03 | 2.4151E+04 | 2.4459E+04 | 2.4445E+04 | 5.6696E−02 |
| 71.Lu | 2.0823E−03 | 3.5358E+04 | 3.6000E+04 | 3.5835E+04 | 4.6143E−01 |
| 72.Hf | 1.7001E−03 | 3.4524E+04 | 3.4784E+04 | 3.5013E+04 | 6.5818E−01 |
| | 2.0942E−03 | 4.2092E+04 | 4.2896E+04 | 4.2691E+04 | 4.7855E−01 |
| 73.Ta | 1.7598E−03 | 3.2209E+04 | 3.2466E+04 | 3.2660E+04 | 5.9857E−01 |
| | 2.1155E−03 | 5.4134E+04 | 5.5225E+04 | 5.4994E+04 | 4.1944E−01 |
| 74.W | 1.8218E−03 | 2.9802E+04 | 3.0057E+04 | 3.0205E+04 | 4.9433E−01 |
| | 2.2300E−03 | 5.7429E+04 | 5.8632E+04 | 5.8413E+04 | 3.7433E−01 |
| | 2.3774E−03 | 5.6515E+04 | 5.7711E+04 | 5.7460E+04 | 4.3714E−01 |
| 75.Re | 1.8874E−03 | 2.7258E+04 | 2.7509E+04 | 2.7623E+04 | 4.1171E−01 |
| | 2.3422E−03 | 5.7175E+04 | 5.8395E+04 | 5.8217E+04 | 3.0581E−01 |
| 78.Pt | 1.0478E−03 | 8.9814E+04 | 9.0103E+04 | 9.0071E+04 | 3.5441E−02 |
| | 2.7149E−03 | 5.3035E+04 | 5.4121E+04 | 5.4186E+04 | 1.2155E−01 |
| | 1.0496E−02 | 2.0814E+03 | 2.1925E+03 | 2.1915E+03 | 4.4706E−02 |
| 91.Pa | 2.0545E−03 | 2.7087E+04 | 2.7488E+04 | 2.7286E+04 | 7.4203E−01 |
| | 5.1598E−03 | 1.2766E+04 | 1.3048E+04 | 1.3224E+04 | 1.3544E+00 |
| | 3.4825E−02 | 3.6644E+02 | 4.2509E+02 | 4.6941E+02 | 1.0425E+01 |
| 92.U | 2.0789E−03 | 3.3458E+04 | 3.4055E+04 | 3.3702E+04 | 1.0476E+00 |
| | 3.8006E−03 | 2.7528E+04 | 2.8052E+04 | 2.8694E+04 | 2.2871E+00 |
| | 4.2526E−03 | 2.0902E+04 | 2.1311E+04 | 2.1730E+04 | 1.9629E+00 |
| 78.PLATINUM | | | | | |
| 28.Ni | 1.2085E−03 | 7.2948E+04 | 7.3205E+04 | 7.3337E+04 | 1.7989E−01 |
| 61.Pm | 2.1123E−03 | 2.0360E+04 | 2.0603E+04 | 2.0477E+04 | 6.1762E−01 |
| 62.Sm | 1.9593E−03 | 2.4509E+04 | 2.4767E+04 | 2.4650E+04 | 4.7283E−01 |
| 64.Gd | 1.6601E−03 | 3.6126E+04 | 3.6384E+04 | 3.6372E+04 | 3.1188E−02 |
| | 2.1327E−03 | 2.4205E+04 | 2.4562E+04 | 2.4376E+04 | 7.6597E−01 |
| 65.Tb | 1.4872E−03 | 4.3683E+04 | 4.3941E+04 | 4.4016E+04 | 1.7076E−01 |
| | 1.5450E−03 | 4.0596E+04 | 4.0853E+04 | 4.0901E+04 | 1.1864E−01 |
| | 2.1421E−03 | 2.6144E+04 | 2.6567E+04 | 2.6342E+04 | 8.5389E−01 |
| | 1.1266E−02 | 1.7234E+03 | 1.8247E+03 | 1.9343E+03 | 6.0077E+00 |
| 66.Dy | 1.4552E−03 | 4.7048E+04 | 4.7306E+04 | 4.7455E+04 | 3.1501E−01 |
| | 2.1476E−03 | 2.7284E+04 | 2.7745E+04 | 2.7519E+04 | 8.2396E−01 |

| Material | $E$, MeV | $\mu_{1en}$, cm$^{-1}$ | $\mu_1$, cm$^{-1}$ | $\mu_2$, cm$^{-1}$ | $R$, % |
|---|---|---|---|---|---|
| | 1.0693E−02 | 1.9899E+03 | 2.0978E+03 | 2.2578E+03 | 7.6267E+00 |
| 67.Ho | 1.4442E−03 | 4.8197E+04 | 4.8454E+04 | 4.8676E+04 | 4.5672E−01 |
| | 2.1513E−03 | 2.8046E+04 | 2.8533E+04 | 2.8307E+04 | 8.0035E−01 |
| | 1.0031E−02 | 2.2977E+03 | 2.4132E+03 | 2.6383E+03 | 9.3282E+00 |
| 68.Er | 1.4622E−03 | 4.6312E+04 | 4.6569E+04 | 4.6822E+04 | 5.4297E−01 |
| 68.Er | 2.1533E−03 | 2.8471E+04 | 2.8972E+04 | 2.8757E+04 | 7.4846E−01 |
| 69.Tm | 2.1616E−03 | 3.0237E+04 | 3.0797E+04 | 3.0575E+04 | 7.2613E−01 |
| 70.Yb | 2.1226E−03 | 2.2098E+04 | 2.2383E+04 | 2.2364E+04 | 8.4319E−02 |
| 71.Lu | 2.1656E−03 | 3.2129E+04 | 3.2739E+04 | 3.2558E+04 | 5.5520E−01 |
| 72.Hf | 1.7002E−03 | 3.4571E+04 | 3.4829E+04 | 3.5061E+04 | 6.6742E−01 |
| | 2.1906E−03 | 4.3861E+04 | 4.4775E+04 | 4.4491E+04 | 6.3660E−01 |
| 73.Ta | 1.7599E−03 | 3.2252E+04 | 3.2510E+04 | 3.2705E+04 | 6.0054E−01 |
| | 2.2720E−03 | 5.2373E+04 | 5.3524E+04 | 5.3187E+04 | 6.3318E−01 |
| 74.W | 1.8219E−03 | 2.9844E+04 | 3.0101E+04 | 3.0248E+04 | 4.8730E−01 |
| | 2.4653E−03 | 5.1748E+04 | 5.2899E+04 | 5.2607E+04 | 5.5481E−01 |
| | 1.3816E−02 | 2.8733E+03 | 3.6545E+03 | 3.4630E+03 | 5.5301E+00 |
| 75.Re | 1.8875E−03 | 2.7298E+04 | 2.7555E+04 | 2.7664E+04 | 3.9339E−01 |
| 76.Os | 3.8107E−03 | 2.6752E+04 | 2.7299E+04 | 2.7248E+04 | 1.8606E−01 |
| | 1.9444E−02 | 1.5091E+03 | 1.8204E+03 | 1.7830E+03 | 2.0960E+00 |
| 77.Ir | 1.0478E−03 | 8.9814E+04 | 9.0071E+04 | 9.0103E+04 | 3.5441E−02 |
| | 2.7149E−03 | 5.3035E+04 | 5.4186E+04 | 5.4121E+04 | 1.2155E−01 |
| | 1.0496E−02 | 2.0814E+03 | 2.1915E+03 | 2.1925E+03 | 4.4706E−02 |
| 91.Pa | 2.1398E−03 | 2.5675E+04 | 2.6082E+04 | 2.5871E+04 | 8.1261E−01 |
| | 5.3028E−03 | 1.1949E+04 | 1.2226E+04 | 1.2376E+04 | 1.2292E+00 |
| | 3.1974E−02 | 4.3563E+02 | 5.0738E+02 | 5.6231E+02 | 1.0826E+01 |
| 92.U | 2.1647E−03 | 3.1681E+04 | 3.2279E+04 | 3.1922E+04 | 1.1165E+00 |
| 79.GOLD | | | | | |
| 28.Ni | 1.3847E−03 | 5.1528E+04 | 5.1780E+04 | 5.1790E+04 | 1.9999E−02 |
| 29.Cu | 1.0313E−03 | 8.6523E+04 | 8.6774E+04 | 8.7156E+04 | 4.4015E−01 |
| | 1.4207E−03 | 4.7961E+04 | 4.8212E+04 | 4.8255E+04 | 8.9595E−02 |
| 61.Pm | 1.9409E−03 | 2.3906E+04 | 2.4140E+04 | 2.4036E+04 | 4.3273E−01 |
| | 2.2062E−03 | 1.9087E+04 | 1.9350E+04 | 1.9199E+04 | 7.8790E−01 |
| 62.Sm | 1.6161E−03 | 3.5843E+04 | 3.6090E+04 | 3.6042E+04 | 1.3397E−01 |
| | 2.2121E−03 | 2.0104E+04 | 2.0402E+04 | 2.0226E+04 | 8.6899E−01 |
| 64.Gd | 2.2270E−03 | 2.2673E+04 | 2.3056E+04 | 2.2835E+04 | 9.6660E−01 |
| | 1.1577E−02 | 1.5193E+03 | 1.6102E+03 | 1.6890E+03 | 4.8942E+00 |
| 65.Tb | 1.4572E−03 | 4.4351E+04 | 4.4602E+04 | 4.4691E+04 | 1.9947E−01 |
| | 2.2375E−03 | 2.4465E+04 | 2.4908E+04 | 2.4652E+04 | 1.0370E+00 |
| | 1.0772E−02 | 1.8542E+03 | 1.9529E+03 | 2.0832E+03 | 6.6749E+00 |

| Material | $E$, MeV | $\mu_{1en}$, cm$^{-1}$ | $\mu_1$, cm$^{-1}$ | $\mu_2$, cm$^{-1}$ | $R$, % |
|---|---|---|---|---|---|
| 66.Dy | 1.4299E−03 | 4.7047E+04 | 4.7298E+04 | 4.7456E+04 | 3.3370E−01 |
| | 2.2438E−03 | 2.5548E+04 | 2.6026E+04 | 2.5769E+04 | 9.9623E−01 |
| | 9.9632E−03 | 2.2064E+03 | 2.3133E+03 | 2.5083E+03 | 8.4289E+00 |
| 67.Ho | 1.4269E−03 | 4.7349E+04 | 4.7600E+04 | 4.7821E+04 | 4.6328E−01 |
| | 2.2481E−03 | 2.6303E+04 | 2.6806E+04 | 2.6548E+04 | 9.6947E−01 |
| | 9.4335E−03 | 2.6532E+03 | 2.7693E+03 | 3.0669E+03 | 1.0745E+01 |
| 68.Er | 1.4543E−03 | 4.4630E+04 | 4.4881E+04 | 4.5122E+04 | 5.3658E−01 |
| | 2.2506E−03 | 2.7269E+04 | 2.7800E+04 | 2.7543E+04 | 9.3305E−01 |
| 69.Tm | 2.2514E−03 | 2.7567E+04 | 2.8105E+04 | 2.7869E+04 | 8.4686E−01 |
| | 9.7395E−03 | 2.3951E+03 | 2.5059E+03 | 2.8096E+03 | 1.2119E+01 |
| 70.Yb | 2.2181E−03 | 2.1136E+04 | 2.1468E+04 | 2.1388E+04 | 3.7530E−01 |
| | 1.1917E−02 | 1.3781E+03 | 1.4657E+03 | 1.6212E+03 | 1.0612E+01 |
| 71.Lu | 2.2555E−03 | 2.9111E+04 | 2.9694E+04 | 2.9490E+04 | 6.9236E−01 |
| 72.Hf | 1.6969E−03 | 3.2875E+04 | 3.3118E+04 | 3.3334E+04 | 6.5226E−01 |
| | 2.2833E−03 | 3.9695E+04 | 4.0577E+04 | 4.0258E+04 | 7.9157E−01 |
| 73.Ta | 1.7556E−03 | 3.0715E+04 | 3.0956E+04 | 3.1136E+04 | 5.7922E−01 |
| | 2.4191E−03 | 4.5005E+04 | 4.6052E+04 | 4.5685E+04 | 8.0445E−01 |
| | 2.4803E−03 | 4.4945E+04 | 4.6003E+04 | 4.5621E+04 | 8.3688E−01 |
| 74.W | 1.8180E−03 | 2.8425E+04 | 2.8664E+04 | 2.8799E+04 | 4.7251E−01 |
| 75.Re | 1.8846E−03 | 2.5975E+04 | 2.6211E+04 | 2.6311E+04 | 3.8293E−01 |
| | 2.7831E−03 | 4.6547E+04 | 4.7609E+04 | 4.7325E+04 | 5.9993E−01 |
| | 3.6848E−03 | 2.6911E+04 | 2.7481E+04 | 2.7378E+04 | 3.7747E−01 |
| | 1.7479E−02 | 1.8853E+03 | 2.3498E+03 | 2.2386E+03 | 4.9698E+00 |
| 76.Os | 1.7059E−03 | 3.2541E+04 | 3.2784E+04 | 3.2789E+04 | 1.5454E−02 |
| | 1.0770E−02 | 1.8552E+03 | 1.9539E+03 | 1.9611E+03 | 3.6789E−01 |
| 90.Th | 2.1739E−03 | 1.8181E+04 | 1.8401E+04 | 1.8329E+04 | 3.9349E−01 |
| | 1.1649E−02 | 1.4896E+03 | 1.5798E+03 | 1.5641E+03 | 1.0025E+00 |
| 91.Pa | 2.2353E−03 | 2.4095E+04 | 2.4525E+04 | 2.4289E+04 | 9.7125E−01 |
| | 2.7908E−02 | 6.2249E+02 | 7.3907E+02 | 8.3571E+02 | 1.3076E+01 |
| 92.U | 2.2572E−03 | 2.9763E+04 | 3.0364E+04 | 3.0002E+04 | 1.2081E+00 |
| 121. | 2.1596E−03 | 1.8472E+04 | 1.8694E+04 | 1.8604E+04 | 4.8463E−01 |
| **80.MERCURY** | | | | | |
| 26.Fe | 1.3487E−03 | 4.0168E+04 | 4.0345E+04 | 4.0307E+04 | 9.2124E−02 |
| 27.Co | 1.9835E−03 | 1.6322E+04 | 1.6485E+04 | 1.6395E+04 | 5.4769E−01 |
| | 2.0320E−03 | 1.5431E+04 | 1.5593E+04 | 1.5501E+04 | 5.8942E−01 |
| 28.Ni | 2.3054E−03 | 1.4523E+04 | 1.4767E+04 | 1.4599E+04 | 1.1558E+00 |
| | 1.1891E−02 | 1.0367E+03 | 1.0999E+03 | 1.3954E+03 | 2.6863E+01 |
| 29.Cu | 2.3116E−03 | 1.5286E+04 | 1.5558E+04 | 1.5376E+04 | 1.1821E+00 |
| | 1.2001E−02 | 1.0050E+03 | 1.0674E+03 | 1.4257E+03 | 3.3568E+01 |

| Material | $E$, MeV | $\mu_{1en}$, cm$^{-1}$ | $\mu_1$, cm$^{-1}$ | $\mu_2$, cm$^{-1}$ | $R$, % |
|---|---|---|---|---|---|
| 30.Zn | 1.0839E−03 | 5.9230E+04 | 5.9406E+04 | 5.9735E+04 | 5.5446E−01 |
| | 2.2975E−03 | 1.3570E+04 | 1.3780E+04 | 1.3664E+04 | 8.5074E−01 |
| 31.Ga | 1.4540E−03 | 3.2591E+04 | 3.2767E+04 | 3.2877E+04 | 3.3547E−01 |
| | 1.6517E−03 | 2.5216E+04 | 2.5388E+04 | 2.5427E+04 | 1.5301E−01 |
| | 2.2538E−03 | 1.2312E+04 | 1.2467E+04 | 1.2407E+04 | 4.7949E−01 |
| 33.As | 1.4918E−03 | 2.9873E+04 | 3.0049E+04 | 3.0239E+04 | 6.3175E−01 |
| | 1.5140E−03 | 2.8907E+04 | 2.9083E+04 | 2.9256E+04 | 5.9533E−01 |
| | 2.2966E−03 | 1.3462E+04 | 1.3669E+04 | 1.3596E+04 | 5.3628E−01 |
| 40.Zr | 2.2980E−03 | 1.3627E+04 | 1.3839E+04 | 1.3951E+04 | 8.0516E−01 |
| | 2.3356E−03 | 1.8205E+04 | 1.8581E+04 | 1.8678E+04 | 5.1811E−01 |
| 44.Ru | 1.3902E−03 | 3.7186E+04 | 3.7362E+04 | 3.7278E+04 | 2.2487E−01 |
| 45.Rh | 1.7251E−03 | 2.3249E+04 | 2.3419E+04 | 2.3336E+04 | 3.5644E−01 |
| | 2.1995E−03 | 1.3075E+04 | 1.3231E+04 | 1.3159E+04 | 5.4742E−01 |
| 46.Pd | 1.8943E−03 | 1.8714E+04 | 1.8880E+04 | 1.8801E+04 | 4.1904E−01 |
| | 2.1029E−03 | 1.4433E+04 | 1.4593E+04 | 1.4517E+04 | 5.2449E−01 |
| 47.Ag | 1.4959E−03 | 2.9577E+04 | 2.9753E+04 | 2.9661E+04 | 3.1009E−01 |
| | 2.2635E−03 | 1.2176E+04 | 1.2331E+04 | 1.2256E+04 | 6.1057E−01 |
| 57.La | 2.1699E−03 | 1.3492E+04 | 1.3649E+04 | 1.3556E+04 | 6.8523E−01 |
| 58.Ce | 1.3251E−03 | 4.1868E+04 | 4.2044E+04 | 4.2015E+04 | 7.0307E−02 |
| | 2.3013E−03 | 1.4031E+04 | 1.4258E+04 | 1.4103E+04 | 1.0993E+00 |
| 59.Pr | 1.0763E−03 | 5.9780E+04 | 5.9956E+04 | 6.0008E+04 | 8.6789E−02 |
| | 2.3087E−03 | 1.4929E+04 | 1.5189E+04 | 1.5008E+04 | 1.2013E+00 |
| | 1.1895E−02 | 1.0355E+03 | 1.0987E+03 | 1.1137E+03 | 1.3682E+00 |
| 60.Nd | 2.3165E−03 | 1.5875E+04 | 1.6168E+04 | 1.5960E+04 | 1.2990E+00 |
| | 1.1175E−02 | 1.2413E+03 | 1.3098E+03 | 1.3426E+03 | 2.5007E+00 |
| 61.Pm | 1.1849E−03 | 5.1959E+04 | 5.2136E+04 | 5.2220E+04 | 1.6161E−01 |
| | 2.3292E−03 | 1.7418E+04 | 1.7766E+04 | 1.7524E+04 | 1.3812E+00 |
| | 7.9561E−03 | 2.8638E+03 | 2.9666E+03 | 3.1630E+03 | 6.6191E+00 |
| 62.Sm | 1.2169E−03 | 4.9657E+04 | 4.9833E+04 | 4.9929E+04 | 1.9281E−01 |
| | 2.3366E−03 | 1.8322E+04 | 1.8703E+04 | 1.8436E+04 | 1.4441E+00 |
| | 7.7398E−03 | 3.1871E+03 | 3.2958E+03 | 3.5604E+03 | 8.0295E+00 |
| 63.Eu | 1.4988E−03 | 2.9368E+04 | 2.9544E+04 | 2.9547E+04 | 9.3543E−03 |
| | 1.5022E−03 | 2.9223E+04 | 2.9399E+04 | 2.9401E+04 | 5.6669E−03 |
| | 1.6406E−03 | 2.5513E+04 | 2.5686E+04 | 2.5666E+04 | 7.6722E−02 |
| | 2.3003E−03 | 1.3912E+04 | 1.4135E+04 | 1.4002E+04 | 9.4401E−01 |
| 64.Gd | 1.3710E−03 | 3.8565E+04 | 3.8741E+04 | 3.8826E+04 | 2.1823E−01 |
| | 2.3488E−03 | 2.0693E+04 | 2.1145E+04 | 2.0845E+04 | 1.4406E+00 |
| | 7.9402E−03 | 2.8875E+03 | 2.9907E+03 | 3.2686E+03 | 9.2914E+00 |
| | 8.2440E−03 | 2.6491E+03 | 2.7478E+03 | 2.9894E+03 | 8.7947E+00 |

| Material | $E$, MeV | $\mu_{1en}$, cm$^{-1}$ | $\mu_1$, cm$^{-1}$ | $\mu_2$, cm$^{-1}$ | $R$, % |
|---|---|---|---|---|---|
| 65.Tb | 2.3566E−03 | 2.2368E+04 | 2.2868E+04 | 2.2541E+04 | 1.4527E+00 |
| 66.Dy | 2.3615E−03 | 2.3422E+04 | 2.3953E+04 | 2.3628E+04 | 1.3769E+00 |
| 67.Ho | 1.3879E−03 | 3.7353E+04 | 3.7529E+04 | 3.7709E+04 | 4.7915E−01 |
| | 2.3651E−03 | 2.4194E+04 | 2.4747E+04 | 2.4422E+04 | 1.3321E+00 |
| 68.Er | 1.4418E−03 | 3.3473E+04 | 3.3649E+04 | 3.3824E+04 | 5.1974E−01 |
| | 2.3694E−03 | 2.5117E+04 | 2.5697E+04 | 2.5370E+04 | 1.2889E+00 |
| 69.Tm | 1.4892E−03 | 3.0060E+04 | 3.0237E+04 | 3.0396E+04 | 5.2585E−01 |
| | 2.3733E−03 | 2.5965E+04 | 2.6570E+04 | 2.6242E+04 | 1.2477E+00 |
| 70.Yb | 2.3396E−03 | 1.8710E+04 | 1.9105E+04 | 1.8933E+04 | 9.0751E−01 |
| 71.Lu | 1.6222E−03 | 2.6006E+04 | 2.6179E+04 | 2.6347E+04 | 6.4030E−01 |
| | 2.3796E−03 | 2.7331E+04 | 2.7975E+04 | 2.7683E+04 | 1.0544E+00 |
| 72.Hf | 1.6761E−03 | 2.4562E+04 | 2.4733E+04 | 2.4866E+04 | 5.3969E−01 |
| | 2.7884E−03 | 2.8073E+04 | 2.8767E+04 | 2.8450E+04 | 1.1152E+00 |
| | 1.4497E−02 | 1.6766E+03 | 2.2671E+03 | 1.9630E+03 | 1.5495E+01 |
| 73.Ta | 3.8667E−03 | 1.7115E+04 | 1.7500E+04 | 1.7388E+04 | 6.4725E−01 |
| | 2.7620E−02 | 4.6321E+02 | 5.5531E+02 | 5.2849E+02 | 5.0761E+00 |
| 85.At | 2.2488E−03 | 1.2382E+04 | 1.2536E+04 | 1.2506E+04 | 2.3966E−01 |
| | 1.1828E−02 | 1.0546E+03 | 1.1182E+03 | 1.1109E+03 | 6.6171E−01 |
| 87.Fr | 2.0801E−03 | 1.4754E+04 | 1.4914E+04 | 1.4882E+04 | 2.1358E−01 |
| | 1.1116E−02 | 1.2582E+03 | 1.3271E+03 | 1.3199E+03 | 5.4782E−01 |
| 89.Ac | 1.4163E−03 | 3.5303E+04 | 3.5479E+04 | 3.5437E+04 | 1.1737E−01 |
| | 2.3005E−03 | 1.3934E+04 | 1.4157E+04 | 1.4059E+04 | 7.0045E−01 |
| | 8.5808E−03 | 2.4435E+03 | 2.5381E+03 | 2.5399E+03 | 7.2297E−02 |
| | 5.8211E−02 | 5.8468E+01 | 7.0292E+01 | 7.1692E+01 | 1.9913E+00 |
| 90.Th | 2.3210E−03 | 1.6419E+04 | 1.6732E+04 | 1.6564E+04 | 1.0119E+00 |
| | 4.4177E−03 | 1.2895E+04 | 1.3190E+04 | 1.3353E+04 | 1.2368E+00 |
| | 4.4411E−03 | 1.2743E+04 | 1.3035E+04 | 1.3195E+04 | 1.2298E+00 |
| | 2.4683E−02 | 6.3178E+02 | 7.6546E+02 | 8.6736E+02 | 1.3311E+01 |
| 91.Pa | 2.3554E−03 | 2.2108E+04 | 2.2601E+04 | 2.2299E+04 | 1.3529E+00 |
| 92.U | 2.3792E−03 | 2.7233E+04 | 2.7875E+04 | 2.7468E+04 | 1.4808E+00 |
| 121. | 1.4573E−03 | 3.2357E+04 | 3.2533E+04 | 3.2573E+04 | 1.2174E−01 |
| | 2.3152E−03 | 1.5717E+04 | 1.6004E+04 | 1.5831E+04 | 1.0950E+00 |
| | 1.0566E−02 | 1.4155E+03 | 1.4886E+03 | 1.5742E+03 | 5.7560E+00 |
| 81.THALLIUM | | | | | |
| 25.Mn | 1.1310E−03 | 5.0101E+04 | 5.0250E+04 | 5.0250E+04 | 4.6642E−05 |
| 26.Fe | 1.5914E−03 | 2.4133E+04 | 2.4274E+04 | 2.4213E+04 | 2.5285E−01 |
| 27.Co | 1.1818E−02 | 9.6793E+02 | 1.0244E+03 | 1.2435E+03 | 2.1390E+01 |
| 28.Ni | 2.3932E−03 | 1.3479E+04 | 1.3740E+04 | 1.3552E+04 | 1.3890E+00 |
| | 1.0711E−02 | 1.2364E+03 | 1.2998E+03 | 1.6856E+03 | 2.9682E+01 |

| Material | $E$, MeV | $\mu_{1en}$, cm$^{-1}$ | $\mu_1$, cm$^{-1}$ | $\mu_2$, cm$^{-1}$ | $R$, % |
|---|---|---|---|---|---|
| 29.Cu | 2.3998E−03 | 1.4181E+04 | 1.4466E+04 | 1.4267E+04 | 1.3988E+00 |
| | 1.0985E−02 | 1.1699E+03 | 1.2316E+03 | 1.6841E+03 | 3.6739E+01 |
| 33.As | 1.3912E−03 | 3.3340E+04 | 3.3483E+04 | 3.3767E+04 | 8.4791E−01 |
| 34.Se | 2.1648E−03 | 1.2327E+04 | 1.2464E+04 | 1.2471E+04 | 6.0426E−02 |
| 40.Zr | 2.4230E−03 | 1.6654E+04 | 1.7025E+04 | 1.7080E+04 | 3.2214E−01 |
| 41.Nb | 2.4254E−03 | 1.6913E+04 | 1.7293E+04 | 1.7362E+04 | 3.9484E−01 |
| | 2.4743E−03 | 2.2247E+04 | 2.2797E+04 | 2.2883E+04 | 3.7723E−01 |
| 43.Tc | 1.2784E−03 | 4.0611E+04 | 4.0757E+04 | 4.0697E+04 | 1.4802E−01 |
| | 2.8551E−03 | 2.3546E+04 | 2.4153E+04 | 2.4323E+04 | 7.0511E−01 |
| | 3.3452E−03 | 1.9358E+04 | 1.9833E+04 | 1.9959E+04 | 6.3688E−01 |
| 44.Ru | 1.8719E−03 | 1.7374E+04 | 1.7515E+04 | 1.7461E+04 | 3.0794E−01 |
| | 2.2073E−03 | 1.1822E+04 | 1.1957E+04 | 1.1905E+04 | 4.4067E−01 |
| | 2.9858E−03 | 2.5310E+04 | 2.5946E+04 | 2.6246E+04 | 1.1550E+00 |
| | 3.7415E−03 | 1.6284E+04 | 1.6662E+04 | 1.6809E+04 | 8.8465E−01 |
| 45.Rh | 4.5171E−03 | 1.0889E+04 | 1.1143E+04 | 1.1240E+04 | 8.7012E−01 |
| | 1.2042E−02 | 9.1362E+02 | 9.6863E+02 | 9.5145E+02 | 1.8053E+00 |
| 46.Pd | 4.8698E−03 | 8.8422E+03 | 9.0547E+03 | 9.1469E+03 | 1.0178E+00 |
| 46.Pd | 1.1759E−02 | 9.8210E+02 | 1.0389E+03 | 1.0219E+03 | 1.6648E+00 |
| 47.Ag | 1.2510E−02 | 8.0010E+02 | 8.5214E+02 | 8.3460E+02 | 2.1014E+00 |
| 48.Cd | 1.4118E−03 | 3.2014E+04 | 3.2156E+04 | 3.2093E+04 | 1.9734E−01 |
| 50.Sn | 1.1503E−03 | 4.8862E+04 | 4.9011E+04 | 4.8948E+04 | 1.2789E−01 |
| 58.Ce | 1.0945E−03 | 5.2456E+04 | 5.2606E+04 | 5.2633E+04 | 5.2513E−02 |
| | 2.3894E−03 | 1.3082E+04 | 1.3328E+04 | 1.3152E+04 | 1.3446E+00 |
| | 1.1569E−02 | 1.0282E+03 | 1.0862E+03 | 1.1003E+03 | 1.2919E+00 |
| 59.Pr | 1.2118E−03 | 4.4897E+04 | 4.5044E+04 | 4.5069E+04 | 5.5093E−02 |
| | 2.3972E−03 | 1.3910E+04 | 1.4185E+04 | 1.3986E+04 | 1.4218E+00 |
| | 1.0511E−02 | 1.2848E+03 | 1.3496E+03 | 1.3829E+03 | 2.4674E+00 |
| 60.Nd | 2.4054E−03 | 1.4782E+04 | 1.5088E+04 | 1.4865E+04 | 1.5014E+00 |
| | 7.7852E−03 | 2.7829E+03 | 2.8786E+03 | 3.0545E+03 | 6.1113E+00 |
| 61.Pm | 1.1016E−03 | 5.1997E+04 | 5.2147E+04 | 5.2262E+04 | 2.1982E−01 |
| | 2.4187E−03 | 1.6203E+04 | 1.6558E+04 | 1.6305E+04 | 1.5557E+00 |
| 62.Sm | 1.1224E−03 | 5.0659E+04 | 5.0808E+04 | 5.0941E+04 | 2.6045E−01 |
| | 2.4265E−03 | 1.7035E+04 | 1.7419E+04 | 1.7143E+04 | 1.6062E+00 |
| 63.Eu | 1.2006E−02 | 9.2226E+02 | 9.7749E+02 | 1.0165E+03 | 3.9924E+00 |
| 64.Gd | 1.3167E−03 | 3.8145E+04 | 3.8289E+04 | 3.8405E+04 | 3.0233E−01 |
| | 2.4458E−03 | 1.9117E+04 | 1.9570E+04 | 1.9260E+04 | 1.6085E+00 |
| 65.Tb | 1.2748E−03 | 4.0843E+04 | 4.0989E+04 | 4.1163E+04 | 4.2369E−01 |
| | 2.4590E−03 | 2.0566E+04 | 2.1063E+04 | 2.0727E+04 | 1.6234E+00 |
| 66.Dy | 1.3282E−03 | 3.7403E+04 | 3.7548E+04 | 3.7728E+04 | 4.8065E−01 |

| Material | $E$, MeV | $\mu_{1en}$, cm$^{-1}$ | $\mu_1$, cm$^{-1}$ | $\mu_2$, cm$^{-1}$ | $R$, % |
|---|---|---|---|---|---|
| | 2.4676E−03 | 2.1506E+04 | 2.2033E+04 | 2.1698E+04 | 1.5452E+00 |
| 67.Ho | 1.3819E−03 | 3.3940E+04 | 3.4084E+04 | 3.4260E+04 | 5.1767E−01 |
| | 2.4742E−03 | 2.2228E+04 | 2.2777E+04 | 2.2440E+04 | 1.5036E+00 |
| | 8.7574E−03 | 2.0852E+03 | 2.1670E+03 | 2.3474E+03 | 8.3239E+00 |
| 68.Er | 1.4355E−03 | 3.0492E+04 | 3.0634E+04 | 3.0807E+04 | 5.6388E−01 |
| | 2.4819E−03 | 2.3078E+04 | 2.3653E+04 | 2.3312E+04 | 1.4642E+00 |
| | 1.3509E−02 | 1.3558E+03 | 1.7607E+03 | 1.5497E+03 | 1.3615E+01 |
| 69.Tm | 1.4844E−03 | 2.7337E+04 | 2.7478E+04 | 2.7635E+04 | 5.7197E−01 |
| | 1.4270E−02 | 1.1868E+03 | 1.4932E+03 | 1.3585E+03 | 9.9176E+00 |
| 70.Yb | 1.5711E−03 | 2.4621E+04 | 2.4762E+04 | 2.4931E+04 | 6.8309E−01 |
| | 2.4352E−03 | 1.7957E+04 | 1.8373E+04 | 1.8167E+04 | 1.1333E+00 |
| 71.Lu | 1.6164E−03 | 2.3529E+04 | 2.3670E+04 | 2.3832E+04 | 6.8579E−01 |
| 72.Hf | 1.6691E−03 | 2.2260E+04 | 2.2400E+04 | 2.2520E+04 | 5.3397E−01 |
| | 3.3751E−03 | 1.8868E+04 | 1.9330E+04 | 1.9128E+04 | 1.0552E+00 |
| 82.Pb | 2.8918E−03 | 2.3127E+04 | 2.3717E+04 | 2.3764E+04 | 1.9931E−01 |
| | 3.3707E−03 | 1.8940E+04 | 1.9405E+04 | 1.9451E+04 | 2.3784E−01 |
| | 5.1678E−03 | 7.5947E+03 | 7.7822E+03 | 7.7887E+03 | 8.4290E−02 |
| | 1.3413E−02 | 1.3821E+03 | 1.7858E+03 | 1.7296E+03 | 3.2508E+00 |
| | 4.1399E−02 | 1.2892E+02 | 1.5232E+02 | 1.5295E+02 | 4.1384E−01 |
| 84.Po | 2.8181E−03 | 2.3969E+04 | 2.4591E+04 | 2.4751E+04 | 6.5104E−01 |
| 84.Po | 1.2570E−02 | 7.8541E+02 | 8.3706E+02 | 8.3168E+02 | 6.4735E−01 |
| 85.At | 1.2060E−03 | 4.5270E+04 | 4.5417E+04 | 4.5410E+04 | 1.6585E−02 |
| | 6.8488E−03 | 4.0268E+03 | 4.1461E+03 | 4.1539E+03 | 1.8956E−01 |
| | 4.9734E−02 | 7.7961E+01 | 9.2746E+01 | 9.3874E+01 | 1.2161E+00 |
| 87.Fr | 1.0671E−03 | 5.4220E+04 | 5.4371E+04 | 5.4360E+04 | 1.9840E−02 |
| | 1.2768E−03 | 4.0714E+04 | 4.0860E+04 | 4.0850E+04 | 2.3112E−02 |
| | 4.8897E−03 | 8.7269E+03 | 8.9370E+03 | 8.9934E+03 | 6.3164E−01 |
| | 3.7226E−02 | 1.7954E+02 | 2.1251E+02 | 2.2088E+02 | 3.9366E+00 |
| 89.Ac | 4.6669E−03 | 1.0019E+04 | 1.0256E+04 | 1.0359E+04 | 1.0113E+00 |
| | 2.6348E−02 | 4.7294E+02 | 5.7579E+02 | 6.3419E+02 | 1.0142E+01 |
| 90.Th | 2.4107E−03 | 1.5345E+04 | 1.5670E+04 | 1.5488E+04 | 1.1792E+00 |
| 91.Pa | 2.4577E−03 | 2.0416E+04 | 2.0909E+04 | 2.0604E+04 | 1.4771E+00 |
| | 1.4109E−02 | 1.2206E+03 | 1.5526E+03 | 1.2981E+03 | 1.9607E+01 |
| 121. | 1.4081E−03 | 3.2255E+04 | 3.2398E+04 | 3.2471E+04 | 2.2521E−01 |
| | 2.4001E−03 | 1.4213E+04 | 1.4499E+04 | 1.4318E+04 | 1.2663E+00 |
| 123. | 1.4668E−03 | 2.8473E+04 | 2.8614E+04 | 2.8774E+04 | 5.5900E−01 |
| 130. | 2.3695E−03 | 9.8926E+03 | 1.0024E+04 | 1.0039E+04 | 1.4195E−01 |
| 82.LEAD | | | | | |
| 25.Mn | 1.0949E−03 | 5.2839E+04 | 5.2985E+04 | 5.2997E+04 | 2.2611E−02 |

| Material | $E$, MeV | $\mu_{1en}$, $cm^{-1}$ | $\mu_1$, $cm^{-1}$ | $\mu_2$, $cm^{-1}$ | $R$, % |
|---|---|---|---|---|---|
| 26.Fe | 1.5205E−03 | 2.6107E+04 | 2.6243E+04 | 2.6192E+04 | 1.9369E−01 |
| 27.Co | 1.2176E−02 | 9.1080E+02 | 9.6483E+02 | 1.1656E+03 | 2.0805E+01 |
| 28.Ni | 1.0937E−02 | 1.1980E+03 | 1.2594E+03 | 1.6299E+03 | 2.9417E+01 |
| 29.Cu | 1.1230E−02 | 1.1301E+03 | 1.1897E+03 | 1.6217E+03 | 3.6309E+01 |
| 32.Ge | 1.9684E−03 | 1.5228E+04 | 1.5354E+04 | 1.5361E+04 | 4.9726E−02 |
| | 2.0714E−03 | 1.3649E+04 | 1.3774E+04 | 1.3766E+04 | 5.8555E−02 |
| 33.As | 1.4014E−03 | 3.2990E+04 | 3.3128E+04 | 3.3411E+04 | 8.5270E−01 |
| 34.Se | 2.2669E−03 | 1.1427E+04 | 1.1552E+04 | 1.1560E+04 | 6.6604E−02 |
| 40.Zr | 2.4864E−03 | 1.5678E+04 | 1.6037E+04 | 1.6068E+04 | 1.9251E−01 |
| 41.Nb | 2.5628E−03 | 2.0436E+04 | 2.0967E+04 | 2.1005E+04 | 1.8082E−01 |
| 42.Mo | 2.5376E−03 | 1.9246E+04 | 1.9749E+04 | 1.9798E+04 | 2.4706E−01 |
| 43.Tc | 1.2446E−03 | 4.3144E+04 | 4.3286E+04 | 4.3231E+04 | 1.2867E−01 |
| | 2.8454E−03 | 2.3733E+04 | 2.4391E+04 | 2.4517E+04 | 5.1873E−01 |
| | 3.2932E−03 | 1.9974E+04 | 2.0522E+04 | 2.0598E+04 | 3.7356E−01 |
| 44.Ru | 1.8155E−03 | 1.8942E+04 | 1.9071E+04 | 1.9029E+04 | 2.2161E−01 |
| | 2.3683E−03 | 1.0276E+04 | 1.0401E+04 | 1.0356E+04 | 4.3829E−01 |
| 45.Rh | 4.5613E−03 | 1.0618E+04 | 1.0882E+04 | 1.0959E+04 | 7.1004E−01 |
| | 1.2497E−02 | 8.3650E+02 | 8.8862E+02 | 8.7226E+02 | 1.8761E+00 |
| 46.Pd | 4.8819E−03 | 8.7673E+03 | 8.9877E+03 | 9.0687E+03 | 9.0059E−01 |
| | 1.2189E−02 | 9.0782E+02 | 9.6177E+02 | 9.4558E+02 | 1.7115E+00 |
| 47.Ag | 1.2987E−02 | 7.2284E+02 | 7.7204E+02 | 7.5511E+02 | 2.2421E+00 |
| 48.Cd | 1.3861E−03 | 3.3981E+04 | 3.4120E+04 | 3.4061E+04 | 1.7311E−01 |
| 50.Sn | 1.0875E−03 | 5.3318E+04 | 5.3463E+04 | 5.3408E+04 | 1.0421E−01 |
| 58.Ce | 1.0853E−03 | 5.3462E+04 | 5.3608E+04 | 5.3643E+04 | 6.6076E−02 |
| | 1.1946E−02 | 9.6423E+02 | 1.0196E+03 | 1.0317E+03 | 1.1817E+00 |
| 59.Pr | 1.2002E−03 | 4.6022E+04 | 4.6165E+04 | 4.6198E+04 | 7.2549E−02 |
| | 1.0744E−02 | 1.2428E+03 | 1.3053E+03 | 1.3375E+03 | 2.4630E+00 |
| 60.Nd | 7.8040E−03 | 2.7652E+03 | 2.8611E+03 | 3.0344E+03 | 6.0582E+00 |
| 61.Pm | 1.1080E−03 | 5.1994E+04 | 5.2140E+04 | 5.2259E+04 | 2.2860E−01 |
| 62.Sm | 1.1298E−03 | 5.0580E+04 | 5.0725E+04 | 5.0861E+04 | 2.6903E−01 |
| | 2.4923E−03 | 1.6094E+04 | 1.6470E+04 | 1.6199E+04 | 1.6743E+00 |
| 63.Eu | 1.2406E−02 | 8.5760E+02 | 9.1027E+02 | 9.4443E+02 | 3.7530E+00 |
| 64.Gd | 1.3213E−03 | 3.8180E+04 | 3.8320E+04 | 3.8441E+04 | 3.1430E−01 |
| | 2.5182E−03 | 1.7942E+04 | 1.8394E+04 | 1.8078E+04 | 1.7450E+00 |
| 65.Tb | 2.5366E−03 | 1.9200E+04 | 1.9702E+04 | 1.9352E+04 | 1.8077E+00 |
| 66.Dy | 1.3286E−03 | 3.7703E+04 | 3.7843E+04 | 3.8031E+04 | 4.9604E−01 |
| | 2.5529E−03 | 1.9966E+04 | 2.0486E+04 | 2.0146E+04 | 1.6881E+00 |
| 67.Ho | 1.3824E−03 | 3.4220E+04 | 3.4359E+04 | 3.4542E+04 | 5.3532E−01 |
| | 2.5658E−03 | 2.0577E+04 | 2.1111E+04 | 2.0774E+04 | 1.6205E+00 |

| Material | $E$, MeV | $\mu_{1en}$, cm$^{-1}$ | $\mu_1$, cm$^{-1}$ | $\mu_2$, cm$^{-1}$ | $R$, % |
|---|---|---|---|---|---|
| | 8.6451E−03 | 2.1535E+03 | 2.2366E+03 | 2.4269E+03 | 8.5055E+00 |
| 68.Er | 1.4360E−03 | 3.0749E+04 | 3.0887E+04 | 3.1067E+04 | 5.8380E−01 |
| | 2.5809E−03 | 2.1285E+04 | 2.1836E+04 | 2.1502E+04 | 1.5534E+00 |
| | 1.3449E−02 | 1.3741E+03 | 1.7190E+03 | 1.5715E+03 | 9.3876E+00 |
| 69.Tm | 1.4849E−03 | 2.7584E+04 | 2.7721E+04 | 2.7886E+04 | 5.9514E−01 |
| | 1.4202E−02 | 1.2085E+03 | 1.4995E+03 | 1.3846E+03 | 8.2986E+00 |
| 70.Yb | 1.5720E−03 | 2.4855E+04 | 2.4990E+04 | 2.5169E+04 | 7.1493E−01 |
| | 2.5060E−03 | 1.7073E+04 | 1.7489E+04 | 1.7273E+04 | 1.2475E+00 |
| 71.Lu | 1.6170E−03 | 2.3763E+04 | 2.3896E+04 | 2.4069E+04 | 7.2371E−01 |
| 72.Hf | 1.6698E−03 | 2.2480E+04 | 2.2613E+04 | 2.2745E+04 | 5.8459E−01 |
| | 3.3863E−03 | 1.8737E+04 | 1.9240E+04 | 1.8996E+04 | 1.2817E+00 |
| | 1.6260E−02 | 1.2857E+03 | 1.6821E+03 | 1.4885E+03 | 1.3005E+01 |
| 81.Tl | 2.8918E−03 | 2.3127E+04 | 2.3764E+04 | 2.3717E+04 | 1.9931E−01 |
| | 3.3707E−03 | 1.8940E+04 | 1.9451E+04 | 1.9405E+04 | 2.3784E−01 |
| | 5.1678E−03 | 7.5947E+03 | 7.7887E+03 | 7.7822E+03 | 8.4290E−02 |
| | 1.3413E−02 | 1.3821E+03 | 1.7296E+03 | 1.7858E+03 | 3.2508E+00 |
| | 4.1399E−02 | 1.2892E+02 | 1.5295E+02 | 1.5232E+02 | 4.1384E−01 |
| 84.Po | 2.8078E−03 | 2.4224E+04 | 2.4899E+04 | 2.5016E+04 | 4.7239E−01 |
| 85.At | 1.3228E−03 | 3.8083E+04 | 3.8224E+04 | 3.8223E+04 | 5.8251E−04 |
| | 3.4632E−03 | 1.7740E+04 | 1.8205E+04 | 1.8277E+04 | 3.9639E−01 |
| | 7.5435E−03 | 3.1109E+03 | 3.2136E+03 | 3.2168E+03 | 9.9773E−02 |
| | 5.3935E−02 | 6.4928E+01 | 7.7778E+01 | 7.8393E+01 | 7.9041E−01 |
| 87.Fr | 1.0594E−03 | 5.5139E+04 | 5.5285E+04 | 5.5279E+04 | 1.1221E−02 |
| | 1.3142E−03 | 3.8637E+04 | 3.8778E+04 | 3.8772E+04 | 1.3057E−02 |
| | 4.8865E−03 | 8.7409E+03 | 8.9606E+03 | 9.0079E+03 | 5.2700E−01 |
| | 3.6400E−02 | 1.9159E+02 | 2.2820E+02 | 2.3622E+02 | 3.5134E+00 |
| 89.Ac | 3.9686E−03 | 1.4130E+04 | 1.4478E+04 | 1.4631E+04 | 1.0548E+00 |
| | 4.0090E−03 | 1.3806E+04 | 1.4146E+04 | 1.4297E+04 | 1.0729E+00 |
| | 4.6574E−03 | 1.0064E+04 | 1.0315E+04 | 1.0406E+04 | 8.8389E−01 |
| | 2.4803E−02 | 5.4517E+02 | 6.7466E+02 | 7.4008E+02 | 9.6963E+00 |
| 90.Th | 1.9956E−02 | 7.8892E+02 | 9.8840E+02 | 1.1006E+03 | 1.1350E+01 |
| | 2.0118E−02 | 7.7721E+02 | 9.7270E+02 | 1.0828E+03 | 1.1321E+01 |
| 91.Pa | 2.5352E−03 | 1.9133E+04 | 1.9633E+04 | 1.9320E+04 | 1.6240E+00 |
| | 1.4038E−02 | 1.2447E+03 | 1.5474E+03 | 1.3229E+03 | 1.6972E+01 |
| 121. | 1.4126E−03 | 3.2264E+04 | 3.2402E+04 | 3.2480E+04 | 2.3942E−01 |
| 123. | 1.4786E−03 | 2.7988E+04 | 2.8125E+04 | 2.8283E+04 | 5.6030E−01 |
| | 1.5262E−03 | 2.5968E+04 | 2.6103E+04 | 2.6239E+04 | 5.1840E−01 |
| | 1.9769E−03 | 1.5020E+04 | 1.5145E+04 | 1.5160E+04 | 9.8209E−02 |
| | 2.0434E−03 | 1.3967E+04 | 1.4092E+04 | 1.4096E+04 | 2.8843E−02 |
| 130. | 2.3767E−03 | 1.0180E+04 | 1.0306E+04 | 1.0335E+04 | 2.8440E−01 |

| Material | $E$, MeV | $\mu_{1en}$, cm$^{-1}$ | $\mu_1$, cm$^{-1}$ | $\mu_2$, cm$^{-1}$ | $R$, % |
|---|---|---|---|---|---|
| 83.BISMUTH | | | | | |
| 24.Cr | 1.0156E−03 | 5.1996E+04 | 5.2132E+04 | 5.2116E+04 | 3.1331E−02 |
| 25.Mn | 1.3995E−03 | 2.9750E+04 | 2.9879E+04 | 2.9840E+04 | 1.3164E−01 |
| 26.Fe | 1.9559E−03 | 1.3985E+04 | 1.4103E+04 | 1.4036E+04 | 4.7811E−01 |
| | 2.2098E−03 | 1.0994E+04 | 1.1109E+04 | 1.1039E+04 | 6.3448E−01 |
| | 1.3189E−02 | 6.3627E+02 | 6.7915E+02 | 7.7314E+02 | 1.3840E+01 |
| 27.Co | 1.0201E−02 | 1.2256E+03 | 1.2849E+03 | 1.5949E+03 | 2.4123E+01 |
| 28.Ni | 9.1166E−03 | 1.6944E+03 | 1.7639E+03 | 2.4284E+03 | 3.7677E+01 |
| 29.Cu | 9.6561E−03 | 1.4323E+03 | 1.4962E+03 | 2.1231E+03 | 4.1896E+01 |
| 30.Zn | 1.2794E−02 | 7.1422E+02 | 7.5927E+02 | 1.0571E+03 | 3.9227E+01 |
| 31.Ga | 1.1788E−03 | 4.2537E+04 | 4.2670E+04 | 4.2954E+04 | 6.6485E−01 |
| 32.Ge | 1.3762E−03 | 3.1104E+04 | 3.1233E+04 | 3.1441E+04 | 6.6781E−01 |
| 42.Mo | 2.6241E−03 | 1.7424E+04 | 1.7913E+04 | 1.7905E+04 | 4.2586E−02 |
| 43.Tc | 1.5212E−03 | 2.3466E+04 | 2.3592E+04 | 2.3546E+04 | 1.9451E−01 |
| | 3.9560E−03 | 1.2125E+04 | 1.2450E+04 | 1.2455E+04 | 3.6535E−02 |
| 44.Ru | 6.4981E−03 | 4.0127E+03 | 4.1309E+03 | 4.1229E+03 | 1.9483E−01 |
| | 1.2347E−02 | 8.0236E+02 | 8.4988E+02 | 8.3579E+02 | 1.6856E+00 |
| | 5.2246E−02 | 6.2392E+01 | 7.4782E+01 | 8.9709E+01 | 1.9960E+01 |
| 45.Rh | 9.8484E−03 | 1.3388E+03 | 1.4008E+03 | 1.3879E+03 | 9.3260E−01 |
| | 1.0200E−02 | 1.2257E+03 | 1.2850E+03 | 1.2719E+03 | 1.0288E+00 |
| | 4.6218E−02 | 8.8713E+01 | 1.0589E+02 | 1.3766E+02 | 2.9996E+01 |
| 46.Pd | 4.7866E−02 | 7.9802E+01 | 9.5336E+01 | 1.2507E+02 | 3.1193E+01 |
| 47.Ag | 7.3199E−03 | 3.0410E+03 | 3.1388E+03 | 3.1455E+03 | 2.1398E−01 |
| | 1.1664E−02 | 9.3699E+02 | 9.8826E+02 | 9.7543E+02 | 1.3155E+00 |
| 48.Cd | 1.8989E−03 | 1.5227E+04 | 1.5346E+04 | 1.5291E+04 | 3.5897E−01 |
| | 2.2114E−03 | 1.0978E+04 | 1.1092E+04 | 1.1038E+04 | 4.9529E−01 |
| 49.In | 1.3937E−03 | 3.0089E+04 | 3.0218E+04 | 3.0159E+04 | 1.9341E−01 |
| 50.Sn | 1.5491E−03 | 2.2857E+04 | 2.2983E+04 | 2.2922E+04 | 2.6473E−01 |
| 50.Sn | 2.4556E−03 | 8.6181E+03 | 8.7289E+03 | 8.6719E+03 | 6.5749E−01 |
| 51.Sb | 1.4371E−03 | 2.7572E+04 | 2.7700E+04 | 2.7642E+04 | 2.0859E−01 |
| | 2.5629E−03 | 7.5811E+03 | 7.6905E+03 | 7.6297E+03 | 7.9636E−01 |
| 52.Te | 1.2580E−03 | 3.7947E+04 | 3.8078E+04 | 3.8028E+04 | 1.3329E−01 |
| 57.La | 1.0524E−03 | 4.9860E+04 | 4.9996E+04 | 5.0004E+04 | 1.6830E−02 |
| | 1.2697E−02 | 7.3340E+02 | 7.7900E+02 | 7.8103E+02 | 2.6121E−01 |
| 58.Ce | 7.6476E−03 | 2.6536E+03 | 2.7433E+03 | 2.8751E+03 | 4.8069E+00 |
| 59.Pr | 7.0547E−03 | 3.3546E+03 | 3.4590E+03 | 3.6772E+03 | 6.3067E+00 |
| 61.Pm | 7.3093E−03 | 3.0536E+03 | 3.1517E+03 | 3.4033E+03 | 7.9853E+00 |
| 63.Eu | 1.4200E−03 | 2.8564E+04 | 2.8692E+04 | 2.8736E+04 | 1.5334E−01 |
| | 1.0519E−02 | 1.1628E+03 | 1.2204E+03 | 1.2848E+03 | 5.2740E+00 |

| Material | $E$, MeV | $\mu_{1en}$, cm$^{-1}$ | $\mu_1$, cm$^{-1}$ | $\mu_2$, cm$^{-1}$ | $R$, % |
|---|---|---|---|---|---|
| 64.Gd | 1.2619E−03 | 3.7721E+04 | 3.7852E+04 | 3.7982E+04 | 3.4172E−01 |
| | 2.5821E−03 | 1.6903E+04 | 1.7354E+04 | 1.7034E+04 | 1.8758E+00 |
| 65.Tb | 1.2698E−03 | 3.7265E+04 | 3.7396E+04 | 3.7555E+04 | 4.2689E−01 |
| | 2.6320E−03 | 1.7521E+04 | 1.8018E+04 | 1.7663E+04 | 2.0097E+00 |
| | 7.8162E−03 | 2.4543E+03 | 2.5398E+03 | 2.7416E+03 | 7.9458E+00 |
| 66.Dy | 1.3232E−03 | 3.4172E+04 | 3.4303E+04 | 3.4468E+04 | 4.8335E−01 |
| | 2.6860E−03 | 1.7563E+04 | 1.8051E+04 | 1.7725E+04 | 1.8374E+00 |
| | 1.3679E−02 | 1.1550E+03 | 1.4564E+03 | 1.2948E+03 | 1.2480E+01 |
| 67.Ho | 1.3769E−03 | 3.1060E+04 | 3.1189E+04 | 3.1349E+04 | 5.1361E−01 |
| | 1.4321E−02 | 1.0369E+03 | 1.2980E+03 | 1.1654E+03 | 1.1383E+01 |
| 68.Er | 1.4301E−03 | 2.7979E+04 | 2.8107E+04 | 2.8263E+04 | 5.5487E−01 |
| | 1.4855E−02 | 9.3872E+02 | 1.1663E+03 | 1.0558E+03 | 1.0471E+01 |
| | 1.5406E−02 | 8.5578E+02 | 1.0566E+03 | 9.5957E+02 | 1.0112E+01 |
| 69.Tm | 1.4805E−03 | 2.5060E+04 | 2.5187E+04 | 2.5327E+04 | 5.5673E−01 |
| | 5.9446E−02 | 4.3555E+01 | 5.2704E+01 | 1.1366E+02 | 1.1567E+02 |
| 70.Yb | 1.5632E−03 | 2.2551E+04 | 2.2677E+04 | 2.2830E+04 | 6.7752E−01 |
| 71.Lu | 1.6106E−03 | 2.1516E+04 | 2.1641E+04 | 2.1786E+04 | 6.6927E−01 |
| 72.Hf | 1.6634E−03 | 2.0365E+04 | 2.0489E+04 | 2.0589E+04 | 4.8831E−01 |
| | 3.9543E−03 | 1.2137E+04 | 1.2464E+04 | 1.2328E+04 | 1.0991E+00 |
| | 2.7365E−02 | 3.6919E+02 | 4.5619E+02 | 4.1915E+02 | 8.8378E+00 |
| 84.Po | 3.3542E−03 | 1.7113E+04 | 1.7604E+04 | 1.7617E+04 | 7.4146E−02 |
| | 3.5232E−03 | 1.5190E+04 | 1.5620E+04 | 1.5635E+04 | 9.4218E−02 |
| | 3.6089E−03 | 1.4319E+04 | 1.4715E+04 | 1.4735E+04 | 1.3458E−01 |
| | 5.4190E−03 | 6.1108E+03 | 6.2754E+03 | 6.2804E+03 | 7.9162E−02 |
| | 4.6219E−02 | 8.8705E+01 | 1.0588E+02 | 1.0630E+02 | 3.9734E−01 |
| 85.At | 2.7981E−03 | 2.2629E+04 | 2.3305E+04 | 2.3357E+04 | 2.2548E−01 |
| 87.Fr | 3.6263E−03 | 1.4143E+04 | 1.4532E+04 | 1.4615E+04 | 5.7104E−01 |
| | 4.2684E−03 | 1.0939E+04 | 1.1225E+04 | 1.1283E+04 | 5.1908E−01 |
| 91.Pa | 2.6323E−03 | 1.7526E+04 | 1.8022E+04 | 1.7710E+04 | 1.7626E+00 |
| 121. | 1.3581E−03 | 3.2151E+04 | 3.2280E+04 | 3.2367E+04 | 2.6729E−01 |
| | 8.3387E−03 | 2.0724E+03 | 2.1498E+03 | 2.3308E+03 | 8.4176E+00 |
| 125. | 2.5034E−03 | 8.1555E+03 | 8.2657E+03 | 8.3513E+03 | 1.0359E+00 |
| 130. | 2.3606E−03 | 9.5365E+03 | 9.6486E+03 | 9.6712E+03 | 2.3427E−01 |

84.POLONIUM

| Material | $E$, MeV | $\mu_{1en}$, cm$^{-1}$ | $\mu_1$, cm$^{-1}$ | $\mu_2$, cm$^{-1}$ | $R$, % |
|---|---|---|---|---|---|
| 25.Mn | 1.3860E−03 | 3.0779E+04 | 3.0902E+04 | 3.0871E+04 | 1.0000E−01 |
| 26.Fe | 1.9325E−03 | 1.4635E+04 | 1.4748E+04 | 1.4688E+04 | 4.1219E−01 |
| | 2.4927E−03 | 8.6182E+03 | 8.7253E+03 | 8.6580E+03 | 7.7686E−01 |
| 27.Co | 1.0435E−02 | 1.1883E+03 | 1.2457E+03 | 1.5440E+03 | 2.3949E+01 |
| 28.Ni | 9.1676E−03 | 1.6749E+03 | 1.7439E+03 | 2.3957E+03 | 3.7377E+01 |

| Material | $E$, MeV | $\mu_{1en}$, cm$^{-1}$ | $\mu_1$, cm$^{-1}$ | $\mu_2$, cm$^{-1}$ | $R$, % |
|---|---|---|---|---|---|
| 29.Cu | 9.6838E−03 | 1.4240E+03 | 1.4872E+03 | 2.1079E+03 | 4.1736E+01 |
| 30.Zn | 1.3261E−02 | 6.5515E+02 | 6.9783E+02 | 9.5596E+02 | 3.6991E+01 |
| 31.Ga | 1.1864E−03 | 4.2382E+04 | 4.2509E+04 | 4.2795E+04 | 6.7443E−01 |
| 32.Ge | 1.4018E−03 | 2.9858E+04 | 2.9981E+04 | 3.0180E+04 | 6.6317E−01 |
| 42.Mo | 2.9339E−03 | 2.1110E+04 | 2.1780E+04 | 2.1718E+04 | 2.8797E−01 |
| 43.Tc | 1.4899E−03 | 2.4735E+04 | 2.4856E+04 | 2.4815E+04 | 1.6367E−01 |
| | 3.9595E−03 | 1.2083E+04 | 1.2417E+04 | 1.2412E+04 | 4.3982E−02 |
| | 4.1137E−03 | 1.1029E+04 | 1.1334E+04 | 1.1323E+04 | 9.8564E−02 |
| 44.Ru | 6.4178E−03 | 4.1122E+03 | 4.2347E+03 | 4.2248E+03 | 2.3503E−01 |
| | 1.3172E−02 | 6.7198E+02 | 7.1512E+02 | 7.0215E+02 | 1.8465E+00 |
| | 5.2989E−02 | 6.0546E+01 | 7.2832E+01 | 8.6846E+01 | 1.9242E+01 |
| 45.Rh | 9.7062E−03 | 1.4131E+03 | 1.4760E+03 | 1.4639E+03 | 8.2857E−01 |
| | 1.0558E−02 | 1.1651E+03 | 1.2218E+03 | 1.2097E+03 | 1.0030E+00 |
| | 4.6218E−02 | 8.8713E+01 | 1.0631E+02 | 1.3766E+02 | 2.9481E+01 |
| 46.Pd | 4.7910E−02 | 7.9603E+01 | 9.5450E+01 | 1.2469E+02 | 3.0632E+01 |
| 47.Ag | 7.2349E−03 | 3.1466E+03 | 3.2482E+03 | 3.2547E+03 | 2.0045E−01 |
| | 1.2388E−02 | 8.1986E+02 | 8.6708E+02 | 8.5493E+02 | 1.4213E+00 |
| 48.Cd | 1.8529E−03 | 1.6385E+04 | 1.6500E+04 | 1.6451E+04 | 2.9752E−01 |
| | 2.4100E−03 | 9.3791E+03 | 9.4870E+03 | 9.4375E+03 | 5.2452E−01 |
| 49.In | 1.3701E−03 | 3.1700E+04 | 3.1824E+04 | 3.1772E+04 | 1.6397E−01 |
| 50.Sn | 1.4907E−03 | 2.4691E+04 | 2.4812E+04 | 2.4757E+04 | 2.2216E−01 |
| | 2.6791E−03 | 6.9034E+03 | 7.0087E+03 | 6.9549E+03 | 7.7389E−01 |
| 51.Sb | 1.4138E−03 | 2.9161E+04 | 2.9284E+04 | 2.9233E+04 | 1.7529E−01 |
| 52.Te | 1.2126E−03 | 4.0855E+04 | 4.0982E+04 | 4.0939E+04 | 1.0342E−01 |
| 57.La | 1.0467E−03 | 5.0500E+04 | 5.0630E+04 | 5.0646E+04 | 3.1594E−02 |
| | 1.3416E−02 | 6.2581E+02 | 6.6768E+02 | 6.6644E+02 | 1.8535E−01 |
| 58.Ce | 7.6762E−03 | 2.6251E+03 | 2.7154E+03 | 2.8434E+03 | 4.7151E+00 |
| 59.Pr | 7.0779E−03 | 3.3321E+03 | 3.4377E+03 | 3.6519E+03 | 6.2302E+00 |
| 61.Pm | 7.3404E−03 | 3.0219E+03 | 3.1208E+03 | 3.3617E+03 | 7.7186E+00 |
| 63.Eu | 1.4321E−03 | 2.8096E+04 | 2.8219E+04 | 2.8266E+04 | 1.6604E−01 |
| | 1.0875E−02 | 1.1052E+03 | 1.1603E+03 | 1.2205E+03 | 5.1898E+00 |
| 64.Gd | 1.2660E−03 | 3.7753E+04 | 3.7878E+04 | 3.8013E+04 | 3.5688E−01 |
| 65.Tb | 1.2702E−03 | 3.7511E+04 | 3.7636E+04 | 3.7803E+04 | 4.4484E−01 |
| | 7.8292E−03 | 2.4442E+03 | 2.5306E+03 | 2.7299E+03 | 7.8778E+00 |
| 66.Dy | 1.3236E−03 | 3.4406E+04 | 3.4531E+04 | 3.4705E+04 | 5.0271E−01 |
| | 1.3896E−02 | 1.0942E+03 | 1.3911E+03 | 1.2247E+03 | 1.3589E+01 |
| 67.Ho | 1.3773E−03 | 3.1281E+04 | 3.1405E+04 | 3.1573E+04 | 5.3562E−01 |
| | 2.7562E−03 | 1.7147E+04 | 1.7657E+04 | 1.7315E+04 | 1.9725E+00 |
| | 1.4442E−02 | 1.0015E+03 | 1.2651E+03 | 1.1240E+03 | 1.2552E+01 |

| Material | $E$, MeV | $\mu_{1en}$, cm$^{-1}$ | $\mu_1$, cm$^{-1}$ | $\mu_2$, cm$^{-1}$ | $R$, % |
|---|---|---|---|---|---|
| 68.Er | 1.4305E−03 | 2.8186E+04 | 2.8308E+04 | 2.8473E+04 | 5.8024E−01 |
| | 2.7049E−03 | 1.9036E+04 | 1.9608E+04 | 1.9232E+04 | 1.9535E+00 |
| | 1.4909E−02 | 9.2213E+02 | 1.1572E+03 | 1.0361E+03 | 1.1681E+01 |
| | 1.5334E−02 | 8.6258E+02 | 1.0776E+03 | 9.6727E+02 | 1.1406E+01 |
| 69.Tm | 1.4808E−03 | 2.5263E+04 | 2.5384E+04 | 2.5533E+04 | 5.8519E−01 |
| | 5.9422E−02 | 4.3747E+01 | 5.3030E+01 | 1.1289E+02 | 1.1288E+02 |
| 70.Yb | 1.5639E−03 | 2.2743E+04 | 2.2863E+04 | 2.3025E+04 | 7.0851E−01 |
| 71.Lu | 1.6113E−03 | 2.1700E+04 | 2.1820E+04 | 2.1973E+04 | 7.0475E−01 |
| 72.Hf | 1.6639E−03 | 2.0543E+04 | 2.0661E+04 | 2.0770E+04 | 5.2704E−01 |
| | 3.9580E−03 | 1.2094E+04 | 1.2429E+04 | 1.2285E+04 | 1.1734E+00 |
| | 4.1038E−03 | 1.1094E+04 | 1.1401E+04 | 1.1274E+04 | 1.1279E+00 |
| | 2.8254E−02 | 3.2775E+02 | 4.0627E+02 | 3.7194E+02 | 9.2293E+00 |
| 81.Tl | 2.8181E−03 | 2.3969E+04 | 2.4751E+04 | 2.4591E+04 | 6.5104E−01 |
| | 1.2570E−02 | 7.8541E+02 | 8.3168E+02 | 8.3706E+02 | 6.4735E−01 |
| 82.Pb | 2.8078E−03 | 2.4224E+04 | 2.5016E+04 | 2.4899E+04 | 4.7239E−01 |
| 83.Bi | 3.3542E−03 | 1.7113E+04 | 1.7617E+04 | 1.7604E+04 | 7.4146E−02 |
| | 3.5232E−03 | 1.5190E+04 | 1.5635E+04 | 1.5620E+04 | 9.4218E−02 |
| | 3.6089E−03 | 1.4319E+04 | 1.4735E+04 | 1.4715E+04 | 1.3458E−01 |
| | 5.4190E−03 | 6.1108E+03 | 6.2804E+03 | 6.2754E+03 | 7.9162E−02 |
| | 4.6219E−02 | 8.8705E+01 | 1.0630E+02 | 1.0588E+02 | 3.9734E−01 |
| 87.Fr | 3.6192E−03 | 1.4228E+04 | 1.4640E+04 | 1.4703E+04 | 4.3538E−01 |
| 92.U | 1.6457E−02 | 9.2458E+02 | 1.2315E+03 | 9.9929E+02 | 2.3237E+01 |
| 121. | 1.3622E−03 | 3.2159E+04 | 3.2283E+04 | 3.2375E+04 | 2.8506E−01 |
| | 8.3021E−03 | 2.0955E+03 | 2.1742E+03 | 2.3579E+03 | 8.4478E+00 |
| 125. | 2.5132E−03 | 8.4300E+03 | 8.5369E+03 | 8.6366E+03 | 1.1679E+00 |
| 130. | 2.3666E−03 | 9.7780E+03 | 9.8863E+03 | 9.9204E+03 | 3.4408E−01 |

85.ASTATINE

| Material | $E$, MeV | $\mu_{1en}$, cm$^{-1}$ | $\mu_1$, cm$^{-1}$ | $\mu_2$, cm$^{-1}$ | $R$, % |
|---|---|---|---|---|---|
| 25.Mn | 1.1460E−03 | 4.8965E+04 | 4.9105E+04 | 4.9111E+04 | 1.2163E−02 |
| 26.Fe | 1.4822E−03 | 2.8269E+04 | 2.8409E+04 | 2.8361E+04 | 1.6643E−01 |
| 27.Co | 1.3920E−02 | 6.3287E+02 | 6.7698E+02 | 7.8650E+02 | 1.6178E+01 |
| 28.Ni | 1.2054E−02 | 1.0091E+03 | 1.0641E+03 | 1.3552E+03 | 2.7360E+01 |
| 29.Cu | 1.2373E−02 | 9.4472E+02 | 9.9786E+02 | 1.3312E+03 | 3.3408E+01 |
| 31.Ga | 1.9845E−03 | 1.5203E+04 | 1.5334E+04 | 1.5320E+04 | 8.9656E−02 |
| | 2.3394E−03 | 1.1495E+04 | 1.1618E+04 | 1.1584E+04 | 2.8946E−01 |
| 32.Ge | 1.8833E−03 | 1.7703E+04 | 1.7835E+04 | 1.7865E+04 | 1.6741E−01 |
| 33.As | 1.4107E−03 | 3.2670E+04 | 3.2810E+04 | 3.3086E+04 | 8.3903E−01 |
| 41.Nb | 2.8648E−03 | 1.8024E+04 | 1.8582E+04 | 1.8496E+04 | 4.6777E−01 |
| 42.Mo | 2.8293E−03 | 2.0121E+04 | 2.0761E+04 | 2.0711E+04 | 2.4548E−01 |
| 43.Tc | 1.2631E−03 | 4.1756E+04 | 4.1896E+04 | 4.1841E+04 | 1.2918E−01 |

| Material | $E$, MeV | $\mu_{1en}$, cm$^{-1}$ | $\mu_1$, cm$^{-1}$ | $\mu_2$, cm$^{-1}$ | $R$, % |
|---|---|---|---|---|---|
| | 3.5796E−03 | 1.6582E+04 | 1.7079E+04 | 1.7079E+04 | 4.9175E−03 |
| 44.Ru | 1.6748E−03 | 2.2853E+04 | 2.2990E+04 | 2.2940E+04 | 2.1637E−01 |
| 45.Rh | 4.9232E−03 | 8.4068E+03 | 8.6445E+03 | 8.6642E+03 | 2.2724E−01 |
| 46.Pd | 5.0987E−03 | 7.7409E+03 | 7.9597E+03 | 7.9993E+03 | 4.9824E−01 |
| 47.Ag | 1.9567E−03 | 1.5889E+04 | 1.6020E+04 | 1.5973E+04 | 2.9339E−01 |
| | 2.3885E−03 | 1.1013E+04 | 1.1135E+04 | 1.1090E+04 | 4.0160E−01 |
| 48.Cd | 1.3725E−03 | 3.5021E+04 | 3.5161E+04 | 3.5101E+04 | 1.7078E−01 |
| 50.Sn | 1.1671E−03 | 4.7670E+04 | 4.7810E+04 | 4.7755E+04 | 1.1463E−01 |
| 51.Sb | 1.0341E−03 | 5.5006E+04 | 5.5152E+04 | 5.5098E+04 | 9.8809E−02 |
| 58.Ce | 1.1032E−03 | 5.1603E+04 | 5.1743E+04 | 5.1778E+04 | 6.7204E−02 |
| | 1.4050E−02 | 6.0671E+02 | 6.5006E+02 | 6.4846E+02 | 2.4692E−01 |
| 59.Pr | 1.2114E−03 | 4.4942E+04 | 4.5082E+04 | 4.5115E+04 | 7.1839E−02 |
| | 1.2158E−02 | 9.8806E+02 | 1.0425E+03 | 1.0625E+03 | 1.9229E+00 |
| 60.Nd | 7.8101E−03 | 2.7593E+03 | 2.8571E+03 | 3.0278E+03 | 5.9743E+00 |
| 61.Pm | 1.0967E−03 | 5.2000E+04 | 5.2140E+04 | 5.2264E+04 | 2.3946E−01 |
| 62.Sm | 1.1177E−03 | 5.0708E+04 | 5.0848E+04 | 5.0991E+04 | 2.7984E−01 |
| 64.Gd | 1.3212E−03 | 3.8180E+04 | 3.8320E+04 | 3.8440E+04 | 3.1498E−01 |
| 66.Dy | 1.3287E−03 | 3.7720E+04 | 3.7860E+04 | 3.8048E+04 | 4.9640E−01 |
| 67.Ho | 1.3827E−03 | 3.4392E+04 | 3.4532E+04 | 3.4716E+04 | 5.3458E−01 |
| | 8.5649E−03 | 2.2023E+03 | 2.2872E+03 | 2.4836E+03 | 8.5856E+00 |
| 68.Er | 1.4367E−03 | 3.1069E+04 | 3.1209E+04 | 3.1391E+04 | 5.8282E−01 |
| 69.Tm | 1.4857E−03 | 2.8052E+04 | 2.8192E+04 | 2.8359E+04 | 5.9552E−01 |
| | 1.4641E−02 | 1.0683E+03 | 1.3621E+03 | 1.2162E+03 | 1.1996E+01 |
| | 1.6341E−02 | 8.1982E+02 | 1.0255E+03 | 9.2550E+02 | 1.0807E+01 |
| 70.Yb | 1.5739E−03 | 2.5345E+04 | 2.5483E+04 | 2.5665E+04 | 7.1408E−01 |
| 71.Lu | 1.6181E−03 | 2.4252E+04 | 2.4390E+04 | 2.4566E+04 | 7.2261E−01 |
| | 2.8369E−03 | 1.9509E+04 | 2.0128E+04 | 1.9760E+04 | 1.8596E+00 |
| 72.Hf | 1.6712E−03 | 2.2942E+04 | 2.3078E+04 | 2.3215E+04 | 5.9323E−01 |
| | 2.9535E−03 | 2.4292E+04 | 2.5114E+04 | 2.4613E+04 | 2.0324E+00 |
| | 3.5253E−03 | 1.7122E+04 | 1.7638E+04 | 1.7365E+04 | 1.5716E+00 |
| | 1.9322E−02 | 8.1635E+02 | 1.0757E+03 | 9.3309E+02 | 1.5286E+01 |
| 73.Ta | 1.0075E−03 | 5.7756E+04 | 5.7896E+04 | 5.7955E+04 | 1.0287E−01 |
| | 1.0913E−03 | 5.2336E+04 | 5.2476E+04 | 5.2533E+04 | 1.0817E−01 |
| 80.Hg | 2.2488E−03 | 1.2382E+04 | 1.2506E+04 | 1.2536E+04 | 2.3966E−01 |
| | 1.1828E−02 | 1.0546E+03 | 1.1109E+03 | 1.1182E+03 | 6.6171E−01 |
| 81.Tl | 1.2060E−03 | 4.5270E+04 | 4.5410E+04 | 4.5417E+04 | 1.6585E−02 |
| | 6.8488E−03 | 4.0268E+03 | 4.1539E+03 | 4.1461E+03 | 1.8956E−01 |
| | 4.9734E−02 | 7.7961E+01 | 9.3874E+01 | 9.2746E+01 | 1.2161E+00 |
| 82.Pb | 1.3228E−03 | 3.8083E+04 | 3.8223E+04 | 3.8224E+04 | 5.8251E−04 |

| Material | $E$, MeV | $\mu_{1en}$, cm$^{-1}$ | $\mu_1$, cm$^{-1}$ | $\mu_2$, cm$^{-1}$ | $R$, % |
|---|---|---|---|---|---|
| | 3.4632E−03 | 1.7740E+04 | 1.8277E+04 | 1.8205E+04 | 3.9639E−01 |
| 82.Pb | 7.5435E−03 | 3.1109E+03 | 3.2168E+03 | 3.2136E+03 | 9.9773E−02 |
| | 5.3935E−02 | 6.4928E+01 | 7.8393E+01 | 7.7778E+01 | 7.9041E−01 |
| 83.Bi | 2.7981E−03 | 2.2629E+04 | 2.3357E+04 | 2.3305E+04 | 2.2548E−01 |
| 87.Fr | 1.0741E−03 | 5.3396E+04 | 5.3536E+04 | 5.3536E+04 | 7.2964E−06 |
| | 1.3097E−03 | 3.8885E+04 | 3.9025E+04 | 3.9021E+04 | 1.1572E−02 |
| | 1.6465E−02 | 8.0242E+02 | 1.0021E+03 | 1.0226E+03 | 2.0488E+00 |
| | 2.5795E−02 | 4.7604E+02 | 6.0749E+02 | 6.2338E+02 | 2.6153E+00 |
| 89.Ac | 4.5138E−03 | 1.0442E+04 | 1.0742E+04 | 1.0799E+04 | 5.3016E−01 |
| 91.Pa | 1.4487E−02 | 1.0941E+03 | 1.3977E+03 | 1.1675E+03 | 1.9716E+01 |
| 121. | 1.4171E−03 | 3.2274E+04 | 3.2414E+04 | 3.2489E+04 | 2.3374E−01 |
| 123. | 1.8725E−03 | 1.7970E+04 | 1.8102E+04 | 1.8144E+04 | 2.3020E−01 |
| 125. | 2.5544E−03 | 9.3882E+03 | 9.5062E+03 | 9.6281E+03 | 1.2819E+00 |
| 130. | 2.4044E−03 | 1.0857E+04 | 1.0979E+04 | 1.1041E+04 | 5.7036E−01 |
| | | | 86.RADON | | |
| 3.Li | 2.4318E−03 | 9.7784E+00 | 9.8820E+00 | 9.9538E+00 | 7.2700E−01 |
| 4.Be | 5.4477E−03 | 6.0351E+00 | 6.2142E+00 | 6.5500E+00 | 5.4033E+00 |
| 104. | 1.8293E−02 | 8.0622E−01 | 1.0928E+00 | 1.1658E+00 | 6.6772E+00 |
| 106. | 1.4940E−02 | 8.9787E−01 | 1.1536E+00 | 1.2226E+00 | 5.9831E+00 |
| | 1.6876E−02 | 6.7403E−01 | 8.4798E−01 | 9.8473E−01 | 1.6127E+01 |
| 107. | 1.9599E−02 | 6.9096E−01 | 9.2005E−01 | 9.7001E−01 | 5.4299E+00 |
| 109. | 1.9284E−02 | 7.1876E−01 | 9.6172E−01 | 9.9259E−01 | 3.2094E+00 |
| 110. | 1.7648E−02 | 7.6231E−01 | 1.1063E+00 | 1.0334E+00 | 7.0567E+00 |
| 111. | 3.8902E−02 | 1.3578E−01 | 1.6499E−01 | 4.5718E−01 | 1.7709E+02 |
| | 4.4425E−02 | 9.8125E−02 | 1.1869E−01 | 4.0537E−01 | 2.4154E+02 |
| 115. | 2.5738E−02 | 4.2299E−01 | 5.4681E−01 | 6.7143E−01 | 2.2792E+01 |
| | 5.6549E−02 | 5.1449E−02 | 6.2427E−02 | 2.4649E−01 | 2.9485E+02 |
| 119. | 1.8279E−02 | 8.0743E−01 | 1.0947E+00 | 1.0908E+00 | 3.5059E−01 |
| 120. | 1.9841E−02 | 6.6962E−01 | 8.8806E−01 | 9.3921E−01 | 5.7602E+00 |
| 128. | 1.9413E−02 | 7.0737E−01 | 9.4465E−01 | 9.8283E−01 | 4.0418E+00 |
| 131. | 1.9265E−02 | 7.2040E−01 | 9.6419E−01 | 9.9616E−01 | 3.3153E+00 |
| 132. | 1.9316E−02 | 7.1593E−01 | 9.5748E−01 | 9.9239E−01 | 3.6462E+00 |
| 143. | 1.9143E−02 | 7.3115E−01 | 9.8030E−01 | 1.0061E+00 | 2.6290E+00 |
| 144. | 1.9378E−02 | 7.1042E−01 | 9.4923E−01 | 9.8784E−01 | 4.0672E+00 |
| 148. | 1.8624E−02 | 7.7699E−01 | 1.0490E+00 | 1.0472E+00 | 1.7294E−01 |
| | | | 87.FRANCIUM | | |
| 25.Mn | 1.0504E−03 | 5.6210E+04 | 5.6350E+04 | 5.6377E+04 | 4.8456E−02 |
| | 1.1951E−03 | 4.5243E+04 | 4.5382E+04 | 4.5378E+04 | 8.3242E−03 |
| 26.Fe | 1.4510E−03 | 3.1049E+04 | 3.1181E+04 | 3.1153E+04 | 8.9290E−02 |

| Material | $E$, MeV | $\mu_{1en}$, cm$^{-1}$ | $\mu_1$, cm$^{-1}$ | $\mu_2$, cm$^{-1}$ | $R$, % |
|---|---|---|---|---|---|
| 27.Co | 2.2339E−03 | 1.3341E+04 | 1.3466E+04 | 1.3405E+04 | 4.5460E−01 |
| 28.Ni | 2.9865E−03 | 6.4287E+03 | 6.5369E+03 | 6.4755E+03 | 9.4862E−01 |
| 29.Cu | 1.4958E−02 | 5.2546E+02 | 5.6560E+02 | 6.7423E+02 | 1.9207E+01 |
| 30.Zn | 2.7589E−03 | 8.5194E+03 | 8.6327E+03 | 8.5832E+03 | 5.7693E−01 |
| 31.Ga | 1.8290E−03 | 1.9882E+04 | 2.0012E+04 | 2.0042E+04 | 1.5310E−01 |
| 32.Ge | 1.6529E−03 | 2.4403E+04 | 2.4533E+04 | 2.4644E+04 | 4.5110E−01 |
| 33.As | 1.4400E−03 | 3.1659E+04 | 3.1791E+04 | 3.2057E+04 | 8.3590E−01 |
| | 2.7640E−03 | 8.4724E+03 | 8.5856E+03 | 8.5554E+03 | 3.5299E−01 |
| 39.Y | 2.1911E−03 | 1.3734E+04 | 1.3860E+04 | 1.4064E+04 | 1.4667E+00 |
| 41.Nb | 3.1110E−03 | 1.5016E+04 | 1.5497E+04 | 1.5393E+04 | 6.7639E−01 |
| 43.Tc | 1.0166E−03 | 6.0257E+04 | 6.0397E+04 | 6.0349E+04 | 8.0165E−02 |
| | 1.2776E−03 | 4.0666E+04 | 4.0802E+04 | 4.0752E+04 | 1.2464E−01 |
| 44.Ru | 1.4799E−03 | 2.9444E+04 | 2.9575E+04 | 2.9532E+04 | 1.4463E−01 |
| 45.Rh | 1.8839E−03 | 1.8472E+04 | 1.8602E+04 | 1.8559E+04 | 2.3239E−01 |
| | 3.0480E−03 | 1.7437E+04 | 1.8019E+04 | 1.8067E+04 | 2.6223E−01 |
| | 4.8211E−03 | 9.0309E+03 | 9.3071E+03 | 9.3120E+03 | 5.2054E−02 |
| 46.Pd | 1.9915E−03 | 1.5707E+04 | 1.5837E+04 | 1.5792E+04 | 2.8912E−01 |
| | 4.8855E−03 | 8.7455E+03 | 9.0126E+03 | 9.0459E+03 | 3.6876E−01 |
| 47.Ag | 1.7525E−03 | 2.1846E+04 | 2.1976E+04 | 2.1930E+04 | 2.0976E−01 |
| 48.Cd | 1.3542E−03 | 3.6417E+04 | 3.6551E+04 | 3.6497E+04 | 1.4750E−01 |
| 50.Sn | 1.0558E−03 | 5.5572E+04 | 5.5712E+04 | 5.5663E+04 | 8.6654E−02 |
| | 1.2231E−03 | 4.3694E+04 | 4.3832E+04 | 4.3776E+04 | 1.2792E−01 |
| 51.Sb | 1.1352E−03 | 4.8126E+04 | 4.8266E+04 | 4.8212E+04 | 1.1110E−01 |
| 57.La | 1.2161E−03 | 4.4079E+04 | 4.4217E+04 | 4.4219E+04 | 3.3217E−03 |
| | 1.8514E−03 | 1.9306E+04 | 1.9436E+04 | 1.9385E+04 | 2.6481E−01 |
| 59.Pr | 1.2260E−03 | 4.3533E+04 | 4.3671E+04 | 4.3700E+04 | 6.6675E−02 |
| 60.Nd | 1.0458E−03 | 5.6769E+04 | 5.6909E+04 | 5.7019E+04 | 1.9306E−01 |
| 61.Pm | 1.0902E−03 | 5.2003E+04 | 5.2143E+04 | 5.2268E+04 | 2.4009E−01 |
| 63.Eu | 1.5733E−03 | 2.6449E+04 | 2.6579E+04 | 2.6610E+04 | 1.1814E−01 |
| 64.Gd | 1.3223E−03 | 3.8188E+04 | 3.8323E+04 | 3.8449E+04 | 3.2768E−01 |
| 65.Tb | 1.2747E−03 | 4.0826E+04 | 4.0963E+04 | 4.1146E+04 | 4.4652E−01 |
| 66.Dy | 1.3288E−03 | 3.7826E+04 | 3.7961E+04 | 3.8155E+04 | 5.1103E−01 |
| 67.Ho | 1.3834E−03 | 3.4797E+04 | 3.4931E+04 | 3.5126E+04 | 5.5985E−01 |
| 68.Er | 1.4381E−03 | 3.1762E+04 | 3.1893E+04 | 3.2092E+04 | 6.2237E−01 |
| 69.Tm | 1.4874E−03 | 2.9030E+04 | 2.9160E+04 | 2.9351E+04 | 6.5438E−01 |
| | 1.6292E−02 | 8.2475E+02 | 1.0537E+03 | 9.3113E+02 | 1.3161E+01 |
| 71.Lu | 1.6204E−03 | 2.5238E+04 | 2.5368E+04 | 2.5567E+04 | 7.8375E−01 |
| | 3.0888E−03 | 1.5872E+04 | 1.6389E+04 | 1.6081E+04 | 1.9155E+00 |
| 72.Hf | 1.6740E−03 | 2.3862E+04 | 2.3992E+04 | 2.4153E+04 | 6.7223E−01 |

| Material | $E$, MeV | $\mu_{1en}$, cm$^{-1}$ | $\mu_1$, cm$^{-1}$ | $\mu_2$, cm$^{-1}$ | $R$, % |
|---|---|---|---|---|---|
| | 3.1511E−03 | 2.1470E+04 | 2.2259E+04 | 2.1758E+04 | 2.3025E+00 |
| | 1.9549E−02 | 7.8164E+02 | 1.0575E+03 | 8.9203E+02 | 1.8554E+01 |
| 73.Ta | 1.0729E−03 | 5.3525E+04 | 5.3665E+04 | 5.3722E+04 | 1.0691E−01 |
| | 1.2356E−03 | 4.2996E+04 | 4.3134E+04 | 4.3188E+04 | 1.2596E−01 |
| | 9.2767E−03 | 1.8750E+03 | 1.9531E+03 | 1.9615E+03 | 4.3211E−01 |
| 80.Hg | 2.0801E−03 | 1.4754E+04 | 1.4882E+04 | 1.4914E+04 | 2.1358E−01 |
| | 1.1116E−02 | 1.2582E+03 | 1.3199E+03 | 1.3271E+03 | 5.4782E−01 |
| 81.Tl | 1.0671E−03 | 5.4220E+04 | 5.4360E+04 | 5.4371E+04 | 1.9840E−02 |
| | 1.2768E−03 | 4.0714E+04 | 4.0850E+04 | 4.0860E+04 | 2.3112E−02 |
| | 4.8897E−03 | 8.7269E+03 | 8.9934E+03 | 8.9370E+03 | 6.3164E−01 |
| | 3.7226E−02 | 1.7954E+02 | 2.2088E+02 | 2.1251E+02 | 3.9366E+00 |
| 82.Pb | 1.0594E−03 | 5.5139E+04 | 5.5279E+04 | 5.5285E+04 | 1.1221E−02 |
| | 1.3142E−03 | 3.8637E+04 | 3.8772E+04 | 3.8778E+04 | 1.3057E−02 |
| | 4.8865E−03 | 8.7409E+03 | 9.0079E+03 | 8.9606E+03 | 5.2700E−01 |
| | 3.6400E−02 | 1.9159E+02 | 2.3622E+02 | 2.2820E+02 | 3.5134E+00 |
| 83.Bi | 3.6263E−03 | 1.4143E+04 | 1.4615E+04 | 1.4532E+04 | 5.7104E−01 |
| | 4.2684E−03 | 1.0939E+04 | 1.1283E+04 | 1.1225E+04 | 5.1908E−01 |
| 84.Po | 3.6192E−03 | 1.4228E+04 | 1.4703E+04 | 1.4640E+04 | 4.3538E−01 |
| 85.At | 1.0741E−03 | 5.3396E+04 | 5.3536E+04 | 5.3536E+04 | 7.2964E−06 |
| | 1.3097E−03 | 3.8885E+04 | 3.9021E+04 | 3.9025E+04 | 1.1572E−02 |
| | 1.6465E−02 | 8.0242E+02 | 1.0226E+03 | 1.0021E+03 | 2.0488E+00 |
| | 2.5795E−02 | 4.7604E+02 | 6.2338E+02 | 6.0749E+02 | 2.6153E+00 |
| 121. | 1.4285E−03 | 3.2297E+04 | 3.2429E+04 | 3.2513E+04 | 2.5809E−01 |
| | 8.9766E−03 | 2.0426E+03 | 2.1249E+03 | 2.2977E+03 | 8.1311E+00 |
| 123. | 1.5617E−03 | 2.6746E+04 | 2.6876E+04 | 2.7022E+04 | 5.4063E−01 |
| 130. | 2.6160E−03 | 9.8324E+03 | 9.9488E+03 | 1.0010E+04 | 6.1410E−01 |
| | | | 88.RADIUM | | |
| 23.V | 1.4827E−03 | 1.5149E+04 | 1.5214E+04 | 1.5187E+04 | 1.8022E−01 |
| 24.Cr | 2.8542E−03 | 3.9717E+03 | 4.0270E+03 | 3.9978E+03 | 7.3078E−01 |
| 30.Zn | 1.0232E−03 | 2.9688E+04 | 2.9758E+04 | 2.9908E+04 | 5.0553E−01 |
| 31.Ga | 1.1208E−03 | 2.5466E+04 | 2.5536E+04 | 2.5697E+04 | 6.2853E−01 |
| 32.Ge | 1.2465E−02 | 5.1701E+02 | 5.4478E+02 | 8.5620E+02 | 5.7163E+01 |
| 34.Se | 1.4730E−02 | 2.9425E+02 | 3.1539E+02 | 4.9374E+02 | 5.6547E+01 |
| 41.Nb | 1.7737E−03 | 1.1048E+04 | 1.1110E+04 | 1.1099E+04 | 9.3464E−02 |
| | 5.5471E−03 | 3.4061E+03 | 3.5149E+03 | 3.4800E+03 | 1.0030E+00 |
| | 3.7478E−02 | 9.0161E+01 | 1.1163E+02 | 1.3600E+02 | 2.1824E+01 |
| 42.Mo | 2.4950E−03 | 5.6827E+03 | 5.7400E+03 | 5.7412E+03 | 2.1343E−02 |
| | 2.5811E−02 | 2.4164E+02 | 3.2073E+02 | 5.1169E+02 | 5.9541E+01 |
| 43.Tc | 2.1761E−02 | 3.3445E+02 | 4.5369E+02 | 8.1901E+02 | 8.0520E+01 |

| Material | $E$, MeV | $\mu_{1en}$, cm$^{-1}$ | $\mu_1$, cm$^{-1}$ | $\mu_2$, cm$^{-1}$ | $R$, % |
|---|---|---|---|---|---|
| 46.Pd | 2.5199E−02 | 2.5567E+02 | 3.4083E+02 | 6.6503E+02 | 9.5121E+01 |
| 47.Ag | 2.7987E−02 | 1.9178E+02 | 2.4929E+02 | 4.7330E+02 | 8.9858E+01 |
| 48.Cd | 3.3666E−02 | 1.1845E+02 | 1.4812E+02 | 2.6267E+02 | 7.7336E+01 |
| 49.In | 3.9698E−02 | 7.3689E+01 | 9.0387E+01 | 1.4149E+02 | 5.6543E+01 |
| 50.Sn | 3.9881E−02 | 7.2336E+01 | 8.8643E+01 | 1.4386E+02 | 6.2294E+01 |
| 51.Sb | 4.7141E−02 | 4.9304E+01 | 6.0184E+01 | 9.2287E+01 | 5.3342E+01 |
| 52.Te | 5.3597E−02 | 3.4956E+01 | 4.2624E+01 | 6.1551E+01 | 4.4405E+01 |
| 53.I | 1.1258E−02 | 6.3572E+02 | 6.6704E+02 | 6.6827E+02 | 1.8517E−01 |
| 56.Ba | 2.1276E−03 | 7.4323E+03 | 7.4916E+03 | 7.4692E+03 | 2.9998E−01 |
| 57.La | 5.0168E−02 | 4.0183E+01 | 4.8940E+01 | 8.8478E+01 | 8.0789E+01 |
| 58.Ce | 4.8282E−02 | 4.5768E+01 | 5.5822E+01 | 1.1453E+02 | 1.0517E+02 |
| 59.Pr | 4.8224E−02 | 4.5949E+01 | 5.6045E+01 | 1.2097E+02 | 1.1584E+02 |
| 60.Nd | 4.8219E−02 | 4.5962E+01 | 5.6061E+01 | 1.2753E+02 | 1.2748E+02 |
| 61.Pm | 1.0399E−03 | 2.8828E+04 | 2.8898E+04 | 2.8977E+04 | 2.7151E−01 |
| | 3.1469E−03 | 7.6931E+03 | 7.9565E+03 | 7.7628E+03 | 2.4954E+00 |
| | 4.7556E−02 | 4.8018E+01 | 5.8597E+01 | 1.4468E+02 | 1.4691E+02 |
| 62.Sm | 1.0907E−03 | 2.6838E+04 | 2.6908E+04 | 2.6987E+04 | 2.9163E−01 |
| | 4.7935E−02 | 4.6843E+01 | 5.7148E+01 | 1.4820E+02 | 1.5933E+02 |
| 63.Eu | 1.1541E−03 | 2.4126E+04 | 2.4195E+04 | 2.4277E+04 | 3.4029E−01 |
| | 5.9688E−02 | 2.5671E+01 | 3.1405E+01 | 6.1694E+01 | 9.6447E+01 |
| 64.Gd | 1.2045E−03 | 2.2204E+04 | 2.2269E+04 | 2.2355E+04 | 3.8484E−01 |
| 65.Tb | 1.2454E−03 | 2.1516E+04 | 2.1586E+04 | 2.1671E+04 | 3.9410E−01 |
| | 3.3554E−03 | 9.0509E+03 | 9.3922E+03 | 9.1409E+03 | 2.7498E+00 |
| 66.Dy | 1.2982E−03 | 2.0101E+04 | 2.0169E+04 | 2.0263E+04 | 4.6309E−01 |
| | 1.9877E−02 | 3.8023E+02 | 5.1993E+02 | 4.1871E+02 | 2.4173E+01 |
| 67.Ho | 1.3520E−03 | 1.8658E+04 | 1.8725E+04 | 1.8810E+04 | 4.5360E−01 |
| | 3.8479E−03 | 7.2821E+03 | 7.5327E+03 | 7.3768E+03 | 2.1138E+00 |
| | 4.4608E−03 | 5.0553E+03 | 5.2206E+03 | 5.1348E+03 | 1.6707E+00 |
| | 2.6423E−02 | 2.2762E+02 | 3.0064E+02 | 2.5277E+02 | 1.8940E+01 |
| 68.Er | 4.7686E−03 | 4.5486E+03 | 4.7010E+03 | 4.6289E+03 | 1.5575E+00 |
| | 2.9673E−02 | 1.5314E+02 | 1.9393E+02 | 1.7152E+02 | 1.3065E+01 |
| 69.Tm | 4.9416E−03 | 4.3601E+03 | 4.4987E+03 | 4.4427E+03 | 1.2602E+00 |
| | 3.9521E−02 | 7.5003E+01 | 9.2082E+01 | 8.5857E+01 | 7.2502E+00 |
| 70.Yb | 1.5321E−03 | 1.4258E+04 | 1.4323E+04 | 1.4416E+04 | 6.5347E−01 |
| | 3.4076E−03 | 8.6727E+03 | 9.0000E+03 | 8.7856E+03 | 2.4403E+00 |
| 71.Lu | 1.4004E−03 | 1.7358E+04 | 1.7425E+04 | 1.7468E+04 | 2.4960E−01 |
| 90.Th | 3.1682E−03 | 7.3923E+03 | 7.6421E+03 | 7.5188E+03 | 1.6396E+00 |
| 112. | 5.7473E−02 | 2.9048E+01 | 3.5485E+01 | 4.7029E+01 | 3.2530E+01 |
| 116. | 5.9806E−03 | 2.7484E+03 | 2.8368E+03 | 2.9331E+03 | 3.3955E+00 |

| Material | $E$, MeV | $\mu_{1en}$, cm$^{-1}$ | $\mu_1$, cm$^{-1}$ | $\mu_2$, cm$^{-1}$ | $R$, % |
|---|---|---|---|---|---|
| | 6.4222E−03 | 2.4268E+03 | 2.5063E+03 | 2.5866E+03 | 3.2008E+00 |
| 121. | 1.2082E−03 | 2.2063E+04 | 2.2128E+04 | 2.2201E+04 | 3.2890E−01 |
| | 1.2090E−03 | 2.2494E+04 | 2.2564E+04 | 2.2635E+04 | 3.1348E−01 |
| | 5.5696E−02 | 3.1756E+01 | 3.8758E+01 | 9.1838E+01 | 1.3695E+02 |
| 123. | 1.2996E−02 | 4.6483E+02 | 4.9106E+02 | 7.4877E+02 | 5.2483E+01 |
| 125. | 1.9904E−03 | 8.1680E+03 | 8.2281E+03 | 8.2811E+03 | 6.4388E−01 |
| | 2.0190E−03 | 7.9497E+03 | 8.0096E+03 | 8.0604E+03 | 6.3451E−01 |
| | 3.6346E−03 | 7.2928E+03 | 7.5596E+03 | 7.4753E+03 | 1.1275E+00 |
| 130. | 3.1646E−03 | 7.4432E+03 | 7.6954E+03 | 7.5872E+03 | 1.4255E+00 |
| | 1.1871E−02 | 5.7549E+02 | 6.0501E+02 | 6.0717E+02 | 3.5778E−01 |
| | 4.8884E−02 | 4.3900E+01 | 5.3517E+01 | 7.0542E+01 | 3.1811E+01 |

89.ACTINIUM

| Material | $E$, MeV | $\mu_{1en}$, cm$^{-1}$ | $\mu_1$, cm$^{-1}$ | $\mu_2$, cm$^{-1}$ | $R$, % |
|---|---|---|---|---|---|
| 26.Fe | 1.3846E−03 | 3.6974E+04 | 3.7110E+04 | 3.7100E+04 | 2.5153E−02 |
| 27.Co | 1.8056E−03 | 2.2373E+04 | 2.2504E+04 | 2.2468E+04 | 1.5796E−01 |
| 28.Ni | 2.6495E−03 | 1.0433E+04 | 1.0552E+04 | 1.0494E+04 | 5.4521E−01 |
| 29.Cu | 2.8959E−03 | 7.9622E+03 | 8.0760E+03 | 8.0200E+03 | 6.9848E−01 |
| 30.Zn | 1.0575E−03 | 5.8764E+04 | 5.8905E+04 | 5.9274E+04 | 6.2766E−01 |
| | 1.9821E−03 | 1.7446E+04 | 1.7577E+04 | 1.7565E+04 | 6.9441E−02 |
| 31.Ga | 1.3687E−03 | 3.7808E+04 | 3.7945E+04 | 3.8154E+04 | 5.5135E−01 |
| 33.As | 1.9299E−03 | 1.8905E+04 | 1.9036E+04 | 1.9105E+04 | 3.5908E−01 |
| 39.Y | 2.6496E−03 | 1.0432E+04 | 1.0551E+04 | 1.0656E+04 | 9.9424E−01 |
| 40.Zr | 2.2583E−03 | 1.4357E+04 | 1.4483E+04 | 1.4706E+04 | 1.5361E+00 |
| 41.Nb | 3.3337E−03 | 1.3181E+04 | 1.3628E+04 | 1.3505E+04 | 9.1507E−01 |
| 44.Ru | 1.4052E−03 | 3.5886E+04 | 3.6021E+04 | 3.5978E+04 | 1.2081E−01 |
| 45.Rh | 1.4780E−03 | 3.2060E+04 | 3.2192E+04 | 3.2148E+04 | 1.3658E−01 |
| 46.Pd | 1.5000E−03 | 3.0907E+04 | 3.1037E+04 | 3.1003E+04 | 1.1209E−01 |
| | 4.7163E−03 | 9.7889E+03 | 1.0120E+04 | 1.0135E+04 | 1.4527E−01 |
| 47.Ag | 1.4537E−03 | 3.3337E+04 | 3.3470E+04 | 3.3423E+04 | 1.4058E−01 |
| 48.Cd | 1.0443E−03 | 6.0104E+04 | 6.0245E+04 | 6.0190E+04 | 9.1787E−02 |
| 58.Ce | 2.4436E−03 | 1.2498E+04 | 1.2621E+04 | 1.2567E+04 | 4.3016E−01 |
| 59.Pr | 1.1231E−03 | 5.3462E+04 | 5.3603E+04 | 5.3667E+04 | 1.1916E−01 |
| 60.Nd | 1.1350E−03 | 5.2410E+04 | 5.2551E+04 | 5.2633E+04 | 1.5585E−01 |
| 61.Pm | 1.1399E−03 | 5.1980E+04 | 5.2121E+04 | 5.2243E+04 | 2.3349E−01 |
| | 7.9397E−03 | 2.8795E+03 | 2.9877E+03 | 3.1809E+03 | 6.4655E+00 |
| 62.Sm | 1.1592E−03 | 5.0269E+04 | 5.0410E+04 | 5.0547E+04 | 2.7198E−01 |
| 63.Eu | 1.9732E−03 | 1.7695E+04 | 1.7826E+04 | 1.7804E+04 | 1.2266E−01 |
| | 2.2553E−03 | 1.4387E+04 | 1.4513E+04 | 1.4480E+04 | 2.2936E−01 |
| 64.Gd | 1.3564E−03 | 3.8452E+04 | 3.8589E+04 | 3.8713E+04 | 3.2013E−01 |
| | 8.2621E−03 | 2.6350E+03 | 2.7365E+03 | 2.9728E+03 | 8.6361E+00 |

| Material | $E$, MeV | $\mu_{1en}$, cm$^{-1}$ | $\mu_1$, cm$^{-1}$ | $\mu_2$, cm$^{-1}$ | $R$, % |
|---|---|---|---|---|---|
| 66.Dy | 1.3318E−03 | 3.9749E+04 | 3.9887E+04 | 4.0095E+04 | 5.2159E−01 |
| 67.Ho | 1.3870E−03 | 3.6847E+04 | 3.6982E+04 | 3.7197E+04 | 5.8077E−01 |
| 68.Er | 1.4427E−03 | 3.3917E+04 | 3.4050E+04 | 3.4273E+04 | 6.5494E−01 |
| 69.Tm | 1.4914E−03 | 3.1355E+04 | 3.1487E+04 | 3.1708E+04 | 7.0311E−01 |
| 70.Yb | 1.0366E−02 | 1.5158E+03 | 1.5871E+03 | 1.7872E+03 | 1.2608E+01 |
| 71.Lu | 1.6254E−03 | 2.7403E+04 | 2.7534E+04 | 2.7765E+04 | 8.3785E−01 |
| | 3.2377E−03 | 1.4633E+04 | 1.5142E+04 | 1.4829E+04 | 2.1112E+00 |
| 72.Hf | 1.6801E−03 | 2.5877E+04 | 2.6008E+04 | 2.6208E+04 | 7.6675E−01 |
| 73.Ta | 1.7377E−03 | 2.4269E+04 | 2.4400E+04 | 2.4555E+04 | 6.3581E−01 |
| | 3.9593E−02 | 1.5517E+02 | 1.9172E+02 | 1.7854E+02 | 7.3862E+00 |
| 74.W | 1.6082E−03 | 2.7885E+04 | 2.8016E+04 | 2.8098E+04 | 2.9050E−01 |
| 80.Hg | 1.4163E−03 | 3.5303E+04 | 3.5437E+04 | 3.5479E+04 | 1.1737E−01 |
| | 2.3005E−03 | 1.3934E+04 | 1.4059E+04 | 1.4157E+04 | 7.0045E−01 |
| | 8.5808E−03 | 2.4435E+03 | 2.5399E+03 | 2.5381E+03 | 7.2297E−02 |
| | 5.8211E−02 | 5.8468E+01 | 7.1692E+01 | 7.0292E+01 | 1.9913E+00 |
| 81.Tl | 4.6669E−03 | 1.0019E+04 | 1.0359E+04 | 1.0256E+04 | 1.0113E+00 |
| 81.Tl | 2.6348E−02 | 4.7294E+02 | 6.3419E+02 | 5.7579E+02 | 1.0142E+01 |
| 82.Pb | 3.9686E−03 | 1.4130E+04 | 1.4631E+04 | 1.4478E+04 | 1.0548E+00 |
| | 4.0090E−03 | 1.3806E+04 | 1.4297E+04 | 1.4146E+04 | 1.0729E+00 |
| | 4.6574E−03 | 1.0064E+04 | 1.0406E+04 | 1.0315E+04 | 8.8389E−01 |
| | 2.4803E−02 | 5.4517E+02 | 7.4008E+02 | 6.7466E+02 | 9.6963E+00 |
| 85.At | 4.5138E−03 | 1.0442E+04 | 1.0799E+04 | 1.0742E+04 | 5.3016E−01 |
| 121. | 1.4718E−03 | 3.2387E+04 | 3.2519E+04 | 3.2603E+04 | 2.5715E−01 |
| | 1.5792E−02 | 4.9262E+02 | 5.3216E+02 | 5.3826E+02 | 1.1468E+00 |
| 125. | 1.5591E−02 | 5.1032E+02 | 5.5053E+02 | 6.6523E+02 | 2.0836E+01 |
| 130. | 2.8026E−03 | 8.8978E+03 | 9.0133E+03 | 9.0655E+03 | 5.7860E−01 |
| | 1.5326E−02 | 5.3360E+02 | 5.7470E+02 | 6.4504E+02 | 1.2240E+01 |
| **90.THORIUM** | | | | | |
| 27.Co | 1.4162E−03 | 4.1818E+04 | 4.1976E+04 | 4.1998E+04 | 5.1462E−02 |
| 28.Ni | 1.6132E−03 | 3.3129E+04 | 3.3281E+04 | 3.3286E+04 | 1.6585E−02 |
| 29.Cu | 1.8486E−03 | 2.5300E+04 | 2.5453E+04 | 2.5443E+04 | 3.7591E−02 |
| 30.Zn | 1.3846E−03 | 4.3678E+04 | 4.3838E+04 | 4.4012E+04 | 3.9596E−01 |
| 45.Rh | 1.0276E−03 | 7.3878E+04 | 7.4042E+04 | 7.3989E+04 | 7.2667E−02 |
| | 1.3222E−03 | 4.6530E+04 | 4.6684E+04 | 4.6626E+04 | 1.2373E−01 |
| | 3.7251E−03 | 1.7163E+04 | 1.7823E+04 | 1.7774E+04 | 2.7833E−01 |
| | 4.0433E−03 | 1.3784E+04 | 1.4289E+04 | 1.4245E+04 | 3.0787E−01 |
| 46.Pd | 1.3353E−03 | 4.6574E+04 | 4.6737E+04 | 4.6674E+04 | 1.3619E−01 |
| | 3.9251E−03 | 1.4977E+04 | 1.5541E+04 | 1.5557E+04 | 1.0281E−01 |
| 47.Ag | 1.1232E−03 | 6.2818E+04 | 6.2983E+04 | 6.2918E+04 | 1.0214E−01 |

| Material | $E$, MeV | $\mu_{1en}$, cm$^{-1}$ | $\mu_1$, cm$^{-1}$ | $\mu_2$, cm$^{-1}$ | $R$, % |
|---|---|---|---|---|---|
| 64.Gd | 1.4599E−03 | 3.9253E+04 | 3.9408E+04 | 3.9513E+04 | 2.6794E−01 |
| | 9.8168E−03 | 2.0232E+03 | 2.1137E+03 | 2.2609E+03 | 6.9614E+00 |
| 65.Tb | 1.3064E−03 | 4.7698E+04 | 4.7853E+04 | 4.8076E+04 | 4.6624E−01 |
| 67.Ho | 9.2919E−03 | 2.3969E+03 | 2.4982E+03 | 2.7609E+03 | 1.0516E+01 |
| 69.Tm | 1.5037E−03 | 3.6770E+04 | 3.6922E+04 | 3.7194E+04 | 7.3634E−01 |
| 70.Yb | 1.8131E−03 | 2.6480E+04 | 2.6633E+04 | 2.6819E+04 | 7.0002E−01 |
| | 1.3678E−02 | 9.9336E+02 | 1.0528E+03 | 1.1537E+03 | 9.5884E+00 |
| 71.Lu | 1.6369E−03 | 3.2341E+04 | 3.2493E+04 | 3.2777E+04 | 8.7396E−01 |
| 72.Hf | 1.6922E−03 | 3.0501E+04 | 3.0653E+04 | 3.0918E+04 | 8.6405E−01 |
| 73.Ta | 1.7497E−03 | 2.8589E+04 | 2.8741E+04 | 2.8965E+04 | 7.7880E−01 |
| | 2.5655E−02 | 5.8127E+02 | 7.9221E+02 | 6.6414E+02 | 1.9283E+01 |
| 74.W | 1.8126E−03 | 2.6499E+04 | 2.6651E+04 | 2.6833E+04 | 6.8118E−01 |
| | 5.6450E−03 | 7.9828E+03 | 8.2558E+03 | 8.1659E+03 | 1.1003E+00 |
| | 4.4348E−02 | 1.4317E+02 | 1.7715E+02 | 1.6632E+02 | 6.5145E+00 |
| 75.Re | 1.4744E−03 | 3.8402E+04 | 3.8556E+04 | 3.8654E+04 | 2.5448E−01 |
| | 1.8560E−03 | 2.5052E+04 | 2.5205E+04 | 2.5340E+04 | 5.3838E−01 |
| 79.Au | 2.1739E−03 | 1.8181E+04 | 1.8329E+04 | 1.8401E+04 | 3.9349E−01 |
| | 1.1649E−02 | 1.4896E+03 | 1.5641E+03 | 1.5798E+03 | 1.0025E+00 |
| 80.Hg | 2.3210E−03 | 1.6420E+04 | 1.6564E+04 | 1.6732E+04 | 1.0119E+00 |
| 80.Hg | 4.4177E−03 | 1.2895E+04 | 1.3353E+04 | 1.3190E+04 | 1.2368E+00 |
| | 4.4411E−03 | 1.2743E+04 | 1.3195E+04 | 1.3035E+04 | 1.2298E+00 |
| | 2.4683E−02 | 6.3178E+02 | 8.6736E+02 | 7.6546E+02 | 1.3311E+01 |
| 81.Tl | 2.4107E−03 | 1.5345E+04 | 1.5488E+04 | 1.5670E+04 | 1.1792E+00 |
| 82.Pb | 1.9956E−02 | 7.8892E+02 | 1.1006E+03 | 9.8840E+02 | 1.1350E+01 |
| | 2.0118E−02 | 7.7721E+02 | 1.0828E+03 | 9.7270E+02 | 1.1321E+01 |
| 88.Ra | 3.1682E−03 | 7.3923E+03 | 7.5188E+03 | 7.6421E+03 | 1.6396E+00 |
| 121. | 2.1807E−03 | 1.8100E+04 | 1.8248E+04 | 1.8229E+04 | 1.0565E−01 |
| | 2.7419E−03 | 1.1377E+04 | 1.1512E+04 | 1.1525E+04 | 1.1433E−01 |
| 125. | 2.7570E−03 | 1.1197E+04 | 1.1331E+04 | 1.1499E+04 | 1.4810E+00 |
| 130. | 2.9706E−03 | 8.6385E+03 | 8.7681E+03 | 8.8024E+03 | 3.9103E−01 |
| | 3.2155E−03 | 7.1413E+03 | 7.2672E+03 | 7.2806E+03 | 1.8495E−01 |
| | | | 91.PROTACTINIUM | | |
| 40.Zr | 3.1430E−03 | 1.0444E+04 | 1.0617E+04 | 1.0671E+04 | 5.1623E−01 |
| 42.Mo | 2.5580E−03 | 1.8755E+04 | 1.8941E+04 | 1.9295E+04 | 1.8673E+00 |
| 44.Ru | 3.5081E−03 | 1.9077E+04 | 1.9769E+04 | 1.9718E+04 | 2.6004E−01 |
| 65.Tb | 2.6225E−03 | 1.7689E+04 | 1.7873E+04 | 1.7831E+04 | 2.3700E−01 |
| | 3.2916E−03 | 9.4087E+03 | 9.5778E+03 | 9.5002E+03 | 8.1663E−01 |
| 67.Ho | 1.5000E−03 | 5.0922E+04 | 5.1137E+04 | 5.1423E+04 | 5.5954E−01 |
| | 1.5001E−03 | 5.0916E+04 | 5.1131E+04 | 5.1417E+04 | 5.5947E−01 |

| Material | $E$, MeV | $\mu_{1en}$, cm$^{-1}$ | $\mu_1$, cm$^{-1}$ | $\mu_2$, cm$^{-1}$ | $R$, % |
|---|---|---|---|---|---|
| 68.Er | 1.4880E−03 | 5.1844E+04 | 5.2059E+04 | 5.2414E+04 | 6.8224E−01 |
| | 1.6932E−03 | 4.2062E+04 | 4.2271E+04 | 4.2509E+04 | 5.6180E−01 |
| | 1.5760E−02 | 8.2253E+02 | 8.8635E+02 | 9.2196E+02 | 4.0174E+00 |
| 69.Tm | 1.8276E−03 | 3.5895E+04 | 3.6100E+04 | 3.6305E+04 | 5.6577E−01 |
| | 1.2992E−02 | 1.5950E+03 | 1.6844E+03 | 1.8487E+03 | 9.7505E+00 |
| 70.Yb | 3.3588E−03 | 8.9398E+03 | 9.1075E+03 | 9.0553E+03 | 5.7650E−01 |
| 71.Lu | 1.8320E−03 | 3.5692E+04 | 3.5897E+04 | 3.6181E+04 | 7.9209E−01 |
| 72.Hf | 1.7130E−03 | 4.1154E+04 | 4.1362E+04 | 4.1761E+04 | 9.6387E−01 |
| | 9.9086E−03 | 2.6866E+03 | 2.8106E+03 | 3.1335E+03 | 1.1489E+01 |
| | 1.0116E−02 | 2.5588E+03 | 2.6790E+03 | 2.9779E+03 | 1.1159E+01 |
| 73.Ta | 1.7722E−03 | 3.8438E+04 | 3.8645E+04 | 3.9010E+04 | 9.4488E−01 |
| 74.W | 1.8376E−03 | 3.5437E+04 | 3.5642E+04 | 3.5958E+04 | 8.8826E−01 |
| | 3.6459E−03 | 2.4524E+04 | 2.5531E+04 | 2.4921E+04 | 2.4480E+00 |
| 75.Re | 1.8991E−03 | 3.2618E+04 | 3.2821E+04 | 3.3101E+04 | 8.5352E−01 |
| | 2.6376E−02 | 7.2427E+02 | 9.8885E+02 | 8.3793E+02 | 1.8011E+01 |
| 76.Os | 2.9761E−02 | 4.9943E+02 | 6.5055E+02 | 5.7621E+02 | 1.2902E+01 |
| 77.Ir | 2.0545E−03 | 2.7087E+04 | 2.7286E+04 | 2.7488E+04 | 7.4203E−01 |
| | 5.1598E−03 | 1.2766E+04 | 1.3224E+04 | 1.3048E+04 | 1.3544E+00 |
| | 3.4825E−02 | 3.6644E+02 | 4.6941E+02 | 4.2509E+02 | 1.0425E+01 |
| 78.Pt | 2.1398E−03 | 2.5675E+04 | 2.5871E+04 | 2.6082E+04 | 8.1261E−01 |
| | 5.3028E−03 | 1.1949E+04 | 1.2376E+04 | 1.2226E+04 | 1.2292E+00 |
| | 3.1974E−02 | 4.3563E+02 | 5.6231E+02 | 5.0738E+02 | 1.0826E+01 |
| 79.Au | 2.2353E−03 | 2.4095E+04 | 2.4289E+04 | 2.4525E+04 | 9.7125E−01 |
| | 2.7908E−02 | 6.2249E+02 | 8.3571E+02 | 7.3907E+02 | 1.3076E+01 |
| 80.Hg | 2.3554E−03 | 2.2108E+04 | 2.2299E+04 | 2.2601E+04 | 1.3529E+00 |
| 81.Tl | 2.4577E−03 | 2.0416E+04 | 2.0604E+04 | 2.0909E+04 | 1.4771E+00 |
| | 1.4109E−02 | 1.2206E+03 | 1.2981E+03 | 1.5526E+03 | 1.9607E+01 |
| 82.Pb | 2.5352E−03 | 1.9133E+04 | 1.9320E+04 | 1.9633E+04 | 1.6240E+00 |
| | 1.4038E−02 | 1.2447E+03 | 1.3229E+03 | 1.5474E+03 | 1.6972E+01 |
| 83.Bi | 2.6323E−03 | 1.7526E+04 | 1.7710E+04 | 1.8022E+04 | 1.7626E+00 |
| 85.At | 1.4487E−02 | 1.0941E+03 | 1.1675E+03 | 1.3977E+03 | 1.9716E+01 |
| 92.URANIUM | | | | | |
| 41.Nb | 2.7011E−03 | 2.0559E+04 | 2.0784E+04 | 2.1114E+04 | 1.5889E+00 |
| 68.Er | 3.4696E−03 | 1.0445E+04 | 1.0648E+04 | 1.0568E+04 | 7.6303E−01 |
| 69.Tm | 2.8799E−03 | 1.6851E+04 | 1.7071E+04 | 1.7040E+04 | 1.8132E−01 |
| 71.Lu | 2.2020E−03 | 3.0907E+04 | 3.1147E+04 | 3.1315E+04 | 5.3951E−01 |
| | 2.4075E−03 | 2.6645E+04 | 2.6879E+04 | 2.6988E+04 | 4.0602E−01 |
| | 1.6884E−02 | 8.5779E+02 | 9.2974E+02 | 9.8278E+02 | 5.7053E+00 |
| 72.Hf | 1.7743E−03 | 4.8066E+04 | 4.8321E+04 | 4.8779E+04 | 9.4867E−01 |

| Material | $E$, MeV | $\mu_{1en}$, cm$^{-1}$ | $\mu_1$, cm$^{-1}$ | $\mu_2$, cm$^{-1}$ | $R$, % |
|---|---|---|---|---|---|
| 73.Ta | 1.7876E−03 | 4.7299E+04 | 4.7554E+04 | 4.8038E+04 | 1.0184E+00 |
| | 1.0427E−02 | 3.0638E+03 | 3.2097E+03 | 3.5929E+03 | 1.1940E+01 |
| 74.W | 1.8523E−03 | 4.3581E+04 | 4.3833E+04 | 4.4271E+04 | 9.9861E−01 |
| 75.Re | 1.9151E−03 | 3.9975E+04 | 4.0225E+04 | 4.0620E+04 | 9.8326E−01 |
| | 2.1414E−02 | 1.1218E+03 | 1.7577E+03 | 1.3039E+03 | 3.4806E+01 |
| 77.Ir | 2.0789E−03 | 3.3458E+04 | 3.3702E+04 | 3.4055E+04 | 1.0476E+00 |
| | 3.8006E−03 | 2.7528E+04 | 2.8694E+04 | 2.8052E+04 | 2.2871E+00 |
| | 4.2526E−03 | 2.0902E+04 | 2.1730E+04 | 2.1311E+04 | 1.9629E+00 |
| 78.Pt | 2.1647E−03 | 3.1681E+04 | 3.1922E+04 | 3.2279E+04 | 1.1165E+00 |
| 79.Au | 2.2572E−03 | 2.9763E+04 | 3.0002E+04 | 3.0364E+04 | 1.2081E+00 |
| 80.Hg | 2.3792E−03 | 2.7233E+04 | 2.7468E+04 | 2.7875E+04 | 1.4808E+00 |
| 84.Po | 1.6457E−02 | 9.2458E+02 | 9.9929E+02 | 1.2315E+03 | 2.3237E+01 |
| 101.A-150 TISSUE−EQUIVALENT PLASTIC | | | | | |
| 5.B | 3.7082E−03 | 6.3582E+01 | 6.4311E+01 | 6.4616E+01 | 4.7445E−01 |
| | 5.4547E−02 | 4.0553E−02 | 2.3798E−01 | 3.8577E−01 | 6.2103E+01 |
| 6.C | 4.6920E−03 | 4.1445E+01 | 4.3826E+01 | 4.2274E+01 | 3.6698E+00 |
| | 5.8524E−02 | 3.6416E−02 | 2.2946E−01 | 3.0097E−01 | 3.1163E+01 |
| 102. | 1.7270E−03 | 6.0949E+02 | 6.1098E+02 | 6.1114E+02 | 2.6872E−02 |
| | 2.0225E−03 | 3.5187E+02 | 3.5311E+02 | 3.5310E+02 | 2.7311E−03 |
| | 2.9683E−03 | 1.1582E+02 | 1.1669E+02 | 1.1679E+02 | 8.4231E−02 |
| 104. | 2.8709E−02 | 2.0225E−01 | 4.4450E−01 | 5.0485E−01 | 1.3578E+01 |
| | 4.2956E−02 | 6.4280E−02 | 2.7661E−01 | 3.2929E−01 | 1.9045E+01 |
| 109. | 5.3734E−02 | 4.1398E−02 | 2.3972E−01 | 2.2817E−01 | 5.0602E+00 |
| 110. | 7.1950E−03 | 1.2688E+01 | 1.3553E+01 | 1.3167E+01 | 2.9359E+00 |
| 119. | 2.8191E−02 | 2.2109E−01 | 4.6544E−01 | 4.5825E−01 | 1.5678E+00 |
| 122. | 4.0871E−03 | 5.8631E+01 | 6.1968E+01 | 5.9437E+01 | 4.2578E+00 |
| 128. | 5.6678E−02 | 3.8336E−02 | 2.3341E−01 | 2.2313E−01 | 4.6075E+00 |
| 131. | 5.3623E−02 | 4.1514E−02 | 2.3996E−01 | 2.2937E−01 | 4.6160E+00 |
| 132. | 5.3623E−02 | 4.1514E−02 | 2.3996E−01 | 2.3007E−01 | 4.2991E+00 |
| 137. | 1.3341E−02 | 2.2432E+00 | 2.6153E+00 | 2.6379E+00 | 8.6649E−01 |
| 138. | 4.2764E−03 | 5.3253E+01 | 5.6291E+01 | 5.3999E+01 | 4.2444E+00 |
| 143. | 4.8196E−02 | 5.0149E−02 | 2.5512E−01 | 2.4356E−01 | 4.7431E+00 |
| 144. | 5.7678E−02 | 3.7296E−02 | 2.3127E−01 | 2.2241E−01 | 3.9879E+00 |
| 145. | 1.8099E−02 | 7.9555E−01 | 1.0910E+00 | 1.0644E+00 | 2.5018E+00 |
| 148. | 3.1255E−02 | 1.4487E−01 | 3.7931E−01 | 3.6213E−01 | 4.7433E+00 |
| 102.ADIPOSE TISSUE (ICRU-44) | | | | | |
| 4.Be | 5.5548E−02 | 2.6577E−02 | 1.9383E−01 | 2.8093E−01 | 4.4932E+01 |
| 5.B | 2.9827E−03 | 1.1404E+02 | 1.1500E+02 | 1.1523E+02 | 1.9988E−01 |
| | 3.5453E−02 | 6.4714E−02 | 2.5643E−01 | 4.5404E−01 | 7.7060E+01 |

| Material | $E$, MeV | $\mu_{1en}$, cm$^{-1}$ | $\mu_1$, cm$^{-1}$ | $\mu_2$, cm$^{-1}$ | $R$, % |
|---|---|---|---|---|---|
| 35.Br | 2.9428E−02 | 1.0271E−01 | 3.0520E−01 | 1.3819E−01 | 1.2085E+02 |
| | 4.1453E−02 | 4.1405E−02 | 2.2385E−01 | 5.2131E−02 | 3.2940E+02 |
| 54.Xe | 3.7543E−02 | 5.4945E−02 | 2.4319E−01 | 1.5042E−01 | 6.1666E+01 |
| 101. | 1.7270E−03 | 6.0949E+02 | 6.1114E+02 | 6.1098E+02 | 2.6872E−02 |
| | 2.0225E−03 | 3.5187E+02 | 3.5310E+02 | 3.5311E+02 | 2.7311E−03 |
| | 2.9683E−03 | 1.1582E+02 | 1.1679E+02 | 1.1669E+02 | 8.4231E−02 |
| 139. | 2.4507E−03 | 2.0155E+02 | 2.0251E+02 | 2.0239E+02 | 5.8662E−02 |
| | 2.6594E−03 | 1.5828E+02 | 1.5931E+02 | 1.5907E+02 | 1.4636E−01 |
| 142. | 3.8631E−03 | 5.6179E+01 | 5.6891E+01 | 5.6866E+01 | 4.4543E−02 |
| | 4.1135E−02 | 4.1857E−02 | 2.2468E−01 | 2.4674E−01 | 9.8209E+00 |
| | | | 103.AIR, DRY (NEAR SEA LEVEL) | | |
| 147. | 3.9990E−03 | 9.2115E−02 | 9.3948E−02 | 9.3302E−02 | 6.9222E−01 |
| | 3.9775E−02 | 8.4655E−05 | 3.0230E−04 | 4.3641E−04 | 4.4363E+01 |
| | | | 104.ALANINE | | |
| 5.B | 5.7150E−02 | 4.0201E−02 | 2.8250E−01 | 3.8071E−01 | 3.4762E+01 |
| 15.P | 1.4971E−03 | 1.4507E+03 | 1.4550E+03 | 1.4562E+03 | 8.2587E−02 |
| | 2.0701E−03 | 6.0367E+02 | 6.0562E+02 | 6.0841E+02 | 4.6073E−01 |
| 86.Rn | 1.8293E−02 | 8.0622E−01 | 1.1658E+00 | 1.0928E+00 | 6.6772E+00 |
| 101. | 2.8709E−02 | 2.0225E−01 | 5.0485E−01 | 4.4450E−01 | 1.3578E+01 |
| | 4.2956E−02 | 6.4280E−02 | 3.2929E−01 | 2.7661E−01 | 1.9045E+01 |
| 107. | 2.9943E−03 | 1.9688E+02 | 1.9817E+02 | 1.9859E+02 | 2.1049E−01 |
| | 3.0584E−03 | 1.8783E+02 | 1.8909E+02 | 1.8949E+02 | 2.0639E−01 |
| | 3.9063E−03 | 9.2773E+01 | 9.3796E+01 | 9.4129E+01 | 3.5449E−01 |
| | 6.6899E−03 | 1.9000E+01 | 1.9651E+01 | 1.9616E+01 | 1.7554E−01 |
| | 7.4671E−03 | 1.3518E+01 | 1.4116E+01 | 1.4158E+01 | 2.9560E−01 |
| | 5.2614E−02 | 4.4283E−02 | 2.9290E−01 | 2.3534E−01 | 2.4458E+01 |
| 109. | 3.9576E−03 | 8.7017E+01 | 8.8026E+01 | 8.8442E+01 | 4.7245E−01 |
| | 4.8090E−02 | 5.1419E−02 | 3.0714E−01 | 2.4508E−01 | 2.5321E+01 |
| 115. | 1.9637E−03 | 6.9259E+02 | 6.9475E+02 | 6.9490E+02 | 2.1014E−02 |
| | 2.0081E−03 | 6.3096E+02 | 6.3294E+02 | 6.3311E+02 | 2.6268E−02 |
| | 2.8518E−03 | 2.5960E+02 | 2.6099E+02 | 2.6221E+02 | 4.6968E−01 |
| 119. | 1.9276E−02 | 6.4889E−01 | 9.9945E−01 | 9.2445E−01 | 8.1130E+00 |
| | 2.3775E−02 | 3.8963E−01 | 7.1563E−01 | 6.4442E−01 | 1.1050E+01 |
| 120. | 2.9241E−03 | 2.2780E+02 | 2.2914E+02 | 2.3008E+02 | 4.1291E−01 |
| | 5.3016E−02 | 4.3921E−02 | 2.9198E−01 | 2.2972E−01 | 2.7106E+01 |
| 128. | 2.9913E−03 | 1.9819E+02 | 1.9948E+02 | 2.0008E+02 | 3.0449E−01 |
| | 3.0875E−03 | 1.8456E+02 | 1.8582E+02 | 1.8636E+02 | 2.9198E−01 |
| | 3.8932E−03 | 9.4239E+01 | 9.5266E+01 | 9.5622E+01 | 3.7442E−01 |
| | 4.9044E−02 | 4.9031E−02 | 3.0302E−01 | 2.4266E−01 | 2.4877E+01 |

| Material | $E$, MeV | $\mu_{1en}$, cm$^{-1}$ | $\mu_1$, cm$^{-1}$ | $\mu_2$, cm$^{-1}$ | $R$, % |
|---|---|---|---|---|---|
| 131. | 3.9544E−03 | 8.7378E+01 | 8.8388E+01 | 8.8838E+01 | 5.0957E−01 |
| | 4.7977E−02 | 5.1702E−02 | 3.0762E−01 | 2.4649E−01 | 2.4800E+01 |
| 132. | 2.9941E−03 | 1.9697E+02 | 1.9826E+02 | 1.9866E+02 | 2.0060E−01 |
| | 3.0601E−03 | 1.8764E+02 | 1.8891E+02 | 1.8928E+02 | 1.9798E−01 |
| | 3.9060E−03 | 9.2799E+01 | 9.3823E+01 | 9.4101E+01 | 2.9706E−01 |
| | 4.7995E−02 | 5.1658E−02 | 3.0755E−01 | 2.4717E−01 | 2.4427E+01 |
| 143. | 3.9533E−03 | 8.7500E+01 | 8.8510E+01 | 8.8745E+01 | 2.6568E−01 |
| | 4.5785E−02 | 5.7193E−02 | 3.1708E−01 | 2.5412E−01 | 2.4778E+01 |
| 144. | 3.9182E−03 | 9.1433E+01 | 9.2453E+01 | 9.2885E+01 | 4.6786E−01 |
| | 4.9196E−02 | 4.8649E−02 | 3.0237E−01 | 2.4360E−01 | 2.4126E+01 |
| 148. | 4.7802E−03 | 5.0677E+01 | 5.1529E+01 | 5.1414E+01 | 2.2368E−01 |
| | 3.5281E−02 | 1.1016E−01 | 3.9285E−01 | 3.1894E−01 | 2.3174E+01 |
| **105.B-100 BONE−EQUIVALENT PLASTIC** | | | | | |
| 16.S | 2.2649E−03 | 5.7668E+02 | 5.7916E+02 | 5.8145E+02 | 3.9530E−01 |
| **106.BAKELITE** | | | | | |
| 5.B | 4.0638E−02 | 4.8866E−02 | 2.7820E−01 | 4.2301E−01 | 5.2049E+01 |
| 54.Xe | 3.9646E−02 | 5.1686E−02 | 2.8271E−01 | 1.2824E−01 | 1.2044E+02 |
| | 5.2499E−02 | 3.3132E−02 | 2.4581E−01 | 6.3059E−02 | 2.8981E+02 |
| 86.Rn | 1.4940E−02 | 8.9787E−01 | 1.2226E+00 | 1.1536E+00 | 5.9831E+00 |
| | 1.6876E−02 | 6.7403E−01 | 9.8473E−01 | 8.4798E−01 | 1.6127E+01 |
| 110. | 1.0593E−03 | 2.8512E+03 | 2.8558E+03 | 2.8587E+03 | 9.9346E−02 |
| | 1.1768E−03 | 2.3577E+03 | 2.3617E+03 | 2.3638E+03 | 9.1385E−02 |
| | 2.2140E−03 | 3.7214E+02 | 3.7353E+02 | 3.7373E+02 | 5.2100E−02 |
| **107.BLOOD, WHOLE (ICRU-44)** | | | | | |
| 5.B | 5.5831E−02 | 4.0379E−02 | 2.2781E−01 | 3.8327E−01 | 6.8244E+01 |
| 6.C | 1.0618E−03 | 3.4381E+03 | 3.4482E+03 | 3.4413E+03 | 2.0062E−01 |
| | 1.1399E−03 | 3.0373E+03 | 3.0460E+03 | 3.0403E+03 | 1.8686E−01 |
| | 2.3463E−03 | 3.8791E+02 | 3.8966E+02 | 3.8944E+02 | 5.7573E−02 |
| | 2.6855E−03 | 2.6572E+02 | 2.6728E+02 | 2.6707E+02 | 8.0045E−02 |
| | 5.9508E−02 | 3.5916E−02 | 2.1919E−01 | 2.9900E−01 | 3.6407E+01 |
| 19.K | 2.1073E−03 | 5.2515E+02 | 5.2708E+02 | 5.2760E+02 | 9.8231E−02 |
| 19.K | 2.9503E−03 | 2.0621E+02 | 2.0797E+02 | 2.0830E+02 | 1.6103E−01 |
| 86.Rn | 1.9599E−02 | 6.9096E−01 | 9.7001E−01 | 9.2005E−01 | 5.4299E+00 |
| 104. | 2.9943E−03 | 1.9688E+02 | 1.9859E+02 | 1.9817E+02 | 2.1049E−01 |
| | 3.0584E−03 | 1.8783E+02 | 1.8949E+02 | 1.8909E+02 | 2.0639E−01 |
| | 3.9063E−03 | 9.2773E+01 | 9.4129E+01 | 9.3796E+01 | 3.5449E−01 |
| | 6.6899E−03 | 1.9000E+01 | 1.9616E+01 | 1.9651E+01 | 1.7554E−01 |
| | 7.4671E−03 | 1.3518E+01 | 1.4158E+01 | 1.4116E+01 | 2.9560E−01 |

| Material | $E$, MeV | $\mu_{1en}$, cm$^{-1}$ | $\mu_1$, cm$^{-1}$ | $\mu_2$, cm$^{-1}$ | $R$, % |
|---|---|---|---|---|---|
| | 5.2614E−02 | 4.4283E−02 | 2.3534E−01 | 2.9290E−01 | 2.4458E+01 |
| 109. | 6.2091E−03 | 2.3437E+01 | 2.4104E+01 | 2.4122E+01 | 7.7160E−02 |
| | 7.8308E−03 | 1.1621E+01 | 1.2222E+01 | 1.2139E+01 | 6.7943E−01 |
| 115. | 1.1190E−03 | 3.1347E+03 | 3.1437E+03 | 3.1444E+03 | 2.2149E−02 |
| | 1.4672E−03 | 1.5079E+03 | 1.5125E+03 | 1.5120E+03 | 3.4797E−02 |
| 119. | 3.4033E−03 | 1.4149E+02 | 1.4290E+02 | 1.4278E+02 | 8.3538E−02 |
| | 3.7533E−03 | 1.0464E+02 | 1.0612E+02 | 1.0576E+02 | 3.3716E−01 |
| | 6.9130E−03 | 1.6941E+01 | 1.7534E+01 | 1.7494E+01 | 2.3185E−01 |
| | 7.2510E−03 | 1.4645E+01 | 1.5309E+01 | 1.5173E+01 | 8.9568E−01 |
| 120. | 5.6039E−02 | 4.0127E−02 | 2.2732E−01 | 2.2257E−01 | 2.1363E+00 |
| 128. | 7.9408E−03 | 1.1047E+01 | 1.1636E+01 | 1.1556E+01 | 6.9023E−01 |
| 131. | 6.2100E−03 | 2.3428E+01 | 2.4095E+01 | 2.4129E+01 | 1.4355E−01 |
| | 7.8284E−03 | 1.1633E+01 | 1.2234E+01 | 1.2158E+01 | 6.3003E−01 |
| 132. | 1.1314E−03 | 3.0769E+03 | 3.0857E+03 | 3.0856E+03 | 2.6981E−03 |
| | 3.3818E−03 | 1.4438E+02 | 1.4581E+02 | 1.4579E+02 | 9.2416E−03 |
| | 3.9515E−03 | 8.9263E+01 | 9.0584E+01 | 9.0540E+01 | 4.8419E−02 |
| | 6.0104E−03 | 2.5270E+01 | 2.5958E+01 | 2.5952E+01 | 2.4621E−02 |
| | 7.9013E−03 | 1.1253E+01 | 1.1846E+01 | 1.1755E+01 | 7.7221E−01 |
| 137. | 1.0030E−03 | 3.9926E+03 | 4.0043E+03 | 4.0009E+03 | 8.5247E−02 |
| | 1.4418E−03 | 1.6264E+03 | 1.6314E+03 | 1.6302E+03 | 7.3145E−02 |
| | 2.0783E−03 | 5.4703E+02 | 5.4899E+02 | 5.4891E+02 | 1.4400E−02 |
| | 2.8991E−03 | 2.1705E+02 | 2.1886E+02 | 2.1836E+02 | 2.3118E−01 |
| | 3.5924E−03 | 1.1607E+02 | 1.1735E+02 | 1.1713E+02 | 1.8809E−01 |
| 141. | 2.3999E−03 | 3.6417E+02 | 3.6585E+02 | 3.6656E+02 | 1.9508E−01 |
| 143. | 6.2560E−03 | 2.3003E+01 | 2.3665E+01 | 2.3656E+01 | 4.0524E−02 |
| | 7.7937E−03 | 1.1814E+01 | 1.2419E+01 | 1.2326E+01 | 7.5713E−01 |
| 144. | 6.0232E−03 | 2.5152E+01 | 2.5839E+01 | 2.5860E+01 | 8.2661E−02 |
| | 7.9052E−03 | 1.1232E+01 | 1.1826E+01 | 1.1756E+01 | 5.9366E−01 |
| 145. | 1.0438E−03 | 3.5957E+03 | 3.6069E+03 | 3.6060E+03 | 2.4252E−02 |
| | 1.3199E−03 | 2.1962E+03 | 2.2026E+03 | 2.2020E+03 | 2.6753E−02 |
| | 2.0905E−03 | 5.3781E+02 | 5.3976E+02 | 5.3964E+02 | 2.2327E−02 |
| | 2.9043E−03 | 2.1596E+02 | 2.1777E+02 | 2.1713E+02 | 2.9183E−01 |
| | 3.5449E−03 | 1.2246E+02 | 1.2377E+02 | 1.2341E+02 | 2.9395E−01 |
| | 3.6118E−03 | 1.1562E+02 | 1.1721E+02 | 1.1656E+02 | 5.5916E−01 |
| 148. | 2.9812E−03 | 1.9966E+02 | 2.0138E+02 | 2.0087E+02 | 2.4965E−01 |
| 148. | 3.1617E−03 | 1.7395E+02 | 1.7553E+02 | 1.7509E+02 | 2.4929E−01 |
| | 3.8885E−03 | 9.4152E+01 | 9.5522E+01 | 9.5058E+01 | 4.8719E−01 |
| | 6.6092E−03 | 1.9744E+01 | 2.0370E+01 | 2.0293E+01 | 3.7569E−01 |
| | 7.5555E−03 | 1.3057E+01 | 1.3687E+01 | 1.3542E+01 | 1.0763E+00 |

| Material | $E$, MeV | $\mu_{1en}$, cm$^{-1}$ | $\mu_1$, cm$^{-1}$ | $\mu_2$, cm$^{-1}$ | $R$, % |
|---|---|---|---|---|---|
| 108.BONE, CORTICAL (ICRU-44) | | | | | |
| 11.Na | 2.1842E−03 | 1.2812E+03 | 1.3094E+03 | 1.2956E+03 | 1.0685E+00 |
| | 2.7365E−03 | 7.4403E+02 | 7.5996E+02 | 7.5174E+02 | 1.0931E+00 |
| 111. | 1.0928E−03 | 5.7873E+03 | 5.8000E+03 | 5.8133E+03 | 2.2893E−01 |
| | 1.4202E−03 | 2.9401E+03 | 2.9486E+03 | 2.9523E+03 | 1.2569E−01 |
| | 2.1410E−03 | 9.2839E+02 | 9.3243E+02 | 9.3294E+02 | 5.4900E−02 |
| 124. | 1.5511E−03 | 2.3400E+03 | 2.3474E+03 | 2.3489E+03 | 6.7043E−02 |
| | 1.6474E−03 | 2.0790E+03 | 2.0857E+03 | 2.0903E+03 | 2.2131E−01 |
| 126. | 3.2478E−03 | 4.8038E+02 | 4.9052E+02 | 4.8377E+02 | 1.3959E+00 |
| 140. | 2.9620E−03 | 5.8330E+02 | 5.9562E+02 | 5.8684E+02 | 1.4966E+00 |
| 109.BRAIN, GREY/WHITE MATTER (ICRU-44) | | | | | |
| 5.B | 5.4459E−02 | 4.0565E−02 | 2.2654E−01 | 3.8594E−01 | 7.0364E+01 |
| 6.C | 1.0180E−03 | 3.6631E+03 | 3.6740E+03 | 3.6664E+03 | 2.0624E−01 |
| | 1.3451E−03 | 1.9836E+03 | 1.9890E+03 | 1.9861E+03 | 1.4690E−01 |
| | 2.2543E−03 | 4.2110E+02 | 4.2317E+02 | 4.2267E+02 | 1.1882E−01 |
| | 2.7677E−03 | 2.3608E+02 | 2.3770E+02 | 2.3739E+02 | 1.3244E−01 |
| | 5.7696E−02 | 3.6837E−02 | 2.1923E−01 | 3.0263E−01 | 3.8042E+01 |
| 14.Si | 1.0402E−03 | 3.4575E+03 | 3.4676E+03 | 3.4643E+03 | 9.3876E−02 |
| | 1.3587E−03 | 1.9230E+03 | 1.9281E+03 | 1.9289E+03 | 4.1816E−02 |
| 19.K | 2.0357E−03 | 5.5222E+02 | 5.5414E+02 | 5.5470E+02 | 1.0098E−01 |
| | 2.9868E−03 | 1.9241E+02 | 1.9429E+02 | 1.9449E+02 | 1.0024E−01 |
| | 3.3308E−03 | 1.4665E+02 | 1.4824E+02 | 1.4858E+02 | 2.2879E−01 |
| 86.Rn | 1.9284E−02 | 7.1876E−01 | 9.9259E−01 | 9.6172E−01 | 3.2094E+00 |
| 101. | 5.3734E−02 | 4.1398E−02 | 2.2817E−01 | 2.3972E−01 | 5.0602E+00 |
| 104. | 3.9576E−03 | 8.7017E+01 | 8.8442E+01 | 8.8026E+01 | 4.7245E−01 |
| | 4.8090E−02 | 5.1419E−02 | 2.4508E−01 | 3.0714E−01 | 2.5321E+01 |
| 107. | 6.2091E−03 | 2.3437E+01 | 2.4122E+01 | 2.4104E+01 | 7.7160E−02 |
| | 7.8308E−03 | 1.1621E+01 | 1.2139E+01 | 1.2222E+01 | 6.7943E−01 |
| 115. | 1.1752E−03 | 2.7415E+03 | 2.7494E+03 | 2.7500E+03 | 2.1871E−02 |
| | 1.4211E−03 | 1.6446E+03 | 1.6488E+03 | 1.6497E+03 | 5.3341E−02 |
| 119. | 3.2317E−03 | 1.5955E+02 | 1.6122E+02 | 1.6093E+02 | 1.8154E−01 |
| | 3.8259E−03 | 9.7003E+01 | 9.8557E+01 | 9.8086E+01 | 4.8039E−01 |
| 120. | 6.8155E−03 | 1.9018E+01 | 1.9641E+01 | 1.9614E+01 | 1.3905E−01 |
| | 7.5237E−03 | 1.3858E+01 | 1.4408E+01 | 1.4398E+01 | 7.0230E−02 |
| 122. | 2.4640E−03 | 3.2488E+02 | 3.2665E+02 | 3.2625E+02 | 1.2221E−01 |
| 131. | 5.9613E−03 | 2.5666E+01 | 2.6382E+01 | 2.6399E+01 | 6.4352E−02 |
| | 5.5777E−02 | 3.9047E−02 | 2.2356E−01 | 2.2453E−01 | 4.3236E−01 |
| 132. | 3.3462E−02 | 1.3696E−01 | 3.5642E−01 | 3.5849E−01 | 5.8083E−01 |
| 132. | 5.5777E−02 | 3.9047E−02 | 2.2356E−01 | 2.2520E−01 | 7.3400E−01 |

| Material | $E$, MeV | $\mu_{1en}$, cm$^{-1}$ | $\mu_1$, cm$^{-1}$ | $\mu_2$, cm$^{-1}$ | $R$, % |
|---|---|---|---|---|---|
| 137. | 2.9330E−03 | 2.0342E+02 | 2.0533E+02 | 2.0471E+02 | 3.0435E−01 |
| | 3.4692E−03 | 1.2864E+02 | 1.3011E+02 | 1.2974E+02 | 2.8577E−01 |
| | 3.6446E−03 | 1.1075E+02 | 1.1248E+02 | 1.1180E+02 | 6.1296E−01 |
| | 5.8815E−02 | 3.5549E−02 | 2.1671E−01 | 2.6027E−01 | 2.0102E+01 |
| 138. | 2.4684E−03 | 3.2302E+02 | 3.2479E+02 | 3.2429E+02 | 1.5546E−01 |
| 141. | 2.2520E−03 | 4.2233E+02 | 4.2441E+02 | 4.2478E+02 | 8.6639E−02 |
| | 2.6446E−03 | 2.6791E+02 | 2.6967E+02 | 2.7022E+02 | 2.0249E−01 |
| 143. | 4.7222E−03 | 5.4465E+01 | 5.5525E+01 | 5.5419E+01 | 1.9183E−01 |
| 145. | 1.0035E−03 | 3.8003E+03 | 3.8116E+03 | 3.8112E+03 | 1.0313E−02 |
| | 1.4841E−03 | 1.3638E+03 | 1.3671E+03 | 1.3670E+03 | 7.1258E−03 |
| | 2.0133E−03 | 5.6832E+02 | 5.7028E+02 | 5.7021E+02 | 1.1839E−02 |
| | 2.9391E−03 | 2.0217E+02 | 2.0408E+02 | 2.0332E+02 | 3.7330E−01 |
| | 3.4140E−03 | 1.3582E+02 | 1.3734E+02 | 1.3681E+02 | 3.8692E−01 |
| | 3.7026E−03 | 1.0635E+02 | 1.0802E+02 | 1.0726E+02 | 7.1266E−01 |
| 148. | 3.9443E−03 | 8.8028E+01 | 8.9466E+01 | 8.8916E+01 | 6.1792E−01 |
| | | | 110.BREAST TISSUE (ICRU-44) | | |
| 5.B | 4.7197E−02 | 4.3472E−02 | 2.3281E−01 | 4.0311E−01 | 7.3151E+01 |
| 6.C | 2.9789E−03 | 1.5998E+02 | 1.6132E+02 | 1.6118E+02 | 8.5221E−02 |
| | 4.4011E−02 | 5.0381E−02 | 2.4399E−01 | 3.3894E−01 | 3.8918E+01 |
| 13.Al | 1.0313E−03 | 3.0608E+03 | 3.0689E+03 | 3.0662E+03 | 8.9529E−02 |
| | 1.4244E−03 | 1.3993E+03 | 1.4031E+03 | 1.4050E+03 | 1.3159E−01 |
| 86.Rn | 1.7648E−02 | 7.6231E−01 | 1.0334E+00 | 1.1063E+00 | 7.0567E+00 |
| 101. | 7.1950E−03 | 1.2688E+01 | 1.3167E+01 | 1.3553E+01 | 2.9359E+00 |
| 106. | 1.0593E−03 | 2.8512E+03 | 2.8587E+03 | 2.8558E+03 | 9.9346E−02 |
| | 1.1768E−03 | 2.3577E+03 | 2.3638E+03 | 2.3617E+03 | 9.1385E−02 |
| | 2.2140E−03 | 3.7214E+02 | 3.7373E+02 | 3.7353E+02 | 5.2100E−02 |
| 122. | 1.4818E−03 | 1.1772E+03 | 1.1805E+03 | 1.1797E+03 | 6.2922E−02 |
| | 2.0428E−03 | 4.6577E+02 | 4.6744E+02 | 4.6731E+02 | 2.7963E−02 |
| | 2.9341E−03 | 1.6765E+02 | 1.6901E+02 | 1.6884E+02 | 9.9591E−02 |
| | 4.9120E−02 | 3.9301E−02 | 2.2606E−01 | 2.7151E−01 | 2.0105E+01 |
| 138. | 1.0006E−03 | 3.3149E+03 | 3.3231E+03 | 3.3221E+03 | 3.0888E−02 |
| | 1.4660E−03 | 1.2384E+03 | 1.2418E+03 | 1.2413E+03 | 3.6955E−02 |
| | 2.0469E−03 | 4.6325E+02 | 4.6492E+02 | 4.6477E+02 | 3.2089E−02 |
| | 2.9367E−03 | 1.6721E+02 | 1.6857E+02 | 1.6820E+02 | 2.2158E−01 |
| | 5.5542E−02 | 3.2956E−02 | 2.1280E−01 | 2.3691E−01 | 1.1333E+01 |
| | | | 111.C-552 AIR-EQUIVALENT PLASTIC | | |
| 86.Rn | 3.8902E−02 | 1.3578E−01 | 4.5718E−01 | 1.6499E−01 | 1.7709E+02 |
| | 4.4425E−02 | 9.8125E−02 | 4.0537E−01 | 1.1869E−01 | 2.4154E+02 |
| 108. | 1.0928E−03 | 5.7873E+03 | 5.8133E+03 | 5.8000E+03 | 2.2893E−01 |

| Material | $E$, MeV | $\mu_{1en}$, cm$^{-1}$ | $\mu_1$, cm$^{-1}$ | $\mu_2$, cm$^{-1}$ | $R$, % |
|---|---|---|---|---|---|
| | 1.4202E−03 | 2.9401E+03 | 2.9523E+03 | 2.9486E+03 | 1.2569E−01 |
| | 2.1410E−03 | 9.2839E+02 | 9.3294E+02 | 9.3243E+02 | 5.4900E−02 |
| 124. | 1.0556E−03 | 6.1113E+03 | 6.1388E+03 | 6.1279E+03 | 1.7882E−01 |
| 112.CADMIUM TELLURIDE | | | | | |
| 24.Cr | 1.3731E−03 | 2.7862E+04 | 2.7929E+04 | 2.7931E+04 | 6.1260E−03 |
| | 7.8641E−03 | 1.5931E+03 | 1.6627E+03 | 1.9335E+03 | 1.6282E+01 |
| 25.Mn | 2.5801E−03 | 6.4986E+03 | 6.5424E+03 | 6.5329E+03 | 1.4639E−01 |
| | 3.4169E−03 | 2.7716E+03 | 2.8094E+03 | 2.7959E+03 | 4.8119E−01 |
| | 7.2832E−03 | 2.0716E+03 | 2.1659E+03 | 2.6860E+03 | 2.4015E+01 |
| 26.Fe | 2.8338E−02 | 7.7179E+01 | 1.5912E+02 | 8.7282E+01 | 8.2311E+01 |
| 29.Cu | 3.6617E−03 | 4.2868E+03 | 4.4347E+03 | 4.3287E+03 | 2.4492E+00 |
| 31.Ga | 2.9051E−02 | 7.3831E+01 | 1.4889E+02 | 9.0454E+01 | 6.4605E+01 |
| 32.Ge | 1.2487E−03 | 3.5228E+04 | 3.5300E+04 | 3.5632E+04 | 9.4240E−01 |
| | 1.3368E−02 | 4.5150E+02 | 4.7400E+02 | 7.2481E+02 | 5.2912E+01 |
| | 2.8484E−02 | 7.6493E+01 | 1.5703E+02 | 9.6613E+01 | 6.2534E+01 |
| 33.As | 1.2782E−02 | 5.1548E+02 | 5.4043E+02 | 8.9178E+02 | 6.5014E+01 |
| | 2.9901E−02 | 6.9842E+01 | 1.3670E+02 | 8.8027E+01 | 5.5297E+01 |
| 34.Se | 1.4859E−02 | 2.8846E+02 | 3.0473E+02 | 4.7991E+02 | 5.7485E+01 |
| | 2.7177E−02 | 8.2629E+01 | 1.7578E+02 | 1.1275E+02 | 5.5905E+01 |
| 38.Sr | 2.9632E−03 | 4.0099E+03 | 4.0499E+03 | 4.0781E+03 | 6.9692E−01 |
| | 2.6551E−02 | 5.6396E+01 | 6.2685E+01 | 9.1832E+01 | 4.6498E+01 |
| 39.Y | 1.7265E−02 | 2.0520E+02 | 2.1816E+02 | 4.4812E+02 | 1.0541E+02 |
| 40.Zr | 3.6867E−02 | 6.8933E+01 | 1.5673E+02 | 1.0154E+02 | 5.4347E+01 |
| 41.Nb | 4.7054E−03 | 5.3035E+03 | 5.5864E+03 | 5.4172E+03 | 3.1239E+00 |
| 42.Mo | 1.1952E−03 | 3.8398E+04 | 3.8472E+04 | 3.8470E+04 | 5.0364E−03 |
| | 1.7414E−02 | 2.0074E+02 | 2.1352E+02 | 2.1540E+02 | 8.7930E−01 |
| 43.Tc | 2.6371E−03 | 6.1286E+03 | 6.1719E+03 | 6.1962E+03 | 3.9262E−01 |
| 52.Te | 4.6785E−03 | 5.3753E+03 | 5.6630E+03 | 5.7227E+03 | 1.0547E+00 |
| | 4.3982E−02 | 5.1329E+01 | 9.8356E+01 | 1.0596E+02 | 7.7319E+00 |
| 53.I | 3.2812E−03 | 3.0969E+03 | 3.1352E+03 | 3.1295E+03 | 1.8379E−01 |
| | 2.2922E−02 | 9.3436E+01 | 1.0160E+02 | 1.0107E+02 | 5.2374E−01 |
| 57.La | 2.8462E−02 | 7.6596E+01 | 1.5734E+02 | 8.4301E+01 | 8.6647E+01 |
| | 4.7944E−02 | 4.2961E+01 | 7.7155E+01 | 1.0337E+02 | 3.3979E+01 |
| 58.Ce | 3.6717E−03 | 4.2584E+03 | 4.4052E+03 | 4.3056E+03 | 2.3133E+00 |
| | 2.9727E−02 | 7.0659E+01 | 1.3920E+02 | 7.8475E+01 | 7.7380E+01 |
| | 4.4479E−02 | 5.0280E+01 | 9.5697E+01 | 1.4407E+02 | 5.0547E+01 |
| 59.Pr | 6.1572E−03 | 2.9990E+03 | 3.1412E+03 | 3.2523E+03 | 3.5382E+00 |
| | 4.4820E−02 | 4.9559E+01 | 9.3870E+01 | 1.4717E+02 | 5.6785E+01 |
| 60.Nd | 4.5157E−02 | 4.8846E+01 | 9.2065E+01 | 1.5105E+02 | 6.4070E+01 |

| Material | $E$, MeV | $\mu_{1en}$, cm$^{-1}$ | $\mu_1$, cm$^{-1}$ | $\mu_2$, cm$^{-1}$ | $R$, % |
|---|---|---|---|---|---|
| 61.Pm | 3.8072E−03 | 4.8865E+03 | 5.0829E+03 | 4.9447E+03 | 2.7948E+00 |
| 63.Eu | 1.2864E−03 | 3.2993E+04 | 3.3063E+04 | 3.3196E+04 | 4.0106E−01 |
| | 2.9834E−02 | 7.0156E+01 | 1.3766E+02 | 7.7985E+01 | 7.6522E+01 |
| 64.Gd | 3.5732E−02 | 7.2261E+01 | 1.7015E+02 | 8.1369E+01 | 1.0910E+02 |
| 65.Tb | 1.2656E−03 | 3.4226E+04 | 3.4297E+04 | 3.4493E+04 | 5.7044E−01 |
| 65.Tb | 3.7797E−02 | 6.6201E+01 | 1.4572E+02 | 7.5093E+01 | 9.4049E+01 |
| 66.Dy | 1.3185E−03 | 3.1097E+04 | 3.1165E+04 | 3.1365E+04 | 6.3947E−01 |
| | 3.9178E−02 | 6.2149E+01 | 1.2938E+02 | 7.0917E+01 | 8.2442E+01 |
| 67.Ho | 1.3715E−03 | 2.7953E+04 | 2.8020E+04 | 2.8210E+04 | 6.7642E−01 |
| | 4.1726E−02 | 5.6092E+01 | 1.1042E+02 | 6.4496E+01 | 7.1211E+01 |
| 68.Er | 1.4232E−03 | 2.4889E+04 | 2.4954E+04 | 2.5133E+04 | 7.1877E−01 |
| | 4.6627E−02 | 4.5742E+01 | 8.4200E+01 | 5.3267E+01 | 5.8071E+01 |
| 69.Tm | 1.4749E−03 | 2.1832E+04 | 2.1895E+04 | 2.2055E+04 | 7.3361E−01 |
| | 4.9842E−02 | 3.8953E+01 | 6.6997E+01 | 4.5933E+01 | 4.5857E+01 |
| 70.Yb | 1.5508E−03 | 1.9319E+04 | 1.9380E+04 | 1.9550E+04 | 8.8021E−01 |
| | 3.7967E−02 | 6.5704E+01 | 1.4371E+02 | 7.4906E+01 | 9.1858E+01 |
| 71.Lu | 1.5989E−03 | 1.8350E+04 | 1.8410E+04 | 1.8560E+04 | 8.1675E−01 |
| 88.Ra | 5.7473E−02 | 2.9048E+01 | 4.7029E+01 | 3.5485E+01 | 3.2530E+01 |
| 116. | 3.4307E−03 | 2.7384E+03 | 2.7761E+03 | 2.7683E+03 | 2.8207E−01 |
| | 2.4128E−02 | 8.1125E+01 | 8.8665E+01 | 8.7970E+01 | 7.9022E−01 |
| 121. | 1.3026E−03 | 3.2036E+04 | 3.2105E+04 | 3.2251E+04 | 4.5579E−01 |
| | 5.5098E−02 | 3.2089E+01 | 5.3106E+01 | 9.4451E+01 | 7.7854E+01 |
| 123. | 1.3629E−02 | 4.2294E+02 | 4.4436E+02 | 6.6688E+02 | 5.0078E+01 |
| | 2.8512E−02 | 7.6363E+01 | 1.5663E+02 | 9.6788E+01 | 6.1831E+01 |
| 125. | 3.9242E−02 | 6.1963E+01 | 1.2863E+02 | 7.3702E+01 | 7.4530E+01 |
| 130. | 1.9091E−03 | 1.2099E+04 | 1.2151E+04 | 1.2165E+04 | 1.1570E−01 |
| | 2.0271E−03 | 1.0091E+04 | 1.0141E+04 | 1.0155E+04 | 1.4070E−01 |
| | 2.3156E−03 | 8.2170E+03 | 8.2635E+03 | 8.3047E+03 | 4.9860E−01 |
| | 1.1106E−02 | 6.9870E+02 | 7.3066E+02 | 7.3511E+02 | 6.0928E−01 |
| 134. | 2.6039E−02 | 6.1627E+01 | 6.8181E+01 | 1.3150E+02 | 9.2875E+01 |
| 113.CALSIUM FLUORIDE | | | | | |
| 12.Mg | 1.3930E−03 | 8.1458E+03 | 8.1769E+03 | 8.3412E+03 | 2.0099E+00 |
| 21.Sc | 3.7403E−03 | 5.1489E+02 | 5.2071E+02 | 5.2156E+02 | 1.6250E−01 |
| 26.Fe | 6.6849E−03 | 4.9889E+02 | 5.4411E+02 | 5.1454E+02 | 5.7481E+00 |
| 34.Se | 1.2595E−02 | 9.9956E+01 | 1.0669E+02 | 1.0653E+02 | 1.4881E−01 |
| 38.Sr | 7.8166E−03 | 3.1491E+02 | 3.3974E+02 | 3.2346E+02 | 5.0349E+00 |
| | 1.4791E−02 | 5.3576E+01 | 5.7210E+01 | 5.7259E+01 | 8.6163E−02 |
| | 1.5025E−02 | 4.9026E+01 | 5.2357E+01 | 5.2600E+01 | 4.6456E−01 |
| 53.I | 4.4109E−03 | 1.3815E+03 | 1.5592E+03 | 1.4092E+03 | 1.0646E+01 |

| Material | $E$, MeV | $\mu_{1en}$, cm$^{-1}$ | $\mu_1$, cm$^{-1}$ | $\mu_2$, cm$^{-1}$ | $R$, % |
|---|---|---|---|---|---|
| 63.Eu | 1.1334E−03 | 1.3748E+04 | 1.3801E+04 | 1.3833E+04 | 2.3320E−01 |
| 116. | 4.2079E−03 | 1.5212E+03 | 1.7228E+03 | 1.5476E+03 | 1.1322E+01 |
| 117. | 1.8604E−03 | 3.5723E+03 | 3.5870E+03 | 3.6707E+03 | 2.3347E+00 |
| 133. | 1.7987E−03 | 3.9599E+03 | 3.9758E+03 | 3.9988E+03 | 5.7685E−01 |
| | 1.4279E−02 | 6.4395E+01 | 6.8753E+01 | 9.5081E+01 | 3.8294E+01 |
| 114.CALSIUM SULFATE | | | | | |
| 12.Mg | 2.4924E−03 | 2.2341E+03 | 2.3313E+03 | 2.2706E+03 | 2.6719E+00 |
| 19.K | 3.7518E−03 | 8.4367E+02 | 8.7387E+02 | 9.4797E+02 | 8.4786E+00 |
| 24.Cr | 4.8907E−03 | 8.2989E+02 | 9.0453E+02 | 8.4672E+02 | 6.8279E+00 |
| 126. | 2.2717E−03 | 1.4313E+03 | 1.4382E+03 | 1.4383E+03 | 7.4608E−03 |
| 129. | 2.1490E−03 | 1.6543E+03 | 1.6615E+03 | 1.6680E+03 | 3.9008E−01 |
| 140. | 2.3403E−03 | 1.3066E+03 | 1.3133E+03 | 1.3128E+03 | 3.3036E−02 |
| 115.0.015 M CERIC AMMONIUM SULFATE SOLUTION | | | | | |
| 6.C | 1.1138E−03 | 3.1708E+03 | 3.1806E+03 | 3.1739E+03 | 2.1030E−01 |
| | 1.3921E−03 | 1.7424E+03 | 1.7475E+03 | 1.7447E+03 | 1.6142E−01 |
| 14.Si | 1.1451E−03 | 2.9522E+03 | 2.9613E+03 | 2.9588E+03 | 8.5007E−02 |
| | 1.4057E−03 | 1.6965E+03 | 1.7017E+03 | 1.7024E+03 | 4.1477E−02 |
| 15.P | 2.1289E−03 | 5.5720E+02 | 5.5922E+02 | 5.6185E+02 | 4.6899E−01 |
| 19.K | 1.2049E−03 | 2.5617E+03 | 2.5695E+03 | 2.5653E+03 | 1.6248E−01 |
| | 1.3651E−03 | 1.8333E+03 | 1.8385E+03 | 1.8364E+03 | 1.1429E−01 |
| | 2.3019E−03 | 4.5150E+02 | 4.5333E+02 | 4.5387E+02 | 1.1827E−01 |
| | 2.6497E−03 | 3.1991E+02 | 3.2300E+02 | 3.2213E+02 | 2.6888E−01 |
| 86.Rn | 2.5738E−02 | 4.2299E−01 | 6.7143E−01 | 5.4681E−01 | 2.2792E+01 |
| | 5.6549E−02 | 5.1449E−02 | 2.4649E−01 | 6.2427E−02 | 2.9485E+02 |
| 104. | 1.9637E−03 | 6.9259E+02 | 6.9490E+02 | 6.9475E+02 | 2.1014E−02 |
| | 2.0081E−03 | 6.3096E+02 | 6.3311E+02 | 6.3294E+02 | 2.6268E−02 |
| | 2.8518E−03 | 2.5960E+02 | 2.6221E+02 | 2.6099E+02 | 4.6968E−01 |
| 107. | 1.1190E−03 | 3.1347E+03 | 3.1444E+03 | 3.1437E+03 | 2.2149E−02 |
| | 1.4672E−03 | 1.5079E+03 | 1.5120E+03 | 1.5125E+03 | 3.4797E−02 |
| 109. | 1.1752E−03 | 2.7415E+03 | 2.7500E+03 | 2.7494E+03 | 2.1871E−02 |
| | 1.4211E−03 | 1.6446E+03 | 1.6497E+03 | 1.6488E+03 | 5.3341E−02 |
| 119. | 1.1765E−03 | 2.7318E+03 | 2.7402E+03 | 2.7399E+03 | 1.3366E−02 |
| | 1.4165E−03 | 1.6600E+03 | 1.6652E+03 | 1.6645E+03 | 4.1304E−02 |
| 120. | 1.0822E−03 | 3.4087E+03 | 3.4192E+03 | 3.4197E+03 | 1.5837E−02 |
| | 1.4928E−03 | 1.4363E+03 | 1.4404E+03 | 1.4395E+03 | 6.3262E−02 |
| | 5.5333E−03 | 3.6247E+01 | 3.7042E+01 | 3.7019E+01 | 6.2415E−02 |
| 128. | 1.1302E−03 | 3.0564E+03 | 3.0658E+03 | 3.0650E+03 | 2.6828E−02 |
| | 1.4607E−03 | 1.5262E+03 | 1.5303E+03 | 1.5299E+03 | 2.5548E−02 |
| 131. | 1.1599E−03 | 2.8482E+03 | 2.8569E+03 | 2.8565E+03 | 1.4359E−02 |

| Material | $E$, MeV | $\mu_{1en}$, cm$^{-1}$ | $\mu_1$, cm$^{-1}$ | $\mu_2$, cm$^{-1}$ | $R$, % |
|---|---|---|---|---|---|
| | 1.4382E−03 | 1.5889E+03 | 1.5930E+03 | 1.5938E+03 | 5.2591E−02 |
| 132. | 1.1190E−03 | 3.1346E+03 | 3.1443E+03 | 3.1435E+03 | 2.4845E−02 |
| | 1.4676E−03 | 1.5067E+03 | 1.5108E+03 | 1.5113E+03 | 3.1576E−02 |
| 137. | 1.0433E−03 | 3.7755E+03 | 3.7874E+03 | 3.7833E+03 | 1.0692E−01 |
| | 1.4602E−03 | 1.5275E+03 | 1.5316E+03 | 1.5311E+03 | 3.5215E−02 |
| | 2.2750E−03 | 4.6794E+02 | 4.6980E+02 | 4.6968E+02 | 2.5704E−02 |
| | 2.6245E−03 | 3.2744E+02 | 3.3058E+02 | 3.2894E+02 | 4.9975E−01 |
| 143. | 1.1355E−03 | 3.0192E+03 | 3.0285E+03 | 3.0286E+03 | 5.8041E−04 |
| | 1.4577E−03 | 1.5345E+03 | 1.5386E+03 | 1.5383E+03 | 1.8220E−02 |
| 144. | 1.1491E−03 | 2.9237E+03 | 2.9327E+03 | 2.9323E+03 | 1.4570E−02 |
| | 1.4467E−03 | 1.5652E+03 | 1.5693E+03 | 1.5701E+03 | 4.9727E−02 |
| 145. | 1.0838E−03 | 3.3930E+03 | 3.4035E+03 | 3.4026E+03 | 2.3886E−02 |
| | 1.4414E−03 | 1.5799E+03 | 1.5840E+03 | 1.5838E+03 | 1.1569E−02 |
| | 2.2895E−03 | 4.5912E+02 | 4.6096E+02 | 4.6078E+02 | 3.8791E−02 |
| | 2.6159E−03 | 3.3002E+02 | 3.3319E+02 | 3.3143E+02 | 5.3040E−01 |
| 148. | 1.0294E−03 | 3.9069E+03 | 3.9192E+03 | 3.9193E+03 | 2.6412E−03 |
| | 1.4829E−03 | 1.4640E+03 | 1.4681E+03 | 1.4683E+03 | 1.2755E−02 |
| | 2.1106E−03 | 5.6835E+02 | 5.7039E+02 | 5.7035E+02 | 7.3412E−03 |
| | 2.8107E−03 | 2.7188E+02 | 2.7459E+02 | 2.7325E+02 | 4.8995E−01 |
| | | | 116.CESIUM IODIDE | | |
| 24.Cr | 1.8332E−03 | 1.2522E+04 | 1.2570E+04 | 1.2562E+04 | 5.9064E−02 |
| 25.Mn | 3.4804E−03 | 2.6480E+03 | 2.6777E+03 | 2.6720E+03 | 2.1381E−01 |
| | 4.5424E−03 | 1.2288E+03 | 1.2541E+03 | 1.2480E+03 | 4.8765E−01 |
| 28.Ni | 3.7740E−02 | 4.5405E+01 | 1.2213E+02 | 5.2499E+01 | 1.3263E+02 |
| 29.Cu | 4.7080E−03 | 2.0816E+03 | 2.1819E+03 | 2.1133E+03 | 3.2478E+00 |
| | 3.8465E−02 | 4.4431E+01 | 1.1618E+02 | 5.1893E+01 | 1.2388E+02 |
| 30.Zn | 1.0343E−03 | 3.8760E+04 | 3.8850E+04 | 3.9072E+04 | 5.7286E−01 |
| | 3.6325E−02 | 4.7304E+01 | 1.3373E+02 | 5.5931E+01 | 1.3909E+02 |
| 31.Ga | 1.1421E−03 | 3.3058E+04 | 3.3135E+04 | 3.3371E+04 | 7.1078E−01 |
| 32.Ge | 1.1494E−02 | 5.8747E+02 | 6.1942E+02 | 9.9753E+02 | 6.1043E+01 |
| 34.Se | 1.4335E−02 | 3.1189E+02 | 3.2997E+02 | 5.3585E+02 | 6.2393E+01 |
| 38.Sr | 2.4616E−03 | 6.7344E+03 | 6.7735E+03 | 6.8677E+03 | 1.3912E+00 |
| | 2.9327E−02 | 4.1530E+01 | 4.6204E+01 | 6.2021E+01 | 3.4235E+01 |
| 39.Y | 3.6467E−02 | 4.7114E+01 | 1.3256E+02 | 6.7569E+01 | 9.6191E+01 |
| 40.Zr | 5.1319E−02 | 2.8553E+01 | 5.5101E+01 | 3.8078E+01 | 4.4705E+01 |
| 41.Nb | 1.2127E−03 | 2.9104E+04 | 2.9172E+04 | 2.9165E+04 | 2.3706E−02 |
| | 5.8568E−03 | 2.8954E+03 | 3.0934E+03 | 2.9592E+03 | 4.5360E+00 |
| 42.Mo | 2.1128E−03 | 8.8160E+03 | 8.8597E+03 | 8.8783E+03 | 2.1029E−01 |
| 59.Pr | 3.6140E−02 | 4.7552E+01 | 1.3524E+02 | 5.3766E+01 | 1.5153E+02 |

| Material | $E$, MeV | $\mu_{1en}$, cm$^{-1}$ | $\mu_1$, cm$^{-1}$ | $\mu_2$, cm$^{-1}$ | $R$, % |
|---|---|---|---|---|---|
| 60.Nd | 3.7382E−02 | 4.5885E+01 | 1.2506E+02 | 5.2114E+01 | 1.3997E+02 |
| 61.Pm | 1.0478E−03 | 3.7739E+04 | 3.7825E+04 | 3.7929E+04 | 2.7548E−01 |
| | 3.8932E−02 | 4.3805E+01 | 1.1235E+02 | 5.0095E+01 | 1.2428E+02 |
| 62.Sm | 1.1003E−03 | 3.5854E+04 | 3.5936E+04 | 3.6052E+04 | 3.2403E−01 |
| | 3.9701E−02 | 4.2773E+01 | 1.0605E+02 | 4.9088E+01 | 1.1604E+02 |
| 64.Gd | 1.2142E−03 | 2.9015E+04 | 2.9083E+04 | 2.9214E+04 | 4.4971E−01 |
| | 4.5612E−02 | 3.5288E+01 | 7.8033E+01 | 4.1098E+01 | 8.9871E+01 |
| 65.Tb | 1.2568E−03 | 2.8015E+04 | 2.8084E+04 | 2.8230E+04 | 5.2000E−01 |
| | 4.8622E−02 | 3.1487E+01 | 6.4319E+01 | 3.7098E+01 | 7.3378E+01 |
| 66.Dy | 1.3097E−03 | 2.5962E+04 | 2.6028E+04 | 2.6182E+04 | 5.9072E−01 |
| | 5.1297E−02 | 2.8572E+01 | 5.5149E+01 | 3.4013E+01 | 6.2141E+01 |
| 67.Ho | 1.3630E−03 | 2.3895E+04 | 2.3958E+04 | 2.4106E+04 | 6.1879E−01 |
| | 5.5315E−02 | 2.4930E+01 | 4.6180E+01 | 3.0064E+01 | 5.3607E+01 |
| 68.Er | 1.4164E−03 | 2.1822E+04 | 2.1881E+04 | 2.2027E+04 | 6.6418E−01 |
| 68.Er | 5.6671E−03 | 2.9162E+03 | 3.1155E+03 | 2.9830E+03 | 4.4445E+00 |
| 69.Tm | 1.4711E−03 | 1.9700E+04 | 1.9756E+04 | 1.9895E+04 | 7.0195E−01 |
| | 5.7324E−03 | 3.0430E+03 | 3.2544E+03 | 3.1139E+03 | 4.5128E+00 |
| 70.Yb | 1.5450E−03 | 1.7762E+04 | 1.7815E+04 | 1.7971E+04 | 8.7311E−01 |
| | 4.9147E−02 | 3.0824E+01 | 6.1928E+01 | 3.6202E+01 | 7.1060E+01 |
| 71.Lu | 1.5934E−03 | 1.6883E+04 | 1.6935E+04 | 1.7065E+04 | 7.6703E−01 |
| 88.Ra | 5.9806E−03 | 2.7484E+03 | 2.9331E+03 | 2.8368E+03 | 3.3955E+00 |
| | 6.4222E−03 | 2.4268E+03 | 2.5866E+03 | 2.5063E+03 | 3.2008E+00 |
| 112. | 3.4307E−03 | 2.7384E+03 | 2.7683E+03 | 2.7761E+03 | 2.8207E−01 |
| | 2.4128E−02 | 8.1125E+01 | 8.7970E+01 | 8.8665E+01 | 7.9022E−01 |
| 113. | 4.2079E−03 | 1.5212E+03 | 1.5476E+03 | 1.7228E+03 | 1.1322E+01 |
| 121. | 3.8599E−02 | 4.4252E+01 | 1.1508E+02 | 5.0523E+01 | 1.2778E+02 |
| 123. | 1.2251E−02 | 5.1408E+02 | 5.4233E+02 | 8.4505E+02 | 5.5818E+01 |
| 125. | 5.6594E−02 | 2.3770E+01 | 4.3326E+01 | 2.8757E+01 | 5.0662E+01 |
| 130. | 2.2314E−03 | 8.1081E+03 | 8.1501E+03 | 8.1717E+03 | 2.6412E−01 |
| | 1.2252E−02 | 5.1393E+02 | 5.4218E+02 | 5.4326E+02 | 1.9877E−01 |
| 134. | 2.7229E−02 | 5.7508E+01 | 6.3058E+01 | 1.1904E+02 | 8.8786E+01 |
| 117.CONCRETE, ORDINARY | | | | | |
| 11.Na | 1.1737E−03 | 5.4061E+03 | 5.4227E+03 | 5.5011E+03 | 1.4457E+00 |
| 20.Ca | 1.0447E−03 | 7.0976E+03 | 7.1165E+03 | 7.1066E+03 | 1.4018E−01 |
| | 1.4501E−03 | 3.1375E+03 | 3.1479E+03 | 3.1440E+03 | 1.2300E−01 |
| 113. | 1.8604E−03 | 3.5723E+03 | 3.6707E+03 | 3.5870E+03 | 2.3347E+00 |
| 124. | 1.1861E−03 | 5.2465E+03 | 5.2625E+03 | 5.2652E+03 | 5.1254E−02 |
| | 1.3764E−03 | 3.6173E+03 | 3.6295E+03 | 3.6301E+03 | 1.8418E−02 |
| 127. | 1.4841E−03 | 2.9166E+03 | 2.9262E+03 | 2.9268E+03 | 2.2243E−02 |

| Material | $E$, MeV | $\mu_{1en}$, cm$^{-1}$ | $\mu_1$, cm$^{-1}$ | $\mu_2$, cm$^{-1}$ | $R$, % |
|---|---|---|---|---|---|
| | 1.5412E−03 | 2.6175E+03 | 2.6267E+03 | 2.6268E+03 | 4.4985E−03 |
| | 1.6927E−03 | 2.1573E+03 | 2.1697E+03 | 2.1650E+03 | 2.1946E−01 |
| | 1.7069E−03 | 2.1139E+03 | 2.1261E+03 | 2.1214E+03 | 2.1908E−01 |
| 129. | 1.1335E−03 | 5.9687E+03 | 5.9879E+03 | 5.9843E+03 | 5.8837E−02 |
| | 1.1518E−03 | 5.7117E+03 | 5.7297E+03 | 5.7267E+03 | 5.2352E−02 |
| | 1.2932E−03 | 4.1859E+03 | 4.1999E+03 | 4.1988E+03 | 2.8305E−02 |
| 133. | 1.9652E−03 | 3.1921E+03 | 3.2771E+03 | 3.2243E+03 | 1.6365E+00 |
| | 2.5628E−03 | 1.9295E+03 | 1.9769E+03 | 1.9499E+03 | 1.3826E+00 |
| | 3.3023E−03 | 8.4079E+02 | 8.5772E+02 | 8.5141E+02 | 7.4130E−01 |
| 141. | 2.9334E−03 | 1.1814E+03 | 1.2069E+03 | 1.2762E+03 | 5.7369E+00 |
| | 5.7198E−03 | 2.2087E+02 | 2.2937E+02 | 2.3128E+02 | 8.3168E−01 |
| | 7.9973E−03 | 8.4951E+01 | 8.9303E+01 | 8.8388E+01 | 1.0348E+00 |
| | 8.1319E−03 | 8.2190E+01 | 8.6415E+01 | 8.5519E+01 | 1.0471E+00 |
| | 5.8920E−02 | 2.3483E−01 | 6.3047E−01 | 4.8623E−01 | 2.9667E+01 |
| | | 118.CONCRETE, BARITE (TYPE AA) | | | |
| 13.Al | 2.9134E−03 | 2.4212E+03 | 2.4669E+03 | 2.4715E+03 | 1.8481E−01 |
| 14.Si | 3.5188E−03 | 1.6021E+03 | 1.6332E+03 | 1.6444E+03 | 6.8979E−01 |
| 21.Sc | 5.9787E−03 | 1.0509E+03 | 1.1284E+03 | 1.1907E+03 | 5.5230E+00 |
| 22.Ti | 1.4833E−03 | 1.0064E+04 | 1.0095E+04 | 1.0087E+04 | 7.6386E−02 |
| | 1.5561E−03 | 8.9288E+03 | 8.9590E+03 | 8.9508E+03 | 9.1188E−02 |
| | 1.5779E−03 | 8.7095E+03 | 8.7392E+03 | 8.7312E+03 | 9.1424E−02 |
| | 2.3736E−03 | 3.3527E+03 | 3.3734E+03 | 3.3677E+03 | 1.6968E−01 |
| 23.V | 3.8119E−03 | 1.2641E+03 | 1.2894E+03 | 1.2795E+03 | 7.7124E−01 |
| | 3.8675E−02 | 1.5403E+01 | 4.3548E+01 | 1.7607E+01 | 1.4733E+02 |
| 24.Cr | 4.6535E−02 | 1.2171E+01 | 2.8359E+01 | 1.4378E+01 | 9.7240E+01 |
| 25.Mn | 4.9761E−02 | 1.0839E+01 | 2.2762E+01 | 1.3011E+01 | 7.4950E+01 |
| 26.Fe | 5.9697E−02 | 7.6866E+00 | 1.4136E+01 | 9.6680E+00 | 4.6213E+01 |
| 29.Cu | 5.8474E−03 | 1.1116E+03 | 1.1947E+03 | 1.1373E+03 | 5.0474E+00 |
| 37.Rb | 2.9374E−03 | 2.3600E+03 | 2.4046E+03 | 2.3968E+03 | 3.2422E−01 |
| | 1.9261E−02 | 6.0246E+01 | 6.5078E+01 | 1.0600E+02 | 6.2883E+01 |
| 38.Sr | 4.9224E−02 | 1.1060E+01 | 2.3693E+01 | 1.4366E+01 | 6.4926E+01 |
| 39.Y | 7.4493E−03 | 7.2496E+02 | 7.8616E+02 | 7.4274E+02 | 5.8464E+00 |
| 55.Cs | 7.5738E−03 | 6.9601E+02 | 7.5421E+02 | 7.4156E+02 | 1.7056E+00 |
| 61.Pm | 1.0274E−03 | 1.9919E+04 | 1.9973E+04 | 2.0022E+04 | 2.4404E−01 |
| 63.Eu | 1.1428E−03 | 1.7678E+04 | 1.7727E+04 | 1.7786E+04 | 3.3054E−01 |
| 64.Gd | 1.1888E−03 | 1.6218E+04 | 1.6264E+04 | 1.6322E+04 | 3.5748E−01 |
| 70.Yb | 1.0412E−03 | 1.9306E+04 | 1.9358E+04 | 1.9379E+04 | 1.0848E−01 |
| | 1.2129E−03 | 1.5455E+04 | 1.5499E+04 | 1.5526E+04 | 1.7854E−01 |
| 121. | 1.1917E−03 | 1.6126E+04 | 1.6172E+04 | 1.6220E+04 | 3.0052E−01 |

| Material | $E$, MeV | $\mu_{1en}$, cm$^{-1}$ | $\mu_1$, cm$^{-1}$ | $\mu_2$, cm$^{-1}$ | $R$, % |
|---|---|---|---|---|---|
| 123. | 1.1330E−03 | 1.7337E+04 | 1.7387E+04 | 1.7471E+04 | 4.8223E−01 |
| | 1.1369E−03 | 1.7866E+04 | 1.7917E+04 | 1.8007E+04 | 5.0199E−01 |
| 133. | 5.0618E−03 | 6.4124E+02 | 6.6570E+02 | 6.6121E+02 | 6.7812E−01 |
| | 2.9471E−02 | 1.8291E+01 | 2.0545E+01 | 3.5212E+01 | 7.1392E+01 |
| 119.EYE LENS (ICRU-44) | | | | | |
| 5.B | 5.1421E−02 | 4.0975E−02 | 2.3338E−01 | 3.9184E−01 | 6.7897E+01 |
| 6.C | 1.0191E−03 | 3.6570E+03 | 3.6677E+03 | 3.6604E+03 | 1.9849E−01 |
| | 1.3519E−03 | 1.9485E+03 | 1.9540E+03 | 1.9510E+03 | 1.5319E−01 |
| | 2.2085E−03 | 4.3760E+02 | 4.3944E+02 | 4.3919E+02 | 5.6186E−02 |
| | 2.8063E−03 | 2.2216E+02 | 2.2378E+02 | 2.2345E+02 | 1.4577E−01 |
| | 5.3386E−02 | 3.9028E−02 | 2.2926E−01 | 3.1128E−01 | 3.5774E+01 |
| 14.Si | 1.0414E−03 | 3.4516E+03 | 3.4610E+03 | 3.4585E+03 | 7.4637E−02 |
| | 1.3719E−03 | 1.8594E+03 | 1.8645E+03 | 1.8653E+03 | 4.3878E−02 |
| 19.K | 2.0255E−03 | 5.5607E+02 | 5.5798E+02 | 5.5856E+02 | 1.0422E−01 |
| | 3.1933E−03 | 1.6358E+02 | 1.6499E+02 | 1.6557E+02 | 3.5501E−01 |
| 86.Rn | 1.8279E−02 | 8.0743E−01 | 1.0908E+00 | 1.0947E+00 | 3.5059E−01 |
| 101. | 2.8191E−02 | 2.2109E−01 | 4.5825E−01 | 4.6544E−01 | 1.5678E+00 |
| 104. | 1.9276E−02 | 6.4889E−01 | 9.2445E−01 | 9.9945E−01 | 8.1130E+00 |
| | 2.3775E−02 | 3.8963E−01 | 6.4442E−01 | 7.1563E−01 | 1.1050E+01 |
| 107. | 3.4033E−03 | 1.4149E+02 | 1.4278E+02 | 1.4290E+02 | 8.3538E−02 |
| 107. | 3.7533E−03 | 1.0464E+02 | 1.0576E+02 | 1.0612E+02 | 3.3716E−01 |
| | 6.9130E−03 | 1.6941E+01 | 1.7494E+01 | 1.7534E+01 | 2.3185E−01 |
| | 7.2510E−03 | 1.4645E+01 | 1.5173E+01 | 1.5309E+01 | 8.9568E−01 |
| 109. | 3.2317E−03 | 1.5955E+02 | 1.6093E+02 | 1.6122E+02 | 1.8154E−01 |
| | 3.8259E−03 | 9.7003E+01 | 9.8086E+01 | 9.8557E+01 | 4.8039E−01 |
| 115. | 1.1765E−03 | 2.7318E+03 | 2.7399E+03 | 2.7402E+03 | 1.3366E−02 |
| | 1.4165E−03 | 1.6600E+03 | 1.6645E+03 | 1.6652E+03 | 4.1304E−02 |
| 122. | 2.3813E−03 | 3.5256E+02 | 3.5417E+02 | 3.5397E+02 | 5.6937E−02 |
| | 2.6585E−03 | 2.5982E+02 | 2.6152E+02 | 2.6112E+02 | 1.5269E−01 |
| 128. | 3.4222E−03 | 1.3949E+02 | 1.4078E+02 | 1.4094E+02 | 1.1820E−01 |
| | 3.7343E−03 | 1.0664E+02 | 1.0777E+02 | 1.0813E+02 | 3.3537E−01 |
| 131. | 3.1905E−03 | 1.6388E+02 | 1.6529E+02 | 1.6540E+02 | 6.8454E−02 |
| | 3.8215E−03 | 9.7462E+01 | 9.8547E+01 | 9.9047E+01 | 5.0707E−01 |
| 132. | 3.4032E−03 | 1.4150E+02 | 1.4279E+02 | 1.4290E+02 | 7.4215E−02 |
| | 3.7521E−03 | 1.0477E+02 | 1.0589E+02 | 1.0616E+02 | 2.5399E−01 |
| 137. | 2.9632E−03 | 1.9129E+02 | 1.9283E+02 | 1.9256E+02 | 1.4279E−01 |
| | 4.9631E−02 | 4.3354E−02 | 2.3787E−01 | 2.8021E−01 | 1.7799E+01 |
| 138. | 2.3876E−03 | 3.4988E+02 | 3.5149E+02 | 3.5120E+02 | 8.2134E−02 |
| | 2.6576E−03 | 2.6005E+02 | 2.6175E+02 | 2.6121E+02 | 2.0929E−01 |

| Material | $E$, MeV | $\mu_{1en}$, cm$^{-1}$ | $\mu_1$, cm$^{-1}$ | $\mu_2$, cm$^{-1}$ | $R$, % |
|---|---|---|---|---|---|
| 141. | 2.1966E−03 | 4.4416E+02 | 4.4602E+02 | 4.4663E+02 | 1.3608E−01 |
| | 2.6774E−03 | 2.5502E+02 | 2.5671E+02 | 2.5732E+02 | 2.3702E−01 |
| 143. | 3.3106E−03 | 1.5124E+02 | 1.5258E+02 | 1.5259E+02 | 3.5801E−03 |
| | 3.8185E−03 | 9.7779E+01 | 9.8865E+01 | 9.9106E+01 | 2.4377E−01 |
| 144. | 3.3286E−03 | 1.4934E+02 | 1.5068E+02 | 1.5086E+02 | 1.2114E−01 |
| | 3.7703E−03 | 1.0286E+02 | 1.0397E+02 | 1.0443E+02 | 4.4037E−01 |
| 145. | 1.0048E−03 | 3.7939E+03 | 3.8054E+03 | 3.8048E+03 | 1.4688E−02 |
| | 1.4930E−03 | 1.3183E+03 | 1.3217E+03 | 1.3215E+03 | 1.5362E−02 |
| | 2.0024E−03 | 5.7265E+02 | 5.7457E+02 | 5.7454E+02 | 4.5361E−03 |
| | 2.9702E−03 | 1.8990E+02 | 1.9144E+02 | 1.9103E+02 | 2.1468E−01 |
| 148. | 4.8393E−02 | 4.6608E−02 | 2.4292E−01 | 2.3355E−01 | 4.0082E+00 |
| 120.FERROUS SULFATE (STANDARD FRICKE) | | | | | |
| 5.B | 5.5839E−02 | 4.0378E−02 | 2.2304E−01 | 3.8326E−01 | 7.1834E+01 |
| 6.C | 5.9315E−02 | 3.6014E−02 | 2.1482E−01 | 2.9938E−01 | 3.9367E+01 |
| 19.K | 2.2780E−03 | 4.6054E+02 | 4.6233E+02 | 4.6292E+02 | 1.2794E−01 |
| | 2.8474E−03 | 2.4512E+02 | 2.4753E+02 | 2.4725E+02 | 1.1314E−01 |
| 86.Rn | 1.9841E−02 | 6.6962E−01 | 9.3921E−01 | 8.8806E−01 | 5.7602E+00 |
| 104. | 2.9241E−03 | 2.2780E+02 | 2.3008E+02 | 2.2914E+02 | 4.1291E−01 |
| | 5.3016E−02 | 4.3921E−02 | 2.2972E−01 | 2.9198E−01 | 2.7106E+01 |
| 107. | 5.6039E−02 | 4.0127E−02 | 2.2257E−01 | 2.2732E−01 | 2.1363E+00 |
| 109. | 6.8155E−03 | 1.9018E+01 | 1.9614E+01 | 1.9641E+01 | 1.3905E−01 |
| | 7.5237E−03 | 1.3858E+01 | 1.4398E+01 | 1.4408E+01 | 7.0230E−02 |
| 115. | 1.0822E−03 | 3.4087E+03 | 3.4197E+03 | 3.4192E+03 | 1.5837E−02 |
| 115. | 1.4928E−03 | 1.4363E+03 | 1.4395E+03 | 1.4404E+03 | 6.3262E−02 |
| | 5.5333E−03 | 3.6247E+01 | 3.7019E+01 | 3.7042E+01 | 6.2415E−02 |
| 128. | 6.6357E−03 | 2.0783E+01 | 2.1399E+01 | 2.1416E+01 | 7.9882E−02 |
| | 7.6761E−03 | 1.3022E+01 | 1.3549E+01 | 1.3556E+01 | 4.9459E−02 |
| 131. | 6.8167E−03 | 1.9006E+01 | 1.9602E+01 | 1.9642E+01 | 2.0143E−01 |
| | 7.5213E−03 | 1.3871E+01 | 1.4411E+01 | 1.4429E+01 | 1.2470E−01 |
| 132. | 6.6975E−03 | 2.0176E+01 | 2.0785E+01 | 2.0793E+01 | 3.6476E−02 |
| | 7.6245E−03 | 1.3305E+01 | 1.3837E+01 | 1.3834E+01 | 2.2322E−02 |
| 137. | 1.0294E−03 | 3.8503E+03 | 3.8628E+03 | 3.8583E+03 | 1.1616E−01 |
| | 1.3489E−03 | 2.1277E+03 | 2.1337E+03 | 2.1325E+03 | 5.8526E−02 |
| | 2.2474E−03 | 4.7903E+02 | 4.8085E+02 | 4.8079E+02 | 1.3958E−02 |
| | 2.7971E−03 | 2.5805E+02 | 2.6055E+02 | 2.5944E+02 | 4.3114E−01 |
| 143. | 6.8494E−03 | 1.8686E+01 | 1.9278E+01 | 1.9284E+01 | 3.1344E−02 |
| | 7.4793E−03 | 1.4101E+01 | 1.4645E+01 | 1.4642E+01 | 2.1709E−02 |
| 144. | 6.7024E−03 | 2.0128E+01 | 2.0737E+01 | 2.0770E+01 | 1.5850E−01 |
| | 7.6264E−03 | 1.3294E+01 | 1.3826E+01 | 1.3845E+01 | 1.3607E−01 |

| Material | $E$, MeV | $\mu_{1en}$, cm$^{-1}$ | $\mu_1$, cm$^{-1}$ | $\mu_2$, cm$^{-1}$ | $R$, % |
|---|---|---|---|---|---|
| 145. | 2.2632E−03 | 4.6950E+02 | 4.7131E+02 | 4.7119E+02 | 2.5123E−02 |
| | 2.7997E−03 | 2.5730E+02 | 2.5980E+02 | 2.5856E+02 | 4.7796E−01 |
| 148. | 1.0178E−03 | 3.9691E+03 | 3.9819E+03 | 3.9818E+03 | 2.9553E−03 |
| | 1.4488E−03 | 1.6478E+03 | 1.6518E+03 | 1.6527E+03 | 5.2631E−02 |
| | 2.0738E−03 | 5.8396E+02 | 5.8601E+02 | 5.8599E+02 | 3.5518E−03 |
| | 2.9041E−03 | 2.3231E+02 | 2.3463E+02 | 2.3360E+02 | 4.4093E−01 |
| | 7.0817E−03 | 1.6405E+01 | 1.6972E+01 | 1.6922E+01 | 2.9289E−01 |
| | 7.1584E−03 | 1.5863E+01 | 1.6433E+01 | 1.6375E+01 | 3.5351E−01 |
| 121.GADOLINIUM OXYSULFIDE | | | | | |
| 22.Ti | 1.2037E−03 | 1.9634E+04 | 1.9755E+04 | 1.9667E+04 | 4.4618E−01 |
| 24.Cr | 1.3110E−03 | 3.2053E+04 | 3.2269E+04 | 3.2130E+04 | 4.3062E−01 |
| 25.Mn | 1.3676E−03 | 3.2171E+04 | 3.2386E+04 | 3.2267E+04 | 3.6956E−01 |
| 26.Fe | 1.4368E−03 | 3.2314E+04 | 3.2530E+04 | 3.2423E+04 | 3.3077E−01 |
| 28.Ni | 1.7936E−03 | 2.6143E+04 | 2.6312E+04 | 2.6268E+04 | 1.6598E−01 |
| 29.Cu | 2.4069E−03 | 1.4092E+04 | 1.4196E+04 | 1.4177E+04 | 1.3395E−01 |
| | 2.9533E−02 | 9.1515E+01 | 1.0175E+02 | 1.0741E+02 | 5.5566E+00 |
| | 3.1133E−02 | 7.8501E+01 | 8.7660E+01 | 9.1691E+01 | 4.5991E+00 |
| 31.Ga | 1.4578E−03 | 3.2358E+04 | 3.2574E+04 | 3.2642E+04 | 2.0767E−01 |
| 32.Ge | 1.3548E−03 | 3.2144E+04 | 3.2360E+04 | 3.2495E+04 | 4.1783E−01 |
| | 1.4306E−03 | 3.2302E+04 | 3.2517E+04 | 3.2642E+04 | 3.8255E−01 |
| 33.As | 1.4219E−03 | 3.2283E+04 | 3.2499E+04 | 3.2692E+04 | 5.9298E−01 |
| 39.Y | 1.1332E−03 | 1.4416E+04 | 1.4487E+04 | 1.4446E+04 | 2.8296E−01 |
| 40.Zr | 1.2052E−03 | 2.0461E+04 | 2.0588E+04 | 2.0504E+04 | 4.0949E−01 |
| | 2.4937E−02 | 1.6850E+02 | 1.8503E+02 | 3.1821E+02 | 7.1983E+01 |
| 41.Nb | 5.6769E−02 | 3.1158E+01 | 8.7146E+01 | 4.1786E+01 | 1.0855E+02 |
| 42.Mo | 1.2985E−03 | 3.2027E+04 | 3.2243E+04 | 3.2099E+04 | 4.4931E−01 |
| 42.Mo | 7.3503E−03 | 2.1442E+03 | 2.3885E+03 | 2.1997E+03 | 8.5799E+00 |
| 43.Tc | 1.3902E−03 | 3.2218E+04 | 3.2433E+04 | 3.2301E+04 | 4.1092E−01 |
| 44.Ru | 1.4464E−03 | 3.2334E+04 | 3.2550E+04 | 3.2424E+04 | 3.8931E−01 |
| 45.Rh | 1.4744E−03 | 3.2393E+04 | 3.2608E+04 | 3.2481E+04 | 3.9291E−01 |
| 46.Pd | 1.4841E−03 | 3.2413E+04 | 3.2629E+04 | 3.2509E+04 | 3.6672E−01 |
| 47.Ag | 1.4646E−03 | 3.2372E+04 | 3.2588E+04 | 3.2458E+04 | 4.0137E−01 |
| 48.Cd | 1.4087E−03 | 3.2256E+04 | 3.2472E+04 | 3.2335E+04 | 4.2160E−01 |
| 49.In | 1.3633E−03 | 3.2162E+04 | 3.2378E+04 | 3.2234E+04 | 4.4666E−01 |
| | 7.8640E−03 | 1.8098E+03 | 2.0048E+03 | 1.8811E+03 | 6.5753E+00 |
| 50.Sn | 1.3848E−03 | 3.2206E+04 | 3.2422E+04 | 3.2279E+04 | 4.4374E−01 |
| 51.Sb | 1.3695E−03 | 3.2175E+04 | 3.2390E+04 | 3.2249E+04 | 4.3991E−01 |
| | 7.8697E−03 | 1.8063E+03 | 2.0004E+03 | 1.8885E+03 | 5.9222E+00 |
| | 5.9389E−02 | 2.9699E+01 | 7.5693E+01 | 4.7793E+01 | 5.8377E+01 |

| Material | $E$, MeV | $\mu_{1en}$, cm$^{-1}$ | $\mu_1$, cm$^{-1}$ | $\mu_2$, cm$^{-1}$ | $R$, % |
|---|---|---|---|---|---|
| 52.Te | 1.3488E−03 | 3.2132E+04 | 3.2347E+04 | 3.2206E+04 | 4.4063E−01 |
| | 7.5699E−03 | 1.9905E+03 | 2.2338E+03 | 2.0912E+03 | 6.8191E+00 |
| | 5.6474E−02 | 3.1323E+01 | 8.8438E+01 | 5.3637E+01 | 6.4882E+01 |
| 53.I | 1.2431E−03 | 3.1912E+04 | 3.2128E+04 | 3.1984E+04 | 4.4952E−01 |
| | 3.6756E−02 | 5.2708E+01 | 5.9692E+01 | 1.4108E+02 | 1.3635E+02 |
| 56.Ba | 1.2117E−03 | 2.3968E+04 | 2.4119E+04 | 2.4038E+04 | 3.3595E−01 |
| | 4.7301E−02 | 2.5049E+01 | 2.9540E+01 | 5.8449E+01 | 9.7866E+01 |
| 57.La | 1.4391E−03 | 3.2319E+04 | 3.2535E+04 | 3.2429E+04 | 3.2605E−01 |
| | 5.9838E−02 | 2.9449E+01 | 7.3734E+01 | 5.5703E+01 | 3.2370E+01 |
| 59.Pr | 1.6016E−03 | 3.1928E+04 | 3.2141E+04 | 3.2059E+04 | 2.5404E−01 |
| | 2.4543E−03 | 1.3253E+04 | 1.3351E+04 | 1.3328E+04 | 1.7738E−01 |
| 60.Nd | 2.2832E−03 | 1.6284E+04 | 1.6401E+04 | 1.6371E+04 | 1.8768E−01 |
| | 8.8558E−03 | 2.1034E+03 | 2.3682E+03 | 2.2952E+03 | 3.1822E+00 |
| 61.Pm | 2.8593E−03 | 1.0226E+04 | 1.0360E+04 | 1.0305E+04 | 5.3942E−01 |
| | 4.2244E−02 | 3.3898E+01 | 3.9246E+01 | 3.9345E+01 | 2.5126E−01 |
| 62.Sm | 2.9953E−03 | 8.8918E+03 | 9.0114E+03 | 8.9667E+03 | 4.9835E−01 |
| | 5.4593E−03 | 2.0330E+03 | 2.0799E+03 | 2.0784E+03 | 7.1573E−02 |
| | 6.0289E−03 | 1.5203E+03 | 1.5617E+03 | 1.5619E+03 | 9.7235E−03 |
| 63.Eu | 1.1349E−03 | 1.4372E+04 | 1.4443E+04 | 1.4461E+04 | 1.2214E−01 |
| | 1.3288E−03 | 3.2090E+04 | 3.2306E+04 | 3.2285E+04 | 6.4937E−02 |
| 64.Gd | 1.1697E−03 | 1.3468E+04 | 1.3537E+04 | 1.3549E+04 | 8.9485E−02 |
| 65.Tb | 1.2625E−03 | 3.1952E+04 | 3.2168E+04 | 3.2200E+04 | 1.0107E−01 |
| 66.Dy | 1.1885E−03 | 1.5422E+04 | 1.5510E+04 | 1.5508E+04 | 1.6600E−02 |
| | 1.3200E−03 | 3.2072E+04 | 3.2287E+04 | 3.2349E+04 | 1.8943E−01 |
| 67.Ho | 1.1931E−03 | 1.6448E+04 | 1.6544E+04 | 1.6536E+04 | 5.2656E−02 |
| | 1.3789E−03 | 3.2194E+04 | 3.2410E+04 | 3.2495E+04 | 2.6400E−01 |
| 68.Er | 1.1982E−03 | 1.7576E+04 | 1.7682E+04 | 1.7676E+04 | 3.6176E−02 |
| | 1.4393E−03 | 3.2320E+04 | 3.2535E+04 | 3.2657E+04 | 3.7279E−01 |
| | 5.0649E−02 | 3.4569E+01 | 1.1390E+02 | 4.0911E+01 | 1.7842E+02 |
| 69.Tm | 1.2023E−03 | 1.8861E+04 | 1.8977E+04 | 1.8963E+04 | 7.0521E−02 |
| | 1.4933E−03 | 3.2432E+04 | 3.2648E+04 | 3.2799E+04 | 4.6418E−01 |
| | 5.3533E−02 | 3.2962E+01 | 1.0129E+02 | 3.9245E+01 | 1.5810E+02 |
| 70.Yb | 1.1909E−03 | 1.5950E+04 | 1.6042E+04 | 1.6021E+04 | 1.3122E−01 |
| | 1.6706E−03 | 2.8957E+04 | 2.9154E+04 | 2.9333E+04 | 6.1389E−01 |
| | 1.7380E−03 | 2.8096E+04 | 2.8281E+04 | 2.8461E+04 | 6.3875E−01 |
| 71.Lu | 1.2116E−03 | 2.3905E+04 | 2.4055E+04 | 2.4019E+04 | 1.5170E−01 |
| | 1.6327E−03 | 3.0541E+04 | 3.0745E+04 | 3.0950E+04 | 6.6499E−01 |
| | 5.7740E−02 | 3.0617E+01 | 8.2902E+01 | 3.6850E+01 | 1.2497E+02 |
| 72.Hf | 1.2506E−03 | 3.1928E+04 | 3.2143E+04 | 3.2074E+04 | 2.1622E−01 |

| Material | $E$, MeV | $\mu_{1en}$, cm$^{-1}$ | $\mu_1$, cm$^{-1}$ | $\mu_2$, cm$^{-1}$ | $R$, % |
|---|---|---|---|---|---|
| | 1.6873E−03 | 2.8260E+04 | 2.8454E+04 | 2.8636E+04 | 6.4269E−01 |
| | 1.6909E−03 | 2.9807E+04 | 3.0007E+04 | 3.0212E+04 | 6.8249E−01 |
| 73.Ta | 1.4018E−03 | 3.2242E+04 | 3.2458E+04 | 3.2428E+04 | 9.0488E−02 |
| | 1.7474E−03 | 2.7756E+04 | 2.7938E+04 | 2.8114E+04 | 6.3262E−01 |
| | 9.0871E−03 | 1.9869E+03 | 2.2331E+03 | 2.0755E+03 | 7.5958E+00 |
| 74.W | 1.4883E−03 | 3.2421E+04 | 3.2637E+04 | 3.2634E+04 | 9.2048E−03 |
| | 1.8101E−03 | 2.5636E+04 | 2.5803E+04 | 2.5952E+04 | 5.7710E−01 |
| 75.Re | 1.5729E−03 | 3.3326E+04 | 3.3548E+04 | 3.3579E+04 | 9.1625E−02 |
| | 1.8428E−03 | 2.4632E+04 | 2.4794E+04 | 2.4898E+04 | 4.1847E−01 |
| 79.Au | 2.1596E−03 | 1.8472E+04 | 1.8604E+04 | 1.8694E+04 | 4.8463E−01 |
| 80.Hg | 1.4573E−03 | 3.2357E+04 | 3.2573E+04 | 3.2533E+04 | 1.2174E−01 |
| | 2.3152E−03 | 1.5717E+04 | 1.5831E+04 | 1.6004E+04 | 1.0950E+00 |
| | 1.0566E−02 | 1.4155E+03 | 1.5742E+03 | 1.4886E+03 | 5.7560E+00 |
| 81.Tl | 1.4081E−03 | 3.2255E+04 | 3.2471E+04 | 3.2398E+04 | 2.2521E−01 |
| | 2.4001E−03 | 1.4213E+04 | 1.4318E+04 | 1.4499E+04 | 1.2663E+00 |
| 82.Pb | 1.4126E−03 | 3.2264E+04 | 3.2480E+04 | 3.2402E+04 | 2.3942E−01 |
| 83.Bi | 1.3581E−03 | 3.2151E+04 | 3.2367E+04 | 3.2280E+04 | 2.6729E−01 |
| | 8.3387E−03 | 2.0724E+03 | 2.3308E+03 | 2.1498E+03 | 8.4176E+00 |
| 84.Po | 1.3622E−03 | 3.2159E+04 | 3.2375E+04 | 3.2283E+04 | 2.8506E−01 |
| | 8.3021E−03 | 2.0955E+03 | 2.3579E+03 | 2.1742E+03 | 8.4478E+00 |
| 85.At | 1.4171E−03 | 3.2274E+04 | 3.2489E+04 | 3.2414E+04 | 2.3374E−01 |
| 87.Fr | 1.4285E−03 | 3.2297E+04 | 3.2513E+04 | 3.2429E+04 | 2.5809E−01 |
| | 8.9766E−03 | 2.0426E+03 | 2.2977E+03 | 2.1249E+03 | 8.1311E+00 |
| 88.Ra | 1.2082E−03 | 2.2063E+04 | 2.2201E+04 | 2.2128E+04 | 3.2890E−01 |
| | 1.2090E−03 | 2.2494E+04 | 2.2635E+04 | 2.2564E+04 | 3.1348E−01 |
| | 5.5696E−02 | 3.1756E+01 | 9.1838E+01 | 3.8758E+01 | 1.3695E+02 |
| 89.Ac | 1.4718E−03 | 3.2387E+04 | 3.2603E+04 | 3.2519E+04 | 2.5715E−01 |
| | 1.5792E−02 | 4.9262E+02 | 5.3826E+02 | 5.3216E+02 | 1.1468E+00 |
| 90.Th | 2.1807E−03 | 1.8100E+04 | 1.8229E+04 | 1.8248E+04 | 1.0565E−01 |
| | 2.7419E−03 | 1.1377E+04 | 1.1525E+04 | 1.1512E+04 | 1.1433E−01 |
| 112. | 1.3026E−03 | 3.2036E+04 | 3.2251E+04 | 3.2105E+04 | 4.5579E−01 |
| | 5.5098E−02 | 3.2089E+01 | 9.4451E+01 | 5.3106E+01 | 7.7854E+01 |
| 116. | 3.8599E−02 | 4.4252E+01 | 5.0523E+01 | 1.1508E+02 | 1.2778E+02 |
| 118. | 1.1917E−03 | 1.6126E+04 | 1.6220E+04 | 1.6172E+04 | 3.0052E−01 |
| 123. | 1.1168E−03 | 1.4841E+04 | 1.4913E+04 | 1.4949E+04 | 2.4292E−01 |
| | 1.2079E−03 | 2.1902E+04 | 2.2038E+04 | 2.2095E+04 | 2.5625E−01 |
| | 1.3761E−03 | 3.2188E+04 | 3.2404E+04 | 3.2544E+04 | 4.3237E−01 |
| 125. | 1.2055E−03 | 2.0618E+04 | 2.0746E+04 | 2.0691E+04 | 2.6712E−01 |
| | 2.7662E−03 | 1.1139E+04 | 1.1284E+04 | 1.1439E+04 | 1.3758E+00 |

| Material | $E$, MeV | $\mu_{1en}$, cm$^{-1}$ | $\mu_1$, cm$^{-1}$ | $\mu_2$, cm$^{-1}$ | $R$, % |
|---|---|---|---|---|---|
| 130. | 1.2552E−03 | 3.1937E+04 | 3.2153E+04 | 3.2024E+04 | 4.0134E−01 |
| | 3.8619E−03 | 4.9548E+03 | 5.0316E+03 | 5.0555E+03 | 4.7604E−01 |
| | 4.4891E−03 | 3.4146E+03 | 3.4755E+03 | 3.4902E+03 | 4.2320E−01 |
| | 1.4869E−02 | 5.6392E+02 | 6.1698E+02 | 6.8332E+02 | 1.0752E+01 |
| | 5.7184E−02 | 3.0927E+01 | 8.5331E+01 | 4.7038E+01 | 8.1408E+01 |
| 134. | 1.1360E−03 | 1.4342E+04 | 1.4413E+04 | 1.4372E+04 | 2.8788E−01 |
| | | | 122.GAFCHROMIC SENSOR | | |
| 5.B | 4.6316E−02 | 4.4196E−02 | 2.8084E−01 | 4.0578E−01 | 4.4488E+01 |
| 6.C | 9.3908E−03 | 4.6532E+00 | 5.0923E+00 | 5.1749E+00 | 1.6236E+00 |
| | 3.4044E−02 | 8.9952E−02 | 3.4995E−01 | 4.0213E−01 | 1.4913E+01 |
| 101. | 4.0871E−03 | 5.8631E+01 | 5.9437E+01 | 6.1968E+01 | 4.2578E+00 |
| 109. | 2.4640E−03 | 3.2488E+02 | 3.2625E+02 | 3.2665E+02 | 1.2221E−01 |
| 110. | 1.4818E−03 | 1.1772E+03 | 1.1797E+03 | 1.1805E+03 | 6.2922E−02 |
| | 2.0428E−03 | 4.6577E+02 | 4.6731E+02 | 4.6744E+02 | 2.7963E−02 |
| | 2.9341E−03 | 1.6765E+02 | 1.6884E+02 | 1.6901E+02 | 9.9591E−02 |
| | 4.9120E−02 | 3.9301E−02 | 2.7151E−01 | 2.2606E−01 | 2.0105E+01 |
| 119. | 2.3813E−03 | 3.5256E+02 | 3.5397E+02 | 3.5417E+02 | 5.6937E−02 |
| | 2.6585E−03 | 2.5982E+02 | 2.6112E+02 | 2.6152E+02 | 1.5269E−01 |
| 138. | 2.6987E−03 | 2.4637E+02 | 2.4766E+02 | 2.4750E+02 | 6.3131E−02 |
| | 3.7154E−02 | 7.1818E−02 | 3.2484E−01 | 3.0275E−01 | 7.2959E+00 |
| 141. | 2.7029E−03 | 2.4499E+02 | 2.4628E+02 | 2.4728E+02 | 4.0791E−01 |
| 145. | 5.6157E−02 | 3.4107E−02 | 2.5729E−01 | 2.1011E−01 | 2.2457E+01 |
| | | | 123.GALLIUM ARSENIDE | | |
| 22.Ti | 1.0799E−02 | 4.0586E+02 | 6.0545E+02 | 4.4829E+02 | 3.5055E+01 |
| 24.Cr | 1.4173E−02 | 3.8695E+02 | 5.9652E+02 | 4.3851E+02 | 3.6032E+01 |
| 25.Mn | 1.4931E−02 | 3.3679E+02 | 4.9847E+02 | 3.8435E+02 | 2.9691E+01 |
| 26.Fe | 1.4910E−03 | 2.7483E+04 | 2.7770E+04 | 2.7573E+04 | 7.1489E−01 |
| | 2.7408E−02 | 8.8421E+01 | 1.1356E+02 | 1.0010E+02 | 1.3442E+01 |
| 27.Co | 6.9351E−03 | 5.8886E+02 | 6.0367E+02 | 6.0697E+02 | 5.4803E−01 |
| 32.Ge | 1.9284E−03 | 1.6390E+04 | 1.6546E+04 | 1.6537E+04 | 5.5723E−02 |
| | 1.0241E−02 | 1.7912E+02 | 1.8835E+02 | 1.8836E+02 | 8.6604E−03 |
| | 1.9082E−02 | 1.9924E+02 | 2.7447E+02 | 2.7291E+02 | 5.7052E−01 |
| 34.Se | 1.0082E−02 | 1.8711E+02 | 1.9652E+02 | 1.9573E+02 | 4.0451E−01 |
| 39.Y | 1.1164E−03 | 1.4772E+04 | 1.4879E+04 | 1.4802E+04 | 5.2377E−01 |
| | 2.4426E−02 | 1.2099E+02 | 1.5886E+02 | 2.1684E+02 | 3.6501E+01 |
| 42.Mo | 1.3539E−03 | 2.8613E+04 | 2.8908E+04 | 2.8685E+04 | 7.7854E−01 |
| | 1.3796E−02 | 4.1187E+02 | 6.4523E+02 | 4.3246E+02 | 4.9199E+01 |
| 43.Tc | 1.4080E−03 | 3.0882E+04 | 3.1219E+04 | 3.0965E+04 | 8.2058E−01 |
| | 1.5232E−02 | 3.2467E+02 | 4.7733E+02 | 3.4483E+02 | 3.8424E+01 |

| Material | $E$, MeV | $\mu_{1en}$, cm$^{-1}$ | $\mu_1$, cm$^{-1}$ | $\mu_2$, cm$^{-1}$ | $R$, % |
|---|---|---|---|---|---|
| 44.Ru | 2.0157E−02 | 1.6762E+02 | 2.2371E+02 | 1.8274E+02 | 2.2417E+01 |
| 45.Rh | 2.1695E−02 | 1.5082E+02 | 2.0035E+02 | 1.6529E+02 | 2.1212E+01 |
| 46.Pd | 2.2575E−02 | 1.4121E+02 | 1.8699E+02 | 1.5495E+02 | 2.0673E+01 |
| 47.Ag | 3.2209E−03 | 4.5036E+03 | 4.5462E+03 | 4.5677E+03 | 4.7392E−01 |
| | 2.1693E−02 | 1.5085E+02 | 2.0038E+02 | 1.6431E+02 | 2.1957E+01 |
| 48.Cd | 1.4482E−03 | 2.9236E+04 | 2.9548E+04 | 2.9315E+04 | 7.9762E−01 |
| | 1.6896E−02 | 2.7045E+02 | 3.8964E+02 | 2.8731E+02 | 3.5616E+01 |
| 49.In | 1.4572E−02 | 3.6057E+02 | 5.4495E+02 | 3.7980E+02 | 4.3484E+01 |
| 50.Sn | 1.3973E−03 | 3.1320E+04 | 3.1663E+04 | 3.1392E+04 | 8.6437E−01 |
| | 1.4848E−02 | 3.4233E+02 | 5.0929E+02 | 3.6139E+02 | 4.0927E+01 |
| 51.Sb | 1.3590E−03 | 3.2889E+04 | 3.3256E+04 | 3.2964E+04 | 8.8487E−01 |
| | 1.4646E−02 | 3.5565E+02 | 5.3534E+02 | 3.7517E+02 | 4.2690E+01 |
| 52.Te | 1.4382E−02 | 3.7311E+02 | 5.6948E+02 | 3.9345E+02 | 4.4738E+01 |
| 53.I | 1.2852E−02 | 4.7435E+02 | 7.6739E+02 | 4.9943E+02 | 5.3655E+01 |
| 55.Cs | 1.1164E−03 | 1.4777E+04 | 1.4885E+04 | 1.4814E+04 | 4.7621E−01 |
| 56.Ba | 3.8674E−02 | 3.1861E+01 | 3.8678E+01 | 9.4372E+01 | 1.4399E+02 |
| 57.La | 2.8180E−02 | 7.9993E+01 | 1.0184E+02 | 8.7896E+01 | 1.5860E+01 |
| 63.Eu | 1.1520E−03 | 2.2844E+04 | 2.3049E+04 | 2.2986E+04 | 2.7340E−01 |
| | 1.5760E−03 | 2.6342E+04 | 2.6612E+04 | 2.6502E+04 | 4.1458E−01 |
| 64.Gd | 1.1162E−03 | 1.4741E+04 | 1.4849E+04 | 1.4826E+04 | 1.5395E−01 |
| | 1.2041E−03 | 2.1965E+04 | 2.2159E+04 | 2.2114E+04 | 2.0211E−01 |
| 65.Tb | 1.1228E−03 | 1.5807E+04 | 1.5925E+04 | 1.5889E+04 | 2.2493E−01 |
| | 1.2444E−03 | 2.0907E+04 | 2.1090E+04 | 2.1056E+04 | 1.5952E−01 |
| 66.Dy | 1.1297E−03 | 1.6888E+04 | 1.7017E+04 | 1.6974E+04 | 2.5285E−01 |
| | 1.2966E−03 | 1.9289E+04 | 1.9454E+04 | 1.9443E+04 | 5.7240E−02 |
| | 1.3005E−03 | 2.1293E+04 | 2.1478E+04 | 2.1467E+04 | 5.1078E−02 |
| 67.Ho | 1.1380E−03 | 1.8025E+04 | 1.8167E+04 | 1.8114E+04 | 2.9107E−01 |
| | 1.3787E−03 | 3.2083E+04 | 3.2437E+04 | 3.2383E+04 | 1.6723E−01 |
| 68.Er | 1.4340E−03 | 2.9816E+04 | 3.0137E+04 | 3.0123E+04 | 4.7812E−02 |
| 69.Tm | 1.4851E−03 | 2.7723E+04 | 2.8013E+04 | 2.8026E+04 | 4.6504E−02 |
| 70.Yb | 1.1324E−03 | 1.7260E+04 | 1.7394E+04 | 1.7333E+04 | 3.5173E−01 |
| 71.Lu | 1.6201E−03 | 2.5097E+04 | 2.5353E+04 | 2.5423E+04 | 2.7773E−01 |
| 72.Hf | 1.6732E−03 | 2.3598E+04 | 2.3837E+04 | 2.3884E+04 | 1.9782E−01 |
| 73.Ta | 1.4485E−03 | 2.9223E+04 | 2.9535E+04 | 2.9408E+04 | 4.3359E−01 |
| 81.Tl | 1.4668E−03 | 2.8473E+04 | 2.8774E+04 | 2.8614E+04 | 5.5900E−01 |
| 82.Pb | 1.4786E−03 | 2.7988E+04 | 2.8283E+04 | 2.8125E+04 | 5.6030E−01 |
| | 1.5262E−03 | 2.5968E+04 | 2.6239E+04 | 2.6103E+04 | 5.1840E−01 |
| | 1.9769E−03 | 1.5020E+04 | 1.5160E+04 | 1.5145E+04 | 9.8209E−02 |
| 82.Pb | 2.0434E−03 | 1.3967E+04 | 1.4096E+04 | 1.4092E+04 | 2.8843E−02 |

| Material | $E$, MeV | $\mu_{1en}$, cm$^{-1}$ | $\mu_1$, cm$^{-1}$ | $\mu_2$, cm$^{-1}$ | $R$, % |
|---|---|---|---|---|---|
| 85.At | 1.8725E−03 | 1.7970E+04 | 1.8144E+04 | 1.8102E+04 | 2.3020E−01 |
| 87.Fr | 1.5617E−03 | 2.6746E+04 | 2.7022E+04 | 2.6876E+04 | 5.4063E−01 |
| 88.Ra | 1.2996E−02 | 4.6483E+02 | 7.4877E+02 | 4.9106E+02 | 5.2483E+01 |
| 112. | 1.3629E−02 | 4.2294E+02 | 6.6688E+02 | 4.4436E+02 | 5.0078E+01 |
| | 2.8512E−02 | 7.6363E+01 | 9.6788E+01 | 1.5663E+02 | 6.1831E+01 |
| 116. | 1.2251E−02 | 5.1408E+02 | 8.4505E+02 | 5.4233E+02 | 5.5818E+01 |
| 118. | 1.1330E−03 | 1.7337E+04 | 1.7471E+04 | 1.7387E+04 | 4.8223E−01 |
| | 1.1369E−03 | 1.7866E+04 | 1.8007E+04 | 1.7917E+04 | 5.0199E−01 |
| 121. | 1.1168E−03 | 1.4841E+04 | 1.4949E+04 | 1.4913E+04 | 2.4292E−01 |
| | 1.2079E−03 | 2.1902E+04 | 2.2095E+04 | 2.2038E+04 | 2.5625E−01 |
| | 1.3761E−03 | 3.2188E+04 | 3.2544E+04 | 3.2404E+04 | 4.3237E−01 |
| 125. | 2.5487E−03 | 9.2857E+03 | 9.3712E+03 | 9.5228E+03 | 1.6175E+00 |
| 130. | 1.2252E−02 | 5.1401E+02 | 8.4492E+02 | 5.4334E+02 | 5.5505E+01 |
| 134. | 1.1162E−03 | 1.4738E+04 | 1.4846E+04 | 1.4768E+04 | 5.2620E−01 |
| | 4.5685E−02 | 2.0273E+01 | 2.4505E+01 | 3.1244E+01 | 2.7499E+01 |
| | | | 124.GLASS, BOROSILICATE ("PYREX") | | |
| 11.Na | 1.1343E−03 | 5.6894E+03 | 5.7097E+03 | 5.7909E+03 | 1.4212E+00 |
| 12.Mg | 3.9818E−03 | 5.2232E+02 | 5.3321E+02 | 5.2891E+02 | 8.1240E−01 |
| 39.Y | 2.0251E−03 | 3.1955E+03 | 3.2897E+03 | 3.2209E+03 | 2.1353E+00 |
| 108. | 1.5511E−03 | 2.3400E+03 | 2.3489E+03 | 2.3474E+03 | 6.7043E−02 |
| | 1.6474E−03 | 2.0790E+03 | 2.0903E+03 | 2.0857E+03 | 2.2131E−01 |
| 111. | 1.0556E−03 | 6.1113E+03 | 6.1279E+03 | 6.1388E+03 | 1.7882E−01 |
| 117. | 1.1861E−03 | 5.2465E+03 | 5.2652E+03 | 5.2625E+03 | 5.1254E−02 |
| | 1.3764E−03 | 3.6173E+03 | 3.6301E+03 | 3.6295E+03 | 1.8418E−02 |
| 129. | 1.2288E−03 | 4.8807E+03 | 4.8981E+03 | 4.8945E+03 | 7.2826E−02 |
| 141. | 2.9881E−03 | 1.1427E+03 | 1.1686E+03 | 1.2329E+03 | 5.5049E+00 |
| | | | 125.GLASS, LEAD | | |
| 23.V | 5.6478E−03 | 2.6993E+03 | 2.7737E+03 | 3.3397E+03 | 2.0408E+01 |
| 26.Fe | 2.5136E−03 | 8.4426E+03 | 8.6498E+03 | 8.4822E+03 | 1.9757E+00 |
| | 1.3917E−02 | 5.3551E+02 | 6.6539E+02 | 6.4308E+02 | 3.4688E+00 |
| 27.Co | 2.5768E−03 | 9.7934E+03 | 1.0044E+04 | 9.8467E+03 | 2.0061E+00 |
| 30.Zn | 1.0220E−03 | 2.8790E+04 | 2.8864E+04 | 2.9001E+04 | 4.7370E−01 |
| 31.Ga | 1.1172E−03 | 2.4072E+04 | 2.4146E+04 | 2.4286E+04 | 5.8033E−01 |
| | 2.5563E−03 | 9.4228E+03 | 9.6637E+03 | 9.4973E+03 | 1.7522E+00 |
| 32.Ge | 2.5470E−03 | 9.2553E+03 | 9.4916E+03 | 9.3358E+03 | 1.6690E+00 |
| 34.Se | 2.5360E−03 | 9.0562E+03 | 9.2872E+03 | 9.1603E+03 | 1.3849E+00 |
| 40.Zr | 3.8254E−03 | 6.4506E+03 | 6.6093E+03 | 6.5813E+03 | 4.2429E−01 |
| 41.Nb | 1.9093E−03 | 8.9628E+03 | 9.0852E+03 | 9.0149E+03 | 7.8028E−01 |
| | 2.5611E−02 | 2.1063E+02 | 2.5975E+02 | 4.1828E+02 | 6.1030E+01 |

| Material | $E$, MeV | $\mu_{1en}$, cm$^{-1}$ | $\mu_1$, cm$^{-1}$ | $\mu_2$, cm$^{-1}$ | $R$, % |
|---|---|---|---|---|---|
| 44.Ru | 2.5252E−03 | 8.7687E+03 | 8.9887E+03 | 8.8462E+03 | 1.6106E+00 |
| | 1.4202E−02 | 5.0898E+02 | 6.3029E+02 | 5.3508E+02 | 1.7794E+01 |
| 45.Rh | 2.5653E−03 | 9.5854E+03 | 9.8306E+03 | 9.6646E+03 | 1.7179E+00 |
| | 1.4705E−02 | 4.6227E+02 | 5.6852E+02 | 4.8794E+02 | 1.6514E+01 |
| 46.Pd | 2.5761E−03 | 9.7801E+03 | 1.0030E+04 | 9.8587E+03 | 1.7427E+00 |
| | 1.4840E−02 | 4.4976E+02 | 5.5197E+02 | 4.7503E+02 | 1.6197E+01 |
| 47.Ag | 2.5574E−03 | 9.4427E+03 | 9.6841E+03 | 9.5168E+03 | 1.7579E+00 |
| | 1.4450E−02 | 4.8597E+02 | 5.9987E+02 | 5.1143E+02 | 1.7293E+01 |
| 48.Cd | 2.5164E−03 | 8.5219E+03 | 8.7322E+03 | 8.5798E+03 | 1.7763E+00 |
| | 2.8775E−02 | 1.4519E+02 | 1.7585E+02 | 3.6756E+02 | 1.0901E+02 |
| 49.In | 2.4938E−03 | 7.8827E+03 | 8.0678E+03 | 7.9358E+03 | 1.6630E+00 |
| | 3.2937E−02 | 1.0146E+02 | 1.2123E+02 | 2.4411E+02 | 1.0135E+02 |
| 50.Sn | 2.5061E−03 | 8.2306E+03 | 8.4294E+03 | 8.2839E+03 | 1.7561E+00 |
| | 3.4270E−02 | 9.3110E+01 | 1.1118E+02 | 2.3323E+02 | 1.0978E+02 |
| 51.Sb | 2.4997E−03 | 8.0509E+03 | 8.2426E+03 | 8.1001E+03 | 1.7592E+00 |
| | 3.7537E−02 | 7.2639E+01 | 8.6549E+01 | 1.7108E+02 | 9.7668E+01 |
| 52.Te | 2.4924E−03 | 7.8440E+03 | 8.0275E+03 | 7.8896E+03 | 1.7478E+00 |
| | 3.9509E−02 | 6.0290E+01 | 7.1689E+01 | 1.3499E+02 | 8.8303E+01 |
| 53.I | 4.9450E−02 | 3.3230E+01 | 3.9795E+01 | 6.3391E+01 | 5.9293E+01 |
| 56.Ba | 7.1315E−03 | 1.5893E+03 | 1.6397E+03 | 1.7086E+03 | 4.2033E+00 |
| 57.La | 2.5716E−03 | 9.6995E+03 | 9.9478E+03 | 9.7556E+03 | 1.9697E+00 |
| | 1.4190E−02 | 5.1015E+02 | 6.3184E+02 | 5.4326E+02 | 1.6306E+01 |
| | 4.3318E−02 | 4.8792E+01 | 5.8088E+01 | 1.3560E+02 | 1.3344E+02 |
| 58.Ce | 4.1198E−02 | 5.4171E+01 | 6.4410E+01 | 1.6955E+02 | 1.6323E+02 |
| 60.Nd | 2.6351E−03 | 1.1962E+04 | 1.2288E+04 | 1.2036E+04 | 2.0898E+00 |
| 61.Pm | 1.0391E−03 | 2.7944E+04 | 2.8019E+04 | 2.8088E+04 | 2.4851E−01 |
| | 2.8142E−03 | 1.0838E+04 | 1.1129E+04 | 1.0919E+04 | 1.9203E+00 |
| 62.Sm | 1.0887E−03 | 2.5484E+04 | 2.5559E+04 | 2.5626E+04 | 2.6219E−01 |
| | 2.8947E−03 | 1.0333E+04 | 1.0608E+04 | 1.0414E+04 | 1.8695E+00 |
| 63.Eu | 1.1513E−03 | 2.2401E+04 | 2.2475E+04 | 2.2540E+04 | 2.8728E−01 |
| | 5.1141E−02 | 3.0439E+01 | 3.6528E+01 | 9.2838E+01 | 1.5416E+02 |
| 64.Gd | 1.2024E−03 | 2.0722E+04 | 2.0794E+04 | 2.0862E+04 | 3.2614E−01 |
| | 1.9281E−02 | 3.6715E+02 | 4.6485E+02 | 4.0117E+02 | 1.5874E+01 |
| 65.Tb | 1.2418E−03 | 1.9426E+04 | 1.9497E+04 | 1.9560E+04 | 3.2515E−01 |
| | 3.8008E−03 | 6.5539E+03 | 6.7156E+03 | 6.6329E+03 | 1.2466E+00 |
| | 2.7970E−02 | 1.6184E+02 | 1.9719E+02 | 1.7914E+02 | 1.0074E+01 |
| 66.Dy | 3.9215E−03 | 6.3370E+03 | 6.4916E+03 | 6.4212E+03 | 1.0963E+00 |
| | 3.8777E−02 | 6.4871E+01 | 7.7202E+01 | 7.3887E+01 | 4.4857E+00 |
| 67.Ho | 7.0737E−03 | 1.6229E+03 | 1.6740E+03 | 1.6739E+03 | 4.6964E−03 |
| | 5.3846E−02 | 2.7130E+01 | 3.2672E+01 | 3.2511E+01 | 4.9748E−01 |

| Material | $E$, MeV | $\mu_{1en}$, cm$^{-1}$ | $\mu_1$, cm$^{-1}$ | $\mu_2$, cm$^{-1}$ | $R$, % |
|---|---|---|---|---|---|
| 70.Yb | 3.7760E−03 | 6.6579E+03 | 6.8226E+03 | 6.7513E+03 | 1.0572E+00 |
| | 2.7086E−02 | 1.8012E+02 | 2.2064E+02 | 2.0251E+02 | 8.9536E+00 |
| 83.Bi | 2.5034E−03 | 8.1555E+03 | 8.3513E+03 | 8.2657E+03 | 1.0359E+00 |
| 84.Po | 2.5132E−03 | 8.4300E+03 | 8.6366E+03 | 8.5369E+03 | 1.1679E+00 |
| 85.At | 2.5544E−03 | 9.3882E+03 | 9.6281E+03 | 9.5062E+03 | 1.2819E+00 |
| 88.Ra | 1.9904E−03 | 8.1680E+03 | 8.2811E+03 | 8.2281E+03 | 6.4388E−01 |
| | 2.0190E−03 | 7.9497E+03 | 8.0604E+03 | 8.0096E+03 | 6.3451E−01 |
| | 3.6346E−03 | 7.2928E+03 | 7.4753E+03 | 7.5596E+03 | 1.1275E+00 |
| 89.Ac | 1.5591E−02 | 5.1032E+02 | 6.6523E+02 | 5.5053E+02 | 2.0836E+01 |
| 90.Th | 2.7570E−03 | 1.1197E+04 | 1.1499E+04 | 1.1331E+04 | 1.4810E+00 |
| 112. | 3.9242E−02 | 6.1963E+01 | 7.3702E+01 | 1.2863E+02 | 7.4530E+01 |
| 116. | 5.6594E−02 | 2.3770E+01 | 2.8757E+01 | 4.3326E+01 | 5.0662E+01 |
| 121. | 1.2055E−03 | 2.0618E+04 | 2.0691E+04 | 2.0746E+04 | 2.6712E−01 |
| | 2.7662E−03 | 1.1139E+04 | 1.1439E+04 | 1.1284E+04 | 1.3758E+00 |
| 123. | 2.5487E−03 | 9.2857E+03 | 9.5228E+03 | 9.3712E+03 | 1.6175E+00 |
| 130. | 1.3107E−02 | 6.1076E+02 | 7.6490E+02 | 7.0279E+02 | 8.8383E+00 |
| | 3.5778E−02 | 8.3662E+01 | 9.9814E+01 | 1.6101E+02 | 6.1314E+01 |

126.LITHIUM FLUORIDE

| Material | $E$, MeV | $\mu_{1en}$, cm$^{-1}$ | $\mu_1$, cm$^{-1}$ | $\mu_2$, cm$^{-1}$ | $R$, % |
|---|---|---|---|---|---|
| 30.Zn | 1.0037E−03 | 1.0949E+04 | 1.1014E+04 | 1.0985E+04 | 2.7187E−01 |
| 33.As | 1.1317E−03 | 9.1174E+03 | 9.1708E+03 | 9.1511E+03 | 2.1545E−01 |
| 108. | 3.2478E−03 | 4.8038E+02 | 4.8377E+02 | 4.9052E+02 | 1.3959E+00 |
| 114. | 2.2717E−03 | 1.4313E+03 | 1.4383E+03 | 1.4382E+03 | 7.4608E−03 |
| 129. | 1.4709E−03 | 4.2636E+03 | 4.2848E+03 | 4.3042E+03 | 4.5248E−01 |

127.LITHIUM TETRABORATE

| Material | $E$, MeV | $\mu_{1en}$, cm$^{-1}$ | $\mu_1$, cm$^{-1}$ | $\mu_2$, cm$^{-1}$ | $R$, % |
|---|---|---|---|---|---|
| 11.Na | 1.4151E−03 | 3.6700E+03 | 3.6823E+03 | 3.7257E+03 | 1.1780E+00 |
| | 5.9638E−02 | 6.5736E−02 | 4.3732E−01 | 2.2211E−01 | 9.6897E+01 |
| 20.Ca | 1.9463E−03 | 1.3867E+03 | 1.3917E+03 | 1.3919E+03 | 1.8920E−02 |
| 117. | 1.4841E−03 | 2.9166E+03 | 2.9268E+03 | 2.9262E+03 | 2.2243E−02 |
| | 1.5412E−03 | 2.6175E+03 | 2.6268E+03 | 2.6267E+03 | 4.4985E−03 |
| | 1.6927E−03 | 2.1573E+03 | 2.1650E+03 | 2.1697E+03 | 2.1946E−01 |
| | 1.7069E−03 | 2.1139E+03 | 2.1214E+03 | 2.1261E+03 | 2.1908E−01 |
| 129. | 1.0124E−03 | 8.0698E+03 | 8.0939E+03 | 8.0920E+03 | 2.3847E−02 |

128.LUNG TISSUE (ICRU-44)

| Material | $E$, MeV | $\mu_{1en}$, cm$^{-1}$ | $\mu_1$, cm$^{-1}$ | $\mu_2$, cm$^{-1}$ | $R$, % |
|---|---|---|---|---|---|
| 5.B | 5.4808E−02 | 4.0517E−02 | 2.2739E−01 | 3.8526E−01 | 6.9424E+01 |
| 6.C | 1.0518E−03 | 3.4893E+03 | 3.4993E+03 | 3.4926E+03 | 1.9388E−01 |
| | 1.1908E−03 | 2.7756E+03 | 2.7833E+03 | 2.7785E+03 | 1.7350E−01 |
| | 2.3310E−03 | 3.9344E+02 | 3.9530E+02 | 3.9497E+02 | 8.2017E−02 |
| | 2.6774E−03 | 2.6863E+02 | 2.7046E+02 | 2.6999E+02 | 1.7512E−01 |

| Material | $E$, MeV | $\mu_{1en}$, cm$^{-1}$ | $\mu_1$, cm$^{-1}$ | $\mu_2$, cm$^{-1}$ | $R$, % |
|---|---|---|---|---|---|
| | 5.8169E−02 | 3.6596E−02 | 2.1974E−01 | 3.0168E−01 | 3.7293E+01 |
| 19.K | 2.0962E−03 | 5.2933E+02 | 5.3118E+02 | 5.3178E+02 | 1.1336E−01 |
| | 2.9461E−03 | 2.0779E+02 | 2.0971E+02 | 2.0988E+02 | 8.1143E−02 |
| 86.Rn | 1.9413E−02 | 7.0737E−01 | 9.8283E−01 | 9.4465E−01 | 4.0418E+00 |
| 101. | 5.6678E−02 | 3.8336E−02 | 2.2313E−01 | 2.3341E−01 | 4.6075E+00 |
| 104. | 2.9913E−03 | 1.9819E+02 | 2.0008E+02 | 1.9948E+02 | 3.0449E−01 |
| | 3.0875E−03 | 1.8456E+02 | 1.8636E+02 | 1.8582E+02 | 2.9198E−01 |
| | 3.8932E−03 | 9.4239E+01 | 9.5622E+01 | 9.5266E+01 | 3.7442E−01 |
| 104. | 4.9044E−02 | 4.9031E−02 | 2.4266E−01 | 3.0302E−01 | 2.4877E+01 |
| 107. | 7.9408E−03 | 1.1047E+01 | 1.1556E+01 | 1.1636E+01 | 6.9023E−01 |
| 115. | 1.1302E−03 | 3.0564E+03 | 3.0650E+03 | 3.0658E+03 | 2.6828E−02 |
| | 1.4607E−03 | 1.5262E+03 | 1.5299E+03 | 1.5303E+03 | 2.5548E−02 |
| 119. | 3.4222E−03 | 1.3949E+02 | 1.4094E+02 | 1.4078E+02 | 1.1820E−01 |
| | 3.7343E−03 | 1.0664E+02 | 1.0813E+02 | 1.0777E+02 | 3.3537E−01 |
| 120. | 6.6357E−03 | 2.0783E+01 | 2.1416E+01 | 2.1399E+01 | 7.9882E−02 |
| | 7.6761E−03 | 1.3022E+01 | 1.3556E+01 | 1.3549E+01 | 4.9459E−02 |
| 137. | 1.4590E−03 | 1.5337E+03 | 1.5374E+03 | 1.5373E+03 | 1.0450E−02 |
| | 2.0659E−03 | 5.5199E+02 | 5.5389E+02 | 5.5387E+02 | 2.4133E−03 |
| | 2.8954E−03 | 2.1855E+02 | 2.2050E+02 | 2.1987E+02 | 2.9002E−01 |
| | 5.9601E−02 | 3.4926E−02 | 2.1647E−01 | 2.5862E−01 | 1.9470E+01 |
| 141. | 2.3760E−03 | 3.7359E+02 | 3.7539E+02 | 3.7599E+02 | 1.6062E−01 |
| 144. | 4.1303E−02 | 7.2546E−02 | 2.7753E−01 | 2.7907E−01 | 5.5710E−01 |
| 145. | 1.0341E−03 | 3.6453E+03 | 3.6559E+03 | 3.6558E+03 | 3.4193E−03 |
| | 1.3612E−03 | 1.9865E+03 | 1.9917E+03 | 1.9918E+03 | 1.3729E−03 |
| | 2.0786E−03 | 5.4251E+02 | 5.4439E+02 | 5.4435E+02 | 8.1627E−03 |
| | 2.9004E−03 | 2.1749E+02 | 2.1944E+02 | 2.1867E+02 | 3.5177E−01 |
| | 3.5608E−03 | 1.2083E+02 | 1.2214E+02 | 1.2178E+02 | 2.9542E−01 |
| 148. | 2.9780E−03 | 2.0102E+02 | 2.0292E+02 | 2.0224E+02 | 3.3783E−01 |
| | 3.1869E−03 | 1.7118E+02 | 1.7287E+02 | 1.7231E+02 | 3.2371E−01 |
| | 3.8742E−03 | 9.5721E+01 | 9.7118E+01 | 9.6633E+01 | 5.0200E−01 |
| | | | 129.MAGNESIUM TETRABORATE | | |
| 11.Na | 1.1930E−03 | 5.2673E+03 | 5.2817E+03 | 5.3592E+03 | 1.4677E+00 |
| 20.Ca | 1.0989E−03 | 6.5683E+03 | 6.5858E+03 | 6.5769E+03 | 1.3395E−01 |
| 114. | 2.1490E−03 | 1.6543E+03 | 1.6680E+03 | 1.6615E+03 | 3.9008E−01 |
| 117. | 1.1335E−03 | 5.9687E+03 | 5.9843E+03 | 5.9879E+03 | 5.8837E−02 |
| | 1.1518E−03 | 5.7117E+03 | 5.7267E+03 | 5.7297E+03 | 5.2352E−02 |
| | 1.2932E−03 | 4.1859E+03 | 4.1988E+03 | 4.1999E+03 | 2.8305E−02 |
| 124. | 1.2288E−03 | 4.8807E+03 | 4.8945E+03 | 4.8981E+03 | 7.2826E−02 |
| 126. | 1.4709E−03 | 4.2636E+03 | 4.3042E+03 | 4.2848E+03 | 4.5248E−01 |

| Material | $E$, MeV | $\mu_{1en}$, cm$^{-1}$ | $\mu_1$, cm$^{-1}$ | $\mu_2$, cm$^{-1}$ | $R$, % |
|---|---|---|---|---|---|
| 127. | 1.0124E−03 | 8.0698E+03 | 8.0920E+03 | 8.0939E+03 | 2.3847E−02 |
| 140. | 1.4503E−03 | 4.4447E+03 | 4.4872E+03 | 4.4668E+03 | 4.5756E−01 |
| | | | 130.MERCURIC IODIDE | | |
| 24.Cr | 1.4645E−03 | 2.1690E+04 | 2.1768E+04 | 2.1745E+04 | 1.0367E−01 |
| | 1.0421E−02 | 8.0924E+02 | 8.4989E+02 | 9.3904E+02 | 1.0490E+01 |
| 25.Mn | 2.3200E−03 | 8.3051E+03 | 8.3966E+03 | 8.3441E+03 | 6.2951E−01 |
| | 7.7583E−03 | 1.7721E+03 | 1.8548E+03 | 2.2539E+03 | 2.1519E+01 |
| 26.Fe | 2.3645E−03 | 9.6946E+03 | 9.8343E+03 | 9.7364E+03 | 1.0058E+00 |
| 27.Co | 2.5351E−03 | 1.0225E+04 | 1.0406E+04 | 1.0280E+04 | 1.2216E+00 |
| | 1.4364E−02 | 5.6219E+02 | 6.7583E+02 | 6.9011E+02 | 2.1135E+00 |
| 28.Ni | 2.7614E−03 | 9.1043E+03 | 9.2742E+03 | 9.1608E+03 | 1.2378E+00 |
| 29.Cu | 2.8337E−03 | 8.7423E+03 | 8.9084E+03 | 8.8035E+03 | 1.1911E+00 |
| 30.Zn | 1.0385E−03 | 4.2418E+04 | 4.2513E+04 | 4.2767E+04 | 5.9666E−01 |
| | 2.6584E−03 | 9.6201E+03 | 9.7954E+03 | 9.6905E+03 | 1.0820E+00 |
| 31.Ga | 2.4078E−03 | 1.0841E+04 | 1.1025E+04 | 1.0925E+04 | 9.0882E−01 |
| | 1.0725E−02 | 7.6019E+02 | 7.9896E+02 | 1.2451E+03 | 5.5844E+01 |
| 32.Ge | 1.2044E−02 | 5.4760E+02 | 5.7822E+02 | 9.1757E+02 | 5.8689E+01 |
| 33.As | 2.6549E−03 | 9.6375E+03 | 9.8129E+03 | 9.7323E+03 | 8.2835E−01 |
| 34.Se | 2.3825E−03 | 1.0409E+04 | 1.0571E+04 | 1.0530E+04 | 3.9497E−01 |
| 38.Sr | 2.2603E−03 | 7.8282E+03 | 7.8918E+03 | 7.9876E+03 | 1.2139E+00 |
| 39.Y | 2.8386E−03 | 8.7176E+03 | 8.8834E+03 | 8.8952E+03 | 1.3296E−01 |
| 40.Zr | 2.8080E−02 | 1.2852E+02 | 1.5014E+02 | 2.2104E+02 | 4.7224E+01 |
| 41.Nb | 1.9175E−02 | 3.1699E+02 | 3.7604E+02 | 7.3565E+02 | 9.5628E+01 |
| | 5.4603E−02 | 3.4581E+01 | 5.3423E+01 | 4.6635E+01 | 1.4555E+01 |
| 42.Mo | 1.4725E−03 | 2.1297E+04 | 2.1375E+04 | 2.1369E+04 | 2.8106E−02 |
| | 7.8016E−03 | 1.7353E+03 | 1.8162E+03 | 1.7828E+03 | 1.8736E+00 |
| | 1.0668E−02 | 7.6939E+02 | 8.0851E+02 | 7.9836E+02 | 1.2708E+00 |
| 43.Tc | 2.3424E−03 | 8.8101E+03 | 8.9219E+03 | 8.8836E+03 | 4.3068E−01 |
| 44.Ru | 2.3770E−03 | 1.0192E+04 | 1.0347E+04 | 1.0272E+04 | 7.3254E−01 |
| 45.Rh | 2.4603E−03 | 1.0587E+04 | 1.0769E+04 | 1.0668E+04 | 9.5318E−01 |
| 46.Pd | 2.5267E−03 | 1.0266E+04 | 1.0447E+04 | 1.0345E+04 | 9.7902E−01 |
| 47.Ag | 2.4062E−03 | 1.0849E+04 | 1.1033E+04 | 1.0926E+04 | 9.8006E−01 |
| 48.Cd | 2.3656E−03 | 9.7367E+03 | 9.8777E+03 | 9.7953E+03 | 8.4108E−01 |
| 49.In | 2.3461E−03 | 8.9578E+03 | 9.0742E+03 | 9.0124E+03 | 6.8525E−01 |
| | 2.8603E−02 | 1.1932E+02 | 1.3925E+02 | 3.2754E+02 | 1.3522E+02 |
| 50.Sn | 2.3566E−03 | 9.3774E+03 | 9.5071E+03 | 9.4323E+03 | 7.9370E−01 |
| 51.Sb | 2.3511E−03 | 9.1571E+03 | 9.2798E+03 | 9.2076E+03 | 7.8484E−01 |
| | 4.2915E−02 | 5.8888E+01 | 1.0122E+02 | 1.1794E+02 | 1.6518E+01 |
| 52.Te | 2.3448E−03 | 8.9048E+03 | 9.0196E+03 | 8.9517E+03 | 7.5814E−01 |

| Material | $E$, MeV | $\mu_{1en}$, cm$^{-1}$ | $\mu_1$, cm$^{-1}$ | $\mu_2$, cm$^{-1}$ | $R$, % |
|---|---|---|---|---|---|
| | 3.2689E−02 | 7.6042E+01 | 8.8573E+01 | 2.2103E+02 | 1.4954E+02 |
| 53.I | 2.1568E−03 | 8.8323E+03 | 8.8959E+03 | 8.8750E+03 | 2.3498E−01 |
| | 2.3016E−03 | 7.9378E+03 | 8.0135E+03 | 7.9791E+03 | 4.3191E−01 |
| | 1.1900E−02 | 5.7069E+02 | 6.0219E+02 | 6.0022E+02 | 3.2735E−01 |
| 57.La | 2.4958E−03 | 1.0416E+04 | 1.0597E+04 | 1.0473E+04 | 1.1804E+00 |
| | 5.2383E−02 | 3.7725E+01 | 5.8915E+01 | 8.0972E+01 | 3.7439E+01 |
| 58.Ce | 2.7567E−03 | 9.1279E+03 | 9.2980E+03 | 9.1881E+03 | 1.1960E+00 |
| | 1.4254E−02 | 5.7207E+02 | 6.8815E+02 | 6.1133E+02 | 1.2565E+01 |
| | 4.8013E−02 | 4.6086E+01 | 7.5017E+01 | 1.1661E+02 | 5.5452E+01 |
| 59.Pr | 1.4677E−02 | 5.3417E+02 | 6.4085E+02 | 5.7254E+02 | 1.1932E+01 |
| | 4.7955E−02 | 4.6234E+01 | 7.5319E+01 | 1.2304E+02 | 6.3358E+01 |
| 60.Nd | 1.0004E−03 | 4.5736E+04 | 4.5837E+04 | 4.5937E+04 | 2.1731E−01 |
| | 6.2196E−03 | 3.0810E+03 | 3.2288E+03 | 3.3625E+03 | 4.1414E+00 |
| | 4.7969E−02 | 4.6197E+01 | 7.5244E+01 | 1.2945E+02 | 7.2040E+01 |
| 61.Pm | 1.0511E−03 | 4.1407E+04 | 4.1500E+04 | 4.1614E+04 | 2.7575E−01 |
| | 2.9833E−03 | 8.5446E+03 | 8.7064E+03 | 8.6177E+03 | 1.0297E+00 |
| | 3.0612E−03 | 8.0574E+03 | 8.2109E+03 | 8.1286E+03 | 1.0121E+00 |
| | 1.7686E−02 | 4.0079E+02 | 4.8012E+02 | 4.3296E+02 | 1.0893E+01 |
| | 4.7084E−02 | 4.8419E+01 | 7.9791E+01 | 1.4843E+02 | 8.6027E+01 |
| 62.Sm | 1.1037E−03 | 3.9352E+04 | 3.9446E+04 | 3.9570E+04 | 3.1528E−01 |
| | 3.8534E−03 | 4.9832E+03 | 5.0844E+03 | 5.0438E+03 | 8.0411E−01 |
| | 4.5039E−03 | 3.3819E+03 | 3.4569E+03 | 3.4352E+03 | 6.3235E−01 |
| | 2.6467E−02 | 1.5686E+02 | 1.8371E+02 | 1.7193E+02 | 6.8545E+00 |
| | 3.1668E−02 | 8.3151E+01 | 9.6769E+01 | 9.2762E+01 | 4.3196E+00 |
| | 4.7631E−02 | 4.7047E+01 | 7.6982E+01 | 1.5054E+02 | 9.5550E+01 |
| 63.Eu | 1.2224E−03 | 3.3540E+04 | 3.3629E+04 | 3.3752E+04 | 3.6537E−01 |
| | 2.7509E−03 | 9.1569E+03 | 9.3273E+03 | 9.2263E+03 | 1.0947E+00 |
| 65.Tb | 1.2620E−03 | 3.1604E+04 | 3.1691E+04 | 3.1849E+04 | 5.0032E−01 |
| | 3.3602E−02 | 9.2659E+01 | 1.8411E+02 | 1.0390E+02 | 7.7210E+01 |
| 66.Dy | 1.3152E−03 | 2.8998E+04 | 2.9082E+04 | 2.9247E+04 | 5.6616E−01 |
| | 3.6373E−02 | 8.1202E+01 | 1.5470E+02 | 9.1707E+01 | 6.8687E+01 |
| 67.Ho | 1.3683E−03 | 2.6400E+04 | 2.6482E+04 | 2.6639E+04 | 5.9256E−01 |
| | 3.8325E−02 | 7.3132E+01 | 1.3398E+02 | 8.3193E+01 | 6.1042E+01 |
| 68.Er | 1.4209E−03 | 2.3825E+04 | 2.3905E+04 | 2.4055E+04 | 6.3045E−01 |
| | 3.9877E−02 | 6.6714E+01 | 1.1750E+02 | 7.6438E+01 | 5.3718E+01 |
| 69.Tm | 1.4738E−03 | 2.1233E+04 | 2.1311E+04 | 2.1449E+04 | 6.4722E−01 |
| | 4.6422E−02 | 5.0082E+01 | 8.3195E+01 | 5.8265E+01 | 4.2787E+01 |
| 70.Yb | 1.5496E−03 | 1.8999E+04 | 1.9074E+04 | 1.9226E+04 | 7.9515E−01 |
| | 3.3754E−02 | 9.2030E+01 | 1.8250E+02 | 1.0405E+02 | 7.5389E+01 |

| Material | $E$, MeV | $\mu_{1en}$, cm$^{-1}$ | $\mu_1$, cm$^{-1}$ | $\mu_2$, cm$^{-1}$ | $R$, % |
|---|---|---|---|---|---|
| 71.Lu | 1.5978E−03 | 1.8073E+04 | 1.8147E+04 | 1.8278E+04 | 7.2128E−01 |
| | 5.9213E−02 | 2.8055E+01 | 4.2020E+01 | 3.3977E+01 | 2.3673E+01 |
| 72.Hf | 1.0407E−03 | 4.2241E+04 | 4.2335E+04 | 4.2387E+04 | 1.2267E−01 |
| 81.Tl | 2.3695E−03 | 9.8926E+03 | 1.0039E+04 | 1.0024E+04 | 1.4195E−01 |
| 82.Pb | 2.3767E−03 | 1.0180E+04 | 1.0335E+04 | 1.0306E+04 | 2.8440E−01 |
| 83.Bi | 2.3606E−03 | 9.5365E+03 | 9.6712E+03 | 9.6486E+03 | 2.3427E−01 |
| 84.Po | 2.3666E−03 | 9.7780E+03 | 9.9204E+03 | 9.8863E+03 | 3.4408E−01 |
| 85.At | 2.4044E−03 | 1.0857E+04 | 1.1041E+04 | 1.0979E+04 | 5.7036E−01 |
| 87.Fr | 2.6160E−03 | 9.8324E+03 | 1.0010E+04 | 9.9488E+03 | 6.1410E−01 |
| 88.Ra | 3.1646E−03 | 7.4432E+03 | 7.5872E+03 | 7.6954E+03 | 1.4255E+00 |
| | 1.1871E−02 | 5.7549E+02 | 6.0717E+02 | 6.0501E+02 | 3.5778E−01 |
| | 4.8884E−02 | 4.3900E+01 | 7.0542E+01 | 5.3517E+01 | 3.1811E+01 |
| 89.Ac | 2.8026E−03 | 8.8978E+03 | 9.0655E+03 | 9.0133E+03 | 5.7860E−01 |
| | 1.5326E−02 | 5.3360E+02 | 6.4504E+02 | 5.7470E+02 | 1.2240E+01 |
| 90.Th | 2.9706E−03 | 8.6385E+03 | 8.8024E+03 | 8.7681E+03 | 3.9103E−01 |
| | 3.2155E−03 | 7.1413E+03 | 7.2806E+03 | 7.2672E+03 | 1.8495E−01 |
| 112. | 1.9091E−03 | 1.2099E+04 | 1.2165E+04 | 1.2151E+04 | 1.1570E−01 |
| 112. | 2.0271E−03 | 1.0091E+04 | 1.0155E+04 | 1.0141E+04 | 1.4070E−01 |
| | 2.3156E−03 | 8.2170E+03 | 8.3047E+03 | 8.2635E+03 | 4.9860E−01 |
| | 1.1106E−02 | 6.9870E+02 | 7.3511E+02 | 7.3066E+02 | 6.0928E−01 |
| 116. | 2.2314E−03 | 8.1081E+03 | 8.1717E+03 | 8.1501E+03 | 2.6412E−01 |
| | 1.2252E−02 | 5.1393E+02 | 5.4326E+02 | 5.4218E+02 | 1.9877E−01 |
| 121. | 1.2552E−03 | 3.1937E+04 | 3.2024E+04 | 3.2153E+04 | 4.0134E−01 |
| | 3.8619E−03 | 4.9548E+03 | 5.0555E+03 | 5.0316E+03 | 4.7604E−01 |
| | 4.4891E−03 | 3.4146E+03 | 3.4902E+03 | 3.4755E+03 | 4.2320E−01 |
| | 1.4869E−02 | 5.6392E+02 | 6.8332E+02 | 6.1698E+02 | 1.0752E+01 |
| | 5.7184E−02 | 3.0927E+01 | 4.7038E+01 | 8.5331E+01 | 8.1408E+01 |
| 123. | 1.2252E−02 | 5.1401E+02 | 5.4334E+02 | 8.4492E+02 | 5.5505E+01 |
| 125. | 1.3107E−02 | 6.1076E+02 | 7.0279E+02 | 7.6490E+02 | 8.8383E+00 |
| | 3.5778E−02 | 8.3662E+01 | 1.6101E+02 | 9.9814E+01 | 6.1314E+01 |

131.MUSCLE, SKELETAL (ICRU-44)

| Material | $E$, MeV | $\mu_{1en}$, cm$^{-1}$ | $\mu_1$, cm$^{-1}$ | $\mu_2$, cm$^{-1}$ | $R$, % |
|---|---|---|---|---|---|
| 5.B | 5.4451E−02 | 4.0566E−02 | 2.2751E−01 | 3.8595E−01 | 6.9644E+01 |
| 6.C | 1.0307E−03 | 3.5976E+03 | 3.6081E+03 | 3.6009E+03 | 1.9948E−01 |
| | 1.3013E−03 | 2.2086E+03 | 2.2152E+03 | 2.2112E+03 | 1.8351E−01 |
| | 2.2608E−03 | 4.1874E+02 | 4.2038E+02 | 4.2031E+02 | 1.7056E−02 |
| | 2.7495E−03 | 2.4264E+02 | 2.4434E+02 | 2.4396E+02 | 1.5744E−01 |
| | 5.7714E−02 | 3.6828E−02 | 2.2018E−01 | 3.0260E−01 | 3.7433E+01 |
| 14.Si | 1.0547E−03 | 3.3874E+03 | 3.3974E+03 | 3.3943E+03 | 9.1636E−02 |
| | 1.2706E−03 | 2.3473E+03 | 2.3543E+03 | 2.3535E+03 | 3.3185E−02 |

| Material | $E$, MeV | $\mu_{1en}$, cm$^{-1}$ | $\mu_1$, cm$^{-1}$ | $\mu_2$, cm$^{-1}$ | $R$, % |
|---|---|---|---|---|---|
| 19.K | 2.0557E−03 | 5.4464E+02 | 5.4662E+02 | 5.4712E+02 | 9.0835E−02 |
| | 2.9932E−03 | 1.8998E+02 | 1.9166E+02 | 1.9205E+02 | 2.0230E−01 |
| | 3.1826E−03 | 1.6490E+02 | 1.6642E+02 | 1.6689E+02 | 2.8176E−01 |
| 86.Rn | 1.9265E−02 | 7.2040E−01 | 9.9616E−01 | 9.6419E−01 | 3.3153E+00 |
| 101. | 5.3623E−02 | 4.1514E−02 | 2.2937E−01 | 2.3996E−01 | 4.6160E+00 |
| 104. | 3.9544E−03 | 8.7378E+01 | 8.8838E+01 | 8.8388E+01 | 5.0957E−01 |
| | 4.7977E−02 | 5.1702E−02 | 2.4649E−01 | 3.0762E−01 | 2.4800E+01 |
| 107. | 6.2100E−03 | 2.3428E+01 | 2.4129E+01 | 2.4095E+01 | 1.4355E−01 |
| | 7.8284E−03 | 1.1633E+01 | 1.2158E+01 | 1.2234E+01 | 6.3003E−01 |
| 109. | 5.9613E−03 | 2.5666E+01 | 2.6399E+01 | 2.6382E+01 | 6.4352E−02 |
| | 5.5777E−02 | 3.9047E−02 | 2.2453E−01 | 2.2356E−01 | 4.3236E−01 |
| 115. | 1.1599E−03 | 2.8482E+03 | 2.8565E+03 | 2.8569E+03 | 1.4359E−02 |
| | 1.4382E−03 | 1.5889E+03 | 1.5938E+03 | 1.5930E+03 | 5.2591E−02 |
| 119. | 3.1905E−03 | 1.6388E+02 | 1.6540E+02 | 1.6529E+02 | 6.8454E−02 |
| | 3.8215E−03 | 9.7462E+01 | 9.9047E+01 | 9.8547E+01 | 5.0707E−01 |
| 120. | 6.8167E−03 | 1.9006E+01 | 1.9642E+01 | 1.9602E+01 | 2.0143E−01 |
| | 7.5213E−03 | 1.3871E+01 | 1.4429E+01 | 1.4411E+01 | 1.2470E−01 |
| 132. | 5.0000E−02 | 4.5664E−02 | 2.3751E−01 | 2.3824E−01 | 3.0945E−01 |
| | 6.0000E−02 | 3.4209E−02 | 2.1504E−01 | 2.1567E−01 | 2.9297E−01 |
| 137. | 1.6685E−03 | 1.0653E+03 | 1.0688E+03 | 1.0681E+03 | 6.8987E−02 |
| 137. | 2.0207E−03 | 5.7017E+02 | 5.7222E+02 | 5.7208E+02 | 2.4026E−02 |
| | 2.9386E−03 | 2.0117E+02 | 2.0288E+02 | 2.0245E+02 | 2.1336E−01 |
| | 3.4370E−03 | 1.3193E+02 | 1.3323E+02 | 1.3304E+02 | 1.4505E−01 |
| | 3.6391E−03 | 1.1131E+02 | 1.1307E+02 | 1.1236E+02 | 6.2956E−01 |
| | 5.8864E−02 | 3.5510E−02 | 2.1759E−01 | 2.6017E−01 | 1.9566E+01 |
| 141. | 2.2599E−03 | 4.1923E+02 | 4.2088E+02 | 4.2168E+02 | 1.9002E−01 |
| | 2.6131E−03 | 2.8031E+02 | 2.8222E+02 | 2.8263E+02 | 1.4655E−01 |
| 143. | 4.2007E−03 | 7.5747E+01 | 7.7070E+01 | 7.6891E+01 | 2.3270E−01 |
| 145. | 1.0166E−03 | 3.7336E+03 | 3.7441E+03 | 3.7444E+03 | 6.2468E−03 |
| | 1.4517E−03 | 1.5281E+03 | 1.5329E+03 | 1.5319E+03 | 6.6564E−02 |
| | 2.0350E−03 | 5.5975E+02 | 5.6178E+02 | 5.6163E+02 | 2.7104E−02 |
| | 2.9449E−03 | 1.9988E+02 | 2.0159E+02 | 2.0102E+02 | 2.8281E−01 |
| | 3.3807E−03 | 1.3923E+02 | 1.4058E+02 | 1.4022E+02 | 2.5229E−01 |
| | 3.6973E−03 | 1.0689E+02 | 1.0859E+02 | 1.0780E+02 | 7.3200E−01 |
| 148. | 3.9408E−03 | 8.8409E+01 | 8.9882E+01 | 8.9298E+01 | 6.5330E−01 |
| | | | 132.OVARY (ICRU-44) | | |
| 5.B | 5.4451E−02 | 4.0566E−02 | 2.2820E−01 | 3.8595E−01 | 6.9132E+01 |
| 6.C | 1.0600E−03 | 3.4470E+03 | 3.4568E+03 | 3.4502E+03 | 1.9008E−01 |
| | 1.1398E−03 | 3.0375E+03 | 3.0461E+03 | 3.0406E+03 | 1.8416E−01 |

| Material | $E$, MeV | $\mu_{1en}$, cm$^{-1}$ | $\mu_1$, cm$^{-1}$ | $\mu_2$, cm$^{-1}$ | $R$, % |
|---|---|---|---|---|---|
| | 2.3749E−03 | 3.7761E+02 | 3.7941E+02 | 3.7912E+02 | 7.6962E−02 |
| | 2.6665E−03 | 2.7253E+02 | 2.7429E+02 | 2.7389E+02 | 1.4449E−01 |
| | 5.7714E−02 | 3.6828E−02 | 2.2083E−01 | 3.0260E−01 | 3.7026E+01 |
| 19.K | 2.1093E−03 | 5.2436E+02 | 5.2630E+02 | 5.2682E+02 | 9.6985E−02 |
| | 2.9499E−03 | 2.0635E+02 | 2.0806E+02 | 2.0844E+02 | 1.8302E−01 |
| 86.Rn | 1.9316E−02 | 7.1593E−01 | 9.9239E−01 | 9.5748E−01 | 3.6462E+00 |
| 101. | 5.3623E−02 | 4.1514E−02 | 2.3007E−01 | 2.3996E−01 | 4.2991E+00 |
| 104. | 2.9941E−03 | 1.9697E+02 | 1.9866E+02 | 1.9826E+02 | 2.0060E−01 |
| | 3.0601E−03 | 1.8764E+02 | 1.8928E+02 | 1.8891E+02 | 1.9798E−01 |
| | 3.9060E−03 | 9.2799E+01 | 9.4101E+01 | 9.3823E+01 | 2.9706E−01 |
| | 4.7995E−02 | 5.1658E−02 | 2.4717E−01 | 3.0755E−01 | 2.4427E+01 |
| 107. | 1.1314E−03 | 3.0769E+03 | 3.0856E+03 | 3.0857E+03 | 2.6981E−03 |
| | 3.3818E−03 | 1.4438E+02 | 1.4579E+02 | 1.4581E+02 | 9.2416E−03 |
| | 3.9515E−03 | 8.9263E+01 | 9.0540E+01 | 9.0584E+01 | 4.8419E−02 |
| | 6.0104E−03 | 2.5270E+01 | 2.5952E+01 | 2.5958E+01 | 2.4621E−02 |
| | 7.9013E−03 | 1.1253E+01 | 1.1755E+01 | 1.1846E+01 | 7.7221E−01 |
| 109. | 3.3462E−02 | 1.3696E−01 | 3.5849E−01 | 3.5642E−01 | 5.8083E−01 |
| | 5.5777E−02 | 3.9047E−02 | 2.2520E−01 | 2.2356E−01 | 7.3400E−01 |
| 115. | 1.1190E−03 | 3.1346E+03 | 3.1435E+03 | 3.1443E+03 | 2.4845E−02 |
| | 1.4676E−03 | 1.5067E+03 | 1.5113E+03 | 1.5108E+03 | 3.1576E−02 |
| 119. | 3.4032E−03 | 1.4150E+02 | 1.4290E+02 | 1.4279E+02 | 7.4215E−02 |
| | 3.7521E−03 | 1.0477E+02 | 1.0616E+02 | 1.0589E+02 | 2.5399E−01 |
| 120. | 6.6975E−03 | 2.0176E+01 | 2.0793E+01 | 2.0785E+01 | 3.6476E−02 |
| 120. | 7.6245E−03 | 1.3305E+01 | 1.3834E+01 | 1.3837E+01 | 2.2322E−02 |
| 131. | 5.0000E−02 | 4.5664E−02 | 2.3824E−01 | 2.3751E−01 | 3.0945E−01 |
| | 6.0000E−02 | 3.4209E−02 | 2.1567E−01 | 2.1504E−01 | 2.9297E−01 |
| 137. | 1.0012E−03 | 4.0026E+03 | 4.0152E+03 | 4.0109E+03 | 1.0627E−01 |
| | 1.4408E−03 | 1.6319E+03 | 1.6368E+03 | 1.6357E+03 | 7.0161E−02 |
| | 2.0805E−03 | 5.4614E+02 | 5.4812E+02 | 5.4801E+02 | 1.9602E−02 |
| | 2.8987E−03 | 2.1722E+02 | 2.1896E+02 | 2.1853E+02 | 1.9585E−01 |
| | 3.5917E−03 | 1.1615E+02 | 1.1742E+02 | 1.1721E+02 | 1.7791E−01 |
| | 5.8864E−02 | 3.5510E−02 | 2.1823E−01 | 2.6017E−01 | 1.9214E+01 |
| 141. | 2.4437E−03 | 3.4692E+02 | 3.4864E+02 | 3.4930E+02 | 1.9044E−01 |
| 144. | 7.4006E−03 | 1.4965E+01 | 1.5515E+01 | 1.5537E+01 | 1.4649E−01 |
| 145. | 1.0422E−03 | 3.6043E+03 | 3.6146E+03 | 3.6146E+03 | 5.1333E−04 |
| | 1.3188E−03 | 2.2018E+03 | 2.2082E+03 | 2.2077E+03 | 2.3721E−02 |
| | 2.0927E−03 | 5.3695E+02 | 5.3892E+02 | 5.3878E+02 | 2.6056E−02 |
| | 2.9038E−03 | 2.1613E+02 | 2.1786E+02 | 2.1730E+02 | 2.5767E−01 |
| | 3.5443E−03 | 1.2252E+02 | 1.2382E+02 | 1.2347E+02 | 2.8397E−01 |

| Material | $E$, MeV | $\mu_{1en}$, cm$^{-1}$ | $\mu_1$, cm$^{-1}$ | $\mu_2$, cm$^{-1}$ | $R$, % |
|---|---|---|---|---|---|
| | 3.6093E−03 | 1.1587E+02 | 1.1734E+02 | 1.1681E+02 | 4.5667E−01 |
| 148. | 2.9810E−03 | 1.9976E+02 | 2.0145E+02 | 2.0098E+02 | 2.3591E−01 |
| | 3.1627E−03 | 1.7383E+02 | 1.7540E+02 | 1.7498E+02 | 2.4071E−01 |
| | 3.8882E−03 | 9.4190E+01 | 9.5502E+01 | 9.5097E+01 | 4.2631E−01 |
| PHOTOGRAPHIC EMULSION (KODAK TYPE AA) | | | | | |
| 13.Al | 3.7107E−03 | 1.2837E+03 | 1.3284E+03 | 1.3068E+03 | 1.6496E+00 |
| 15.P | 3.8882E−03 | 1.2566E+03 | 1.2997E+03 | 1.2993E+03 | 2.9181E−02 |
| 16.S | 6.6514E−03 | 3.3566E+02 | 3.4622E+02 | 3.4702E+02 | 2.2902E−01 |
| | 1.1817E−02 | 7.2444E+01 | 7.5883E+01 | 7.5075E+01 | 1.0764E+00 |
| 21.Sc | 2.6056E−02 | 2.2650E+01 | 4.8359E+01 | 2.4591E+01 | 9.6655E+01 |
| 22.Ti | 3.7305E−02 | 1.1806E+01 | 2.0261E+01 | 1.3426E+01 | 5.0911E+01 |
| 31.Ga | 1.1025E−03 | 7.9472E+03 | 7.9617E+03 | 7.9767E+03 | 1.8870E−01 |
| 32.Ge | 1.1101E−03 | 7.8597E+03 | 7.8742E+03 | 7.8913E+03 | 2.1812E−01 |
| 34.Se | 1.1879E−03 | 6.9657E+03 | 6.9794E+03 | 6.9924E+03 | 1.8655E−01 |
| | 1.2465E−03 | 6.2922E+03 | 6.3054E+03 | 6.3186E+03 | 2.0967E−01 |
| 37.Rb | 5.7569E−02 | 4.1608E+00 | 6.0765E+00 | 5.2861E+00 | 1.4952E+01 |
| 38.Sr | 1.4544E−03 | 3.9030E+03 | 3.9144E+03 | 3.9184E+03 | 1.0398E−01 |
| | 1.4264E−02 | 6.4542E+01 | 9.5331E+01 | 6.8482E+01 | 3.9205E+01 |
| 55.Cs | 2.9173E−02 | 1.8672E+01 | 3.6361E+01 | 2.0707E+01 | 7.5602E+01 |
| 113. | 1.7987E−03 | 3.9599E+03 | 3.9988E+03 | 3.9758E+03 | 5.7685E−01 |
| | 1.4279E−02 | 6.4395E+01 | 9.5081E+01 | 6.8753E+01 | 3.8294E+01 |
| 117. | 1.9652E−03 | 3.1921E+03 | 3.2243E+03 | 3.2771E+03 | 1.6365E+00 |
| | 2.5628E−03 | 1.9295E+03 | 1.9499E+03 | 1.9769E+03 | 1.3826E+00 |
| | 3.3023E−03 | 8.4079E+02 | 8.5141E+02 | 8.5772E+02 | 7.4130E−01 |
| 118. | 5.0618E−03 | 6.4124E+02 | 6.6121E+02 | 6.6570E+02 | 6.7812E−01 |
| | 2.9471E−02 | 1.8291E+01 | 3.5212E+01 | 2.0545E+01 | 7.1392E+01 |
| 141. | 2.9515E−03 | 1.1686E+03 | 1.1819E+03 | 1.2619E+03 | 6.7720E+00 |
| 134.PHOTOGRAPHIC EMULSION (STANDARD NUCLEAR) | | | | | |
| 13.Al | 1.5711E−03 | 1.0220E+04 | 1.0312E+04 | 1.0561E+04 | 2.4069E+00 |
| 14.Si | 2.4655E−03 | 4.3560E+03 | 4.4022E+03 | 4.5196E+03 | 2.6661E+00 |
| | 2.4767E−03 | 4.3113E+03 | 4.3607E+03 | 4.4727E+03 | 2.5687E+00 |
| 16.S | 3.2070E−03 | 2.2575E+03 | 2.2862E+03 | 2.3861E+03 | 4.3722E+00 |
| 21.Sc | 1.0086E−02 | 2.7107E+02 | 2.8199E+02 | 2.9401E+02 | 4.2608E+00 |
| 22.Ti | 1.4886E−02 | 1.5724E+02 | 2.2825E+02 | 1.7058E+02 | 3.3809E+01 |
| 23.V | 1.8634E−03 | 8.7931E+03 | 8.8885E+03 | 8.8208E+03 | 7.6688E−01 |
| | 2.3072E−03 | 5.3616E+03 | 5.4181E+03 | 5.3842E+03 | 6.2911E−01 |
| | 2.7061E−03 | 3.5808E+03 | 3.6226E+03 | 3.6009E+03 | 6.0232E−01 |
| 24.Cr | 2.8863E−02 | 5.1852E+01 | 1.0194E+02 | 5.7581E+01 | 7.7032E+01 |
| 25.Mn | 2.9936E−02 | 4.8138E+01 | 9.0704E+01 | 5.3862E+01 | 6.8401E+01 |

| Material | $E$, MeV | $\mu_{1en}$, cm$^{-1}$ | $\mu_1$, cm$^{-1}$ | $\mu_2$, cm$^{-1}$ | $R$, % |
|---|---|---|---|---|---|
| 26.Fe | 3.8850E−02 | 2.8552E+01 | 4.6648E+01 | 3.2693E+01 | 4.2683E+01 |
| 27.Co | 3.6822E−03 | 3.4183E+03 | 3.5374E+03 | 3.4517E+03 | 2.4825E+00 |
| | 5.3760E−02 | 1.3511E+01 | 1.9681E+01 | 1.6304E+01 | 2.0710E+01 |
| 28.Ni | 3.8616E−03 | 3.3556E+03 | 3.4744E+03 | 3.3912E+03 | 2.4542E+00 |
| 29.Cu | 3.9996E−03 | 3.0764E+03 | 3.1833E+03 | 3.1131E+03 | 2.2521E+00 |
| | 4.0037E−03 | 3.0699E+03 | 3.1765E+03 | 3.1066E+03 | 2.2493E+00 |
| 31.Ga | 4.7908E−02 | 1.7893E+01 | 2.7023E+01 | 2.1433E+01 | 2.6078E+01 |
| 32.Ge | 4.5236E−02 | 2.0755E+01 | 3.2098E+01 | 2.5036E+01 | 2.8209E+01 |
| 34.Se | 3.9738E−02 | 2.6861E+01 | 4.3091E+01 | 3.3363E+01 | 2.9158E+01 |
| 38.Sr | 1.7184E−02 | 1.2084E+02 | 1.7103E+02 | 2.4840E+02 | 4.5243E+01 |
| 39.Y | 1.0656E−03 | 1.5848E+04 | 1.5879E+04 | 1.5879E+04 | 1.1193E−03 |
| | 1.1472E−03 | 1.4119E+04 | 1.4148E+04 | 1.4149E+04 | 5.5634E−03 |
| 40.Zr | 1.4889E−02 | 1.5717E+02 | 2.2814E+02 | 1.6742E+02 | 3.6266E+01 |
| 41.Nb | 2.3691E−03 | 4.9686E+03 | 5.0211E+03 | 5.0184E+03 | 5.4176E−02 |
| 48.Cd | 3.5095E−03 | 3.1248E+03 | 3.2193E+03 | 3.1752E+03 | 1.3876E+00 |
| 49.In | 2.7802E−02 | 5.5525E+01 | 1.1305E+02 | 6.2333E+01 | 8.1361E+01 |
| 50.Sn | 2.9139E−02 | 5.0897E+01 | 9.9049E+01 | 5.7392E+01 | 7.2583E+01 |
| 51.Sb | 2.9555E−02 | 4.9458E+01 | 9.4697E+01 | 5.5544E+01 | 7.0490E+01 |
| 52.Te | 2.9259E−02 | 5.0480E+01 | 9.7788E+01 | 5.6338E+01 | 7.3575E+01 |
| 53.I | 2.7666E−02 | 5.5994E+01 | 1.1446E+02 | 6.1614E+01 | 8.5778E+01 |
| 55.Cs | 1.1217E−03 | 1.4628E+04 | 1.4658E+04 | 1.4665E+04 | 4.9382E−02 |
| 57.La | 3.8663E−02 | 2.8909E+01 | 4.7397E+01 | 3.3386E+01 | 4.1966E+01 |
| 63.Eu | 1.1348E−03 | 1.4366E+04 | 1.4395E+04 | 1.4454E+04 | 4.1028E−01 |
| | 6.6531E−03 | 8.9358E+02 | 9.2167E+02 | 9.2171E+02 | 4.2382E−03 |
| 64.Gd | 1.0306E−03 | 1.7114E+04 | 1.7145E+04 | 1.7196E+04 | 2.9867E−01 |
| | 1.1171E−03 | 1.4719E+04 | 1.4749E+04 | 1.4804E+04 | 3.7192E−01 |
| 112. | 2.6039E−02 | 6.1627E+01 | 1.3150E+02 | 6.8181E+01 | 9.2875E+01 |
| 116. | 2.7229E−02 | 5.7508E+01 | 1.1904E+02 | 6.3058E+01 | 8.8786E+01 |
| 121. | 1.1360E−03 | 1.4342E+04 | 1.4372E+04 | 1.4413E+04 | 2.8788E−01 |
| 123. | 1.1162E−03 | 1.4738E+04 | 1.4768E+04 | 1.4846E+04 | 5.2620E−01 |
| | 4.5685E−02 | 2.0273E+01 | 3.1244E+01 | 2.4505E+01 | 2.7499E+01 |
| 135.PLASTIC SCINTILLATOR (VINYLTOLUENE) | | | | | |
| 4.Be | 4.8893E−02 | 2.5966E−02 | 2.0834E−01 | 2.8894E−01 | 3.8685E+01 |
| 35.Br | 1.8527E−02 | 3.0670E−01 | 5.5150E−01 | 4.9583E−01 | 1.1228E+01 |
| | 4.9345E−02 | 2.5578E−02 | 2.0742E−01 | 3.1840E−02 | 5.5145E+02 |
| 136.POLYETHYLENE | | | | | |
| 4.Be | 4.4975E−02 | 2.6234E−02 | 2.0274E−01 | 2.9516E−01 | 4.5590E+01 |
| 35.Br | 1.5107E−02 | 4.4379E−01 | 6.8679E−01 | 7.8238E−01 | 1.3919E+01 |
| | 5.2011E−02 | 2.2325E−02 | 1.9168E−01 | 2.7762E−02 | 5.9043E+02 |

| Material | $E$, MeV | $\mu_{1en}$, cm$^{-1}$ | $\mu_1$, cm$^{-1}$ | $\mu_2$, cm$^{-1}$ | $R$, % |
|---|---|---|---|---|---|
| 137.POLYETHYLENE TEREPHTHALATE, "MYLAR" | | | | | |
| 5.B | 5.2077E−02 | 4.0886E−02 | 2.7440E−01 | 3.9057E−01 | 4.2334E+01 |
| 6.C | 5.6281E−02 | 3.7557E−02 | 2.6559E−01 | 3.0547E−01 | 1.5018E+01 |
| 19.K | 2.5395E−03 | 3.6163E+02 | 3.6319E+02 | 3.6389E+02 | 1.9482E−01 |
| | 3.5146E−03 | 1.2400E+02 | 1.2509E+02 | 1.2585E+02 | 6.1071E−01 |
| 101. | 1.3341E−02 | 2.2432E+00 | 2.6379E+00 | 2.6153E+00 | 8.6649E−01 |
| 107. | 1.0030E−03 | 3.9926E+03 | 4.0009E+03 | 4.0043E+03 | 8.5247E−02 |
| | 1.4418E−03 | 1.6264E+03 | 1.6302E+03 | 1.6314E+03 | 7.3145E−02 |
| | 2.0783E−03 | 5.4703E+02 | 5.4891E+02 | 5.4899E+02 | 1.4400E−02 |
| | 2.8991E−03 | 2.1705E+02 | 2.1836E+02 | 2.1886E+02 | 2.3118E−01 |
| | 3.5924E−03 | 1.1607E+02 | 1.1713E+02 | 1.1735E+02 | 1.8809E−01 |
| 109. | 2.9330E−03 | 2.0342E+02 | 2.0471E+02 | 2.0533E+02 | 3.0435E−01 |
| | 3.4692E−03 | 1.2864E+02 | 1.2974E+02 | 1.3011E+02 | 2.8577E−01 |
| | 3.6446E−03 | 1.1075E+02 | 1.1180E+02 | 1.1248E+02 | 6.1296E−01 |
| | 5.8815E−02 | 3.5549E−02 | 2.6027E−01 | 2.1671E−01 | 2.0102E+01 |
| 115. | 1.0433E−03 | 3.7755E+03 | 3.7833E+03 | 3.7874E+03 | 1.0692E−01 |
| | 1.4602E−03 | 1.5275E+03 | 1.5311E+03 | 1.5316E+03 | 3.5215E−02 |
| | 2.2750E−03 | 4.6794E+02 | 4.6968E+02 | 4.6980E+02 | 2.5704E−02 |
| | 2.6245E−03 | 3.2744E+02 | 3.2894E+02 | 3.3058E+02 | 4.9975E−01 |
| 119. | 2.9632E−03 | 1.9129E+02 | 1.9256E+02 | 1.9283E+02 | 1.4279E−01 |
| | 4.9631E−02 | 4.3354E−02 | 2.8021E−01 | 2.3787E−01 | 1.7799E+01 |
| 120. | 1.0294E−03 | 3.8503E+03 | 3.8583E+03 | 3.8628E+03 | 1.1616E−01 |
| | 1.3489E−03 | 2.1277E+03 | 2.1325E+03 | 2.1337E+03 | 5.8526E−02 |
| | 2.2474E−03 | 4.7903E+02 | 4.8079E+02 | 4.8085E+02 | 1.3958E−02 |
| | 2.7971E−03 | 2.5805E+02 | 2.5944E+02 | 2.6055E+02 | 4.3114E−01 |
| 128. | 1.4590E−03 | 1.5337E+03 | 1.5373E+03 | 1.5374E+03 | 1.0450E−02 |
| | 2.0659E−03 | 5.5199E+02 | 5.5387E+02 | 5.5389E+02 | 2.4133E−03 |
| | 2.8954E−03 | 2.1855E+02 | 2.1987E+02 | 2.2050E+02 | 2.9002E−01 |
| | 5.9601E−02 | 3.4926E−02 | 2.5862E−01 | 2.1647E−01 | 1.9470E+01 |
| 131. | 1.6685E−03 | 1.0653E+03 | 1.0681E+03 | 1.0688E+03 | 6.8987E−02 |
| | 2.0207E−03 | 5.7017E+02 | 5.7208E+02 | 5.7222E+02 | 2.4026E−02 |
| | 2.9386E−03 | 2.0117E+02 | 2.0245E+02 | 2.0288E+02 | 2.1336E−01 |
| 131. | 3.4370E−03 | 1.3193E+02 | 1.3304E+02 | 1.3323E+02 | 1.4505E−01 |
| | 3.6391E−03 | 1.1131E+02 | 1.1236E+02 | 1.1307E+02 | 6.2956E−01 |
| | 5.8864E−02 | 3.5510E−02 | 2.6017E−01 | 2.1759E−01 | 1.9566E+01 |
| 132. | 1.0012E−03 | 4.0026E+03 | 4.0109E+03 | 4.0152E+03 | 1.0627E−01 |
| | 1.4408E−03 | 1.6319E+03 | 1.6357E+03 | 1.6368E+03 | 7.0161E−02 |
| | 2.0805E−03 | 5.4614E+02 | 5.4801E+02 | 5.4812E+02 | 1.9602E−02 |
| | 2.8987E−03 | 2.1722E+02 | 2.1853E+02 | 2.1896E+02 | 1.9585E−01 |

| Material | $E$, MeV | $\mu_{1en}$, cm$^{-1}$ | $\mu_1$, cm$^{-1}$ | $\mu_2$, cm$^{-1}$ | $R$, % |
|---|---|---|---|---|---|
| | 3.5917E−03 | 1.1615E+02 | 1.1721E+02 | 1.1742E+02 | 1.7791E−01 |
| | 5.8864E−02 | 3.5510E−02 | 2.6017E−01 | 2.1823E−01 | 1.9214E+01 |
| 143. | 1.4659E−03 | 1.4966E+03 | 1.5001E+03 | 1.5003E+03 | 1.1848E−02 |
| | 2.0606E−03 | 5.5414E+02 | 5.5603E+02 | 5.5613E+02 | 1.8573E−02 |
| | 2.9184E−03 | 2.0931E+02 | 2.1061E+02 | 2.1097E+02 | 1.6964E−01 |
| | 3.5234E−03 | 1.2311E+02 | 1.2419E+02 | 1.2431E+02 | 9.5351E−02 |
| | 3.6331E−03 | 1.1192E+02 | 1.1297E+02 | 1.1336E+02 | 3.4572E−01 |
| | 5.7194E−02 | 3.6833E−02 | 2.6367E−01 | 2.1973E−01 | 1.9998E+01 |
| 144. | 1.4891E−03 | 1.3717E+03 | 1.3750E+03 | 1.3760E+03 | 7.9246E−02 |
| | 2.0379E−03 | 5.6328E+02 | 5.6518E+02 | 5.6524E+02 | 9.3845E−03 |
| | 2.9155E−03 | 2.1046E+02 | 2.1176E+02 | 2.1236E+02 | 2.8454E−01 |
| | 3.5388E−03 | 1.2153E+02 | 1.2261E+02 | 1.2287E+02 | 2.0669E−01 |
| | 5.9968E−02 | 3.4636E−02 | 2.5785E−01 | 2.1716E−01 | 1.8737E+01 |
| 145. | 2.7539E−03 | 2.7542E+02 | 2.7683E+02 | 2.7672E+02 | 4.1533E−02 |
| | 3.9918E−02 | 6.5386E−02 | 3.1875E−01 | 2.6171E−01 | 2.1793E+01 |
| 148. | 4.9394E−02 | 4.3880E−02 | 2.8113E−01 | 2.2941E−01 | 2.2548E+01 |
| | | | 138.POLYMETHYL METHACRYLATE | | |
| 5.B | 4.5334E−02 | 4.5004E−02 | 2.6213E−01 | 4.0876E−01 | 5.5937E+01 |
| 6.C | 7.1765E−03 | 1.1620E+01 | 1.2116E+01 | 1.2241E+01 | 1.0292E+00 |
| | 3.5264E−02 | 8.3165E−02 | 3.1809E−01 | 3.9205E−01 | 2.3252E+01 |
| 101. | 4.2764E−03 | 5.3253E+01 | 5.3999E+01 | 5.6291E+01 | 4.2444E+00 |
| 109. | 2.4684E−03 | 3.2302E+02 | 3.2429E+02 | 3.2479E+02 | 1.5546E−01 |
| 110. | 1.0006E−03 | 3.3149E+03 | 3.3221E+03 | 3.3231E+03 | 3.0888E−02 |
| | 1.4660E−03 | 1.2384E+03 | 1.2413E+03 | 1.2418E+03 | 3.6955E−02 |
| | 2.0469E−03 | 4.6325E+02 | 4.6477E+02 | 4.6492E+02 | 3.2089E−02 |
| | 2.9367E−03 | 1.6721E+02 | 1.6820E+02 | 1.6857E+02 | 2.2158E−01 |
| | 5.5542E−02 | 3.2956E−02 | 2.3691E−01 | 2.1280E−01 | 1.1333E+01 |
| 119. | 2.3876E−03 | 3.4988E+02 | 3.5120E+02 | 3.5149E+02 | 8.2134E−02 |
| | 2.6576E−03 | 2.6005E+02 | 2.6121E+02 | 2.6175E+02 | 2.0929E−01 |
| 122. | 2.6987E−03 | 2.4637E+02 | 2.4750E+02 | 2.4766E+02 | 6.3131E−02 |
| | 3.7154E−02 | 7.1818E−02 | 3.0275E−01 | 3.2484E−01 | 7.2959E+00 |
| 141. | 2.7027E−03 | 2.4504E+02 | 2.4617E+02 | 2.4733E+02 | 4.7190E−01 |
| | | | 139.POLYSTYRENE | | |
| 4.Be | 4.9724E−02 | 2.5909E−02 | 2.1109E−01 | 2.8762E−01 | 3.6252E+01 |
| 35.Br | 1.8941E−02 | 2.9011E−01 | 5.3825E−01 | 4.6115E−01 | 1.6720E+01 |
| 35.Br | 4.8742E−02 | 2.6786E−02 | 2.1314E−01 | 3.3389E−02 | 5.3836E+02 |
| 102. | 2.4507E−03 | 2.0155E+02 | 2.0239E+02 | 2.0251E+02 | 5.8662E−02 |
| | 2.6594E−03 | 1.5828E+02 | 1.5907E+02 | 1.5931E+02 | 1.4636E−01 |

| Material | $E$, MeV | $\mu_{1en}$, cm$^{-1}$ | $\mu_1$, cm$^{-1}$ | $\mu_2$, cm$^{-1}$ | $R$, % |
|---|---|---|---|---|---|
| 140.POLYTETRAFLUOROETHYLENE, "TEFLON" | | | | | |
| 11.Na | 9.1808E−03 | 2.0290E+01 | 2.1269E+01 | 2.0929E+01 | 1.6255E+00 |
| | 4.2036E−02 | 1.7807E−01 | 5.7198E−01 | 3.6236E−01 | 5.7850E+01 |
| 33.As | 1.2624E−03 | 7.0932E+03 | 7.1304E+03 | 7.1238E+03 | 9.2374E−02 |
| 108. | 2.9620E−03 | 5.8330E+02 | 5.8684E+02 | 5.9562E+02 | 1.4966E+00 |
| 114. | 2.3403E−03 | 1.3066E+03 | 1.3128E+03 | 1.3133E+03 | 3.3036E−02 |
| 129. | 1.4503E−03 | 4.4447E+03 | 4.4668E+03 | 4.4872E+03 | 4.5756E−01 |
| 141.POLYVINYL CHLORIDE | | | | | |
| 6.C | 1.8961E−03 | 6.5312E+02 | 6.5574E+02 | 6.5489E+02 | 1.2946E−01 |
| | 2.2653E−03 | 4.1711E+02 | 4.1955E+02 | 4.1868E+02 | 2.0909E−01 |
| 12.Mg | 2.9976E−03 | 1.1361E+03 | 1.2254E+03 | 1.1511E+03 | 6.4526E+00 |
| 14.Si | 1.8032E−03 | 7.7074E+02 | 7.7344E+02 | 7.7592E+02 | 3.2042E−01 |
| 107. | 2.3999E−03 | 3.6417E+02 | 3.6656E+02 | 3.6585E+02 | 1.9508E−01 |
| 109. | 2.2520E−03 | 4.2233E+02 | 4.2478E+02 | 4.2441E+02 | 8.6639E−02 |
| | 2.6446E−03 | 2.6791E+02 | 2.7022E+02 | 2.6967E+02 | 2.0249E−01 |
| 117. | 2.9334E−03 | 1.1814E+03 | 1.2762E+03 | 1.2069E+03 | 5.7369E+00 |
| | 5.7198E−03 | 2.2087E+02 | 2.3128E+02 | 2.2937E+02 | 8.3168E−01 |
| | 7.9973E−03 | 8.4951E+01 | 8.8388E+01 | 8.9303E+01 | 1.0348E+00 |
| | 8.1319E−03 | 8.2190E+01 | 8.5519E+01 | 8.6415E+01 | 1.0471E+00 |
| | 5.8920E−02 | 2.3483E−01 | 4.8623E−01 | 6.3047E−01 | 2.9667E+01 |
| 119. | 2.1966E−03 | 4.4416E+02 | 4.4663E+02 | 4.4602E+02 | 1.3608E−01 |
| | 2.6774E−03 | 2.5502E+02 | 2.5732E+02 | 2.5671E+02 | 2.3702E−01 |
| 122. | 2.7029E−03 | 2.4499E+02 | 2.4728E+02 | 2.4628E+02 | 4.0791E−01 |
| 124. | 2.9881E−03 | 1.1427E+03 | 1.2329E+03 | 1.1686E+03 | 5.5049E+00 |
| 128. | 2.3760E−03 | 3.7359E+02 | 3.7599E+02 | 3.7539E+02 | 1.6062E−01 |
| 131. | 2.2599E−03 | 4.1923E+02 | 4.2168E+02 | 4.2088E+02 | 1.9002E−01 |
| | 2.6131E−03 | 2.8031E+02 | 2.8263E+02 | 2.8222E+02 | 1.4655E−01 |
| 132. | 2.4437E−03 | 3.4692E+02 | 3.4930E+02 | 3.4864E+02 | 1.9044E−01 |
| 133. | 2.9515E−03 | 1.1686E+03 | 1.2619E+03 | 1.1819E+03 | 6.7720E+00 |
| 138. | 2.7027E−03 | 2.4504E+02 | 2.4733E+02 | 2.4617E+02 | 4.7190E−01 |
| 143. | 2.3115E−03 | 3.9894E+02 | 4.0137E+02 | 4.0070E+02 | 1.6641E−01 |
| | 2.5429E−03 | 3.0790E+02 | 3.1025E+02 | 3.0969E+02 | 1.8091E−01 |
| 144. | 2.2950E−03 | 4.0544E+02 | 4.0787E+02 | 4.0736E+02 | 1.2419E−01 |
| | 2.5333E−03 | 3.1170E+02 | 3.1405E+02 | 3.1381E+02 | 7.5688E−02 |
| 142.RADIOCHROMIC DYE FILM (NYLON BASE) | | | | | |
| 4.Be | 5.7849E−02 | 2.6862E−02 | 2.1222E−01 | 2.7833E−01 | 3.1150E+01 |
| 5.B | 2.6061E−03 | 2.1484E+02 | 2.1583E+02 | 2.1612E+02 | 1.3286E−01 |
| | 3.4251E−02 | 6.8765E−02 | 2.8558E−01 | 4.6173E−01 | 6.1679E+01 |

| Material | $E$, MeV | $\mu_{1en}$, cm$^{-1}$ | $\mu_1$, cm$^{-1}$ | $\mu_2$, cm$^{-1}$ | $R$, % |
|---|---|---|---|---|---|
| 35.Br | 2.8871E−02 | 1.1128E−01 | 3.3946E−01 | 1.5203E−01 | 1.2329E+02 |
| | 4.1404E−02 | 4.1504E−02 | 2.4604E−01 | 5.2258E−02 | 3.7082E+02 |
| 54.Xe | 3.7286E−02 | 5.5344E−02 | 2.6664E−01 | 1.5314E−01 | 7.4113E+01 |
| | 5.8457E−02 | 2.6599E−02 | 2.1134E−01 | 4.7062E−02 | 3.4906E+02 |
| 102. | 3.8631E−03 | 5.6179E+01 | 5.6866E+01 | 5.6891E+01 | 4.4543E−02 |
| | 4.1135E−02 | 4.1857E−02 | 2.4674E−01 | 2.2468E−01 | 9.8209E+00 |
| 143.TESTIS (ICRU-44) | | | | | |
| 5.B | 5.3774E−02 | 4.0657E−02 | 2.2730E−01 | 3.8727E−01 | 7.0375E+01 |
| 6.C | 1.0480E−03 | 3.5087E+03 | 3.5187E+03 | 3.5119E+03 | 1.9284E−01 |
| | 1.2124E−03 | 2.6648E+03 | 2.6728E+03 | 2.6676E+03 | 1.9457E−01 |
| | 2.2989E−03 | 4.0500E+02 | 4.0677E+02 | 4.0654E+02 | 5.5534E−02 |
| | 2.7168E−03 | 2.5443E+02 | 2.5605E+02 | 2.5576E+02 | 1.1192E−01 |
| | 5.6769E−02 | 3.7308E−02 | 2.2067E−01 | 3.0449E−01 | 3.7985E+01 |
| 14.Si | 1.0711E−03 | 3.3085E+03 | 3.3179E+03 | 3.3153E+03 | 7.8324E−02 |
| 19.K | 2.0914E−03 | 5.3116E+02 | 5.3310E+02 | 5.3362E+02 | 9.5874E−02 |
| | 2.9712E−03 | 1.9831E+02 | 1.9990E+02 | 2.0039E+02 | 2.4387E−01 |
| | 3.5442E−03 | 1.2037E+02 | 1.2156E+02 | 1.2221E+02 | 5.3458E−01 |
| 86.Rn | 1.9143E−02 | 7.3115E−01 | 1.0061E+00 | 9.8030E−01 | 2.6290E+00 |
| 101. | 4.8196E−02 | 5.0149E−02 | 2.4356E−01 | 2.5512E−01 | 4.7431E+00 |
| 104. | 3.9533E−03 | 8.7500E+01 | 8.8745E+01 | 8.8510E+01 | 2.6568E−01 |
| | 4.5785E−02 | 5.7193E−02 | 2.5412E−01 | 3.1708E−01 | 2.4778E+01 |
| 107. | 6.2560E−03 | 2.3003E+01 | 2.3656E+01 | 2.3665E+01 | 4.0524E−02 |
| | 7.7937E−03 | 1.1814E+01 | 1.2326E+01 | 1.2419E+01 | 7.5713E−01 |
| 109. | 4.7222E−03 | 5.4465E+01 | 5.5419E+01 | 5.5525E+01 | 1.9183E−01 |
| 115. | 1.1355E−03 | 3.0192E+03 | 3.0286E+03 | 3.0285E+03 | 5.8041E−04 |
| | 1.4577E−03 | 1.5345E+03 | 1.5383E+03 | 1.5386E+03 | 1.8220E−02 |
| 119. | 3.3106E−03 | 1.5124E+02 | 1.5259E+02 | 1.5258E+02 | 3.5801E−03 |
| | 3.8185E−03 | 9.7779E+01 | 9.9106E+01 | 9.8865E+01 | 2.4377E−01 |
| 120. | 6.8494E−03 | 1.8686E+01 | 1.9284E+01 | 1.9278E+01 | 3.1344E−02 |
| | 7.4793E−03 | 1.4101E+01 | 1.4642E+01 | 1.4645E+01 | 2.1709E−02 |
| 131. | 4.2007E−03 | 7.5747E+01 | 7.6891E+01 | 7.7070E+01 | 2.3270E−01 |
| 137. | 1.4659E−03 | 1.4966E+03 | 1.5003E+03 | 1.5001E+03 | 1.1848E−02 |
| | 2.0606E−03 | 5.5414E+02 | 5.5613E+02 | 5.5603E+02 | 1.8573E−02 |
| | 2.9184E−03 | 2.0931E+02 | 2.1097E+02 | 2.1061E+02 | 1.6964E−01 |
| | 3.5234E−03 | 1.2311E+02 | 1.2431E+02 | 1.2419E+02 | 9.5351E−02 |
| | 3.6331E−03 | 1.1192E+02 | 1.1336E+02 | 1.1297E+02 | 3.4572E−01 |
| | 5.7194E−02 | 3.6833E−02 | 2.1973E−01 | 2.6367E−01 | 1.9998E+01 |
| 141. | 2.3115E−03 | 3.9894E+02 | 4.0070E+02 | 4.0137E+02 | 1.6641E−01 |
| | 2.5429E−03 | 3.0790E+02 | 3.0969E+02 | 3.1025E+02 | 1.8091E−01 |

| Material | $E$, MeV | $\mu_{1en}$, cm$^{-1}$ | $\mu_1$, cm$^{-1}$ | $\mu_2$, cm$^{-1}$ | $R$, % |
|---|---|---|---|---|---|
| 145. | 1.0311E−03 | 3.6602E+03 | 3.6709E+03 | 3.6707E+03 | 4.1037E−03 |
| | 1.3776E−03 | 1.9035E+03 | 1.9087E+03 | 1.9084E+03 | 1.2786E−02 |
| | 2.0734E−03 | 5.4456E+02 | 5.4654E+02 | 5.4640E+02 | 2.4474E−02 |
| | 2.9241E−03 | 2.0812E+02 | 2.0977E+02 | 2.0928E+02 | 2.3326E−01 |
| 145. | 3.4722E−03 | 1.2988E+02 | 1.3111E+02 | 1.3085E+02 | 2.0183E−01 |
| | 3.6922E−03 | 1.0741E+02 | 1.0882E+02 | 1.0833E+02 | 4.5348E−01 |
| 148. | 2.9972E−03 | 1.9287E+02 | 1.9444E+02 | 1.9408E+02 | 1.8589E−01 |
| | 3.0266E−03 | 1.8878E+02 | 1.9032E+02 | 1.8997E+02 | 1.8452E−01 |
| | 3.9395E−03 | 8.8553E+01 | 8.9806E+01 | 8.9443E+01 | 4.0665E−01 |
| | | 144.TISSUE, SOFT (ICRU-44) | | | |
| 5.B | 5.4918E−02 | 4.0503E−02 | 2.2872E−01 | 3.8505E−01 | 6.8346E+01 |
| 6.C | 1.0369E−03 | 3.5659E+03 | 3.5764E+03 | 3.5692E+03 | 2.0214E−01 |
| | 1.2651E−03 | 2.3941E+03 | 2.4013E+03 | 2.3968E+03 | 1.8650E−01 |
| | 2.2903E−03 | 4.0810E+02 | 4.1004E+02 | 4.0965E+02 | 9.3150E−02 |
| | 2.7107E−03 | 2.5662E+02 | 2.5845E+02 | 2.5796E+02 | 1.8968E−01 |
| | 5.8366E−02 | 3.6496E−02 | 2.2083E−01 | 3.0129E−01 | 3.6435E+01 |
| 14.Si | 1.0615E−03 | 3.3549E+03 | 3.3640E+03 | 3.3617E+03 | 6.7700E−02 |
| | 1.1843E−03 | 2.7630E+03 | 2.7712E+03 | 2.7695E+03 | 6.0500E−02 |
| 19.K | 2.0710E−03 | 5.3887E+02 | 5.4078E+02 | 5.4134E+02 | 1.0332E−01 |
| | 2.9680E−03 | 1.9949E+02 | 2.0133E+02 | 2.0157E+02 | 1.2041E−01 |
| | 3.5952E−03 | 1.1408E+02 | 1.1537E+02 | 1.1590E+02 | 4.6178E−01 |
| 86.Rn | 1.9378E−02 | 7.1042E−01 | 9.8784E−01 | 9.4923E−01 | 4.0672E+00 |
| 101. | 5.7678E−02 | 3.7296E−02 | 2.2241E−01 | 2.3127E−01 | 3.9879E+00 |
| 104. | 3.9182E−03 | 9.1433E+01 | 9.2885E+01 | 9.2453E+01 | 4.6786E−01 |
| | 4.9196E−02 | 4.8649E−02 | 2.4360E−01 | 3.0237E−01 | 2.4126E+01 |
| 107. | 6.0232E−03 | 2.5152E+01 | 2.5860E+01 | 2.5839E+01 | 8.2661E−02 |
| | 7.9052E−03 | 1.1232E+01 | 1.1756E+01 | 1.1826E+01 | 5.9366E−01 |
| 115. | 1.1491E−03 | 2.9237E+03 | 2.9323E+03 | 2.9327E+03 | 1.4570E−02 |
| | 1.4467E−03 | 1.5652E+03 | 1.5701E+03 | 1.5693E+03 | 4.9727E−02 |
| 119. | 3.3286E−03 | 1.4934E+02 | 1.5086E+02 | 1.5068E+02 | 1.2114E−01 |
| | 3.7703E−03 | 1.0286E+02 | 1.0443E+02 | 1.0397E+02 | 4.4037E−01 |
| 120. | 6.7024E−03 | 2.0128E+01 | 2.0770E+01 | 2.0737E+01 | 1.5850E−01 |
| | 7.6264E−03 | 1.3294E+01 | 1.3845E+01 | 1.3826E+01 | 1.3607E−01 |
| 128. | 4.1303E−02 | 7.2546E−02 | 2.7907E−01 | 2.7753E−01 | 5.5710E−01 |
| 132. | 7.4006E−03 | 1.4965E+01 | 1.5537E+01 | 1.5515E+01 | 1.4649E−01 |
| 137. | 1.4891E−03 | 1.3717E+03 | 1.3760E+03 | 1.3750E+03 | 7.9246E−02 |
| | 2.0379E−03 | 5.6328E+02 | 5.6524E+02 | 5.6518E+02 | 9.3845E−03 |
| | 2.9155E−03 | 2.1046E+02 | 2.1236E+02 | 2.1176E+02 | 2.8454E−01 |
| | 3.5388E−03 | 1.2153E+02 | 1.2287E+02 | 1.2261E+02 | 2.0669E−01 |

| Material | $E$, MeV | $\mu_{1en}$, cm$^{-1}$ | $\mu_1$, cm$^{-1}$ | $\mu_2$, cm$^{-1}$ | $R$, % |
|---|---|---|---|---|---|
| | 5.9968E−02 | 3.4636E−02 | 2.1716E−01 | 2.5785E−01 | 1.8737E+01 |
| 141. | 2.2950E−03 | 4.0544E+02 | 4.0736E+02 | 4.0787E+02 | 1.2419E−01 |
| | 2.5333E−03 | 3.1170E+02 | 3.1381E+02 | 3.1405E+02 | 7.5688E−02 |
| 145. | 1.0226E−03 | 3.7036E+03 | 3.7146E+03 | 3.7142E+03 | 9.3075E−03 |
| | 1.4231E−03 | 1.6731E+03 | 1.6783E+03 | 1.6774E+03 | 5.7347E−02 |
| | 2.0515E−03 | 5.5323E+02 | 5.5517E+02 | 5.5509E+02 | 1.4437E−02 |
| | 2.9211E−03 | 2.0929E+02 | 2.1118E+02 | 2.1045E+02 | 3.4833E−01 |
| 145. | 3.4878E−03 | 1.2828E+02 | 1.2966E+02 | 1.2925E+02 | 3.1570E−01 |
| | 3.6330E−03 | 1.1345E+02 | 1.1513E+02 | 1.1438E+02 | 6.5294E−01 |
| 148. | 2.9948E−03 | 1.9390E+02 | 1.9571E+02 | 1.9510E+02 | 3.0934E−01 |
| | 3.0495E−03 | 1.8626E+02 | 1.8802E+02 | 1.8745E+02 | 3.0683E−01 |
| | 3.9015E−03 | 9.2723E+01 | 9.4189E+01 | 9.3626E+01 | 6.0157E−01 |
| 145.TISSUE, SOFT (ICRU FOUR-COMPONENT) | | | | | |
| 5.B | 4.9221E−02 | 4.1808E−02 | 2.2531E−01 | 3.9697E−01 | 7.6190E+01 |
| 6.C | 4.9000E−02 | 4.2358E−02 | 2.2616E−01 | 3.2156E−01 | 4.2180E+01 |
| 19.K | 2.4584E−03 | 3.9231E+02 | 3.9385E+02 | 3.9462E+02 | 1.9524E−01 |
| | 3.4415E−03 | 1.3302E+02 | 1.3400E+02 | 1.3490E+02 | 6.7168E−01 |
| 101. | 1.8099E−02 | 7.9555E−01 | 1.0644E+00 | 1.0910E+00 | 2.5018E+00 |
| 107. | 1.0438E−03 | 3.5957E+03 | 3.6060E+03 | 3.6069E+03 | 2.4252E−02 |
| | 1.3199E−03 | 2.1962E+03 | 2.2020E+03 | 2.2026E+03 | 2.6753E−02 |
| | 2.0905E−03 | 5.3781E+02 | 5.3964E+02 | 5.3976E+02 | 2.2327E−02 |
| | 2.9043E−03 | 2.1596E+02 | 2.1713E+02 | 2.1777E+02 | 2.9183E−01 |
| | 3.5449E−03 | 1.2246E+02 | 1.2341E+02 | 1.2377E+02 | 2.9395E−01 |
| | 3.6118E−03 | 1.1562E+02 | 1.1656E+02 | 1.1721E+02 | 5.5916E−01 |
| 109. | 1.0035E−03 | 3.8003E+03 | 3.8112E+03 | 3.8116E+03 | 1.0313E−02 |
| | 1.4841E−03 | 1.3638E+03 | 1.3670E+03 | 1.3671E+03 | 7.1258E−03 |
| | 2.0133E−03 | 5.6832E+02 | 5.7021E+02 | 5.7028E+02 | 1.1839E−02 |
| | 2.9391E−03 | 2.0217E+02 | 2.0332E+02 | 2.0408E+02 | 3.7330E−01 |
| | 3.4140E−03 | 1.3582E+02 | 1.3681E+02 | 1.3734E+02 | 3.8692E−01 |
| | 3.7026E−03 | 1.0635E+02 | 1.0726E+02 | 1.0802E+02 | 7.1266E−01 |
| 115. | 1.0838E−03 | 3.3930E+03 | 3.4026E+03 | 3.4035E+03 | 2.3886E−02 |
| | 1.4414E−03 | 1.5799E+03 | 1.5838E+03 | 1.5840E+03 | 1.1569E−02 |
| | 2.2895E−03 | 4.5912E+02 | 4.6078E+02 | 4.6096E+02 | 3.8791E−02 |
| | 2.6159E−03 | 3.3002E+02 | 3.3143E+02 | 3.3319E+02 | 5.3040E−01 |
| 119. | 1.0048E−03 | 3.7939E+03 | 3.8048E+03 | 3.8054E+03 | 1.4688E−02 |
| | 1.4930E−03 | 1.3183E+03 | 1.3215E+03 | 1.3217E+03 | 1.5362E−02 |
| | 2.0024E−03 | 5.7265E+02 | 5.7454E+02 | 5.7457E+02 | 4.5361E−03 |
| | 2.9702E−03 | 1.8990E+02 | 1.9103E+02 | 1.9144E+02 | 2.1468E−01 |
| 120. | 2.2632E−03 | 4.6950E+02 | 4.7119E+02 | 4.7131E+02 | 2.5123E−02 |

| Material | $E$, MeV | $\mu_{1en}$, cm$^{-1}$ | $\mu_1$, cm$^{-1}$ | $\mu_2$, cm$^{-1}$ | $R$, % |
|---|---|---|---|---|---|
| | 2.7997E−03 | 2.5730E+02 | 2.5856E+02 | 2.5980E+02 | 4.7796E−01 |
| 122. | 5.6157E−02 | 3.4107E−02 | 2.1011E−01 | 2.5729E−01 | 2.2457E+01 |
| 128. | 1.0341E−03 | 3.6453E+03 | 3.6558E+03 | 3.6559E+03 | 3.4193E−03 |
| | 1.3612E−03 | 1.9865E+03 | 1.9918E+03 | 1.9917E+03 | 1.3729E−03 |
| | 2.0786E−03 | 5.4251E+02 | 5.4435E+02 | 5.4439E+02 | 8.1627E−03 |
| | 2.9004E−03 | 2.1749E+02 | 2.1867E+02 | 2.1944E+02 | 3.5177E−01 |
| | 3.5608E−03 | 1.2083E+02 | 1.2178E+02 | 1.2214E+02 | 2.9542E−01 |
| 131. | 1.0166E−03 | 3.7336E+03 | 3.7444E+03 | 3.7441E+03 | 6.2468E−03 |
| | 1.4517E−03 | 1.5281E+03 | 1.5319E+03 | 1.5329E+03 | 6.6564E−02 |
| | 2.0350E−03 | 5.5975E+02 | 5.6163E+02 | 5.6178E+02 | 2.7104E−02 |
| 131. | 2.9449E−03 | 1.9988E+02 | 2.0102E+02 | 2.0159E+02 | 2.8281E−01 |
| | 3.3807E−03 | 1.3923E+02 | 1.4022E+02 | 1.4058E+02 | 2.5229E−01 |
| | 3.6973E−03 | 1.0689E+02 | 1.0780E+02 | 1.0859E+02 | 7.3200E−01 |
| 132. | 1.0422E−03 | 3.6043E+03 | 3.6146E+03 | 3.6146E+03 | 5.1333E−04 |
| | 1.3188E−03 | 2.2018E+03 | 2.2077E+03 | 2.2082E+03 | 2.3721E−02 |
| | 2.0927E−03 | 5.3695E+02 | 5.3878E+02 | 5.3892E+02 | 2.6056E−02 |
| | 2.9038E−03 | 2.1613E+02 | 2.1730E+02 | 2.1786E+02 | 2.5767E−01 |
| | 3.5443E−03 | 1.2252E+02 | 1.2347E+02 | 1.2382E+02 | 2.8397E−01 |
| | 3.6093E−03 | 1.1587E+02 | 1.1681E+02 | 1.1734E+02 | 4.5667E−01 |
| 137. | 2.7539E−03 | 2.7542E+02 | 2.7672E+02 | 2.7683E+02 | 4.1533E−02 |
| | 3.9918E−02 | 6.5386E−02 | 2.6171E−01 | 3.1875E−01 | 2.1793E+01 |
| 143. | 1.0311E−03 | 3.6602E+03 | 3.6707E+03 | 3.6709E+03 | 4.1037E−03 |
| | 1.3776E−03 | 1.9035E+03 | 1.9084E+03 | 1.9087E+03 | 1.2786E−02 |
| | 2.0734E−03 | 5.4456E+02 | 5.4640E+02 | 5.4654E+02 | 2.4474E−02 |
| | 2.9241E−03 | 2.0812E+02 | 2.0928E+02 | 2.0977E+02 | 2.3326E−01 |
| | 3.4722E−03 | 1.2988E+02 | 1.3085E+02 | 1.3111E+02 | 2.0183E−01 |
| | 3.6922E−03 | 1.0741E+02 | 1.0833E+02 | 1.0882E+02 | 4.5348E−01 |
| 144. | 1.0226E−03 | 3.7036E+03 | 3.7142E+03 | 3.7146E+03 | 9.3075E−03 |
| | 1.4231E−03 | 1.6731E+03 | 1.6774E+03 | 1.6783E+03 | 5.7347E−02 |
| | 2.0515E−03 | 5.5323E+02 | 5.5509E+02 | 5.5517E+02 | 1.4437E−02 |
| | 2.9211E−03 | 2.0929E+02 | 2.1045E+02 | 2.1118E+02 | 3.4833E−01 |
| | 3.4878E−03 | 1.2828E+02 | 1.2925E+02 | 1.2966E+02 | 3.1570E−01 |
| | 3.6330E−03 | 1.1345E+02 | 1.1438E+02 | 1.1513E+02 | 6.5294E−01 |
| 147.TISSUE−EQUIVALENT GAS (PROPANE BASED) | | | | | |
| 8.O | 5.4610E−02 | 5.1383E−05 | 3.7165E−04 | 2.7017E−04 | 3.7563E+01 |
| 10.Ne | 5.8652E−02 | 4.7604E−05 | 3.6065E−04 | 1.8593E−04 | 9.3976E+01 |
| 103. | 3.9990E−03 | 9.2115E−02 | 9.3302E−02 | 9.3948E−02 | 6.9222E−01 |
| | 3.9775E−02 | 8.4655E−05 | 4.3641E−04 | 3.0230E−04 | 4.4363E+01 |

| Material | $E$, MeV | $\mu_{1en}$, cm$^{-1}$ | $\mu_1$, cm$^{-1}$ | $\mu_2$, cm$^{-1}$ | $R$, % |
|---|---|---|---|---|---|
| 148.WATER, LIQUID | | | | | |
| 5.B | 5.1184E−02 | 4.1007E−02 | 2.2441E−01 | 3.9230E−01 | 7.4813E+01 |
| 6.C | 5.2823E−02 | 3.9314E−02 | 2.2097E−01 | 3.1241E−01 | 4.1379E+01 |
| 15.P | 2.1196E−03 | 5.6456E+02 | 5.6655E+02 | 5.6922E+02 | 4.7071E−01 |
| 86.Rn | 1.8624E−02 | 7.7699E−01 | 1.0472E+00 | 1.0490E+00 | 1.7294E−01 |
| 101. | 3.1255E−02 | 1.4487E−01 | 3.6213E−01 | 3.7931E−01 | 4.7433E+00 |
| 104. | 4.7802E−03 | 5.0677E+01 | 5.1414E+01 | 5.1529E+01 | 2.2368E−01 |
| | 3.5281E−02 | 1.1016E−01 | 3.1894E−01 | 3.9285E−01 | 2.3174E+01 |
| 107. | 2.9812E−03 | 1.9966E+02 | 2.0087E+02 | 2.0138E+02 | 2.4965E−01 |
| | 3.1617E−03 | 1.7395E+02 | 1.7509E+02 | 1.7553E+02 | 2.4929E−01 |
| | 3.8885E−03 | 9.4152E+01 | 9.5058E+01 | 9.5522E+01 | 4.8719E−01 |
| | 6.6092E−03 | 1.9744E+01 | 2.0293E+01 | 2.0370E+01 | 3.7569E−01 |
| | 7.5555E−03 | 1.3057E+01 | 1.3542E+01 | 1.3687E+01 | 1.0763E+00 |
| 109. | 3.9443E−03 | 8.8028E+01 | 8.8916E+01 | 8.9466E+01 | 6.1792E−01 |
| 115. | 1.0294E−03 | 3.9069E+03 | 3.9193E+03 | 3.9192E+03 | 2.6412E−03 |
| | 1.4829E−03 | 1.4640E+03 | 1.4683E+03 | 1.4681E+03 | 1.2755E−02 |
| | 2.1106E−03 | 5.6835E+02 | 5.7035E+02 | 5.7039E+02 | 7.3412E−03 |
| | 2.8107E−03 | 2.7188E+02 | 2.7325E+02 | 2.7459E+02 | 4.8995E−01 |
| 119. | 4.8393E−02 | 4.6608E−02 | 2.3355E−01 | 2.4292E−01 | 4.0082E+00 |
| 120. | 1.0178E−03 | 3.9691E+03 | 3.9818E+03 | 3.9819E+03 | 2.9553E−03 |
| | 1.4488E−03 | 1.6478E+03 | 1.6527E+03 | 1.6518E+03 | 5.2631E−02 |
| | 2.0738E−03 | 5.8396E+02 | 5.8599E+02 | 5.8601E+02 | 3.5518E−03 |
| | 2.9041E−03 | 2.3231E+02 | 2.3360E+02 | 2.3463E+02 | 4.4093E−01 |
| | 7.0817E−03 | 1.6405E+01 | 1.6922E+01 | 1.6972E+01 | 2.9289E−01 |
| | 7.1584E−03 | 1.5863E+01 | 1.6375E+01 | 1.6433E+01 | 3.5351E−01 |
| 128. | 2.9780E−03 | 2.0102E+02 | 2.0224E+02 | 2.0292E+02 | 3.3783E−01 |
| | 3.1869E−03 | 1.7118E+02 | 1.7231E+02 | 1.7287E+02 | 3.2371E−01 |
| | 3.8742E−03 | 9.5721E+01 | 9.6633E+01 | 9.7118E+01 | 5.0200E−01 |
| 131. | 3.9408E−03 | 8.8409E+01 | 8.9298E+01 | 8.9882E+01 | 6.5330E−01 |
| 132. | 2.9810E−03 | 1.9976E+02 | 2.0098E+02 | 2.0145E+02 | 2.3591E−01 |
| | 3.1627E−03 | 1.7383E+02 | 1.7498E+02 | 1.7540E+02 | 2.4071E−01 |
| | 3.8882E−03 | 9.4190E+01 | 9.5097E+01 | 9.5502E+01 | 4.2631E−01 |
| 137. | 4.9394E−02 | 4.3880E−02 | 2.2941E−01 | 2.8113E−01 | 2.2548E+01 |
| 143. | 2.9972E−03 | 1.9287E+02 | 1.9408E+02 | 1.9444E+02 | 1.8589E−01 |
| | 3.0266E−03 | 1.8878E+02 | 1.8997E+02 | 1.9032E+02 | 1.8452E−01 |
| | 3.9395E−03 | 8.8553E+01 | 8.9443E+01 | 8.9806E+01 | 4.0665E−01 |
| 144. | 2.9948E−03 | 1.9390E+02 | 1.9510E+02 | 1.9571E+02 | 3.0934E−01 |
| | 3.0495E−03 | 1.8626E+02 | 1.8745E+02 | 1.8802E+02 | 3.0683E−01 |
| | 3.9015E−03 | 9.2723E+01 | 9.3626E+01 | 9.4189E+01 | 6.0157E−01 |

## 2.2. THE TABLES OF POORLY VISIBLE PAIRS AT THE POINTS OF THEIR ABSORPTION EDGES

For the most part of the substances subjected to comparison there are energy values $E > 1$ keV where their coefficients $\mu(E)$ and $\mu_{en}(E)$ undergo a jump (have absorption edges). As this takes place at the point of discontinuity $E$ the limit on the left $\mu_{en}(E-0)$ and the limit on the right $\mu_{en}(E+0)$ obey the inequality $\mu_{en}(E-0) < \mu_{en}(E+0)$, with the value $\mu_{en}(E+0)$ being usually several times more than $\mu_{en}(E-0)$. The same is valid for the total attenuation coefficient $\mu$. Now let us consider two cases, which may occur for a given pair of substances. The first case is that for the first substance for some energy $E$ the coefficient $\mu_{1en}(E)$ is continuous, whereas $\mu_{2en}(E)$ has a jump and inequalities $\mu_{2en}(E-0) \leq \mu_{1en}(E) \leq \mu_{2en}(E+0)$ take place.

The second case is that both coefficients $\mu_{1en}(E)$ and $\mu_{2en}(E)$ are discontinuous at $E$ and the segments $[\mu_{1en}(E-0), \mu_{1en}(E+0)]$, $[\mu_{2en}(E-0), \mu_{2en}(E+0)]$ have nonempty intersection. In both cases the contact boundary for such substances will be poorly visible for a given photon energy $E$. All such pairs of substances for the energy range from 1 to 60 keV are collected at the table of this section. In contradistinction to the pairs adduced at the table of Section 2.1 the condition of a poor visibility for substances at the points of discontinuity of their coefficient $\mu_{en}$ may be easily broken through a little shift to higher or lower energy levels.

The table of this section is organized in a different way than the table from Section 2.1. The first column here gives energy levels for which a poor visibility of the contact boundary of substances takes place for some pairs. The second column lists all such pairs for each energy level. If a bracketed pair is marked by asterisk for example as $(132, 107)^*$ then for a given energy $E$ the absorption coefficients for both substances have a jump. If a pair is not marked by asterisk, then the coefficient $\mu_{1en}(E)$ (the first substance in the brackets) is continuous, whereas the coefficient $\mu_{2en}(E)$ is discontinuous; such pairs constitute the main body of the table of this section. Other information for pairs (the left- and right-hand limiting values of the coefficients $\mu, \mu_{en}$ at the point $E$) is not presented, because it would require essential increase of space. These data are not difficult to get from the tables of Hubbell and Seltzer (1995).

| $E$, MeV | List of poorly visible pairs for this energy) |
|---|---|
| 1.0050E−03 | (24.Cr,60.Nd), (42.Mo,60.Nd), (49.In,60.Nd), (51.Sb,60.Nd), (52.Te,60.Nd), (57.La,60.Nd), (73.Ta,60.Nd), (81.Tl,60.Nd), (82.Pb,60.Nd), (83.Bi,60.Nd), (84.Po,60.Nd), (85.At,60.Nd), (112,60.Nd) |
| 1.0060E−03 | (84.Po,52.Te), (24.Cr,52.Te), (83.Bi,52.Te) |
| 1.0081E−03 | (76.Os,28.Ni), (77.Ir,28.Ni), (78.Pt,28.Ni), (79.Au,28.Ni), (27.Co,28.Ni), (29.Cu,28.Ni) |
| 1.0197E−03 | (69.Tm,30.Zn), (70.Yb,30.Zn), (113,30.Zn), (114,30.Zn), (118,30.Zn), (121,30.Zn), (126,30.Zn), (134,30.Zn), (21.Sc,30.Zn), (22.Ti,30.Zn), (33.As,30.Zn), (39.Y,30.Zn), (40.Zr,30.Zn), (55.Cs,30.Zn), (61.Pm,30.Zn), (62.Sm,30.Zn), (63.Eu,30.Zn), (64.Gd,30.Zn), (65.Tb,30.Zn), (66.Dy,30.Zn), (67.Ho,30.Zn), (68.Er,30.Zn) |
| 1.0269E−03 | (55.Cs,61.Pm), (21.Sc,61.Pm), (39.Y,61.Pm), (62.Sm,61.Pm), (64.Gd,61.Pm), (65.Tb,61.Pm), (113,61.Pm), (121,61.Pm), (134,61.Pm) |
| 1.0420E−03 | (51.Sb,85.At) |
| 1.0428E−03 | (81.Tl,30.Zn), (82.Pb,30.Zn), (83.Bi,30.Zn), (84.Po,30.Zn), (85.At,30.Zn), (87.Fr,30.Zn), (112,30.Zn), (24.Cr,30.Zn), (42.Mo,30.Zn), (43.Tc,30.Zn), (49.In,30.Zn), (50.Sn,30.Zn), (51.Sb,30.Zn), (52.Te,30.Zn), (25.Mn,30.Zn), (57.La,30.Zn), (60.Nd,30.Zn), (73.Ta,30.Zn) |
| 1.0515E−03 | (52.Te,61.Pm), (83.Bi,61.Pm), (84.Po,61.Pm), (112,61.Pm), (24.Cr,61.Pm), (57.La,61.Pm), (42.Mo,61.Pm) |
| 1.0622E−03 | (71.Lu,56.Ba), (88.Ra,56.Ba), (125,56.Ba), (66.Dy,118), (70.Yb,118) |
| 1.0650E−03 | (134,55.Cs), (39.Y,55.Cs), (64.Gd,55.Cs) |
| 1.0721E−03 | (16.S,11.Na), (19.K,11.Na), (37.Rb,11.Na), (101,11.Na), (102,11.Na)*, (104,11.Na), (105,11.Na), (106,11.Na), (107,11.Na)*, (108,11.Na)*, (109,11.Na)*, (110,11.Na)*, (111,11.Na), (115,11.Na), (130,53.I)*, (119,11.Na)*, (120,11.Na), (122,11.Na), (124,11.Na)*, (128,11.Na)*, (131,11.Na)*, (132,11.Na)*, (135,11.Na), (136,11.Na), (137,11.Na), (138,11.Na), (139,11.Na), (141,11.Na), (142,11.Na), (143,11.Na)*, (144,11.Na)*, (145,11.Na), (148,11.Na), (14.Si,143), (4.Be,11.Na), (5.B,11.Na), (6.C,11.Na), (12.Mg,11.Na), (13.Al,11.Na), (14.Si,11.Na), (15.P,11.Na), (72.Hf,130), (132,107)*, (124,108)*, (119,109)*, (111,124) |
| 1.0802E−03 | (113,62.Sm), (118,62.Sm), (121,62.Sm), (134,62.Sm), (55.Cs,62.Sm), (39.Y,62.Sm), (21.Sc,62.Sm), (64.Gd,62.Sm), (65.Tb,62.Sm), (66.Dy,62.Sm), (70.Yb,62.Sm) |
| 1.0961E−03 | (79.Au,29.Cu), (27.Co,29.Cu), (76.Os,29.Cu) |

| $E$, MeV | List of poorly visible pairs for this energy) |
|---|---|
| 1.1060E−03 | (51.Sb,62.Sm), (24.Cr,62.Sm), (57.La,62.Sm), (49.In,62.Sm), (42.Mo,62.Sm), (83.Bi,62.Sm), (84.Po,62.Sm), (87.Fr,62.Sm), (112,62.Sm), (52.Te,62.Sm) |
| 1.1154E−03 | (63.Eu,31.Ga), (64.Gd,31.Ga), (65.Tb,31.Ga), (66.Dy,31.Ga), (67.Ho,31.Ga), (68.Er,31.Ga), (69.Tm,31.Ga), (70.Yb,31.Ga), (113,31.Ga), (114,31.Ga), (118,31.Ga), (121,31.Ga), (123,31.Ga)*, (126,31.Ga), (133,31.Ga), (134,31.Ga), (140,31.Ga), (33.As,123), (34.Se,123), (21.Sc,123), (63.Eu,123), (21.Sc,31.Ga), (22.Ti,31.Ga), (32.Ge,31.Ga), (33.As,31.Ga), (34.Se,31.Ga), (39.Y,31.Ga), (55.Cs,31.Ga), (113,123), (114,123), (126,123), (140,123) |
| 1.1234E−03 | (84.Po,57.La), (87.Fr,57.La), (24.Cr,57.La), (49.In,57.La), (51.Sb,57.La), (52.Te,57.La), (83.Bi,57.La) |
| 1.1309E−03 | (114,63.Eu) |
| 1.1367E−03 | (71.Lu,56.Ba), (123,118) |
| 1.1423E−03 | (112,31.Ga), (22.Ti,123), (130,31.Ga), (42.Mo,31.Ga), (53.I,31.Ga), (68.Er,123), (69.Tm,123), (125,123), (40.Zr,123), (72.Hf,31.Ga) |
| 1.1530E−03 | (51.Sb,87.Fr), (57.La,87.Fr), (58.Ce,87.Fr) |
| 1.1606E−03 | (23.V,63.Eu), (116,63.Eu), (41.Nb,63.Eu) |
| 1.1683E−03 | (47.Ag,90.Th) |
| 1.1852E−03 | (121,64.Gd)*, (134,64.Gd), (65.Tb,121), (134,121), (39.Y,64.Gd), (39.Y,121), (65.Tb,64.Gd) |
| 1.1854E−03 | (51.Sb,58.Ce), (49.In,58.Ce), (57.La,58.Ce), (59.Pr,58.Ce), (60.Nd,58.Ce), (62.Sm,58.Ce), (73.Ta,58.Ce), (81.Tl,58.Ce), (82.Pb,58.Ce), (85.At,58.Ce), (25.Mn,58.Ce), (87.Fr,58.Ce), (89.Ac,58.Ce), (48.Cd,58.Ce), (50.Sn,58.Ce), (43.Tc,58.Ce) |
| 1.1936E−03 | (47.Ag,30.Zn), (26.Fe,30.Zn), (44.Ru,30.Zn), (74.W,30.Zn), (45.Rh,30.Zn), (90.Th,30.Zn) |
| 1.2044E−03 | (51.Sb,57.La), (49.In,57.La), (87.Fr,57.La), (25.Mn,57.La) |
| 1.2084E−03 | (121,88.Ra) |
| 1.2167E−03 | (123,32.Ge), (125,32.Ge), (126,32.Ge), (133,32.Ge), (134,32.Ge), (140,32.Ge), (22.Ti,32.Ge), (21.Sc,32.Ge), (33.As,32.Ge), (34.Se,32.Ge), (38.Sr,32.Ge), (39.Y,32.Ge), (40.Zr,32.Ge), (55.Cs,32.Ge), (65.Tb,32.Ge), (66.Dy,32.Ge), (67.Ho,32.Ge), (68.Er,32.Ge), (69.Tm,32.Ge), (70.Yb,32.Ge), (88.Ra,32.Ge), (113,32.Ge), (114,32.Ge), (118,32.Ge) |
| 1.2171E−03 | (39.Y,55.Cs), (41.Nb,116), (134,55.Cs) |
| 1.2172E−03 | (41.Nb,121), (53.I,64.Gd), (23.V,121), (72.Hf,64.Gd), (116,121), (112,64.Gd), (63.Eu,64.Gd), (121,64.Gd)*, (130,64.Gd), (42.Mo,64.Gd) |
| 1.2412E−03 | (70.Yb,65.Tb), (118,65.Tb), (22.Ti,65.Tb), (66.Dy,65.Tb), (67.Ho,65.Tb), (68.Er,65.Tb), (69.Tm,65.Tb) |

| *E*, MeV | List of poorly visible pairs for this energy) |
|---|---|
| 1.2422E−03 | (89.Ac,59.Pr), (58.Ce,59.Pr), (50.Sn,59.Pr), (43.Tc,59.Pr), (57.La,59.Pr), (48.Cd,59.Pr), (60.Nd,59.Pr), (73.Ta,59.Pr), (80.Hg,59.Pr), (81.Tl,59.Pr), (82.Pb,59.Pr), (85.At,59.Pr), (87.Fr,59.Pr) |
| 1.2478E−03 | (121,32.Ge), (41.Nb,32.Ge), (72.Hf,32.Ge), (42.Mo,32.Ge), (130,32.Ge), (53.I,32.Ge), (23.V,32.Ge), (116,32.Ge), (63.Eu,32.Ge) |
| 1.2690E−03 | (48.Cd,89.Ac), (60.Nd,89.Ac) |
| 1.2750E−03 | (80.Hg,65.Tb), (82.Pb,65.Tb), (85.At,65.Tb), (89.Ac,65.Tb), (59.Pr,65.Tb), (26.Fe,65.Tb), (48.Cd,65.Tb), (61.Pm,65.Tb), (60.Nd,65.Tb), (62.Sm,65.Tb), (44.Ru,65.Tb), (58.Ce,65.Tb) |
| 1.2928E−03 | (71.Lu,56.Ba), (70.Yb,118) |
| 1.2949E−03 | (68.Er,66.Dy), (69.Tm,66.Dy), (70.Yb,66.Dy), (40.Zr,66.Dy), (118,66.Dy), (125,66.Dy), (22.Ti,66.Dy), (67.Ho,66.Dy) |
| 1.2974E−03 | (89.Ac,60.Nd), (80.Hg,60.Nd), (44.Ru,60.Nd), (59.Pr,60.Nd), (61.Pm,60.Nd), (62.Sm,60.Nd), (26.Fe,60.Nd), (58.Ce,60.Nd) |
| 1.2977E−03 | (85.At,31.Ga), (87.Fr,31.Ga), (88.Ra,123), (89.Ac,31.Ga), (43.Tc,31.Ga), (57.La,31.Ga), (48.Cd,31.Ga), (50.Sn,31.Ga), (66.Dy,123), (64.Gd,31.Ga), (25.Mn,31.Ga), (73.Ta,31.Ga), (81.Tl,31.Ga), (82.Pb,31.Ga), (71.Lu,123) |
| 1.3050E−03 | (37.Rb,12.Mg), (38.Sr,12.Mg), (101,12.Mg), (102,12.Mg), (104,12.Mg), (105,12.Mg), (106,12.Mg), (107,12.Mg), (108,12.Mg)*, (109,12.Mg), (110,12.Mg), (111,12.Mg), (114,12.Mg), (115,12.Mg), (117,12.Mg)*, (119,12.Mg), (120,12.Mg), (122,12.Mg), (124,12.Mg), (126,12.Mg), (127,12.Mg), (128,12.Mg), (129,12.Mg)*, (131,12.Mg), (132,12.Mg), (133,12.Mg), (135,12.Mg), (136,12.Mg), (137,12.Mg), (138,12.Mg), (139,12.Mg), (140,12.Mg), (141,12.Mg), (142,12.Mg), (143,12.Mg), (34.Se,129), (38.Sr,129), (144,12.Mg), (145,12.Mg), (148,12.Mg), (11.Na,12.Mg), (20.Ca,129), (6.C,12.Mg), (11.Na,129), (5.B,12.Mg), (13.Al,12.Mg), (14.Si,12.Mg), (15.P,12.Mg), (129,117)*, (16.S,12.Mg), (19.K,12.Mg), (20.Ca,12.Mg), (33.As,12.Mg), (34.Se,12.Mg), (124,129), (127,129), (133,129) |
| 1.3231E−03 | (118,33.As), (23.V,33.As), (123,33.As)*, (125,33.As)*, (53.I,123), (126,33.As), (134,33.As), (140,33.As), (21.Sc,33.As), (72.Hf,123), (22.Ti,33.As), (23.V,123), (12.Mg,33.As), (39.Y,33.As), (40.Zr,33.As), (41.Nb,33.As), (56.Ba,123), (55.Cs,33.As), (56.Ba,33.As), (67.Ho,33.As), (116,123), (68.Er,33.As), (69.Tm,33.As), (70.Yb,33.As), (71.Lu,33.As), (41.Nb,123), (130,123), (88.Ra,33.As), (113,33.As), (114,33.As), (116,33.As) |
| 1.3325E−03 | (60.Nd,66.Dy), (44.Ru,66.Dy), (45.Rh,66.Dy), (46.Pd,66.Dy), (59.Pr,66.Dy), (74.W,66.Dy), (80.Hg,66.Dy), (90.Th,66.Dy), (47.Ag,66.Dy), (58.Ce,66.Dy), (61.Pm,66.Dy), (26.Fe,66.Dy), (62.Sm,66.Dy) |
| 1.3374E−03 | (44.Ru,59.Pr), (26.Fe,59.Pr), (61.Pm,59.Pr) |

| $E$, MeV | List of poorly visible pairs for this energy) |
|---|---|
| 1.3514E−03 | (68.Er,67.Ho), (69.Tm,67.Ho), (125,67.Ho), (40.Zr,67.Ho), (22.Ti,67.Ho) |
| 1.3569E−03 | (65.Tb,61.Pm), (60.Nd,61.Pm), (66.Dy,61.Pm), (74.W,61.Pm), (47.Ag,61.Pm), (30.Zn,61.Pm), (90.Th,61.Pm), (62.Sm,61.Pm), (46.Pd,61.Pm), (45.Rh,61.Pm), (59.Pr,61.Pm) |
| 1.3586E−03 | (25.Mn,123), (42.Mo,33.As), (49.In,123), (83.Bi,123), (84.Po,123), (72.Hf,33.As), (83.Bi,33.As), (84.Po,33.As), (49.In,33.As), (112,33.As), (50.Sn,33.As), (112,123), (63.Eu,123), (51.Sb,33.As), (52.Te,33.As), (53.I,33.As), (121,33.As), (25.Mn,33.As), (121,123), (24.Cr,33.As), (123,33.As)*, (63.Eu,33.As), (32.Ge,123), (52.Te,123), (130,33.As), (24.Cr,123), (32.Ge,33.As) |
| 1.3613E−03 | (81.Tl,57.La), (82.Pb,57.La), (48.Cd,57.La), (87.Fr,57.La), (73.Ta,57.La), (85.At,57.La) |
| 1.3915E−03 | (62.Sm,67.Ho), (61.Pm,67.Ho), (27.Co,67.Ho), (30.Zn,67.Ho), (59.Pr,67.Ho), (46.Pd,67.Ho), (74.W,67.Ho), (90.Th,67.Ho), (45.Rh,67.Ho), (60.Nd,67.Ho) |
| 1.4028E−03 | (46.Pd,60.Nd), (62.Sm,60.Nd), (59.Pr,60.Nd) |
| 1.4093E−03 | (56.Ba,68.Er), (69.Tm,68.Er), (71.Lu,68.Er), (88.Ra,68.Er), (40.Zr,68.Er), (125,68.Er) |
| 1.4143E−03 | (48.Cd,32.Ge), (50.Sn,32.Ge), (33.As,32.Ge), (43.Tc,32.Ge), (73.Ta,32.Ge), (81.Tl,32.Ge), (121,32.Ge), (82.Pb,32.Ge), (85.At,32.Ge), (123,32.Ge), (87.Fr,32.Ge) |
| 1.4198E−03 | (75.Re,62.Sm), (60.Nd,62.Sm), (61.Pm,62.Sm), (27.Co,62.Sm), (90.Th,62.Sm), (30.Zn,62.Sm) |
| 1.4358E−03 | (22.Ti,34.Se), (129,34.Se), (134,34.Se), (140,34.Se), (23.V,34.Se), (21.Sc,34.Se), (39.Y,34.Se), (40.Zr,34.Se), (41.Nb,34.Se), (55.Cs,34.Se), (56.Ba,34.Se), (69.Tm,34.Se), (70.Yb,34.Se), (71.Lu,34.Se), (88.Ra,34.Se), (113,34.Se), (114,34.Se), (118,34.Se), (12.Mg,34.Se), (125,34.Se), (126,34.Se) |
| 1.4366E−03 | (45.Rh,58.Ce), (74.W,58.Ce) |
| 1.4533E−03 | (75.Re,68.Er), (28.Ni,68.Er), (90.Th,68.Er), (60.Nd,68.Er), (62.Sm,68.Er), (61.Pm,68.Er), (64.Gd,68.Er) |
| 1.4677E−03 | (34.Se,69.Tm), (23.V,69.Tm), (71.Lu,69.Tm), (88.Ra,69.Tm), (41.Nb,69.Tm), (125,69.Tm), (56.Ba,69.Tm) |
| 1.4714E−03 | (64.Gd,61.Pm), (62.Sm,61.Pm), (28.Ni,61.Pm) |
| 1.4762E−03 | (53.I,34.Se), (72.Hf,34.Se), (24.Cr,34.Se), (112,34.Se), (69.Tm,34.Se), (42.Mo,34.Se), (130,34.Se), (116,34.Se) |
| 1.4806E−03 | (81.Tl,63.Eu), (82.Pb,63.Eu), (85.At,63.Eu), (87.Fr,63.Eu), (44.Ru,63.Eu), (48.Cd,63.Eu), (57.La,63.Eu), (33.As,63.Eu), (123,63.Eu), (26.Fe,63.Eu), (32.Ge,63.Eu), (73.Ta,63.Eu) |
| 1.5110E−03 | (30.Zn,59.Pr) |

| $E$, MeV | List of poorly visible pairs for this energy) |
|---|---|
| 1.5146E−03 | (76.Os,69.Tm), (77.Ir,69.Tm), (78.Pt,69.Tm), (79.Au,69.Tm), (64.Gd,69.Tm), (61.Pm,69.Tm), (29.Cu,69.Tm), (65.Tb,69.Tm), (62.Sm,69.Tm) |
| 1.5265E−03 | (27.Co,33.As), (82.Pb,123), (31.Ga,33.As), (44.Ru,123), (85.At,123), (87.Fr,123), (89.Ac,33.As), (57.La,33.As), (45.Rh,33.As), (46.Pd,33.As), (74.W,33.As), (80.Hg,33.As), (47.Ag,33.As), (121,33.As) |
| 1.5278E−03 | (118,70.Yb), (125,70.Yb), (22.Ti,70.Yb), (40.Zr,70.Yb) |
| 1.5407E−03 | (76.Os,62.Sm), (79.Au,62.Sm), (29.Cu,62.Sm), (61.Pm,62.Sm) |
| 1.5440E−03 | (77.Ir,64.Gd), (78.Pt,64.Gd), (75.Re,121), (79.Au,64.Gd), (62.Sm,64.Gd), (29.Cu,64.Gd), (30.Zn,121), (58.Ce,121), (59.Pr,121), (27.Co,121), (65.Tb,64.Gd), (60.Nd,121), (61.Pm,64.Gd), (33.As,121), (76.Os,64.Gd) |
| 1.5499E−03 | (38.Sr,133), (114,133), (54.Xe,35.Br), (86.Rn,35.Br), (22.Ti,134), (55.Cs,134), (126,133), (118,134), (40.Zr,134), (129,133), (140,133) |
| 1.5596E−03 | (105,13.Al), (107,13.Al), (108,13.Al), (22.Ti,118), (109,13.Al), (110,13.Al), (111,13.Al), (113,13.Al), (114,13.Al), (115,13.Al), (117,13.Al)*, (118,13.Al)*, (119,13.Al), (120,13.Al), (122,13.Al), (124,13.Al)*, (126,13.Al), (127,13.Al), (128,13.Al), (129,13.Al), (131,13.Al), (132,13.Al), (133,13.Al), (137,13.Al), (108,124), (138,13.Al), (140,13.Al), (141,13.Al), (143,13.Al), (144,13.Al), (145,13.Al), (148,13.Al), (12.Mg,13.Al), (127,117), (6.C,13.Al), (11.Na,13.Al), (14.Si,13.Al), (15.P,13.Al), (16.S,13.Al), (19.K,13.Al), (20.Ca,13.Al), (21.Sc,13.Al), (22.Ti,13.Al), (37.Rb,13.Al), (38.Sr,13.Al), (39.Y,13.Al), (40.Zr,13.Al), (55.Cs,13.Al), (104,13.Al) |
| 1.5753E−03 | (59.Pr,60.Nd), (75.Re,60.Nd), (121,60.Nd) |
| 1.5763E−03 | (45.Rh,70.Yb), (74.W,70.Yb), (80.Hg,70.Yb), (87.Fr,70.Yb), (89.Ac,70.Yb), (47.Ag,70.Yb), (32.Ge,70.Yb), (63.Eu,70.Yb), (123,70.Yb), (46.Pd,70.Yb), (57.La,70.Yb), (31.Ga,70.Yb) |
| 1.5885E−03 | (41.Nb,71.Lu), (88.Ra,71.Lu), (23.V,71.Lu), (56.Ba,71.Lu) |
| 1.5960E−03 | (125,134), (3.Li,35.Br), (13.Al,134) |
| 1.6113E−03 | (77.Ir,65.Tb), (78.Pt,65.Tb), (66.Dy,65.Tb), (64.Gd,65.Tb) |
| 1.6139E−03 | (31.Ga,63.Eu), (123,63.Eu), (87.Fr,63.Eu), (80.Hg,63.Eu), (57.La,63.Eu), (32.Ge,63.Eu), (47.Ag,63.Eu) |
| 1.6394E−03 | (64.Gd,71.Lu), (29.Cu,71.Lu), (62.Sm,71.Lu), (66.Dy,71.Lu), (76.Os,71.Lu), (77.Ir,71.Lu), (78.Pt,71.Lu), (79.Au,71.Lu) |
| 1.6530E−03 | (29.Cu,61.Pm) |
| 1.6539E−03 | (51.Sb,34.Se), (43.Tc,34.Se), (48.Cd,34.Se), (49.In,34.Se), (50.Sn,34.Se), (73.Ta,34.Se), (83.Bi,34.Se), (84.Po,34.Se) |
| 1.6617E−03 | (52.Te,72.Hf), (42.Mo,72.Hf), (24.Cr,72.Hf), (49.In,72.Hf), (51.Sb,72.Hf), (112,72.Hf), (53.I,72.Hf), (25.Mn,72.Hf), (130,72.Hf) |

| *E*, MeV | List of poorly visible pairs for this energy) |
|---|---|
| 1.6756E−03 | (67.Ho,66.Dy), (71.Lu,66.Dy), (69.Tm,66.Dy), (65.Tb,66.Dy) |
| 1.6883E−03 | (75.Re,121), (72.Hf,121), (78.Pt,64.Gd), (77.Ir,64.Gd), (70.Yb,121), (59.Pr,121) |
| 1.7228E−03 | (61.Pm,62.Sm), (79.Au,62.Sm), (76.Os,62.Sm) |
| 1.7351E−03 | (57.La,73.Ta), (31.Ga,73.Ta), (63.Eu,73.Ta), (48.Cd,73.Ta), (47.Ag,73.Ta), (80.Hg,73.Ta), (81.Tl,73.Ta), (82.Pb,73.Ta), (85.At,73.Ta), (87.Fr,73.Ta), (123,73.Ta), (44.Ru,73.Ta), (32.Ge,73.Ta), (45.Rh,73.Ta), (34.Se,73.Ta), (26.Fe,73.Ta) |
| 1.7412E−03 | (71.Lu,67.Ho), (66.Dy,67.Ho), (68.Er,67.Ho), (91.Pa,67.Ho), (65.Tb,67.Ho), (69.Tm,67.Ho) |
| 1.7677E−03 | (73.Ta,65.Tb) |
| 1.7820E−03 | (21.Sc,133) |
| 1.8000E−03 | (45.Rh,63.Eu), (46.Pd,63.Eu), (74.W,63.Eu), (31.Ga,63.Eu), (80.Hg,63.Eu), (57.La,63.Eu) |
| 1.8044E−03 | (39.Y,37.Rb), (108,37.Rb), (111,37.Rb), (113,37.Rb), (114,37.Rb), (117,37.Rb), (124,37.Rb), (126,37.Rb), (127,37.Rb), (129,37.Rb), (133,37.Rb), (140,37.Rb), (21.Sc,37.Rb), (11.Na,37.Rb), (20.Ca,37.Rb), (38.Sr,37.Rb) |
| 1.8092E−03 | (33.As,74.W), (63.Eu,74.W), (30.Zn,74.W), (58.Ce,74.W), (27.Co,74.W), (46.Pd,74.W), (75.Re,74.W), (89.Ac,74.W), (59.Pr,74.W) |
| 1.8118E−03 | (67.Ho,68.Er), (69.Tm,68.Er), (66.Dy,68.Er), (91.Pa,68.Er), (71.Lu,68.Er) |
| 1.8389E−03 | (39.Y,14.Si), (40.Zr,14.Si), (55.Cs,14.Si), (104,14.Si), (105,14.Si), (107,14.Si), (108,14.Si), (38.Sr,117), (38.Sr,124), (109,14.Si), (111,14.Si)*, (113,14.Si), (22.Ti,118), (114,14.Si), (115,14.Si), (117,14.Si)*, (118,14.Si)*, (119,14.Si), (120,14.Si), (124,14.Si)*, (126,14.Si), (127,14.Si), (128,14.Si), (23.V,125), (129,14.Si), (131,14.Si), (108,124), (132,14.Si), (133,14.Si), (137,14.Si), (140,14.Si), (113,124), (114,117), (141,14.Si), (114,124), (6.C,14.Si), (143,14.Si), (144,14.Si), (124,117)*, (126,117), (145,14.Si), (148,14.Si), (129,117), (140,117), (11.Na,124), (20.Ca,124), (11.Na,14.Si), (11.Na,117), (12.Mg,14.Si), (15.P,14.Si), (16.S,14.Si), (19.K,14.Si), (126,124), (127,124), (20.Ca,14.Si), (129,124), (133,124), (140,124), (21.Sc,14.Si), (134,125), (22.Ti,14.Si), (21.Sc,117), (37.Rb,14.Si), (21.Sc,124), (38.Sr,14.Si) |
| 1.8418E−03 | (91.Pa,66.Dy) |
| 1.8639E−03 | (118,37.Rb), (55.Cs,37.Rb), (22.Ti,37.Rb) |
| 1.8716E−03 | (73.Ta,74.W) |
| 1.8808E−03 | (29.Cu,121), (60.Nd,121), (90.Th,121) |
| 1.8845E−03 | (71.Lu,69.Tm), (68.Er,69.Tm), (67.Ho,69.Tm) |

| $E$, MeV | List of poorly visible pairs for this energy) |
|---|---|
| 1.9210E−03 | (54.Xe,36.Kr) |
| 1.9228E−03 | (66.Dy,67.Ho) |
| 1.9396E−03 | (113,38.Sr), (114,38.Sr), (21.Sc,38.Sr), (117,38.Sr), (118,38.Sr), (22.Ti,38.Sr), (124,38.Sr), (126,38.Sr), (14.Si,38.Sr), (129,38.Sr), (37.Rb,38.Sr), (133,38.Sr), (140,38.Sr), (13.Al,38.Sr), (12.Mg,38.Sr), (39.Y,38.Sr), (40.Zr,38.Sr), (55.Cs,38.Sr) |
| 1.9489E−03 | (74.W,75.Re), (73.Ta,75.Re) |
| 1.9498E−03 | (78.Pt,70.Yb), (79.Au,70.Yb), (62.Sm,70.Yb), (61.Pm,70.Yb), (77.Ir,70.Yb) |
| 1.9601E−03 | (64.Gd,76.Os), (71.Lu,76.Os), (61.Pm,76.Os), (62.Sm,76.Os), (68.Er,76.Os), (77.Ir,76.Os), (78.Pt,76.Os), (79.Au,76.Os), (91.Pa,76.Os), (92.U,76.Os), (65.Tb,76.Os), (70.Yb,76.Os), (69.Tm,76.Os), (66.Dy,76.Os), (67.Ho,76.Os) |
| 1.9675E−03 | (91.Pa,65.Tb) |
| 2.0058E−03 | (71.Lu,68.Er) |
| 2.0068E−03 | (88.Ra,38.Sr), (41.Nb,38.Sr), (23.V,38.Sr), (56.Ba,38.Sr), (125,38.Sr), (134,38.Sr) |
| 2.0236E−03 | (92.U,71.Lu), (68.Er,71.Lu), (69.Tm,71.Lu) |
| 2.0308E−03 | (73.Ta,76.Os) |
| 2.0404E−03 | (62.Sm,77.Ir), (78.Pt,77.Ir) |
| 2.0651E−03 | (40.Zr,37.Rb) |
| 2.0800E−03 | (22.Ti,39.Y), (24.Cr,39.Y), (55.Cs,39.Y), (56.Ba,39.Y), (23.V,39.Y), (12.Mg,39.Y), (13.Al,39.Y), (88.Ra,39.Y), (112,39.Y), (116,39.Y), (118,39.Y), (14.Si,39.Y), (124,39.Y), (125,39.Y), (130,39.Y), (134,39.Y), (38.Sr,39.Y), (37.Rb,39.Y), (25.Mn,39.Y), (40.Zr,39.Y), (41.Nb,39.Y), (42.Mo,39.Y), (43.Tc,39.Y), (49.In,39.Y), (51.Sb,39.Y), (52.Te,39.Y), (53.I,39.Y) |
| 2.1216E−03 | (62.Sm,78.Pt), (61.Pm,78.Pt) |
| 2.1283E−03 | (66.Dy,67.Ho) |
| 2.1455E−03 | (40.Zr,15.P), (55.Cs,15.P), (104,15.P), (105,15.P), (108,15.P)*, (111,15.P), (113,15.P), (114,15.P), (115,15.P), (117,15.P), (118,15.P), (124,15.P), (126,15.P), (127,15.P), (129,15.P), (133,15.P), (140,15.P), (128,107)*, (148,15.P), (132,107)*, (111,108), (11.Na,15.P), (20.Ca,108), (11.Na,108), (127,108), (12.Mg,15.P), (131,109)*, (16.S,15.P), (20.Ca,15.P), (143,128)*, (21.Sc,15.P), (22.Ti,15.P), (37.Rb,15.P) |
| 2.1555E−03 | (34.Se,39.Y), (52.Te,39.Y), (31.Ga,39.Y), (27.Co,39.Y), (43.Tc,39.Y), (44.Ru,39.Y), (45.Rh,39.Y), (57.La,39.Y), (46.Pd,39.Y), (47.Ag,39.Y), (48.Cd,39.Y), (80.Hg,39.Y), (81.Tl,39.Y), (82.Pb,39.Y), (83.Bi,39.Y), (84.Po,39.Y), (85.At,39.Y), (87.Fr,39.Y), (26.Fe,39.Y), (49.In,39.Y), (50.Sn,39.Y), (32.Ge,39.Y), (51.Sb,39.Y), (123,39.Y) |

| $E$, MeV | List of poorly visible pairs for this energy) |
|---|---|
| 2.2057E−03 | (90.Th,79.Au), (121,79.Au) |
| 2.2065E−03 | (67.Ho,68.Er) |
| 2.2163E−03 | (24.Cr,38.Sr), (42.Mo,38.Sr) |
| 2.2223E−03 | (48.Cd,40.Zr), (49.In,40.Zr), (50.Sn,40.Zr), (51.Sb,40.Zr), (52.Te,40.Zr), (53.I,40.Zr), (56.Ba,40.Zr), (57.La,40.Zr), (58.Ce,40.Zr), (63.Eu,40.Zr), (31.Ga,40.Zr), (26.Fe,40.Zr), (14.Si,40.Zr), (15.P,40.Zr), (80.Hg,40.Zr), (81.Tl,40.Zr), (82.Pb,40.Zr), (83.Bi,40.Zr), (84.Po,40.Zr), (85.At,40.Zr), (87.Fr,40.Zr), (88.Ra,40.Zr), (89.Ac,40.Zr), (112,40.Zr), (116,40.Zr), (30.Zn,40.Zr), (123,40.Zr), (125,40.Zr), (130,40.Zr), (39.Y,40.Zr), (134,40.Zr), (13.Al,40.Zr), (34.Se,40.Zr), (33.As,40.Zr), (27.Co,40.Zr), (32.Ge,40.Zr), (37.Rb,40.Zr), (24.Cr,40.Zr), (23.V,40.Zr), (38.Sr,40.Zr), (25.Mn,40.Zr), (41.Nb,40.Zr), (42.Mo,40.Zr), (43.Tc,40.Zr), (44.Ru,40.Zr), (45.Rh,40.Zr), (46.Pd,40.Zr), (47.Ag,40.Zr) |
| 2.2635E−03 | (92.U,71.Lu) |
| 2.2810E−03 | (76.Os,74.W), (77.Ir,74.W), (75.Re,74.W) |
| 2.2949E−03 | (45.Rh,80.Hg), (27.Co,80.Hg), (31.Ga,80.Hg), (47.Ag,80.Hg), (116,130), (85.At,80.Hg), (87.Fr,80.Hg), (57.La,80.Hg), (46.Pd,80.Hg), (39.Y,80.Hg), (38.Sr,130) |
| 2.3067E−03 | (61.Pm,40.Zr), (80.Hg,40.Zr), (89.Ac,40.Zr), (90.Th,40.Zr), (28.Ni,40.Zr), (63.Eu,40.Zr), (121,40.Zr), (29.Cu,40.Zr), (58.Ce,40.Zr), (59.Pr,40.Zr), (60.Nd,40.Zr) |
| 2.3068E−03 | (68.Er,69.Tm) |
| 2.3673E−03 | (74.W,75.Re), (76.Os,75.Re), (77.Ir,75.Re) |
| 2.3705E−03 | (112,41.Nb), (32.Ge,41.Nb), (116,41.Nb), (30.Zn,41.Nb), (121,41.Nb), (25.Mn,41.Nb), (123,41.Nb), (125,41.Nb), (130,41.Nb), (134,41.Nb), (29.Cu,41.Nb), (33.As,41.Nb), (23.V,41.Nb), (31.Ga,41.Nb), (27.Co,41.Nb), (39.Y,41.Nb), (26.Fe,41.Nb), (40.Zr,41.Nb), (34.Se,41.Nb), (42.Mo,41.Nb), (43.Tc,41.Nb), (44.Ru,41.Nb), (45.Rh,41.Nb), (46.Pd,41.Nb), (47.Ag,41.Nb), (48.Cd,41.Nb), (49.In,41.Nb), (50.Sn,41.Nb), (51.Sb,41.Nb), (52.Te,41.Nb), (53.I,41.Nb), (56.Ba,41.Nb), (57.La,41.Nb), (58.Ce,41.Nb), (59.Pr,41.Nb), (60.Nd,41.Nb), (61.Pm,41.Nb), (62.Sm,41.Nb), (38.Sr,41.Nb), (63.Eu,41.Nb), (24.Cr,41.Nb), (70.Yb,41.Nb), (28.Ni,41.Nb), (81.Tl,41.Nb), (82.Pb,41.Nb), (83.Bi,41.Nb), (84.Po,41.Nb), (85.At,41.Nb), (87.Fr,41.Nb), (88.Ra,41.Nb), (89.Ac,41.Nb), (90.Th,41.Nb) |
| 2.3725E−03 | (87.Fr,39.Y), (57.La,39.Y), (30.Zn,39.Y), (27.Co,39.Y), (45.Rh,39.Y), (33.As,39.Y), (46.Pd,39.Y) |
| 2.3849E−03 | (123,130), (32.Ge,130) |

| $E$, MeV | List of poorly visible pairs for this energy) |
|---|---|
| 2.3893E−03 | (63.Eu,81.Tl), (31.Ga,81.Tl), (44.Ru,81.Tl), (27.Co,81.Tl), (46.Pd,81.Tl), (45.Rh,81.Tl), (32.Ge,81.Tl), (34.Se,81.Tl), (30.Zn,81.Tl), (33.As,81.Tl), (39.Y,81.Tl), (57.La,81.Tl), (82.Pb,81.Tl), (85.At,81.Tl), (87.Fr,81.Tl), (89.Ac,81.Tl), (123,81.Tl), (130,81.Tl), (47.Ag,81.Tl) |
| 2.4572E−03 | (75.Re,76.Os) |
| 2.4647E−03 | (70.Yb,41.Nb), (65.Tb,41.Nb), (66.Dy,41.Nb), (81.Tl,41.Nb), (67.Ho,41.Nb), (91.Pa,41.Nb), (62.Sm,41.Nb), (64.Gd,41.Nb) |
| 2.4687E−03 | (79.Au,73.Ta) |
| 2.4720E−03 | (124,114), (126,114), (129,114), (113,16.S), (133,114), (140,114), (120,115)*, (29.Cu,121), (114,16.S)*, (117,16.S), (22.Ti,118), (118,16.S)*, (21.Sc,114), (124,16.S), (128,107)*, (126,16.S), (127,16.S), (132,107)*, (141,107), (144,107)*, (129,16.S), (133,16.S), (140,16.S), (11.Na,16.S), (12.Mg,16.S), (20.Ca,16.S), (122,109), (21.Sc,16.S), (131,109)*, (138,109), (22.Ti,16.S), (55.Cs,16.S), (113,114), (59.Pr,121), (60.Nd,121), (132,128)*, (141,128), (105,16.S), (143,128)*, (144,128)*, (117,114), (108,16.S)*, (144,131)*, (141,132), (111,16.S), (144,143)* |
| 2.4840E−03 | (61.Pm,82.Pb), (57.La,82.Pb), (43.Tc,125), (32.Ge,82.Pb), (29.Cu,82.Pb), (34.Se,82.Pb), (56.Ba,125), (45.Rh,82.Pb), (47.Ag,82.Pb), (53.I,125), (33.As,82.Pb), (31.Ga,82.Pb), (30.Zn,82.Pb), (27.Co,82.Pb), (44.Ru,82.Pb), (24.Cr,125), (85.At,82.Pb), (112,125), (87.Fr,82.Pb), (89.Ac,82.Pb), (90.Th,82.Pb), (121,82.Pb), (28.Ni,82.Pb), (123,82.Pb), (130,82.Pb), (60.Nd,82.Pb), (38.Sr,125), (42.Mo,125), (59.Pr,82.Pb), (46.Pd,82.Pb), (39.Y,82.Pb), (88.Ra,125), (63.Eu,82.Pb), (58.Ce,82.Pb), (116,125), (25.Mn,125) |
| 2.4851E−03 | (92.U,81.Tl), (71.Lu,81.Tl), (69.Tm,81.Tl) |
| 2.4912E−03 | (92.U,71.Lu) |
| 2.5202E−03 | (57.La,42.Mo), (58.Ce,42.Mo), (59.Pr,42.Mo), (38.Sr,42.Mo), (60.Nd,42.Mo), (40.Zr,42.Mo), (61.Pm,42.Mo), (33.As,42.Mo), (62.Sm,42.Mo), (63.Eu,42.Mo), (39.Y,42.Mo), (64.Gd,42.Mo), (65.Tb,42.Mo), (70.Yb,42.Mo), (31.Ga,42.Mo), (82.Pb,42.Mo), (83.Bi,42.Mo), (84.Po,42.Mo), (85.At,42.Mo), (87.Fr,42.Mo), (88.Ra,42.Mo), (89.Ac,42.Mo), (90.Th,42.Mo), (91.Pa,42.Mo), (112,42.Mo), (116,42.Mo), (121,42.Mo), (123,42.Mo), (34.Se,42.Mo), (125,42.Mo), (130,42.Mo), (26.Fe,42.Mo), (30.Zn,42.Mo), (29.Cu,42.Mo), (28.Ni,42.Mo), (32.Ge,42.Mo), (25.Mn,42.Mo), (27.Co,42.Mo), (24.Cr,42.Mo), (43.Tc,42.Mo), (44.Ru,42.Mo), (45.Rh,42.Mo), (46.Pd,42.Mo), (47.Ag,42.Mo), (48.Cd,42.Mo), (49.In,42.Mo), (50.Sn,42.Mo), (51.Sb,42.Mo), (52.Te,42.Mo), (53.I,42.Mo) |
| 2.5316E−03 | (70.Yb,40.Zr), (62.Sm,40.Zr) |
| 2.5507E−03 | (75.Re,77.Ir), (76.Os,77.Ir) |

| $E$, MeV | List of poorly visible pairs for this energy) |
|---|---|
| 2.5796E−03 | (61.Pm,83.Bi), (32.Ge,83.Bi), (63.Eu,83.Bi), (30.Zn,83.Bi), (47.Ag,83.Bi), (29.Cu,83.Bi), (62.Sm,83.Bi), (34.Se,83.Bi), (50.Sn,83.Bi), (28.Ni,83.Bi), (57.La,83.Bi), (58.Ce,83.Bi), (59.Pr,83.Bi), (33.As,83.Bi), (84.Po,83.Bi), (85.At,83.Bi), (87.Fr,83.Bi), (89.Ac,83.Bi), (90.Th,83.Bi), (121,83.Bi), (60.Nd,83.Bi), (123,83.Bi), (125,83.Bi), (130,83.Bi), (26.Fe,83.Bi), (46.Pd,83.Bi), (31.Ga,83.Bi), (70.Yb,83.Bi), (48.Cd,83.Bi), (51.Sb,83.Bi), (27.Co,83.Bi), (45.Rh,83.Bi), (44.Ru,83.Bi), (40.Zr,83.Bi), (39.Y,83.Bi) |
| 2.5856E−03 | (81.Tl,82.Pb), (59.Pr,125), (30.Zn,125), (58.Ce,125), (28.Ni,125), (87.Fr,125), (71.Lu,82.Pb), (63.Eu,125), (33.As,125), (89.Ac,125), (69.Tm,82.Pb), (29.Cu,125), (39.Y,125), (92.U,82.Pb), (130,125) |
| 2.6251E−03 | (69.Tm,42.Mo), (41.Nb,42.Mo), (71.Lu,42.Mo), (65.Tb,42.Mo), (66.Dy,42.Mo), (67.Ho,42.Mo), (91.Pa,42.Mo), (92.U,42.Mo), (83.Bi,42.Mo), (68.Er,42.Mo) |
| 2.6454E−03 | (76.Os,78.Pt), (75.Re,78.Pt) |
| 2.6769E−03 | (87.Fr,43.Tc), (89.Ac,43.Tc), (90.Th,43.Tc), (91.Pa,43.Tc), (112,43.Tc), (121,43.Tc), (123,43.Tc), (26.Fe,43.Tc), (125,43.Tc), (130,43.Tc), (41.Nb,43.Tc), (39.Y,43.Tc), (30.Zn,43.Tc), (25.Mn,43.Tc), (27.Co,43.Tc), (32.Ge,43.Tc), (28.Ni,43.Tc), (33.As,43.Tc), (31.Ga,43.Tc), (34.Se,43.Tc), (44.Ru,43.Tc), (45.Rh,43.Tc), (46.Pd,43.Tc), (47.Ag,43.Tc), (48.Cd,43.Tc), (49.In,43.Tc), (50.Sn,43.Tc), (51.Sb,43.Tc), (52.Te,43.Tc), (57.La,43.Tc), (40.Zr,43.Tc), (58.Ce,43.Tc), (29.Cu,43.Tc), (59.Pr,43.Tc), (60.Nd,43.Tc), (61.Pm,43.Tc), (62.Sm,43.Tc), (63.Eu,43.Tc), (64.Gd,43.Tc), (65.Tb,43.Tc), (66.Dy,43.Tc), (67.Ho,43.Tc), (68.Er,43.Tc), (70.Yb,43.Tc), (83.Bi,43.Tc), (84.Po,43.Tc), (85.At,43.Tc) |
| 2.6830E−03 | (60.Nd,84.Po), (29.Cu,84.Po), (70.Yb,84.Po), (28.Ni,84.Po), (26.Fe,84.Po), (66.Dy,84.Po), (33.As,84.Po), (68.Er,84.Po), (47.Ag,84.Po), (39.Y,84.Po), (41.Nb,84.Po), (32.Ge,84.Po), (50.Sn,84.Po), (65.Tb,84.Po), (34.Se,84.Po), (40.Zr,84.Po), (61.Pm,84.Po), (46.Pd,84.Po), (57.La,84.Po), (64.Gd,84.Po), (83.Bi,84.Po), (63.Eu,84.Po), (58.Ce,84.Po), (27.Co,84.Po), (67.Ho,84.Po), (30.Zn,84.Po), (62.Sm,84.Po), (59.Pr,84.Po), (48.Cd,84.Po), (45.Rh,84.Po), (85.At,84.Po), (87.Fr,84.Po), (89.Ac,84.Po), (90.Th,84.Po), (91.Pa,84.Po), (121,84.Po), (44.Ru,84.Po), (123,84.Po), (125,84.Po), (130,84.Po), (31.Ga,84.Po) |
| 2.6876E−03 | (92.U,83.Bi), (71.Lu,83.Bi), (41.Nb,83.Bi), (68.Er,83.Bi), (84.Po,83.Bi), (43.Tc,83.Bi), (69.Tm,83.Bi), (67.Ho,83.Bi), (42.Mo,83.Bi) |
| 2.6977E−03 | (43.Tc,41.Nb), (69.Tm,41.Nb), (67.Ho,41.Nb), (68.Er,41.Nb), (84.Po,41.Nb) |
| 2.7430E−03 | (74.W,79.Au) |

| $E$, MeV | List of poorly visible pairs for this energy) |
|---|---|
| 2.7867E−03 | (47.Ag,85.At), (61.Pm,85.At), (43.Tc,85.At), (58.Ce,85.At), (68.Er,85.At), (83.Bi,85.At), (60.Nd,85.At), (70.Yb,85.At), (45.Rh,85.At), (46.Pd,85.At), (30.Zn,85.At), (27.Co,85.At), (33.As,85.At), (40.Zr,85.At), (29.Cu,85.At), (62.Sm,85.At), (84.Po,85.At), (67.Ho,85.At), (59.Pr,85.At), (28.Ni,85.At), (63.Eu,85.At), (39.Y,85.At), (57.La,85.At), (66.Dy,85.At), (69.Tm,85.At), (71.Lu,85.At), (87.Fr,85.At), (89.Ac,85.At), (90.Th,85.At), (91.Pa,85.At), (92.U,85.At), (121,85.At), (42.Mo,85.At), (125,85.At), (130,85.At), (64.Gd,85.At), (65.Tb,85.At), (41.Nb,85.At), (31.Ga,85.At) |
| 2.7922E−03 | (78.Pt,76.Os), (77.Ir,76.Os) |
| 2.7932E−03 | (41.Nb,43.Tc), (69.Tm,43.Tc), (83.Bi,43.Tc), (92.U,43.Tc), (42.Mo,43.Tc), (71.Lu,43.Tc), (81.Tl,43.Tc), (85.At,43.Tc), (82.Pb,43.Tc) |
| 2.7980E−03 | (71.Lu,84.Po), (69.Tm,84.Po), (92.U,84.Po), (83.Bi,84.Po), (67.Ho,84.Po), (42.Mo,84.Po), (68.Er,84.Po), (82.Pb,84.Po), (85.At,84.Po), (81.Tl,84.Po), (41.Nb,84.Po) |
| 2.8224E−03 | (141,109)*, (115,141), (141,107)*, (111,141), (143,107)*, (104,141), (144,107)*, (105,141), (106,110), (113,141), (20.Ca,141), (126,141), (6.C,141), (127,141), (128,107)*, (132,128)*, (108,141), (141,128)*, (141,119)*, (120,141), (11.Na,141), (144,128)*, (9.F,17.Cl), (122,141), (129,141), (141,131)*, (19.K,141), (132,107)*, (141,132)*, (131,109)*, (137,141), (138,141), (140,141), (143,141)*, (144,141)*, (145,141), (148,141), (21.Sc,141), (144,143)* |
| 2.8379E−03 | (62.Sm,44.Ru), (32.Ge,44.Ru), (63.Eu,44.Ru), (64.Gd,44.Ru), (29.Cu,44.Ru), (65.Tb,44.Ru), (28.Ni,44.Ru), (66.Dy,44.Ru), (67.Ho,44.Ru), (68.Er,44.Ru), (69.Tm,44.Ru), (70.Yb,44.Ru), (71.Lu,44.Ru), (31.Ga,44.Ru), (33.As,44.Ru), (41.Nb,44.Ru), (30.Zn,44.Ru), (27.Co,44.Ru), (85.At,44.Ru), (87.Fr,44.Ru), (89.Ac,44.Ru), (90.Th,44.Ru), (91.Pa,44.Ru), (92.U,44.Ru), (121,44.Ru), (39.Y,44.Ru), (123,44.Ru), (125,44.Ru), (130,44.Ru), (45.Rh,44.Ru), (46.Pd,44.Ru), (47.Ag,44.Ru), (48.Cd,44.Ru), (57.La,44.Ru), (58.Ce,44.Ru), (34.Se,44.Ru), (59.Pr,44.Ru), (40.Zr,44.Ru), (60.Nd,44.Ru), (61.Pm,44.Ru) |
| 2.8471E−03 | (59.Pr,130), (60.Nd,130) |
| 2.8655E−03 | (83.Bi,42.Mo) |
| 2.8924E−03 | (35.Br,86.Rn) |
| 2.9087E−03 | (42.Mo,85.At), (76.Os,77.Ir), (82.Pb,85.At), (78.Pt,77.Ir), (81.Tl,85.At), (41.Nb,85.At), (71.Lu,85.At), (83.Bi,85.At), (72.Hf,85.At), (84.Po,85.At), (44.Ru,85.At), (43.Tc,85.At) |
| 2.9317E−03 | (79.Au,75.Re) |
| 2.9566E−03 | (72.Hf,81.Tl), (85.At,81.Tl) |

| $E$, MeV | List of poorly visible pairs for this energy) |
|---|---|
| 2.9669E−03 | (83.Bi,44.Ru), (43.Tc,44.Ru), (84.Po,44.Ru), (81.Tl,44.Ru), (72.Hf,44.Ru), (85.At,44.Ru), (82.Pb,44.Ru), (42.Mo,44.Ru) |
| 2.9999E−03 | (65.Tb,87.Fr), (40.Zr,87.Fr), (29.Cu,87.Fr), (89.Ac,87.Fr), (90.Th,87.Fr), (91.Pa,87.Fr), (92.U,87.Fr), (121,87.Fr), (59.Pr,87.Fr), (41.Nb,87.Fr), (125,87.Fr), (130,87.Fr), (67.Ho,87.Fr), (58.Ce,87.Fr), (63.Eu,87.Fr), (39.Y,87.Fr), (68.Er,87.Fr), (60.Nd,87.Fr), (70.Yb,87.Fr), (62.Sm,87.Fr), (71.Lu,87.Fr), (66.Dy,87.Fr), (69.Tm,87.Fr), (64.Gd,87.Fr), (61.Pm,87.Fr) |
| 3.0038E−03 | (69.Tm,45.Rh), (30.Zn,45.Rh), (70.Yb,45.Rh), (71.Lu,45.Rh), (41.Nb,45.Rh), (46.Pd,45.Rh), (57.La,45.Rh), (39.Y,45.Rh), (58.Ce,45.Rh), (59.Pr,45.Rh), (60.Nd,45.Rh), (89.Ac,45.Rh), (90.Th,45.Rh), (91.Pa,45.Rh), (92.U,45.Rh), (121,45.Rh), (125,45.Rh), (130,45.Rh), (28.Ni,45.Rh), (61.Pm,45.Rh), (62.Sm,45.Rh), (40.Zr,45.Rh), (63.Eu,45.Rh), (64.Gd,45.Rh), (65.Tb,45.Rh), (29.Cu,45.Rh), (66.Dy,45.Rh), (33.As,45.Rh), (67.Ho,45.Rh), (68.Er,45.Rh) |
| 3.0265E−03 | (76.Os,78.Pt) |
| 3.0425E−03 | (85.At,43.Tc), (82.Pb,43.Tc), (44.Ru,43.Tc), (72.Hf,43.Tc) |
| 3.0485E−03 | (77.Ir,76.Os), (78.Pt,76.Os) |
| 3.0664E−03 | (85.At,82.Pb), (43.Tc,82.Pb), (44.Ru,82.Pb), (72.Hf,82.Pb), (64.Gd,125) |
| 3.1049E−03 | (47.Ag,88.Ra), (59.Pr,88.Ra), (27.Co,88.Ra), (63.Eu,88.Ra), (51.Sb,88.Ra), (46.Pd,88.Ra), (49.In,88.Ra), (29.Cu,88.Ra), (60.Nd,88.Ra), (89.Ac,88.Ra), (90.Th,88.Ra), (112,88.Ra), (116,88.Ra), (38.Sr,88.Ra), (28.Ni,88.Ra), (123,88.Ra), (26.Fe,88.Ra), (130,88.Ra), (39.Y,88.Ra), (52.Te,88.Ra), (50.Sn,88.Ra), (34.Se,88.Ra), (32.Ge,88.Ra), (53.I,88.Ra), (48.Cd,88.Ra), (25.Mn,88.Ra), (33.As,88.Ra), (61.Pm,88.Ra), (31.Ga,88.Ra), (30.Zn,88.Ra), (58.Ce,88.Ra), (57.La,88.Ra) |
| 3.1362E−03 | (72.Hf,87.Fr), (44.Ru,87.Fr), (71.Lu,87.Fr), (42.Mo,87.Fr), (84.Po,87.Fr), (83.Bi,87.Fr), (41.Nb,87.Fr), (85.At,87.Fr), (45.Rh,87.Fr) |
| 3.1461E−03 | (72.Hf,45.Rh), (87.Fr,45.Rh), (43.Tc,45.Rh), (83.Bi,45.Rh), (44.Ru,45.Rh), (84.Po,45.Rh), (42.Mo,45.Rh), (85.At,45.Rh) |
| 3.1733E−03 | (66.Dy,46.Pd), (33.As,46.Pd), (67.Ho,46.Pd), (68.Er,46.Pd), (69.Tm,46.Pd), (40.Zr,46.Pd), (70.Yb,46.Pd), (71.Lu,46.Pd), (30.Zn,46.Pd), (27.Co,46.Pd), (57.La,46.Pd), (58.Ce,46.Pd), (59.Pr,46.Pd), (41.Nb,46.Pd), (60.Nd,46.Pd), (39.Y,46.Pd), (88.Ra,46.Pd), (89.Ac,46.Pd), (90.Th,46.Pd), (91.Pa,46.Pd), (92.U,46.Pd), (121,46.Pd), (125,46.Pd), (130,46.Pd), (61.Pm,46.Pd), (62.Sm,46.Pd), (28.Ni,46.Pd), (63.Eu,46.Pd), (64.Gd,46.Pd), (65.Tb,46.Pd), (29.Cu,46.Pd) |
| 3.1737E−03 | (76.Os,77.Ir) |

| $E$, MeV | List of poorly visible pairs for this energy) |
|---|---|
| 3.1769E−03 | (42.Mo,83.Bi), (85.At,83.Bi), (84.Po,83.Bi) |
| 3.2029E−03 | (8.O,18.Ar), (9.F,18.Ar), (10.Ne,18.Ar) |
| 3.2190E−03 | (130,89.Ac), (59.Pr,89.Ac), (68.Er,89.Ac), (66.Dy,89.Ac), (62.Sm,89.Ac), (71.Lu,89.Ac), (67.Ho,89.Ac), (88.Ra,89.Ac), (41.Nb,89.Ac), (64.Gd,89.Ac), (40.Zr,89.Ac), (60.Nd,89.Ac), (69.Tm,89.Ac), (65.Tb,89.Ac), (70.Yb,89.Ac), (61.Pm,89.Ac), (90.Th,89.Ac), (91.Pa,89.Ac), (92.U,89.Ac), (121,89.Ac), (39.Y,89.Ac), (125,89.Ac) |
| 3.2240E−03 | (81.Tl,44.Ru), (43.Tc,44.Ru), (45.Rh,44.Ru), (72.Hf,44.Ru), (87.Fr,44.Ru), (82.Pb,44.Ru) |
| 3.2484E−03 | (90.Th,88.Ra), (125,88.Ra), (91.Pa,88.Ra), (130,88.Ra), (64.Gd,88.Ra), (62.Sm,88.Ra), (61.Pm,88.Ra), (121,88.Ra), (70.Yb,88.Ra), (65.Tb,88.Ra) |
| 3.2785E−03 | (90.Th,130) |
| 3.3019E−03 | (42.Mo,84.Po), (85.At,84.Po) |
| 3.3303E−03 | (83.Bi,46.Pd), (85.At,46.Pd), (87.Fr,46.Pd), (42.Mo,46.Pd), (84.Po,46.Pd) |
| 3.3320E−03 | (92.U,90.Th), (41.Nb,90.Th), (121,90.Th), (125,90.Th), (68.Er,90.Th), (130,90.Th), (61.Pm,90.Th), (69.Tm,90.Th), (66.Dy,90.Th), (65.Tb,90.Th), (67.Ho,90.Th), (89.Ac,90.Th), (88.Ra,90.Th), (40.Zr,90.Th), (64.Gd,90.Th), (62.Sm,90.Th), (71.Lu,90.Th), (70.Yb,90.Th), (91.Pa,90.Th) |
| 3.3511E−03 | (66.Dy,47.Ag), (67.Ho,47.Ag), (68.Er,47.Ag), (49.In,134), (69.Tm,47.Ag), (25.Mn,134), (70.Yb,47.Ag), (32.Ge,47.Ag), (31.Ga,47.Ag), (34.Se,47.Ag), (22.Ti,133), (40.Zr,47.Ag), (112,134), (124,133), (56.Ba,134), (39.Y,47.Ag), (27.Co,47.Ag), (33.As,47.Ag), (88.Ra,47.Ag), (29.Cu,47.Ag), (91.Pa,47.Ag), (92.U,47.Ag), (121,47.Ag), (123,47.Ag), (125,47.Ag), (130,47.Ag), (30.Zn,47.Ag), (114,133), (24.Cr,134), (28.Ni,47.Ag), (57.La,47.Ag), (58.Ce,47.Ag), (52.Te,134), (59.Pr,47.Ag), (60.Nd,47.Ag), (116,134), (12.Mg,133), (61.Pm,47.Ag), (141,133), (62.Sm,47.Ag), (16.S,134), (53.I,134), (117,133), (63.Eu,47.Ag), (64.Gd,47.Ag), (65.Tb,47.Ag), (55.Cs,133), (38.Sr,134) |
| 3.3702E−03 | (90.Th,89.Ac), (41.Nb,89.Ac), (87.Fr,89.Ac), (42.Mo,89.Ac), (84.Po,89.Ac), (83.Bi,89.Ac), (85.At,89.Ac), (71.Lu,89.Ac) |
| 3.4119E−03 | (43.Tc,45.Rh), (46.Pd,45.Rh), (44.Ru,45.Rh), (81.Tl,45.Rh), (72.Hf,45.Rh), (82.Pb,45.Rh) |
| 3.4157E−03 | (43.Tc,81.Tl), (72.Hf,81.Tl), (82.Pb,81.Tl) |
| 3.4260E−03 | (46.Pd,85.At), (89.Ac,85.At), (83.Bi,85.At), (87.Fr,85.At), (84.Po,85.At) |
| 3.4418E−03 | (41.Nb,91.Pa), (82.Pb,91.Pa), (85.At,91.Pa), (90.Th,91.Pa), (44.Ru,91.Pa), (88.Ra,91.Pa), (46.Pd,91.Pa), (42.Mo,91.Pa), |

| $E$, MeV | List of poorly visible pairs for this energy) |
|---|---|
| | (83.Bi,91.Pa), (84.Po,91.Pa), (92.U,91.Pa), (40.Zr,91.Pa), (72.Hf,91.Pa), (81.Tl,91.Pa), (69.Tm,91.Pa), (87.Fr,91.Pa), (67.Ho,91.Pa), (43.Tc,91.Pa), (68.Er,91.Pa), (71.Lu,91.Pa), (47.Ag,91.Pa), (89.Ac,91.Pa), (65.Tb,91.Pa), (70.Yb,91.Pa), (66.Dy,91.Pa) |
| 3.4908E−03 | (82.Pb,90.Th), (83.Bi,90.Th), (85.At,90.Th), (87.Fr,90.Th), (81.Tl,90.Th), (43.Tc,90.Th), (84.Po,90.Th), (44.Ru,90.Th), (91.Pa,90.Th), (42.Mo,90.Th), (72.Hf,90.Th), (89.Ac,90.Th), (46.Pd,90.Th) |
| 3.5237E−03 | (34.Se,134), (32.Ge,134), (26.Fe,134), (51.Sb,134), (50.Sn,134), (31.Ga,134), (83.Bi,47.Ag), (42.Mo,47.Ag), (84.Po,47.Ag), (71.Lu,47.Ag), (123,134), (87.Fr,47.Ag), (41.Nb,47.Ag) |
| 3.5375E−03 | (32.Ge,48.Cd), (49.In,112), (32.Ge,112), (25.Mn,112), (26.Fe,112), (30.Zn,112), (50.Sn,48.Cd), (51.Sb,48.Cd), (27.Co,112), (50.Sn,112), (57.La,48.Cd), (34.Se,48.Cd), (58.Ce,48.Cd), (28.Ni,112), (116,112), (59.Pr,48.Cd), (123,112), (60.Nd,48.Cd), (61.Pm,48.Cd), (134,112), (62.Sm,48.Cd), (38.Sr,112), (63.Eu,48.Cd), (64.Gd,48.Cd), (51.Sb,112), (39.Y,48.Cd), (65.Tb,48.Cd), (66.Dy,48.Cd), (67.Ho,48.Cd), (70.Yb,48.Cd), (40.Zr,48.Cd), (33.As,48.Cd), (33.As,112), (28.Ni,48.Cd), (52.Te,112), (88.Ra,48.Cd), (31.Ga,112), (112,48.Cd)*, (121,48.Cd), (123,48.Cd), (53.I,112), (125,48.Cd), (130,48.Cd), (57.La,112), (134,48.Cd), (31.Ga,48.Cd), (34.Se,112), (26.Fe,48.Cd), (29.Cu,48.Cd), (27.Co,48.Cd), (30.Zn,48.Cd) |
| 3.5517E−03 | (41.Nb,92.U), (81.Tl,92.U), (80.Hg,92.U), (42.Mo,92.U), (68.Er,92.U), (44.Ru,92.U), (90.Th,92.U), (87.Fr,92.U), (46.Pd,92.U), (83.Bi,92.U), (45.Rh,92.U), (43.Tc,92.U), (72.Hf,92.U), (91.Pa,92.U), (69.Tm,92.U), (85.At,92.U), (84.Po,92.U), (71.Lu,92.U), (47.Ag,92.U), (89.Ac,92.U), (73.Ta,92.U), (82.Pb,92.U) |
| 3.5542E−03 | (43.Tc,82.Pb), (85.At,82.Pb), (72.Hf,82.Pb) |
| 3.5616E−03 | (61.Pm,130) |
| 3.6043E−03 | (43.Tc,46.Pd), (91.Pa,46.Pd), (82.Pb,46.Pd), (44.Ru,46.Pd), (72.Hf,46.Pd), (85.At,46.Pd), (81.Tl,46.Pd) |
| 3.6074E−03 | (131,19.K)*, (144,107)*, (132,19.K)*, (137,19.K), (140,19.K), (11.Na,19.K), (141,19.K), (143,19.K)*, (144,19.K)*, (145,19.K), (148,19.K), (12.Mg,19.K), (132,128)*, (20.Ca,19.K), (131,109)*, (21.Sc,19.K), (104,19.K), (143,109)*, (144,109)*, (144,128)*, (145,128), (105,19.K), (107,19.K)*, (108,19.K), (109,19.K)*, (143,131)*, (111,19.K), (144,131)*, (137,132), (113,19.K), (115,19.K), (144,132)*, (128,107)*, (117,19.K)*, (119,19.K), (137,144), (120,19.K), (124,19.K)*, (132,107)*, (137,107), (126,19.K), (127,19.K), (128,19.K)*, (129,19.K), (144,143)* |
| 3.6112E−03 | (44.Ru,91.Pa), (90.Th,91.Pa), (45.Rh,91.Pa), (80.Hg,91.Pa), (46.Pd,91.Pa), (92.U,91.Pa), (73.Ta,91.Pa) |

| $E$, MeV | List of poorly visible pairs for this energy) |
|---|---|
| 3.6630E−03 | (89.Ac,87.Fr), (84.Po,87.Fr), (72.Hf,87.Fr), (85.At,87.Fr), (47.Ag,87.Fr), (43.Tc,87.Fr), (83.Bi,87.Fr) |
| 3.6963E−03 | (47.Ag,83.Bi), (84.Po,83.Bi) |
| 3.7270E−03 | (68.Er,48.Cd), (63.Eu,112), (69.Tm,48.Cd), (41.Nb,48.Cd), (59.Pr,112), (71.Lu,48.Cd), (39.Y,112), (60.Nd,112) |
| 3.7276E−03 | (74.W,92.U), (75.Re,92.U), (78.Pt,92.U), (91.Pa,92.U), (76.Os,92.U), (79.Au,92.U) |
| 3.7301E−03 | (64.Gd,49.In), (65.Tb,49.In), (70.Yb,49.In), (31.Ga,49.In), (28.Ni,49.In), (88.Ra,49.In), (34.Se,49.In), (112,49.In), (121,49.In), (26.Fe,49.In), (123,49.In), (125,49.In), (130,49.In), (30.Zn,49.In), (134,49.In), (33.As,49.In), (50.Sn,49.In), (51.Sb,49.In), (52.Te,49.In), (32.Ge,49.In), (29.Cu,49.In), (57.La,49.In), (39.Y,49.In), (58.Ce,49.In), (59.Pr,49.In), (27.Co,49.In), (60.Nd,49.In), (61.Pm,49.In), (40.Zr,49.In), (62.Sm,49.In), (63.Eu,49.In) |
| 3.7918E−03 | (70.Yb,88.Ra), (66.Dy,88.Ra), (49.In,88.Ra), (65.Tb,88.Ra), (125,88.Ra), (40.Zr,88.Ra) |
| 3.8058E−03 | (89.Ac,47.Ag), (83.Bi,47.Ag), (37.Rb,133), (118,133), (43.Tc,47.Ag), (33.As,134), (57.La,134), (85.At,47.Ag), (14.Si,133), (23.V,133), (87.Fr,47.Ag), (30.Zn,134), (72.Hf,47.Ag) |
| 3.8507E−03 | (44.Ru,82.Pb) |
| 3.9090E−03 | (87.Fr,89.Ac), (44.Ru,89.Ac), (85.At,89.Ac), (43.Tc,89.Ac), (47.Ag,89.Ac), (72.Hf,89.Ac) |
| 3.9288E−03 | (63.Eu,50.Sn), (64.Gd,50.Sn), (65.Tb,50.Sn), (66.Dy,50.Sn), (70.Yb,50.Sn), (29.Cu,50.Sn), (33.As,50.Sn), (34.Se,50.Sn), (28.Ni,50.Sn), (112,50.Sn), (121,50.Sn), (123,50.Sn), (125,50.Sn), (130,50.Sn), (30.Zn,50.Sn), (134,50.Sn), (32.Ge,50.Sn), (40.Zr,50.Sn), (39.Y,50.Sn), (51.Sb,50.Sn), (57.La,50.Sn), (31.Ga,50.Sn), (58.Ce,50.Sn), (27.Co,50.Sn), (59.Pr,50.Sn), (60.Nd,50.Sn), (61.Pm,50.Sn), (62.Sm,50.Sn) |
| 3.9380E−03 | (41.Nb,49.In), (88.Ra,49.In), (67.Ho,49.In), (68.Er,49.In), (69.Tm,49.In) |
| 4.0080E−03 | (87.Fr,85.At) |
| 4.0180E−03 | (121,112), (130,112), (62.Sm,112), (42.Mo,48.Cd) |
| 4.0381E−03 | (105,20.Ca)*, (19.K,113), (108,20.Ca)*, (113,20.Ca)*, (22.Ti,113), (124,117), (22.Ti,114), (114,20.Ca)*, (117,20.Ca)*, (118,20.Ca)*, (19.K,114), (124,20.Ca), (141,117), (126,20.Ca), (16.S,114), (133,118), (25.Mn,113), (55.Cs,113), (55.Cs,114), (129,20.Ca), (133,20.Ca), (113,108)*, (117,108)*, (140,20.Ca), (11.Na,20.Ca), (141,20.Ca), (124,108), (13.Al,20.Ca), (129,108), (12.Mg,117), (141,108), (37.Rb,113), (12.Mg,20.Ca), (37.Rb,114), (12.Mg,113), (56.Ba,113), (23.V,113), (23.V,114), (12.Mg,108), (13.Al,113), (14.Si,113), (16.S,20.Ca), (11.Na,105), (21.Sc,108), (21.Sc,113), (19.K,20.Ca), (15.P,113), (14.Si,114), (15.P,114), (15.P,20.Ca), (13.Al,114), |

| $E$, MeV | List of poorly visible pairs for this energy) |
|---|---|
| | (14.Si,20.Ca), (114,113)*, (117,113)*, (118,113)*, (16.S,113), (21.Sc,20.Ca), (124,113), (133,113), (22.Ti,20.Ca), (141,113), (23.V,20.Ca), (24.Cr,113), (118,114)*, (15.P,118), (102,101), (106,101), (142,101), (37.Rb,20.Ca), (108,105)*, (111,105), (126,105), (133,114), (127,105), (129,105), (140,105), (55.Cs,20.Ca) |
| 4.0461E−03 | (45.Rh,90.Th), (80.Hg,90.Th), (73.Ta,90.Th), (46.Pd,90.Th) |
| 4.1322E−03 | (123,51.Sb), (130,51.Sb), (29.Cu,51.Sb), (134,51.Sb), (57.La,51.Sb), (30.Zn,51.Sb), (58.Ce,51.Sb), (59.Pr,51.Sb), (31.Ga,51.Sb), (60.Nd,51.Sb), (61.Pm,51.Sb), (33.As,51.Sb), (62.Sm,51.Sb), (63.Eu,51.Sb), (64.Gd,51.Sb), (65.Tb,51.Sb), (70.Yb,51.Sb), (32.Ge,51.Sb), (40.Zr,51.Sb), (39.Y,51.Sb), (34.Se,51.Sb), (27.Co,51.Sb), (28.Ni,51.Sb), (112,51.Sb), (121,51.Sb) |
| 4.1494E−03 | (72.Hf,84.Po), (43.Tc,84.Po) |
| 4.1561E−03 | (49.In,50.Sn), (71.Lu,50.Sn), (41.Nb,50.Sn), (68.Er,50.Sn), (69.Tm,50.Sn), (88.Ra,50.Sn) |
| 4.1738E−03 | (79.Au,91.Pa), (75.Re,91.Pa) |
| 4.2375E−03 | (71.Lu,49.In), (50.Sn,49.In) |
| 4.3034E−03 | (77.Ir,92.U) |
| 4.3170E−03 | (44.Ru,85.At), (47.Ag,85.At) |
| 4.3270E−03 | (83.Bi,87.Fr) |
| 4.3414E−03 | (40.Zr,112), (57.La,52.Te), (58.Ce,52.Te), (59.Pr,52.Te), (32.Ge,52.Te), (60.Nd,52.Te), (30.Zn,52.Te), (88.Ra,112), (61.Pm,52.Te), (28.Ni,52.Te), (70.Yb,112), (67.Ho,112), (62.Sm,52.Te), (63.Eu,52.Te), (64.Gd,52.Te), (65.Tb,52.Te), (70.Yb,52.Te), (39.Y,52.Te), (66.Dy,112), (64.Gd,112), (27.Co,52.Te), (29.Cu,52.Te), (65.Tb,112), (51.Sb,112), (40.Zr,52.Te), (112,52.Te)*, (121,52.Te), (33.As,52.Te), (123,52.Te), (130,52.Te), (34.Se,52.Te), (134,52.Te), (26.Fe,52.Te), (125,112), (31.Ga,52.Te) |
| 4.3804E−03 | (69.Tm,51.Sb), (41.Nb,51.Sb), (112,51.Sb), (67.Ho,51.Sb), (88.Ra,51.Sb), (125,51.Sb), (68.Er,51.Sb) |
| 4.4647E−03 | (49.In,50.Sn), (42.Mo,50.Sn) |
| 4.4895E−03 | (67.Ho,88.Ra), (112,88.Ra) |
| 4.4928E−03 | (32.Ge,21.Sc), (14.Si,21.Sc), (16.S,21.Sc), (34.Se,21.Sc), (15.P,21.Sc), (37.Rb,21.Sc), (20.Ca,21.Sc), (38.Sr,21.Sc), (53.I,21.Sc), (55.Cs,21.Sc), (56.Ba,21.Sc), (22.Ti,21.Sc), (23.V,21.Sc), (24.Cr,21.Sc), (108,21.Sc), (25.Mn,21.Sc), (113,21.Sc), (26.Fe,21.Sc), (114,21.Sc), (116,21.Sc), (27.Co,21.Sc), (117,21.Sc), (118,21.Sc), (19.K,21.Sc), (123,21.Sc), (13.Al,21.Sc), (124,21.Sc), (31.Ga,21.Sc), (133,21.Sc), (12.Mg,21.Sc), (141,21.Sc) |
| 4.5571E−03 | (113,53.I), (116,53.I)*, (121,53.I), (26.Fe,116), (67.Ho,130), (64.Gd,130), (123,53.I), (32.Ge,116), (125,130), (40.Zr,130), (130,53.I)*, (31.Ga,53.I), (134,53.I)*, (32.Ge,53.I), (38.Sr,116), |

| $E$, MeV | List of poorly visible pairs for this energy) |
|---|---|
| | (25.Mn,116), (30.Zn,53.I), (33.As,116), (34.Se,53.I), (26.Fe,53.I), (123,116), (39.Y,53.I), (28.Ni,116), (21.Sc,116), (134,116)*, (27.Co,116), (57.La,116), (66.Dy,130), (34.Se,116), (33.As,53.I), (30.Zn,116), (52.Te,130), (31.Ga,116), (70.Yb,130), (27.Co,53.I), (62.Sm,130), (57.La,53.I), (58.Ce,53.I), (59.Pr,53.I), (60.Nd,53.I), (61.Pm,53.I), (121,130), (65.Tb,130), (113,116), (62.Sm,53.I), (63.Eu,53.I), (38.Sr,53.I), (28.Ni,53.I), (21.Sc,53.I), (29.Cu,53.I) |
| 4.6120E−03 | (69.Tm,52.Te), (69.Tm,112), (66.Dy,52.Te), (88.Ra,112), (88.Ra,52.Te), (125,52.Te), (67.Ho,52.Te), (68.Er,52.Te), (68.Er,112), (130,52.Te), (112,52.Te)* |
| 4.6520E−03 | (89.Ac,87.Fr), (44.Ru,87.Fr), (47.Ag,87.Fr), (85.At,87.Fr) |
| 4.6560E−03 | (87.Fr,89.Ac), (85.At,89.Ac), (45.Rh,89.Ac) |
| 4.6983E−03 | (71.Lu,51.Sb) |
| 4.7822E−03 | (35.Br,54.Xe), (17.Cl,54.Xe), (36.Kr,54.Xe) |
| 4.8521E−03 | (39.Y,116), (41.Nb,130), (52.Te,130), (112,130), (64.Gd,53.I), (65.Tb,53.I), (66.Dy,53.I), (67.Ho,53.I), (88.Ra,130), (68.Er,130), (60.Nd,116), (125,53.I), (58.Ce,116), (70.Yb,53.I), (29.Cu,134), (40.Zr,53.I), (69.Tm,130), (59.Pr,116), (63.Eu,116) |
| 4.9392E−03 | (71.Lu,52.Te), (112,52.Te)*, (130,52.Te), (71.Lu,112), (130,112) |
| 4.9664E−03 | (19.K,22.Ti), (30.Zn,22.Ti), (13.Al,22.Ti), (118,22.Ti), (121,22.Ti), (31.Ga,22.Ti), (123,22.Ti), (20.Ca,22.Ti), (133,22.Ti), (32.Ge,22.Ti), (134,22.Ti), (16.S,22.Ti), (33.As,22.Ti), (14.Si,22.Ti), (34.Se,22.Ti), (15.P,22.Ti), (37.Rb,22.Ti), (21.Sc,22.Ti), (38.Sr,22.Ti), (23.V,22.Ti), (39.Y,22.Ti), (55.Cs,22.Ti), (56.Ba,22.Ti), (57.La,22.Ti), (58.Ce,22.Ti), (59.Pr,22.Ti), (60.Nd,22.Ti), (61.Pm,22.Ti), (62.Sm,22.Ti), (63.Eu,22.Ti), (24.Cr,22.Ti), (25.Mn,22.Ti), (26.Fe,22.Ti), (27.Co,22.Ti), (28.Ni,22.Ti), (113,22.Ti), (29.Cu,22.Ti), (114,22.Ti), (116,22.Ti) |
| 5.0009E−03 | (78.Pt,91.Pa), (77.Ir,91.Pa), (76.Os,91.Pa) |
| 5.0020E−03 | (73.Ta,89.Ac) |
| 5.0119E−03 | (118,55.Cs), (40.Zr,116), (133,55.Cs), (23.V,55.Cs), (26.Fe,55.Cs), (16.S,55.Cs), (37.Rb,55.Cs), (64.Gd,116), (15.P,55.Cs), (14.Si,55.Cs), (20.Ca,55.Cs), (56.Ba,55.Cs), (62.Sm,116), (70.Yb,116), (121,116), (61.Pm,116), (38.Sr,55.Cs), (24.Cr,55.Cs), (13.Al,55.Cs), (25.Mn,55.Cs), (113,55.Cs), (22.Ti,116), (65.Tb,116), (114,55.Cs) |
| 5.1881E−03 | (112,130), (69.Tm,53.I), (88.Ra,53.I), (41.Nb,53.I), (71.Lu,130), (68.Er,53.I), (66.Dy,116) |
| 5.2470E−03 | (26.Fe,56.Ba), (29.Cu,56.Ba), (34.Se,56.Ba), (55.Cs,56.Ba), (133,118), (114,118), (113,56.Ba), (118,56.Ba)*, (32.Ge,56.Ba), (123,56.Ba), (31.Ga,56.Ba), (16.S,118), (24.Cr,118), (134,56.Ba), (21.Sc,56.Ba), (38.Sr,56.Ba), (26.Fe,118), (28.Ni,56.Ba), (55.Cs,118), (20.Ca,118), (27.Co,56.Ba), (39.Y,56.Ba), (25.Mn,56.Ba), (20.Ca,56.Ba), |

| $E$, MeV | List of poorly visible pairs for this energy) |
|---|---|
| | (57.La,56.Ba), (58.Ce,56.Ba), (59.Pr,56.Ba), (60.Nd,56.Ba), (113,118), (63.Eu,56.Ba), (30.Zn,56.Ba), (33.As,56.Ba), (25.Mn,118), (38.Sr,118) |
| 5.3594E−03 | (30.Zn,55.Cs), (67.Ho,116), (33.As,55.Cs), (118,55.Cs), (123,55.Cs), (32.Ge,55.Cs), (27.Co,55.Cs), (31.Ga,55.Cs), (125,116), (34.Se,55.Cs), (57.La,55.Cs) |
| 5.3669E−03 | (78.Pt,91.Pa), (77.Ir,91.Pa) |
| 5.4651E−03 | (55.Cs,23.V), (56.Ba,23.V), (57.La,23.V), (58.Ce,23.V), (59.Pr,23.V), (60.Nd,23.V), (61.Pm,23.V), (62.Sm,23.V), (26.Fe,23.V), (63.Eu,23.V), (64.Gd,23.V), (65.Tb,23.V), (66.Dy,23.V), (27.Co,23.V), (70.Yb,23.V), (28.Ni,23.V), (29.Cu,23.V), (113,23.V), (30.Zn,23.V), (114,23.V), (118,23.V), (31.Ga,23.V), (121,23.V), (20.Ca,23.V), (123,23.V), (32.Ge,23.V), (22.Ti,23.V), (133,23.V), (134,23.V), (33.As,23.V), (15.P,23.V), (34.Se,23.V), (37.Rb,23.V), (21.Sc,23.V), (38.Sr,23.V), (16.S,23.V), (39.Y,23.V), (14.Si,23.V), (40.Zr,23.V), (24.Cr,23.V), (25.Mn,23.V) |
| 5.4827E−03 | (60.Nd,57.La), (29.Cu,57.La), (61.Pm,57.La), (21.Sc,57.La), (62.Sm,57.La), (23.V,57.La), (33.As,57.La), (28.Ni,57.La), (63.Eu,57.La), (64.Gd,57.La), (65.Tb,57.La), (66.Dy,57.La), (67.Ho,57.La), (68.Er,57.La), (116,57.La), (121,57.La), (125,57.La), (40.Zr,57.La), (134,57.La), (70.Yb,57.La), (56.Ba,57.La), (55.Cs,57.La), (58.Ce,57.La), (22.Ti,57.La), (59.Pr,57.La), (39.Y,57.La) |
| 5.6236E−03 | (31.Ga,118), (28.Ni,118), (32.Ge,118), (123,118), (30.Zn,118), (55.Cs,118), (27.Co,118), (33.As,118), (61.Pm,56.Ba), (62.Sm,56.Ba), (121,56.Ba), (34.Se,118), (64.Gd,56.Ba), (22.Ti,56.Ba) |
| 5.7143E−03 | (58.Ce,55.Cs), (57.La,116), (21.Sc,55.Cs), (134,55.Cs), (29.Cu,55.Cs), (118,55.Cs) |
| 5.7234E−03 | (55.Cs,58.Ce), (62.Sm,58.Ce), (63.Eu,58.Ce), (64.Gd,58.Ce), (39.Y,58.Ce), (88.Ra,58.Ce), (65.Tb,58.Ce), (56.Ba,58.Ce), (116,58.Ce), (66.Dy,58.Ce), (121,58.Ce), (67.Ho,58.Ce), (125,58.Ce), (68.Er,58.Ce), (69.Tm,58.Ce), (70.Yb,58.Ce), (120,115), (23.V,58.Ce), (57.La,58.Ce), (53.I,58.Ce), (41.Nb,58.Ce), (59.Pr,58.Ce), (40.Zr,58.Ce), (22.Ti,58.Ce), (60.Nd,58.Ce), (61.Pm,58.Ce) |
| 5.8906E−03 | (88.Ra,57.La), (53.I,57.La), (112,57.La), (52.Te,57.La), (71.Lu,57.La), (58.Ce,57.La), (116,57.La), (42.Mo,57.La), (41.Nb,57.La), (130,57.La), (69.Tm,57.La) |
| 5.9643E−03 | (70.Yb,59.Pr), (71.Lu,59.Pr), (58.Ce,59.Pr), (121,59.Pr), (23.V,59.Pr), (125,59.Pr), (41.Nb,59.Pr), (60.Nd,59.Pr), (22.Ti,59.Pr), (56.Ba,59.Pr), (61.Pm,59.Pr), (62.Sm,59.Pr), (64.Gd,59.Pr), (39.Y,59.Pr), (65.Tb,59.Pr), (40.Zr,59.Pr), (66.Dy,59.Pr), (88.Ra,59.Pr), (53.I,59.Pr), (67.Ho,59.Pr), (68.Er,59.Pr), (112,59.Pr), (69.Tm,59.Pr), (116,59.Pr) |
| 5.9888E−03 | (70.Yb,56.Ba), (65.Tb,56.Ba), (134,118), (63.Eu,118), (66.Dy,56.Ba) |

| $E$, MeV | List of poorly visible pairs for this energy) |
|---|---|
| 5.9892E−03 | (60.Nd,24.Cr), (32.Ge,24.Cr), (61.Pm,24.Cr), (23.V,24.Cr), (62.Sm,24.Cr), (63.Eu,24.Cr), (64.Gd,24.Cr), (65.Tb,24.Cr), (66.Dy,24.Cr), (67.Ho,24.Cr), (68.Er,24.Cr), (69.Tm,24.Cr), (70.Yb,24.Cr), (33.As,24.Cr), (88.Ra,24.Cr), (22.Ti,24.Cr), (113,24.Cr), (114,24.Cr), (116,24.Cr), (34.Se,24.Cr), (118,24.Cr), (121,24.Cr), (20.Ca,24.Cr), (123,24.Cr), (38.Sr,24.Cr), (125,24.Cr), (25.Mn,24.Cr), (134,24.Cr), (39.Y,24.Cr), (26.Fe,24.Cr), (40.Zr,24.Cr), (27.Co,24.Cr), (41.Nb,24.Cr), (28.Ni,24.Cr), (29.Cu,24.Cr), (53.I,24.Cr), (21.Sc,24.Cr), (55.Cs,24.Cr), (56.Ba,24.Cr), (30.Zn,24.Cr), (31.Ga,24.Cr) |
| 6.1642E−03 | (49.In,58.Ce), (57.La,58.Ce), (52.Te,58.Ce), (59.Pr,58.Ce), (50.Sn,58.Ce), (130,58.Ce), (51.Sb,58.Ce), (71.Lu,58.Ce), (112,58.Ce), (42.Mo,58.Ce) |
| 6.2079E−03 | (69.Tm,60.Nd), (70.Yb,60.Nd), (71.Lu,60.Nd), (53.I,60.Nd), (112,60.Nd), (61.Pm,60.Nd), (116,60.Nd), (41.Nb,60.Nd), (22.Ti,60.Nd), (40.Zr,60.Nd), (62.Sm,60.Nd), (121,60.Nd), (125,60.Nd), (64.Gd,60.Nd), (130,60.Nd), (59.Pr,60.Nd), (65.Tb,60.Nd), (24.Cr,60.Nd), (66.Dy,60.Nd), (56.Ba,60.Nd), (67.Ho,60.Nd), (23.V,60.Nd), (88.Ra,60.Nd), (68.Er,60.Nd) |
| 6.2663E−03 | (51.Sb,57.La), (50.Sn,57.La), (49.In,57.La), (58.Ce,57.La) |
| 6.4404E−03 | (112,59.Pr), (52.Te,59.Pr), (50.Sn,59.Pr), (60.Nd,59.Pr), (58.Ce,59.Pr), (49.In,59.Pr), (57.La,59.Pr), (42.Mo,59.Pr), (48.Cd,59.Pr), (51.Sb,59.Pr), (130,59.Pr) |
| 6.4593E−03 | (69.Tm,61.Pm), (112,61.Pm), (42.Mo,61.Pm), (70.Yb,61.Pm), (116,61.Pm), (71.Lu,61.Pm), (121,61.Pm), (125,61.Pm), (52.Te,61.Pm), (130,61.Pm), (22.Ti,61.Pm), (64.Gd,61.Pm), (56.Ba,61.Pm), (41.Nb,61.Pm), (40.Zr,61.Pm), (65.Tb,61.Pm), (60.Nd,61.Pm), (24.Cr,61.Pm), (66.Dy,61.Pm), (23.V,61.Pm), (67.Ho,61.Pm), (88.Ra,61.Pm), (53.I,61.Pm), (68.Er,61.Pm), (62.Sm,61.Pm) |
| 6.5390E−03 | (27.Co,25.Mn), (28.Ni,25.Mn), (53.I,25.Mn), (29.Cu,25.Mn), (55.Cs,25.Mn), (23.V,25.Mn), (56.Ba,25.Mn), (30.Zn,25.Mn), (24.Cr,25.Mn), (62.Sm,25.Mn), (63.Eu,25.Mn), (64.Gd,25.Mn), (65.Tb,25.Mn), (66.Dy,25.Mn), (67.Ho,25.Mn), (68.Er,25.Mn), (69.Tm,25.Mn), (70.Yb,25.Mn), (31.Ga,25.Mn), (32.Ge,25.Mn), (88.Ra,25.Mn), (22.Ti,25.Mn), (33.As,25.Mn), (113,25.Mn), (34.Se,25.Mn), (116,25.Mn), (38.Sr,25.Mn), (118,25.Mn), (121,25.Mn), (21.Sc,25.Mn), (123,25.Mn), (39.Y,25.Mn), (125,25.Mn), (20.Ca,25.Mn), (134,25.Mn), (40.Zr,25.Mn), (26.Fe,25.Mn), (41.Nb,25.Mn) |
| 6.5488E−03 | (72.Hf,58.Ce), (57.La,58.Ce), (48.Cd,58.Ce), (59.Pr,58.Ce), (43.Tc,58.Ce) |
| 6.7162E−03 | (52.Te,62.Sm), (53.I,62.Sm), (66.Dy,62.Sm), (41.Nb,62.Sm), (67.Ho,62.Sm), (49.In,62.Sm), (68.Er,62.Sm), (61.Pm,62.Sm), (88.Ra,62.Sm), (69.Tm,62.Sm), (23.V,62.Sm), (60.Nd,62.Sm), |

| $E$, MeV | List of poorly visible pairs for this energy) |
|---|---|
| | (70.Yb,62.Sm), (42.Mo,62.Sm), (112,62.Sm), (71.Lu,62.Sm), (24.Cr,62.Sm), (116,62.Sm), (56.Ba,62.Sm), (40.Zr,62.Sm), (121,62.Sm), (125,62.Sm), (51.Sb,62.Sm), (130,62.Sm), (64.Gd,62.Sm), (22.Ti,62.Sm), (25.Mn,62.Sm), (65.Tb,62.Sm) |
| 6.7215E−03 | (43.Tc,60.Nd), (48.Cd,60.Nd), (61.Pm,60.Nd), (51.Sb,60.Nd), (49.In,60.Nd), (52.Te,60.Nd), (50.Sn,60.Nd), (42.Mo,60.Nd), (130,60.Nd), (62.Sm,60.Nd), (59.Pr,60.Nd), (57.La,60.Nd) |
| 6.8348E−03 | (48.Cd,59.Pr), (60.Nd,59.Pr), (72.Hf,59.Pr), (57.La,59.Pr), (58.Ce,59.Pr), (43.Tc,59.Pr) |
| 6.9769E−03 | (134,63.Eu), (23.V,63.Eu), (40.Zr,63.Eu), (55.Cs,63.Eu), (56.Ba,63.Eu), (64.Gd,63.Eu), (65.Tb,63.Eu), (66.Dy,63.Eu), (67.Ho,63.Eu), (118,63.Eu), (121,63.Eu), (68.Er,63.Eu), (21.Sc,63.Eu), (70.Yb,63.Eu), (22.Ti,63.Eu), (39.Y,63.Eu), (125,63.Eu) |
| 7.0128E−03 | (49.In,61.Pm), (62.Sm,61.Pm), (51.Sb,61.Pm), (57.La,61.Pm), (72.Hf,61.Pm), (48.Cd,61.Pm), (50.Sn,61.Pm), (43.Tc,61.Pm), (60.Nd,61.Pm), (58.Ce,61.Pm) |
| 7.1120E−03 | (88.Ra,26.Fe), (22.Ti,26.Fe), (112,26.Fe), (113,26.Fe), (27.Co,26.Fe), (116,26.Fe), (28.Ni,26.Fe), (118,26.Fe)*, (121,26.Fe), (123,26.Fe), (125,26.Fe), (130,26.Fe), (29.Cu,26.Fe), (134,26.Fe), (25.Mn,26.Fe), (30.Zn,26.Fe), (53.I,26.Fe), (31.Ga,26.Fe), (55.Cs,26.Fe), (32.Ge,26.Fe), (56.Ba,26.Fe), (33.As,26.Fe), (34.Se,26.Fe), (38.Sr,26.Fe), (63.Eu,26.Fe), (64.Gd,26.Fe), (24.Cr,26.Fe), (65.Tb,26.Fe), (39.Y,26.Fe), (66.Dy,26.Fe), (67.Ho,26.Fe), (68.Er,26.Fe), (69.Tm,26.Fe), (70.Yb,26.Fe), (71.Lu,26.Fe), (23.V,26.Fe), (40.Zr,26.Fe), (21.Sc,26.Fe), (41.Nb,26.Fe) |
| 7.1260E−03 | (72.Hf,60.Nd), (44.Ru,60.Nd), (61.Pm,60.Nd), (83.Bi,60.Nd), (59.Pr,60.Nd), (47.Ag,60.Nd), (84.Po,60.Nd), (58.Ce,60.Nd) |
| 7.2428E−03 | (71.Lu,121), (52.Te,64.Gd), (56.Ba,64.Gd), (63.Eu,64.Gd), (66.Dy,121), (23.V,64.Gd), (40.Zr,64.Gd), (53.I,64.Gd), (40.Zr,121), (88.Ra,64.Gd), (42.Mo,64.Gd), (63.Eu,121), (43.Tc,64.Gd), (24.Cr,64.Gd), (68.Er,121), (112,64.Gd), (116,121), (26.Fe,64.Gd), (65.Tb,121), (116,64.Gd), (24.Cr,121), (70.Yb,121), (25.Mn,121), (121,64.Gd)*, (112,121), (23.V,121), (125,64.Gd), (41.Nb,64.Gd), (49.In,64.Gd), (130,64.Gd), (22.Ti,64.Gd), (56.Ba,121), (88.Ra,121), (65.Tb,64.Gd), (66.Dy,64.Gd), (67.Ho,64.Gd), (67.Ho,121), (22.Ti,121), (68.Er,64.Gd), (50.Sn,64.Gd), (69.Tm,64.Gd), (70.Yb,64.Gd), (69.Tm,121), (125,121), (53.I,121), (130,121), (71.Lu,64.Gd), (48.Cd,64.Gd), (51.Sb,64.Gd), (25.Mn,64.Gd), (41.Nb,121), (62.Sm,64.Gd) |
| 7.3118E−03 | (59.Pr,62.Sm), (50.Sn,62.Sm), (47.Ag,62.Sm), (44.Ru,62.Sm), (83.Bi,62.Sm), (72.Hf,62.Sm), (43.Tc,62.Sm), (84.Po,62.Sm), (48.Cd,62.Sm), (64.Gd,62.Sm), (58.Ce,62.Sm), (61.Pm,62.Sm), (57.La,62.Sm) |

| $E$, MeV | List of poorly visible pairs for this energy) |
|---|---|
| 7.4279E−03 | (46.Pd,61.Pm), (81.Tl,61.Pm), (85.At,61.Pm), (62.Sm,61.Pm), (87.Fr,61.Pm), (82.Pb,61.Pm), (60.Nd,61.Pm), (59.Pr,61.Pm), (45.Rh,61.Pm) |
| 7.5140E−03 | (53.I,65.Tb), (64.Gd,65.Tb), (25.Mn,65.Tb), (43.Tc,65.Tb), (51.Sb,65.Tb), (23.V,65.Tb), (40.Zr,65.Tb), (88.Ra,65.Tb), (66.Dy,65.Tb), (26.Fe,65.Tb), (24.Cr,65.Tb), (67.Ho,65.Tb), (41.Nb,65.Tb), (68.Er,65.Tb), (112,65.Tb), (63.Eu,65.Tb), (116,65.Tb), (56.Ba,65.Tb), (69.Tm,65.Tb), (52.Te,65.Tb), (121,65.Tb), (125,65.Tb), (70.Yb,65.Tb), (130,65.Tb), (71.Lu,65.Tb), (72.Hf,65.Tb), (57.La,65.Tb), (50.Sn,65.Tb), (48.Cd,65.Tb), (49.In,65.Tb), (42.Mo,65.Tb) |
| 7.6171E−03 | (130,63.Eu), (24.Cr,63.Eu), (116,63.Eu), (51.Sb,63.Eu), (52.Te,63.Eu), (25.Mn,63.Eu), (53.I,63.Eu), (121,63.Eu), (71.Lu,63.Eu), (88.Ra,63.Eu), (49.In,63.Eu), (112,63.Eu), (26.Fe,63.Eu), (42.Mo,63.Eu) |
| 7.7089E−03 | (33.As,27.Co), (50.Sn,27.Co), (34.Se,27.Co), (51.Sb,27.Co), (23.V,27.Co), (52.Te,27.Co), (26.Fe,27.Co), (53.I,27.Co), (39.Y,27.Co), (55.Cs,27.Co), (24.Cr,27.Co), (56.Ba,27.Co), (40.Zr,27.Co), (63.Eu,27.Co), (66.Dy,27.Co), (25.Mn,27.Co), (67.Ho,27.Co), (68.Er,27.Co), (69.Tm,27.Co), (70.Yb,27.Co), (71.Lu,27.Co), (41.Nb,27.Co), (28.Ni,27.Co), (42.Mo,27.Co), (22.Ti,27.Co), (43.Tc,27.Co), (29.Cu,27.Co), (30.Zn,27.Co), (31.Ga,27.Co), (88.Ra,27.Co), (32.Ge,27.Co), (112,27.Co), (48.Cd,27.Co), (116,27.Co), (21.Sc,27.Co), (118,27.Co), (49.In,27.Co), (121,27.Co), (123,27.Co), (125,27.Co), (130,27.Co), (134,27.Co) |
| 7.7368E−03 | (82.Pb,62.Sm), (73.Ta,62.Sm), (61.Pm,62.Sm), (89.Ac,62.Sm), (85.At,62.Sm), (60.Nd,62.Sm), (81.Tl,62.Sm), (87.Fr,62.Sm) |
| 7.7901E−03 | (112,66.Dy), (23.V,66.Dy), (116,66.Dy), (53.I,66.Dy), (65.Tb,66.Dy), (67.Ho,66.Dy), (121,66.Dy), (41.Nb,66.Dy), (26.Fe,66.Dy), (125,66.Dy), (68.Er,66.Dy), (130,66.Dy), (64.Gd,66.Dy), (52.Te,66.Dy), (69.Tm,66.Dy), (51.Sb,66.Dy), (49.In,66.Dy), (25.Mn,66.Dy), (71.Lu,66.Dy), (72.Hf,66.Dy), (50.Sn,66.Dy), (48.Cd,66.Dy), (57.La,66.Dy), (83.Bi,66.Dy), (45.Rh,66.Dy), (84.Po,66.Dy), (42.Mo,66.Dy), (58.Ce,66.Dy), (24.Cr,66.Dy), (88.Ra,66.Dy), (47.Ag,66.Dy), (27.Co,66.Dy), (63.Eu,66.Dy), (44.Ru,66.Dy), (56.Ba,66.Dy), (43.Tc,66.Dy) |
| 7.9303E−03 | (63.Eu,121), (58.Ce,64.Gd), (72.Hf,121), (84.Po,121), (89.Ac,64.Gd), (59.Pr,64.Gd), (60.Nd,64.Gd), (57.La,121), (44.Ru,64.Gd), (61.Pm,64.Gd), (48.Cd,121), (83.Bi,121), (73.Ta,64.Gd), (27.Co,121), (43.Tc,121), (121,64.Gd)*, (47.Ag,121), (45.Rh,64.Gd), (47.Ag,64.Gd), (26.Fe,121), (65.Tb,64.Gd), (81.Tl,64.Gd), (82.Pb,64.Gd), (83.Bi,64.Gd), (50.Sn,121), (84.Po,64.Gd), (44.Ru,121), (85.At,64.Gd), (66.Dy,64.Gd), (87.Fr,64.Gd), (46.Pd,64.Gd) |

| $E$, MeV | List of poorly visible pairs for this energy) |
|---|---|
| 8.0520E−03 | (48.Cd,63.Eu), (27.Co,63.Eu), (72.Hf,63.Eu), (57.La,63.Eu), (43.Tc,63.Eu) |
| 8.0711E−03 | (69.Tm,67.Ho), (45.Rh,67.Ho), (71.Lu,67.Ho), (72.Hf,67.Ho), (58.Ce,67.Ho), (51.Sb,67.Ho), (81.Tl,67.Ho), (82.Pb,67.Ho), (47.Ag,67.Ho), (83.Bi,67.Ho), (46.Pd,67.Ho), (66.Dy,67.Ho), (84.Po,67.Ho), (60.Nd,67.Ho), (85.At,67.Ho), (50.Sn,67.Ho), (56.Ba,67.Ho), (88.Ra,67.Ho), (42.Mo,67.Ho), (49.In,67.Ho), (65.Tb,67.Ho), (25.Mn,67.Ho), (26.Fe,67.Ho), (23.V,67.Ho), (112,67.Ho), (48.Cd,67.Ho), (116,67.Ho), (59.Pr,67.Ho), (121,67.Ho), (53.I,67.Ho), (125,67.Ho), (41.Nb,67.Ho), (130,67.Ho), (43.Tc,67.Ho), (24.Cr,67.Ho), (27.Co,67.Ho), (52.Te,67.Ho), (68.Er,67.Ho), (57.La,67.Ho), (63.Eu,67.Ho), (44.Ru,67.Ho) |
| 8.2516E−03 | (60.Nd,65.Tb), (62.Sm,65.Tb), (58.Ce,65.Tb), (89.Ac,65.Tb), (61.Pm,65.Tb), (80.Hg,65.Tb), (81.Tl,65.Tb), (66.Dy,65.Tb), (82.Pb,65.Tb), (59.Pr,65.Tb), (64.Gd,65.Tb), (46.Pd,65.Tb), (85.At,65.Tb), (45.Rh,65.Tb), (87.Fr,65.Tb), (67.Ho,65.Tb), (73.Ta,65.Tb) |
| 8.3328E−03 | (48.Cd,28.Ni), (39.Y,28.Ni), (49.In,28.Ni), (88.Ra,28.Ni), (23.V,28.Ni), (112,28.Ni), (50.Sn,28.Ni), (116,28.Ni), (40.Zr,28.Ni), (118,28.Ni), (51.Sb,28.Ni), (125,28.Ni), (130,28.Ni), (134,28.Ni), (25.Mn,28.Ni), (52.Te,28.Ni), (41.Nb,28.Ni), (53.I,28.Ni), (55.Cs,28.Ni), (24.Cr,28.Ni), (56.Ba,28.Ni), (42.Mo,28.Ni), (57.La,28.Ni), (27.Co,28.Ni), (63.Eu,28.Ni), (43.Tc,28.Ni), (68.Er,28.Ni), (69.Tm,28.Ni), (70.Yb,28.Ni), (71.Lu,28.Ni), (72.Hf,28.Ni), (26.Fe,28.Ni), (44.Ru,28.Ni), (21.Sc,28.Ni), (22.Ti,28.Ni), (29.Cu,28.Ni), (33.As,28.Ni) |
| 8.3579E−03 | (49.In,68.Er), (87.Fr,68.Er), (67.Ho,68.Er), (88.Ra,68.Er), (57.La,68.Er), (41.Nb,68.Er), (25.Mn,68.Er), (23.V,68.Er), (52.Te,68.Er), (58.Ce,68.Er), (24.Cr,68.Er), (112,68.Er), (116,68.Er), (47.Ag,68.Er), (121,68.Er), (66.Dy,68.Er), (44.Ru,68.Er), (48.Cd,68.Er), (130,68.Er), (63.Eu,68.Er), (51.Sb,68.Er), (42.Mo,68.Er), (69.Tm,68.Er), (28.Ni,68.Er), (26.Fe,68.Er), (60.Nd,68.Er), (46.Pd,68.Er), (71.Lu,68.Er), (72.Hf,68.Er), (73.Ta,68.Er), (50.Sn,68.Er), (27.Co,68.Er), (81.Tl,68.Er), (82.Pb,68.Er), (53.I,68.Er), (83.Bi,68.Er), (43.Tc,68.Er), (59.Pr,68.Er), (84.Po,68.Er), (45.Rh,68.Er), (85.At,68.Er) |
| 8.3756E−03 | (46.Pd,121), (85.At,121), (83.Bi,121), (82.Pb,121), (89.Ac,64.Gd), (45.Rh,121), (58.Ce,121), (62.Sm,64.Gd), (61.Pm,64.Gd), (67.Ho,121), (66.Dy,121), (84.Po,121), (80.Hg,64.Gd), (74.W,64.Gd), (65.Tb,64.Gd), (81.Tl,121), (59.Pr,121) |
| 8.5806E−03 | (73.Ta,66.Dy), (87.Fr,66.Dy), (67.Ho,66.Dy), (62.Sm,66.Dy), (59.Pr,66.Dy), (121,66.Dy), (89.Ac,66.Dy), (80.Hg,66.Dy), (81.Tl,66.Dy), (82.Pb,66.Dy), (65.Tb,66.Dy), (60.Nd,66.Dy), (68.Er,66.Dy), (61.Pm,66.Dy), (85.At,66.Dy) |

| $E$, MeV | List of poorly visible pairs for this energy) |
|---|---|
| 8.6480E−03 | (24.Cr,69.Tm), (71.Lu,69.Tm), (72.Hf,69.Tm), (73.Ta,69.Tm), (46.Pd,69.Tm), (41.Nb,69.Tm), (57.La,69.Tm), (44.Ru,69.Tm), (47.Ag,69.Tm), (80.Hg,69.Tm), (27.Co,69.Tm), (81.Tl,69.Tm), (28.Ni,69.Tm), (82.Pb,69.Tm), (25.Mn,69.Tm), (83.Bi,69.Tm), (45.Rh,69.Tm), (84.Po,69.Tm), (68.Er,69.Tm), (85.At,69.Tm), (43.Tc,69.Tm), (87.Fr,69.Tm), (59.Pr,69.Tm), (88.Ra,69.Tm), (60.Nd,69.Tm), (89.Ac,69.Tm), (53.I,69.Tm), (58.Ce,69.Tm), (42.Mo,69.Tm), (49.In,69.Tm), (112,69.Tm), (116,69.Tm), (52.Te,69.Tm), (121,69.Tm), (51.Sb,69.Tm), (67.Ho,69.Tm), (50.Sn,69.Tm), (130,69.Tm), (63.Eu,69.Tm), (26.Fe,69.Tm), (48.Cd,69.Tm) |
| 8.7080E−03 | (62.Sm,65.Tb), (90.Th,65.Tb), (66.Dy,65.Tb), (64.Gd,65.Tb), (74.W,65.Tb) |
| 8.9178E−03 | (60.Nd,67.Ho), (61.Pm,67.Ho), (73.Ta,67.Ho), (64.Gd,67.Ho), (74.W,67.Ho), (66.Dy,67.Ho), (85.At,67.Ho), (80.Hg,67.Ho), (87.Fr,67.Ho), (121,67.Ho), (62.Sm,67.Ho), (81.Tl,67.Ho), (69.Tm,67.Ho), (89.Ac,67.Ho), (82.Pb,67.Ho), (68.Er,67.Ho) |
| 8.9436E−03 | (71.Lu,70.Yb), (72.Hf,70.Yb), (49.In,70.Yb), (112,70.Yb), (23.V,70.Yb), (116,70.Yb), (43.Tc,70.Yb), (42.Mo,70.Yb), (51.Sb,70.Yb), (26.Fe,70.Yb), (48.Cd,70.Yb), (24.Cr,70.Yb), (41.Nb,70.Yb), (125,70.Yb), (52.Te,70.Yb), (130,70.Yb), (50.Sn,70.Yb), (53.I,70.Yb), (57.La,70.Yb), (88.Ra,70.Yb), (25.Mn,70.Yb), (56.Ba,70.Yb) |
| 8.9789E−03 | (116,29.Cu), (118,29.Cu), (53.I,29.Cu), (43.Tc,29.Cu), (55.Cs,29.Cu), (125,29.Cu), (130,29.Cu), (24.Cr,29.Cu), (134,29.Cu), (56.Ba,29.Cu), (22.Ti,29.Cu), (57.La,29.Cu), (39.Y,29.Cu), (21.Sc,29.Cu), (40.Zr,29.Cu), (48.Cd,29.Cu), (70.Yb,29.Cu), (23.V,29.Cu), (71.Lu,29.Cu), (72.Hf,29.Cu), (49.In,29.Cu), (41.Nb,29.Cu), (50.Sn,29.Cu), (25.Mn,29.Cu), (51.Sb,29.Cu), (42.Mo,29.Cu), (52.Te,29.Cu), (26.Fe,29.Cu), (88.Ra,29.Cu), (112,29.Cu) |
| 9.0458E−03 | (65.Tb,66.Dy), (64.Gd,66.Dy), (90.Th,66.Dy), (67.Ho,66.Dy), (74.W,66.Dy) |
| 9.2441E−03 | (25.Mn,71.Lu), (45.Rh,71.Lu), (70.Yb,71.Lu), (112,71.Lu), (27.Co,71.Lu), (121,71.Lu), (59.Pr,71.Lu), (62.Sm,71.Lu), (130,71.Lu), (58.Ce,71.Lu), (26.Fe,71.Lu), (72.Hf,71.Lu), (73.Ta,71.Lu), (68.Er,71.Lu), (60.Nd,71.Lu), (29.Cu,71.Lu), (44.Ru,71.Lu), (42.Mo,71.Lu), (80.Hg,71.Lu), (46.Pd,71.Lu), (81.Tl,71.Lu), (48.Cd,71.Lu), (82.Pb,71.Lu), (49.In,71.Lu), (83.Bi,71.Lu), (63.Eu,71.Lu), (84.Po,71.Lu), (61.Pm,71.Lu), (28.Ni,71.Lu), (85.At,71.Lu), (69.Tm,71.Lu), (43.Tc,71.Lu), (87.Fr,71.Lu), (50.Sn,71.Lu), (57.La,71.Lu), (24.Cr,71.Lu), (89.Ac,71.Lu), (51.Sb,71.Lu), (53.I,71.Lu), (47.Ag,71.Lu), (52.Te,71.Lu) |
| 9.2643E−03 | (74.W,68.Er), (65.Tb,68.Er), (90.Th,68.Er), (64.Gd,68.Er), (80.Hg,68.Er), (62.Sm,68.Er), (69.Tm,68.Er), (71.Lu,68.Er), (67.Ho,68.Er), (61.Pm,68.Er), (89.Ac,68.Er) |

| $E$, MeV | List of poorly visible pairs for this energy) |
|---|---|
| 9.3942E−03 | (75.Re,67.Ho), (65.Tb,67.Ho), (66.Dy,67.Ho), (68.Er,67.Ho) |
| 9.5607E−03 | (70.Yb,72.Hf), (121,72.Hf), (46.Pd,72.Hf), (69.Tm,72.Hf), (62.Sm,72.Hf), (64.Gd,72.Hf), (29.Cu,72.Hf), (60.Nd,72.Hf), (27.Co,72.Hf), (73.Ta,72.Hf), (74.W,72.Hf), (75.Re,72.Hf), (76.Os,72.Hf), (77.Ir,72.Hf), (78.Pt,72.Hf), (79.Au,72.Hf), (80.Hg,72.Hf), (57.La,72.Hf), (66.Dy,72.Hf), (81.Tl,72.Hf), (44.Ru,72.Hf), (65.Tb,72.Hf), (82.Pb,72.Hf), (83.Bi,72.Hf), (59.Pr,72.Hf), (84.Po,72.Hf), (71.Lu,72.Hf), (85.At,72.Hf), (63.Eu,72.Hf), (28.Ni,72.Hf), (87.Fr,72.Hf), (45.Rh,72.Hf), (89.Ac,72.Hf), (67.Ho,72.Hf), (90.Th,72.Hf), (58.Ce,72.Hf), (68.Er,72.Hf), (47.Ag,72.Hf), (61.Pm,72.Hf) |
| 9.6169E−03 | (65.Tb,69.Tm), (74.W,69.Tm), (90.Th,69.Tm), (75.Re,69.Tm), (62.Sm,69.Tm), (64.Gd,69.Tm), (71.Lu,69.Tm), (68.Er,69.Tm), (66.Dy,69.Tm) |
| 9.6586E−03 | (22.Ti,30.Zn), (116,30.Zn), (50.Sn,30.Zn), (40.Zr,30.Zn), (118,30.Zn), (21.Sc,30.Zn), (51.Sb,30.Zn), (41.Nb,30.Zn), (125,30.Zn), (33.As,30.Zn), (130,30.Zn), (52.Te,30.Zn), (24.Cr,30.Zn), (134,30.Zn), (53.I,30.Zn), (42.Mo,30.Zn), (23.V,30.Zn), (88.Ra,30.Zn), (55.Cs,30.Zn), (39.Y,30.Zn), (56.Ba,30.Zn), (112,30.Zn), (49.In,30.Zn), (25.Mn,30.Zn) |
| 9.7513E−03 | (76.Os,68.Er), (77.Ir,68.Er), (78.Pt,68.Er), (79.Au,68.Er), (67.Ho,68.Er), (69.Tm,68.Er), (66.Dy,68.Er) |
| 9.8811E−03 | (76.Os,73.Ta), (77.Ir,73.Ta), (78.Pt,73.Ta), (66.Dy,73.Ta), (79.Au,73.Ta), (65.Tb,73.Ta), (80.Hg,73.Ta), (69.Tm,73.Ta), (68.Er,73.Ta), (61.Pm,73.Ta), (62.Sm,73.Ta), (87.Fr,73.Ta), (72.Hf,73.Ta), (89.Ac,73.Ta), (60.Nd,73.Ta), (90.Th,73.Ta), (71.Lu,73.Ta), (91.Pa,73.Ta), (74.W,73.Ta), (92.U,73.Ta), (121,73.Ta), (64.Gd,73.Ta), (75.Re,73.Ta), (67.Ho,73.Ta) |
| 9.9782E−03 | (89.Ac,70.Yb), (80.Hg,70.Yb), (81.Tl,70.Yb), (82.Pb,70.Yb), (63.Eu,70.Yb), (83.Bi,70.Yb), (45.Rh,70.Yb), (84.Po,70.Yb), (61.Pm,70.Yb), (85.At,70.Yb), (28.Ni,70.Yb), (46.Pd,70.Yb), (121,70.Yb), (87.Fr,70.Yb), (29.Cu,70.Yb), (60.Nd,70.Yb), (58.Ce,70.Yb), (27.Co,70.Yb), (59.Pr,70.Yb) |
| 1.0116E−02 | (67.Ho,69.Tm), (78.Pt,69.Tm), (68.Er,69.Tm), (77.Ir,69.Tm) |
| 1.0207E−02 | (72.Hf,74.W), (79.Au,74.W), (67.Ho,74.W), (90.Th,74.W), (91.Pa,74.W), (71.Lu,74.W), (92.U,74.W), (65.Tb,74.W), (73.Ta,74.W), (66.Dy,74.W), (69.Tm,74.W), (75.Re,74.W), (64.Gd,74.W), (76.Os,74.W), (68.Er,74.W), (77.Ir,74.W), (78.Pt,74.W) |
| 1.0349E−02 | (75.Re,71.Lu), (79.Au,71.Lu), (66.Dy,71.Lu), (65.Tb,71.Lu), (90.Th,71.Lu), (76.Os,71.Lu), (64.Gd,71.Lu), (77.Ir,71.Lu), (67.Ho,71.Lu), (78.Pt,71.Lu) |
| 1.0367E−02 | (41.Nb,31.Ga), (22.Ti,123), (116,31.Ga), (33.As,31.Ga), (134,123), (21.Sc,123), (118,31.Ga), (34.Se,31.Ga), (33.As,123), (53.I,31.Ga), |

| *E*, MeV | List of poorly visible pairs for this energy) |
|---|---|
| | (123,31.Ga)*, (125,31.Ga), (21.Sc,31.Ga), (118,123), (22.Ti,31.Ga), (55.Cs,31.Ga), (39.Y,31.Ga), (88.Ra,31.Ga), (134,31.Ga), (56.Ba,31.Ga), (32.Ge,31.Ga), (32.Ge,123), (40.Zr,31.Ga), (34.Se,123), (112,31.Ga), (23.V,31.Ga), (39.Y,123), (55.Cs,123) |
| 1.0486E−02 | (61.Pm,70.Yb), (89.Ac,70.Yb), (62.Sm,70.Yb) |
| 1.0535E−02 | (79.Au,75.Re), (66.Dy,75.Re), (91.Pa,75.Re), (74.W,75.Re), (92.U,75.Re), (64.Gd,75.Re), (72.Hf,75.Re), (67.Ho,75.Re), (71.Lu,75.Re), (76.Os,75.Re), (69.Tm,75.Re), (68.Er,75.Re), (77.Ir,75.Re), (65.Tb,75.Re), (78.Pt,75.Re), (73.Ta,75.Re) |
| 1.0739E−02 | (69.Tm,72.Hf), (73.Ta,72.Hf), (68.Er,72.Hf), (91.Pa,72.Hf) |
| 1.0870E−02 | (91.Pa,71.Lu), (67.Ho,71.Lu), (69.Tm,71.Lu), (68.Er,71.Lu) |
| 1.0871E−02 | (72.Hf,76.Os), (67.Ho,76.Os), (65.Tb,76.Os), (68.Er,76.Os), (78.Pt,76.Os), (74.W,76.Os), (79.Au,76.Os), (69.Tm,76.Os), (66.Dy,76.Os), (91.Pa,76.Os), (73.Ta,76.Os), (71.Lu,76.Os), (92.U,76.Os), (77.Ir,76.Os), (75.Re,76.Os) |
| 1.1103E−02 | (22.Ti,32.Ge), (41.Nb,32.Ge), (123,32.Ge), (33.As,32.Ge), (125,32.Ge), (55.Cs,32.Ge), (39.Y,32.Ge), (56.Ba,32.Ge), (118,32.Ge), (21.Sc,32.Ge), (34.Se,32.Ge), (134,32.Ge), (40.Zr,32.Ge), (23.V,32.Ge) |
| 1.1136E−02 | (72.Hf,73.Ta), (92.U,73.Ta), (74.W,73.Ta) |
| 1.1215E−02 | (78.Pt,77.Ir), (74.W,77.Ir), (65.Tb,77.Ir), (91.Pa,77.Ir), (69.Tm,77.Ir), (92.U,77.Ir), (67.Ho,77.Ir), (68.Er,77.Ir), (76.Os,77.Ir), (71.Lu,77.Ir), (66.Dy,77.Ir), (75.Re,77.Ir), (72.Hf,77.Ir), (73.Ta,77.Ir) |
| 1.1271E−02 | (92.U,72.Hf) |
| 1.1544E−02 | (75.Re,74.W), (77.Ir,74.W), (76.Os,74.W), (73.Ta,74.W), (72.Hf,74.W) |
| 1.1564E−02 | (91.Pa,78.Pt), (71.Lu,78.Pt), (92.U,78.Pt), (76.Os,78.Pt), (68.Er,78.Pt), (69.Tm,78.Pt), (72.Hf,78.Pt), (67.Ho,78.Pt), (75.Re,78.Pt), (65.Tb,78.Pt), (66.Dy,78.Pt), (73.Ta,78.Pt) |
| 1.1681E−02 | (78.Pt,73.Ta), (77.Ir,73.Ta), (75.Re,73.Ta), (76.Os,73.Ta) |
| 1.1867E−02 | (23.V,33.As), (39.Y,33.As), (41.Nb,123), (130,33.As), (116,33.As), (53.I,33.As), (40.Zr,123), (134,33.As), (21.Sc,33.As), (118,33.As), (32.Ge,33.As), (55.Cs,33.As), (125,123)*, (40.Zr,33.As), (88.Ra,33.As), (22.Ti,123), (56.Ba,33.As), (56.Ba,123), (23.V,123), (123,33.As)*, (41.Nb,33.As), (22.Ti,33.As), (125,33.As)* |
| 1.1919E−02 | (71.Lu,79.Au), (75.Re,79.Au), (66.Dy,79.Au), (67.Ho,79.Au), (72.Hf,79.Au), (90.Th,79.Au), (69.Tm,79.Au), (91.Pa,79.Au), (64.Gd,79.Au), (92.U,79.Au), (65.Tb,79.Au), (68.Er,79.Au), (70.Yb,79.Au) |
| 1.1959E−02 | (78.Pt,75.Re), (77.Ir,75.Re), (74.W,75.Re), (76.Os,75.Re), (79.Au,75.Re), (73.Ta,75.Re) |
| 1.2100E−02 | (75.Re,74.W) |

| $E$, MeV | List of poorly visible pairs for this energy) |
|---|---|
| 1.2284E−02 | (43.Tc,130), (70.Yb,80.Hg), (33.As,130), (60.Nd,80.Hg), (85.At,80.Hg), (48.Cd,130), (87.Fr,80.Hg), (89.Ac,80.Hg), (29.Cu,80.Hg), (90.Th,80.Hg), (71.Lu,80.Hg), (91.Pa,80.Hg), (53.I,130), (121,80.Hg), (65.Tb,80.Hg), (25.Mn,130), (24.Cr,130), (69.Tm,80.Hg), (112,130), (49.In,130), (123,130), (50.Sn,130), (28.Ni,80.Hg), (31.Ga,130), (116,130), (64.Gd,80.Hg), (51.Sb,130), (66.Dy,80.Hg), (62.Sm,80.Hg), (61.Pm,80.Hg), (59.Pr,80.Hg), (67.Ho,80.Hg), (42.Mo,130), (88.Ra,130), (32.Ge,130), (68.Er,80.Hg), (52.Te,130) |
| 1.2385E−02 | (78.Pt,76.Os), (77.Ir,76.Os), (74.W,76.Os), (73.Ta,76.Os), (75.Re,76.Os) |
| 1.2527E−02 | (74.W,75.Re), (76.Os,75.Re) |
| 1.2657E−02 | (63.Eu,81.Tl), (89.Ac,81.Tl), (28.Ni,81.Tl), (90.Th,81.Tl), (66.Dy,81.Tl), (27.Co,81.Tl), (64.Gd,81.Tl), (45.Rh,81.Tl), (121,81.Tl), (29.Cu,81.Tl), (61.Pm,81.Tl), (47.Ag,81.Tl), (60.Nd,81.Tl), (62.Sm,81.Tl), (70.Yb,81.Tl), (82.Pb,81.Tl), (58.Ce,81.Tl), (84.Po,81.Tl), (59.Pr,81.Tl), (46.Pd,81.Tl), (67.Ho,81.Tl), (85.At,81.Tl), (65.Tb,81.Tl), (87.Fr,81.Tl) |
| 1.2658E−02 | (38.Sr,34.Se), (118,34.Se), (21.Sc,34.Se), (134,34.Se), (113,34.Se), (40.Zr,34.Se), (125,34.Se), (22.Ti,34.Se), (55.Cs,34.Se), (39.Y,34.Se) |
| 1.2824E−02 | (76.Os,77.Ir), (74.W,77.Ir), (73.Ta,77.Ir) |
| 1.2968E−02 | (77.Ir,76.Os), (75.Re,76.Os) |
| 1.3035E−02 | (70.Yb,82.Pb), (63.Eu,82.Pb), (29.Cu,82.Pb), (60.Nd,82.Pb), (33.As,125), (65.Tb,82.Pb), (25.Mn,125), (61.Pm,82.Pb), (27.Co,82.Pb), (59.Pr,82.Pb), (31.Ga,125), (56.Ba,125), (50.Sn,125), (85.At,82.Pb), (28.Ni,82.Pb), (87.Fr,82.Pb), (32.Ge,125), (89.Ac,82.Pb), (43.Tc,125), (66.Dy,82.Pb), (90.Th,82.Pb), (24.Cr,125), (58.Ce,82.Pb), (48.Cd,125), (64.Gd,82.Pb), (88.Ra,125), (52.Te,125), (121,82.Pb), (123,125), (42.Mo,125), (45.Rh,82.Pb), (41.Nb,125), (49.In,125), (67.Ho,82.Pb), (34.Se,125), (47.Ag,82.Pb), (112,125), (62.Sm,82.Pb), (46.Pd,82.Pb), (116,125), (23.V,125), (53.I,125), (51.Sb,125) |
| 1.3273E−02 | (73.Ta,78.Pt) |
| 1.3419E−02 | (75.Re,77.Ir), (76.Os,77.Ir) |
| 1.3419E−02 | (87.Fr,83.Bi), (61.Pm,83.Bi), (64.Gd,83.Bi), (89.Ac,83.Bi), (29.Cu,83.Bi), (44.Ru,83.Bi), (90.Th,83.Bi), (47.Ag,83.Bi), (27.Co,83.Bi), (63.Eu,83.Bi), (62.Sm,83.Bi), (46.Pd,83.Bi), (70.Yb,83.Bi), (121,83.Bi), (84.Po,83.Bi), (26.Fe,83.Bi), (65.Tb,83.Bi), (30.Zn,83.Bi), (59.Pr,83.Bi), (58.Ce,83.Bi), (85.At,83.Bi), (57.La,83.Bi), (60.Nd,83.Bi), (28.Ni,83.Bi), (45.Rh,83.Bi) |
| 1.3474E−02 | (55.Cs,134), (114,133), (54.Xe,35.Br), (118,134), (21.Sc,134), (20.Ca,133), (39.Y,134), (16.S,133), (4.Be,35.Br) |
| 1.3734E−02 | (73.Ta,79.Au) |

| $E$, MeV | List of poorly visible pairs for this energy) |
|---|---|
| 1.3814E−02 | (60.Nd,84.Po), (90.Th,84.Po), (44.Ru,84.Po), (29.Cu,84.Po), (45.Rh,84.Po), (58.Ce,84.Po), (46.Pd,84.Po), (47.Ag,84.Po), (57.La,84.Po), (121,84.Po), (62.Sm,84.Po), (30.Zn,84.Po), (61.Pm,84.Po), (65.Tb,84.Po), (85.At,84.Po), (63.Eu,84.Po), (70.Yb,84.Po), (27.Co,84.Po), (87.Fr,84.Po), (28.Ni,84.Po), (64.Gd,84.Po), (89.Ac,84.Po), (59.Pr,84.Po) |
| 1.3880E−02 | (75.Re,78.Pt) |
| 1.4209E−02 | (44.Ru,130), (63.Eu,130), (125,130), (92.U,80.Hg), (57.La,130), (26.Fe,130), (47.Ag,130), (46.Pd,130), (30.Zn,130), (45.Rh,130), (85.At,130) |
| 1.4213E−02 | (27.Co,85.At), (59.Pr,85.At), (58.Ce,85.At), (121,85.At), (61.Pm,85.At), (62.Sm,85.At), (65.Tb,85.At), (87.Fr,85.At), (130,85.At), (29.Cu,85.At), (28.Ni,85.At), (64.Gd,85.At), (84.Po,85.At), (83.Bi,85.At), (89.Ac,85.At), (68.Er,85.At), (70.Yb,85.At), (90.Th,85.At), (60.Nd,85.At), (66.Dy,85.At), (67.Ho,85.At) |
| 1.4326E−02 | (17.Cl,36.Kr) |
| 1.4353E−02 | (74.W,79.Au) |
| 1.4619E−02 | (5.B,86.Rn), (102,86.Rn), (135,86.Rn), (136,86.Rn), (139,86.Rn), (142,86.Rn) |
| 1.4698E−02 | (92.U,81.Tl), (82.Pb,81.Tl), (71.Lu,81.Tl) |
| 1.4839E−02 | (87.Fr,130), (29.Cu,130), (60.Nd,130), (28.Ni,130) |
| 1.5031E−02 | (83.Bi,87.Fr), (121,87.Fr), (29.Cu,87.Fr), (62.Sm,87.Fr), (69.Tm,87.Fr), (65.Tb,87.Fr), (70.Yb,87.Fr), (130,87.Fr), (89.Ac,87.Fr), (66.Dy,87.Fr), (67.Ho,87.Fr), (90.Th,87.Fr), (84.Po,87.Fr), (68.Er,87.Fr), (91.Pa,87.Fr), (64.Gd,87.Fr), (61.Pm,87.Fr) |
| 1.5200E−02 | (133,37.Rb), (113,37.Rb), (16.S,37.Rb), (38.Sr,37.Rb), (114,37.Rb), (20.Ca,37.Rb), (21.Sc,37.Rb) |
| 1.5200E−02 | (121,125), (63.Eu,125), (30.Zn,125), (59.Pr,125), (60.Nd,125), (29.Cu,125), (27.Co,125), (71.Lu,82.Pb), (92.U,82.Pb), (58.Ce,125), (28.Ni,125) |
| 1.5347E−02 | (72.Hf,81.Tl) |
| 1.5444E−02 | (25.Mn,88.Ra), (51.Sb,88.Ra), (123,88.Ra), (33.As,88.Ra), (58.Ce,88.Ra), (26.Fe,88.Ra), (50.Sn,88.Ra), (59.Pr,88.Ra), (30.Zn,88.Ra), (47.Ag,88.Ra), (43.Tc,88.Ra), (45.Rh,88.Ra), (49.In,88.Ra), (63.Eu,88.Ra), (46.Pd,88.Ra), (31.Ga,88.Ra), (32.Ge,88.Ra), (44.Ru,88.Ra), (27.Co,88.Ra), (57.La,88.Ra), (52.Te,88.Ra), (112,88.Ra), (24.Cr,88.Ra), (34.Se,88.Ra), (42.Mo,88.Ra), (48.Cd,88.Ra) |
| 1.5711E−02 | (85.At,83.Bi), (91.Pa,83.Bi), (71.Lu,83.Bi), (68.Er,83.Bi), (92.U,83.Bi), (87.Fr,83.Bi), (69.Tm,83.Bi) |

| $E$, MeV | List of poorly visible pairs for this energy) |
|---|---|
| 1.5861E−02 | (130,125), (61.Pm,125), (62.Sm,125) |
| 1.5871E−02 | (66.Dy,89.Ac), (70.Yb,89.Ac), (64.Gd,89.Ac), (121,89.Ac), (65.Tb,89.Ac), (85.At,89.Ac), (125,89.Ac), (62.Sm,89.Ac), (130,89.Ac), (84.Po,89.Ac), (61.Pm,89.Ac), (67.Ho,89.Ac), (69.Tm,89.Ac), (90.Th,89.Ac), (87.Fr,89.Ac), (68.Er,89.Ac), (91.Pa,89.Ac) |
| 1.6105E−02 | (40.Zr,38.Sr), (21.Sc,38.Sr), (39.Y,38.Sr), (55.Cs,38.Sr), (118,38.Sr), (113,38.Sr), (37.Rb,38.Sr), (133,38.Sr), (22.Ti,38.Sr) |
| 1.6244E−02 | (69.Tm,84.Po), (68.Er,84.Po), (85.At,84.Po), (71.Lu,84.Po), (91.Pa,84.Po), (89.Ac,84.Po), (87.Fr,84.Po) |
| 1.6300E−02 | (91.Pa,90.Th), (67.Ho,90.Th), (65.Tb,90.Th), (92.U,90.Th), (83.Bi,90.Th), (84.Po,90.Th), (85.At,90.Th), (66.Dy,90.Th), (69.Tm,90.Th), (64.Gd,90.Th), (68.Er,90.Th), (89.Ac,90.Th), (71.Lu,90.Th), (70.Yb,90.Th), (87.Fr,90.Th) |
| 1.6387E−02 | (90.Th,83.Bi) |
| 1.6733E−02 | (69.Tm,91.Pa), (83.Bi,91.Pa), (82.Pb,91.Pa), (68.Er,91.Pa), (85.At,91.Pa), (89.Ac,91.Pa), (72.Hf,91.Pa), (84.Po,91.Pa), (71.Lu,91.Pa), (90.Th,91.Pa), (92.U,91.Pa), (87.Fr,91.Pa), (81.Tl,91.Pa) |
| 1.6785E−02 | (90.Th,85.At), (89.Ac,85.At), (87.Fr,85.At), (69.Tm,85.At), (71.Lu,85.At), (84.Po,85.At), (92.U,85.At) |
| 1.6939E−02 | (85.At,84.Po), (90.Th,84.Po) |
| 1.7038E−02 | (134,39.Y), (116,39.Y), (38.Sr,39.Y), (118,39.Y), (53.I,39.Y), (22.Ti,39.Y), (40.Zr,39.Y), (21.Sc,39.Y), (55.Cs,39.Y), (37.Rb,39.Y), (41.Nb,39.Y), (56.Ba,39.Y), (23.V,39.Y) |
| 1.7166E−02 | (91.Pa,92.U), (84.Po,92.U), (83.Bi,92.U), (72.Hf,92.U), (71.Lu,92.U), (85.At,92.U), (81.Tl,92.U), (80.Hg,92.U), (73.Ta,92.U), (82.Pb,92.U), (90.Th,92.U) |
| 1.7337E−02 | (122,86.Rn), (6.C,86.Rn), (106,86.Rn), (138,86.Rn) |
| 1.7493E−02 | (84.Po,85.At), (83.Bi,85.At) |
| 1.7907E−02 | (71.Lu,87.Fr), (90.Th,87.Fr), (69.Tm,87.Fr), (89.Ac,87.Fr) |
| 1.7998E−02 | (134,40.Zr), (22.Ti,40.Zr), (43.Tc,40.Zr), (50.Sn,40.Zr), (25.Mn,40.Zr), (33.As,40.Zr), (51.Sb,40.Zr), (44.Ru,40.Zr), (26.Fe,40.Zr), (52.Te,40.Zr), (23.V,40.Zr), (31.Ga,40.Zr), (53.I,40.Zr), (112,40.Zr), (32.Ge,40.Zr), (56.Ba,40.Zr), (116,40.Zr), (24.Cr,40.Zr), (41.Nb,40.Zr), (57.La,40.Zr), (47.Ag,40.Zr), (39.Y,40.Zr), (123,40.Zr), (38.Sr,40.Zr), (48.Cd,40.Zr), (42.Mo,40.Zr), (34.Se,40.Zr), (49.In,40.Zr) |
| 1.8049E−02 | (101,86.Rn), (145,86.Rn), (137,86.Rn) |
| 1.8484E−02 | (130,88.Ra), (121,88.Ra), (60.Nd,88.Ra), (61.Pm,88.Ra), (29.Cu,88.Ra), (62.Sm,88.Ra), (28.Ni,88.Ra) |
| 1.8639E−02 | (83.Bi,87.Fr), (84.Po,87.Fr) |

| $E$, MeV | List of poorly visible pairs for this energy) |
|---|---|
| 1.8986E−02 | (58.Ce,41.Nb), (46.Pd,41.Nb), (123,41.Nb), (34.Se,41.Nb), (59.Pr,41.Nb), (40.Zr,41.Nb), (47.Ag,41.Nb), (60.Nd,41.Nb), (31.Ga,41.Nb), (29.Cu,41.Nb), (48.Cd,41.Nb), (42.Mo,41.Nb), (23.V,41.Nb), (49.In,41.Nb), (32.Ge,41.Nb), (63.Eu,41.Nb), (27.Co,41.Nb), (50.Sn,41.Nb), (39.Y,41.Nb), (43.Tc,41.Nb), (51.Sb,41.Nb), (33.As,41.Nb), (52.Te,41.Nb), (25.Mn,41.Nb), (44.Ru,41.Nb), (53.I,41.Nb), (26.Fe,41.Nb), (112,41.Nb), (56.Ba,41.Nb), (28.Ni,41.Nb), (116,41.Nb), (45.Rh,41.Nb), (57.La,41.Nb), (24.Cr,41.Nb), (121,41.Nb), (30.Zn,41.Nb) |
| 1.9083E−02 | (90.Th,89.Ac), (71.Lu,89.Ac) |
| 1.9237E−02 | (125,88.Ra), (65.Tb,88.Ra), (70.Yb,88.Ra), (64.Gd,88.Ra) |
| 1.9693E−02 | (87.Fr,90.Th), (72.Hf,90.Th), (89.Ac,90.Th), (83.Bi,90.Th), (84.Po,90.Th), (85.At,90.Th) |
| 1.9840E−02 | (87.Fr,89.Ac), (84.Po,89.Ac), (83.Bi,89.Ac), (85.At,89.Ac), (72.Hf,89.Ac) |
| 2.0000E−02 | (33.As,42.Mo), (125,42.Mo), (60.Nd,42.Mo), (41.Nb,42.Mo), (130,42.Mo), (47.Ag,42.Mo), (29.Cu,42.Mo), (61.Pm,42.Mo), (39.Y,42.Mo), (48.Cd,42.Mo), (31.Ga,42.Mo), (62.Sm,42.Mo), (49.In,42.Mo), (30.Zn,42.Mo), (63.Eu,42.Mo), (28.Ni,42.Mo), (50.Sn,42.Mo), (40.Zr,42.Mo), (64.Gd,42.Mo), (51.Sb,42.Mo), (43.Tc,42.Mo), (52.Te,42.Mo), (34.Se,42.Mo), (24.Cr,42.Mo), (44.Ru,42.Mo), (57.La,42.Mo), (27.Co,42.Mo), (25.Mn,42.Mo), (58.Ce,42.Mo), (112,42.Mo), (45.Rh,42.Mo), (32.Ge,42.Mo), (121,42.Mo), (59.Pr,42.Mo), (123,42.Mo), (26.Fe,42.Mo), (46.Pd,42.Mo) |
| 2.0314E−02 | (92.U,91.Pa), (73.Ta,91.Pa), (80.Hg,91.Pa) |
| 2.0472E−02 | (81.Tl,90.Th), (82.Pb,90.Th) |
| 2.0948E−02 | (91.Pa,92.U), (75.Re,92.U), (74.W,92.U) |
| 2.1044E−02 | (45.Rh,43.Tc), (121,43.Tc), (59.Pr,43.Tc), (123,43.Tc), (30.Zn,43.Tc), (32.Ge,43.Tc), (60.Nd,43.Tc), (125,43.Tc), (46.Pd,43.Tc), (34.Se,43.Tc), (130,43.Tc), (61.Pm,43.Tc), (29.Cu,43.Tc), (47.Ag,43.Tc), (62.Sm,43.Tc), (28.Ni,43.Tc), (48.Cd,43.Tc), (63.Eu,43.Tc), (39.Y,43.Tc), (40.Zr,43.Tc), (64.Gd,43.Tc), (50.Sn,43.Tc), (33.As,43.Tc), (65.Tb,43.Tc), (51.Sb,43.Tc), (26.Fe,43.Tc), (66.Dy,43.Tc), (31.Ga,43.Tc), (57.La,43.Tc), (42.Mo,43.Tc), (44.Ru,43.Tc), (27.Co,43.Tc), (58.Ce,43.Tc), (25.Mn,43.Tc), (41.Nb,43.Tc), (70.Yb,43.Tc) |
| 2.1105E−02 | (74.W,91.Pa) |
| 2.1757E−02 | (79.Au,92.U), (76.Os,92.U), (78.Pt,92.U), (77.Ir,92.U), (75.Re,92.U) |
| 2.2117E−02 | (123,44.Ru), (47.Ag,44.Ru), (125,44.Ru), (65.Tb,44.Ru), (29.Cu,44.Ru), (130,44.Ru), (41.Nb,44.Ru), (57.La,44.Ru), (66.Dy,44.Ru), (27.Co,44.Ru), (58.Ce,44.Ru), (43.Tc,44.Ru), |

| $E$, MeV | List of poorly visible pairs for this energy) |
|---|---|
| | (30.Zn,44.Ru), (59.Pr,44.Ru), (33.As,44.Ru), (32.Ge,44.Ru), (70.Yb,44.Ru), (34.Se,44.Ru), (88.Ra,44.Ru), (60.Nd,44.Ru), (31.Ga,44.Ru), (61.Pm,44.Ru), (39.Y,44.Ru), (42.Mo,44.Ru), (62.Sm,44.Ru), (45.Rh,44.Ru), (40.Zr,44.Ru), (63.Eu,44.Ru), (26.Fe,44.Ru), (46.Pd,44.Ru), (121,44.Ru), (64.Gd,44.Ru), (28.Ni,44.Ru) |
| 2.3220E−02 | (130,45.Rh), (42.Mo,45.Rh), (66.Dy,45.Rh), (58.Ce,45.Rh), (29.Cu,45.Rh), (59.Pr,45.Rh), (33.As,45.Rh), (60.Nd,45.Rh), (26.Fe,45.Rh), (28.Ni,45.Rh), (41.Nb,45.Rh), (61.Pm,45.Rh), (27.Co,45.Rh), (88.Ra,45.Rh), (70.Yb,45.Rh), (62.Sm,45.Rh), (31.Ga,45.Rh), (32.Ge,45.Rh), (63.Eu,45.Rh), (30.Zn,45.Rh), (46.Pd,45.Rh), (64.Gd,45.Rh), (47.Ag,45.Rh), (39.Y,45.Rh), (121,45.Rh), (123,45.Rh), (65.Tb,45.Rh), (125,45.Rh), (57.La,45.Rh), (40.Zr,45.Rh) |
| 2.4350E−02 | (29.Cu,46.Pd), (63.Eu,46.Pd), (34.Se,46.Pd), (39.Y,46.Pd), (64.Gd,46.Pd), (57.La,46.Pd), (40.Zr,46.Pd), (65.Tb,46.Pd), (58.Ce,46.Pd), (31.Ga,46.Pd), (66.Dy,46.Pd), (59.Pr,46.Pd), (33.As,46.Pd), (30.Zn,46.Pd), (121,46.Pd), (123,46.Pd), (60.Nd,46.Pd), (125,46.Pd), (32.Ge,46.Pd), (28.Ni,46.Pd), (130,46.Pd), (26.Fe,46.Pd), (61.Pm,46.Pd), (27.Co,46.Pd), (62.Sm,46.Pd), (70.Yb,46.Pd), (41.Nb,46.Pd) |
| 2.5514E−02 | (62.Sm,47.Ag), (38.Sr,134), (32.Ge,47.Ag), (63.Eu,47.Ag), (25.Mn,47.Ag), (33.As,47.Ag), (64.Gd,47.Ag), (41.Nb,47.Ag), (27.Co,47.Ag), (29.Cu,47.Ag), (121,47.Ag), (57.La,47.Ag), (123,47.Ag), (39.Y,47.Ag), (125,47.Ag), (58.Ce,47.Ag), (23.V,134), (130,47.Ag), (59.Pr,47.Ag), (40.Zr,47.Ag), (28.Ni,47.Ag), (60.Nd,47.Ag), (34.Se,47.Ag), (31.Ga,47.Ag), (61.Pm,47.Ag), (30.Zn,47.Ag), (56.Ba,134), (26.Fe,47.Ag) |
| 2.6711E−02 | (130,48.Cd), (116,112), (24.Cr,48.Cd), (58.Ce,48.Cd), (25.Mn,48.Cd), (28.Ni,48.Cd), (39.Y,48.Cd), (50.Sn,112), (38.Sr,112), (59.Pr,48.Cd), (32.Ge,48.Cd), (31.Ga,48.Cd), (60.Nd,48.Cd), (26.Fe,48.Cd), (40.Zr,48.Cd), (61.Pm,48.Cd), (134,112), (30.Zn,48.Cd), (52.Te,112), (33.As,48.Cd), (62.Sm,48.Cd), (50.Sn,48.Cd), (34.Se,48.Cd), (51.Sb,48.Cd), (49.In,112), (112,48.Cd)*, (63.Eu,48.Cd), (52.Te,48.Cd), (121,48.Cd), (24.Cr,112), (123,48.Cd), (29.Cu,48.Cd), (53.I,112), (51.Sb,112), (57.La,48.Cd), (25.Mn,112), (27.Co,48.Cd) |
| 2.7940E−02 | (30.Zn,49.In), (60.Nd,49.In), (51.Sb,49.In), (134,49.In), (33.As,49.In), (52.Te,49.In), (31.Ga,49.In), (39.Y,49.In), (28.Ni,49.In), (29.Cu,49.In), (63.Eu,49.In), (57.La,49.In), (27.Co,49.In), (26.Fe,49.In), (32.Ge,49.In), (112,49.In), (58.Ce,49.In), (121,49.In), (24.Cr,49.In), (34.Se,49.In), (123,49.In), (59.Pr,49.In), (25.Mn,49.In), (50.Sn,49.In) |
| 2.9200E−02 | (34.Se,50.Sn), (39.Y,50.Sn), (112,50.Sn), (33.As,50.Sn), (58.Ce,50.Sn), (121,50.Sn), (30.Zn,50.Sn), (123,50.Sn), (32.Ge,50.Sn), (27.Co,50.Sn), (59.Pr,50.Sn), (25.Mn,50.Sn), (130,50.Sn), (28.Ni,50.Sn), (60.Nd,50.Sn), (134,50.Sn), (31.Ga,50.Sn), (51.Sb,50.Sn), |

| $E$, MeV | List of poorly visible pairs for this energy) |
|---|---|
| | (61.Pm,50.Sn), (52.Te,50.Sn), (26.Fe,50.Sn), (62.Sm,50.Sn), (29.Cu,50.Sn), (63.Eu,50.Sn), (57.La,50.Sn) |
| 3.0491E−02 | (26.Fe,51.Sb), (39.Y,51.Sb), (60.Nd,51.Sb), (31.Ga,51.Sb), (112,51.Sb), (29.Cu,51.Sb), (121,51.Sb), (61.Pm,51.Sb), (123,51.Sb), (25.Mn,51.Sb), (57.La,51.Sb), (28.Ni,51.Sb), (62.Sm,51.Sb), (130,51.Sb), (30.Zn,51.Sb), (32.Ge,51.Sb), (134,51.Sb), (63.Eu,51.Sb), (58.Ce,51.Sb), (33.As,51.Sb), (34.Se,51.Sb), (59.Pr,51.Sb), (27.Co,51.Sb) |
| 3.1814E−02 | (123,52.Te), (25.Mn,52.Te), (59.Pr,52.Te), (26.Fe,52.Te), (39.Y,112), (24.Cr,52.Te), (60.Nd,52.Te), (28.Ni,112), (32.Ge,52.Te), (29.Cu,112), (61.Pm,52.Te), (134,52.Te), (30.Zn,112), (27.Co,52.Te), (62.Sm,112), (27.Co,112), (31.Ga,52.Te), (39.Y,52.Te), (60.Nd,112), (121,112), (63.Eu,52.Te), (61.Pm,112), (29.Cu,52.Te), (59.Pr,112), (30.Zn,52.Te), (57.La,52.Te), (33.As,52.Te), (112,52.Te)*, (28.Ni,52.Te), (121,52.Te), (130,112), (58.Ce,52.Te), (34.Se,52.Te) |
| 3.3169E−02 | (62.Sm,130), (38.Sr,53.I), (57.La,53.I), (24.Cr,53.I), (116,53.I)*, (31.Ga,53.I), (58.Ce,53.I), (38.Sr,116), (40.Zr,130), (123,53.I), (134,116)*, (26.Fe,53.I), (25.Mn,116), (112,130), (33.As,53.I), (34.Se,53.I), (25.Mn,53.I), (64.Gd,130), (52.Te,130), (24.Cr,116), (51.Sb,130), (134,53.I)*, (63.Eu,53.I), (27.Co,53.I), (32.Ge,53.I) |
| 3.4561E−02 | (136,54.Xe), (139,54.Xe), (36.Kr,54.Xe), (4.Be,54.Xe), (135,54.Xe) |
| 3.5985E−02 | (123,116), (37.Rb,55.Cs), (57.La,116), (133,55.Cs), (22.Ti,55.Cs), (27.Co,116), (31.Ga,116), (58.Ce,116), (32.Ge,116), (118,55.Cs), (33.As,116), (26.Fe,116), (63.Eu,116), (34.Se,116) |
| 3.7441E−02 | (23.V,56.Ba), (24.Cr,56.Ba), (38.Sr,56.Ba), (55.Cs,56.Ba), (25.Mn,56.Ba), (22.Ti,118), (133,118), (134,56.Ba), (37.Rb,118) |
| 3.8925E−02 | (58.Ce,57.La), (62.Sm,57.La), (27.Co,57.La), (29.Cu,57.La), (32.Ge,57.La), (134,57.La), (33.As,57.La), (59.Pr,57.La), (63.Eu,57.La), (30.Zn,57.La), (64.Gd,57.La), (28.Ni,57.La), (34.Se,57.La), (60.Nd,57.La), (39.Y,57.La), (53.I,57.La), (56.Ba,57.La), (61.Pm,57.La), (116,57.La), (26.Fe,57.La), (31.Ga,57.La), (121,57.La), (123,57.La) |
| 4.0443E−02 | (59.Pr,58.Ce), (70.Yb,58.Ce), (57.La,58.Ce), (64.Gd,58.Ce), (39.Y,58.Ce), (30.Zn,58.Ce), (27.Co,58.Ce), (65.Tb,58.Ce), (60.Nd,58.Ce), (53.I,58.Ce), (56.Ba,58.Ce), (61.Pm,58.Ce), (29.Cu,58.Ce), (28.Ni,58.Ce), (116,58.Ce), (40.Zr,58.Ce), (62.Sm,58.Ce), (33.As,58.Ce), (121,58.Ce), (63.Eu,58.Ce) |
| 4.1991E−02 | (65.Tb,59.Pr), (40.Zr,59.Pr), (30.Zn,59.Pr), (57.La,59.Pr), (66.Dy,59.Pr), (121,59.Pr), (61.Pm,59.Pr), (29.Cu,59.Pr), (33.As,59.Pr), (125,59.Pr), (62.Sm,59.Pr), (56.Ba,59.Pr), (39.Y,59.Pr), (64.Gd,59.Pr), (53.I,59.Pr), (60.Nd,59.Pr), (70.Yb,59.Pr), (28.Ni,59.Pr), (116,59.Pr) |
| 4.3569E−02 | (61.Pm,60.Nd), (53.I,60.Nd), (121,60.Nd), (64.Gd,60.Nd), (56.Ba,60.Nd), (125,60.Nd), (40.Zr,60.Nd), (29.Cu,60.Nd), |

| $E$, MeV | List of poorly visible pairs for this energy) |
|---|---|
| | (65.Tb,60.Nd), (57.La,60.Nd), (28.Ni,60.Nd), (39.Y,60.Nd), (116,60.Nd), (70.Yb,60.Nd), (66.Dy,60.Nd), (62.Sm,60.Nd) |
| 4.5184E−02 | (125,61.Pm), (52.Te,61.Pm), (67.Ho,61.Pm), (62.Sm,61.Pm), (60.Nd,61.Pm), (57.La,61.Pm), (65.Tb,61.Pm), (58.Ce,61.Pm), (112,61.Pm), (40.Zr,61.Pm), (53.I,61.Pm), (59.Pr,61.Pm), (116,61.Pm), (66.Dy,61.Pm), (70.Yb,61.Pm), (121,61.Pm), (64.Gd,61.Pm), (29.Cu,61.Pm) |
| 4.6834E−02 | (60.Nd,62.Sm), (65.Tb,62.Sm), (125,62.Sm), (57.La,62.Sm), (68.Er,62.Sm), (52.Te,62.Sm), (64.Gd,62.Sm), (40.Zr,62.Sm), (112,62.Sm), (66.Dy,62.Sm), (58.Ce,62.Sm), (59.Pr,62.Sm), (116,62.Sm), (53.I,62.Sm), (70.Yb,62.Sm), (67.Ho,62.Sm) |
| 4.8519E−02 | (121,63.Eu), (33.As,63.Eu), (39.Y,63.Eu), (116,63.Eu), (64.Gd,63.Eu), (29.Cu,63.Eu), (28.Ni,63.Eu), (56.Ba,63.Eu), (27.Co,63.Eu), (30.Zn,63.Eu) |
| 5.0239E−02 | (57.La,64.Gd), (51.Sb,64.Gd), (130,64.Gd), (65.Tb,121), (88.Ra,64.Gd), (69.Tm,64.Gd), (40.Zr,121), (70.Yb,121), (70.Yb,64.Gd), (60.Nd,64.Gd), (65.Tb,64.Gd), (41.Nb,64.Gd), (71.Lu,64.Gd), (59.Pr,64.Gd), (58.Ce,64.Gd), (112,64.Gd), (40.Zr,64.Gd), (66.Dy,64.Gd), (116,64.Gd), (63.Eu,64.Gd), (67.Ho,121), (53.I,121), (67.Ho,64.Gd), (53.I,64.Gd), (121,64.Gd)*, (52.Te,64.Gd), (63.Eu,121), (125,64.Gd), (116,121), (68.Er,64.Gd), (66.Dy,121), (56.Ba,121), (125,121) |
| 5.1996E−02 | (53.I,65.Tb), (112,65.Tb), (40.Zr,65.Tb), (52.Te,65.Tb), (116,65.Tb), (69.Tm,65.Tb), (66.Dy,65.Tb), (50.Sn,65.Tb), (70.Yb,65.Tb), (51.Sb,65.Tb), (121,65.Tb), (60.Nd,65.Tb), (125,65.Tb), (88.Ra,65.Tb), (71.Lu,65.Tb), (130,65.Tb), (49.In,65.Tb), (41.Nb,65.Tb), (59.Pr,65.Tb), (67.Ho,65.Tb), (63.Eu,65.Tb), (58.Ce,65.Tb), (57.La,65.Tb), (68.Er,65.Tb), (64.Gd,65.Tb) |
| 5.3789E−02 | (41.Nb,66.Dy), (50.Sn,66.Dy), (63.Eu,66.Dy), (51.Sb,66.Dy), (68.Er,66.Dy), (53.I,66.Dy), (62.Sm,66.Dy), (121,66.Dy), (88.Ra,66.Dy), (61.Pm,66.Dy), (57.La,66.Dy), (125,66.Dy), (69.Tm,66.Dy), (52.Te,66.Dy), (130,66.Dy), (58.Ce,66.Dy), (60.Nd,66.Dy), (64.Gd,66.Dy), (65.Tb,66.Dy), (71.Lu,66.Dy), (40.Zr,66.Dy), (67.Ho,66.Dy), (112,66.Dy), (59.Pr,66.Dy), (49.In,66.Dy), (116,66.Dy) |
| 5.5618E−02 | (130,67.Ho), (71.Lu,67.Ho), (41.Nb,67.Ho), (61.Pm,67.Ho), (62.Sm,67.Ho), (52.Te,67.Ho), (59.Pr,67.Ho), (68.Er,67.Ho), (60.Nd,67.Ho), (53.I,67.Ho), (112,67.Ho), (50.Sn,67.Ho), (57.La,67.Ho), (116,67.Ho), (64.Gd,67.Ho), (42.Mo,67.Ho), (49.In,67.Ho), (69.Tm,67.Ho), (58.Ce,67.Ho), (121,67.Ho), (63.Eu,67.Ho), (51.Sb,67.Ho), (125,67.Ho), (88.Ra,67.Ho), (65.Tb,67.Ho) |
| 5.7485E−02 | (62.Sm,68.Er), (57.La,68.Er), (52.Te,68.Er), (63.Eu,68.Er), (60.Nd,68.Er), (58.Ce,68.Er), (69.Tm,68.Er), (61.Pm,68.Er), (49.In,68.Er), (112,68.Er), (48.Cd,68.Er), (50.Sn,68.Er), (53.I,68.Er), |

| *E*, MeV | List of poorly visible pairs for this energy) |
|---|---|
| | (121,68.Er), (41.Nb,68.Er), (64.Gd,68.Er), (65.Tb,68.Er), (88.Ra,68.Er), (130,68.Er), (71.Lu,68.Er), (59.Pr,68.Er), (42.Mo,68.Er), (51.Sb,68.Er) |
| 5.9390E−02 | (52.Te,69.Tm), (50.Sn,69.Tm), (112,69.Tm), (83.Bi,69.Tm), (68.Er,69.Tm), (67.Ho,69.Tm), (121,69.Tm), (43.Tc,69.Tm), (84.Po,69.Tm), (42.Mo,69.Tm), (65.Tb,69.Tm), (130,69.Tm), (62.Sm,69.Tm), (48.Cd,69.Tm), (60.Nd,69.Tm), (64.Gd,69.Tm), (66.Dy,69.Tm), (57.La,69.Tm), (47.Ag,69.Tm), (88.Ra,69.Tm), (59.Pr,69.Tm), (41.Nb,69.Tm), (58.Ce,69.Tm), (71.Lu,69.Tm), (51.Sb,69.Tm), (49.In,69.Tm), (61.Pm,69.Tm), (72.Hf,69.Tm), (63.Eu,69.Tm) |

## 2.3. EXTENSION OF THE APPROACH ONTO ARBITRARY SUBSTANCES

Being rather voluminous the tables of Sections 2.1 and 2.2 do not cover all the cases of poor visibility on the contact boundary an investigator may meet with in his practice. In this section we explain in brief how to overcome this difficulty. Let we have a substance of an arbitrary chemical composition and we know the elements constituting the substance, the fractions by weight $w_i$, $i = 1, \ldots, n$ of the elements and the density $\rho$ of the substance. Let $\rho_i$, $\mu_{ien}(E)$, $\mu_i(E)$ be the density, energy-absorption coefficient and the total attenuation coefficient of the $i$-th component of the substance. Then the coefficients $\nu_{en}(E)$, $\mu(E)$ of the substance satisfy the next equalities (see tables of Hubbell and Seltzer, 1995).

$$\frac{\mu_a(E)}{\rho} = \sum_{i=1}^{n} w_i \frac{\mu_{ia}(E)}{\rho_i}, \qquad \frac{\mu(E)}{\rho} = \sum_{i=1}^{n} w_i \frac{\mu_i(E)}{\rho_i}.$$

In this case by use of the tables listing the dependence $\mu_i(E)/\rho_i$ and $\mu_{ien}(E)/\rho_i$ for 92 elements one can easy obtain dependence $\mu_{en}(E)$ and $\mu(E)$ practically for any needed substance. When the coefficients $\mu_{en}(E)$ for a desired pair of substances and energy range $[E_1, E_2]$ are found, it rests to find the points $E \in [E_1, E_2]$ at which the coefficients $\mu_{1en}(E)$ and $\mu_{2en}(E)$ of the pair are the same. For the users's convenience we list in the table of this section densities of the elements and the substances used while preparing the tables of Sections 2.1 and 2.2. For the substances we also list the weight fractions of the elements composing the substances. These data have been borrowed from the tables of Hubbell and Seltzer (1995).

| Element | Density, g/sm$^3$ | Element | Density, g/sm$^3$ |
|---|---|---|---|
| 1.H (Hydrogen) | 8.375E−05 | 47.Ag (Silver) | 1.050E+01 |
| 2.He (Helium) | 1.663E−04 | 48.Cd (Cadmium) | 8.650E+00 |
| 3.Li (Lithium) | 5.340E−01 | 49.In (Indium) | 7.310E+00 |
| 4.Be (Beryllium) | 1.848E+00 | 50.Sn (Tin) | 7.310E+00 |
| 5.B (Boron) | 2.370E+00 | 51.Sb (Antimony) | 6.691E+00 |
| 6.C (Carbon) | 1.700E+00 | 52.Te (Tellurium) | 6.240E+00 |
| 7.N (Nitrogen) | 1.165E−03 | 53.I (Iodine) | 4.930E+00 |
| 8.O (Oxygen) | 1.332E−03 | 54.Xe (Xenon) | 5.485E−03 |
| 9.F (Fluorine) | 1.580E−03 | 55.Cs (Cesium) | 1.873E+00 |
| 10.Ne (Neon) | 8.385E−04 | 56.Ba (Barium) | 3.500E+00 |
| 11.Na (Sodium) | 9.710E−01 | 57.La (Lanthanum) | 6.154E+00 |
| 12.Mg (Magnesium) | 1.740E+00 | 58.Ce (Cerium) | 6.657E+00 |
| 13.Al (Aluminum) | 2.699E+00 | 59.Pr (Praseodymium) | 6.710E+00 |
| 14.Si (Silicon) | 2.330E+00 | 60.Nd (Neodymium) | 6.900E+00 |
| 15.P (Phosphorus) | 2.200E+00 | 61.Pm (Promethium) | 7.220E+00 |
| 16.S (Sulfur) | 2.000E+00 | 62.Sm (Samarium) | 7.460E+00 |
| 17.Cl (Chlorine) | 2.995E−03 | 63.Eu (Europium) | 5.243E+00 |
| 18.Ar (Argon) | 1.662E−03 | 64.Gd (Gadolinium) | 7.900E+00 |
| 19.K (Potassium) | 8.620E−01 | 65.Tb (Terbium) | 8.229E+00 |
| 20.Ca (Calcium) | 1.550E+00 | 66.Dy (Dysprosium) | 8.550E+00 |
| 21.Sc (Scandium) | 2.989E+00 | 67.Ho (Holmium) | 8.795E+00 |
| 22.Ti (Titanium) | 4.540E+00 | 68.Er (Erbium) | 9.066E+00 |
| 23.V (Vanadium) | 6.110E+00 | 69.Tm (Thulium) | 9.321E+00 |
| 24.Cr (Chromium) | 7.180E+00 | 70.Yb (Ytterbium) | 6.730E+00 |
| 25.Mn (Manganese) | 7.440E+00 | 71.Lu (Lutetium) | 9.840E+00 |
| 26.Fe (Iron) | 7.874E+00 | 72.Hf (Hafnium) | 1.331E+01 |
| 27.Co (Cobalt) | 8.900E+00 | 73.Ta (Tantalum) | 1.665E+01 |
| 28.Ni (Nickel) | 8.902E+00 | 74.W (Tungsten) | 1.930E+01 |
| 29.Cu (Copper) | 8.960E+00 | 75.Re (Rhenium) | 2.102E+01 |
| 30.Zn (Zinc) | 7.133E+00 | 76.Os (Osmium) | 2.257E+01 |
| 31.Ga (Gallium) | 5.904E+00 | 77.Ir (Iridium) | 2.242E+01 |
| 32.Ge (Germanium) | 5.323E+00 | 78.Pt (Platinum) | 2.145E+01 |
| 33.As (Arsenic) | 5.730E+00 | 79.Au (Gold) | 1.932E+01 |
| 34.Se (Selenium) | 4.500E+00 | 80.Hg (Mercury) | 1.355E+01 |
| 35.Br (Bromine) | 7.072E−03 | 81.Tl (Thallium) | 1.172E+01 |
| 36.Kr (Krypton) | 3.478E−03 | 82.Pb (Lead) | 1.135E+01 |
| 37.Rb (Rubidium) | 1.532E+00 | 83.Bi (Bismuth) | 9.747E+00 |
| 38.Sr (Strontium) | 2.540E+00 | 84.Po (Polonium) | 9.320E+00 |
| 39.Y (Yttrium) | 4.469E+00 | 85.At (Astatine) | 1.000E+01 |
| 40.Zr (Zirconium) | 6.506E+00 | 86.Rn (Radon) | 9.066E−03 |
| 41.Nb (Niobium) | 8.570E+00 | 87.Fr (Francium) | 1.000E+01 |
| 42.Mo (Molybdenum) | 1.022E+01 | 88.Ra (Radium) | 5.000E+00 |
| 43.Tc (Technetium) | 1.150E+01 | 89.Ac (Actinium) | 1.007E+01 |
| 44.Ru (Ruthenium) | 1.241E+01 | 90.Th (Thorium) | 1.172E+01 |
| 45.Rh (Rhodium) | 1.241E+01 | 91.Pa (Protactinium) | 1.537E+01 |
| 46.Pd (Palladium) | 1.202E+01 | 92.U (Uranium) | 1.895E+01 |

| Material and the weight fractions of its components | Density, g/sm$^3$ |
|---|---|
| 101.A-150 tissue-equivalent plastic<br>1.H: 0.101330, 6.C: 0.775498, 7.N: 0.035057, 8.O: 0.052315,<br>9.F: 0.017423, 20.Ca: 0.018377 | 1.127E+00 |
| 102.Adipose tissue (ICRU-44)<br>1.H: 0.114000, 6.C: 0.598000, 7.N: 0.007000, 8.O: 0.278000,<br>11.Na: 0.001000, 16.S: 0.001000, 17.Cl: 0.001000 | 9.500E−01 |
| 103.Air, dry (near sea level)<br>6.C: 0.000124, 7.N: 0.755268, 8.O: 0.231781, 18.Ar: 0.012827 | 1.205E−03 |
| 104.Alanine<br>1.H: 0.079192, 6.C: 0.404437, 7.N: 0.157213, 8.O: 0.359157 | 1.424E+00 |
| 105.B-100 bone-equivalent plastic<br>1.H: 0.065473, 6.C: 0.536942, 7.N: 0.021500, 8.O: 0.032084,<br>9.F: 0.167415, 20.Ca: 0.176585 | 1.450E+00 |
| 106.Bakelite<br>1.H: 0.057444, 6.C: 0.774589, 8.O: 0.167968 | 1.250E+00 |
| 107.Blood, whole (ICRU-44)<br>1.H: 0.102000, 6.C: 0.110000, 7.N: 0.033000, 8.O: 0.745000,<br>11.Na: 0.001000, 15.P: 0.001000, 16.S: 0.002000,<br>17.Cl: 0.003000, 19.K: 0.002000, 26.Fe: 0.001000 | 1.060E+00 |
| 108.Bone, cortical (ICRU-44)<br>1.H: 0.034000, 6.C: 0.155000, 7.N: 0.042000, 8.O: 0.435000,<br>11.Na: 0.001000, 12.Mg: 0.002000, 15.P: 0.103000,<br>16.S: 0.003000, 20.Ca: 0.225000 | 1.920E+00 |
| 109.Brain, grey/white matter (ICRU-44)<br>1.H: 0.107000, 6.C: 0.145000, 7.N: 0.022000, 8.O: 0.712000,<br>11.Na: 0.002000, 15.P: 0.004000, 16.S: 0.002000,<br>17.Cl: 0.003000, 19.K: 0.003000 | 1.040E+00 |
| 110.Breast tissue (ICRU-44)<br>1.H: 0.106000, 6.C: 0.332000, 7.N: 0.030000, 8.O: 0.527000,<br>11.Na: 0.001000, 15.P: 0.001000, 16.S: 0.002000,<br>17.Cl: 0.001000 | 1.020E+00 |
| 111.C-552 air-equivalent plastic<br>1.H: 0.024681, 6.C: 0.501610, 8.O: 0.004527, 9.F: 0.465209,<br>14.Si: 0.003973 | 1.760E+00 |
| 112.Cadmium telluride<br>48.Cd: 0.468358, 52.Te: 0.531642 | 6.200E+00 |
| 113.Calcium fluoride<br>9.F: 0.486672, 20.Ca: 0.513328 | 3.180E+00 |
| 114.Calcium sulfate<br>8.O: 0.470081, 16.S: 0.235534, 20.Ca: 0.294385 | 2.960E+00 |
| 115.0.015 m ceric ammonium sulfate solution<br>1.H: 0.107694, 7.N: 0.000816, 8.O: 0.875172, 16.S: 0.014279,<br>58.Ce: 0.002040 | 1.030E+00 |

| Material and the weight fractions of its components | Density, g/sm$^3$ |
|---|---|
| 116.Cesium iodide<br>53.I: 0.488451, 55: 0.511549 | 4.510E+00 |
| 117.Concrete, ordinary<br>1.H: 0.022100, 6.C: 0.002484, 8.O: 0.574930, 11.Na: 0.015208, 12.Mg: 0.001266, 13.Al: 0.019953, 14.Si: 0.304627, 19.K: 0.010045, 20.Ca: 0.042951, 26.Fe: 0.006435 | 2.300E+00 |
| 118.Concrete, barite (type BA)<br>1.H: 0.003585, 8.O: 0.311622, 12.Mg: 0.001195, 13.Al: 0.004183, 14.Si: 0.010457, 16.S: 0.107858, 20.Ca: 0.050194, 26.Fe: 0.047505, 56.Ba: 0.463400 | 3.350E+00 |
| 119.Eye lens (ICRU-44)<br>1.H: 0.096000, 6.C: 0.195000, 7.N: 0.057000, 8.O: 0.646000, 11.Na: 0.001000, 15.P: 0.001000, 16.S: 0.003000, 17.Cl: 0.001000 | 1.070E+00 |
| 120.Ferrous sulfate (standard fricke)<br>1.H: 0.108376, 8.O: 0.878959, 11.Na: 0.000022, 16.S: 0.012553, 17.Cl: 0.000035, 26.Fe: 0.000055 | 1.024E+00 |
| 121.Gadolinium oxysulfide<br>8.O: 0.084527, 16.S: 0.084704, 64.Gd: 0.830769 | 7.440E+00 |
| 122.Gafchromic sensor<br>1.H: 0.089700, 6.C: 0.605800, 7.N: 0.112200, 8.O: 0.192300 | 1.300E+00 |
| 123.Gallium arsenide<br>31.Ga: 0.482030, 33.As: 0.517970 | 5.310E+00 |
| 124.Glass, borosilicate ("pyrex")<br>5.B: 0.040066, 8.O: 0.539559, 11.Na: 0.028191, 13.Al: 0.011644, 14.Si: 0.377220, 19.K: 0.003321 | 2.230E+00 |
| 125.Glass, lead<br>8.O: 0.156453, 14.Si: 0.080866, 22.Ti: 0.008092, 33.As: 0.002651, 82.Pb: 0.751938 | 6.220E+00 |
| 126.Lithium fluoride<br>3.Li: 0.267585, 9.F: 0.732415 | 2.635E+00 |
| 127.Lithium tetraborate<br>3.Li: 0.082081, 5.B: 0.255715, 8.O: 0.662204 | 2.440E+00 |
| 128.Lung tissue (ICRU-44)<br>1.H: 0.103000, 6.C: 0.105000, 7.N: 0.031000, 8.O: 0.749000, 11.Na: 0.002000, 15.P: 0.002000, 16.S: 0.003000, 17.Cl: 0.003000, 19.K: 0.002000 | 1.050E+00 |
| 129.Magnesium tetraborate<br>5.B: 0.240870, 8.O: 0.623762, 12.Mg: 0.135367 | 2.530E+00 |
| 130.Mercuric iodide<br>53.I: 0.558560, 80: 0.441440 | 6.360E+00 |

| Material and the weight fractions of its components | Density, g/sm$^3$ |
|---|---|
| 131.Muscle, skeletal (ICRU-44)<br>1.H: 0.102000, 6.C: 0.143000, 7.N: 0.034000, 8.O: 0.710000,<br>11.Na: 0.001000, 15.P: 0.002000, 16.S: 0.003000,<br>17.Cl: 0.001000, 19.K: 0.004000 | 1.050E+00 |
| 132.Ovary (ICRU-44)<br>1.H: 0.105000, 6.C: 0.093000, 7.N: 0.024000, 8.O: 0.768000,<br>11.Na: 0.002000, 15.P: 0.002000, 16.S: 0.002000,<br>17.Cl: 0.002000, 19.K: 0.002000 | 1.050E+00 |
| 133.Photographic emulsion (Kodak type AA)<br>1.H: 0.030500, 6.C: 0.210700, 7.N: 0.072100, 8.O: 0.163200,<br>35.Br: 0.222800, 47.Ag: 0.300700 | 2.200E+00 |
| 134.Photographic emulsion (standard nuclear)<br>1.H: 0.014100, 6.C: 0.072261, 7.N: 0.019320, 8.O: 0.066101,<br>16.S: 0.001890, 35.Br: 0.349104, 47.Ag: 0.474105, 53.I: 0.003120 | 3.815E+00 |
| 135.Plastic scintillator (vinyltoluene)<br>1.H: 0.085000, 6.C: 0.915000 | 1.032E+00 |
| 136.Polyethylene<br>1.H: 0.143716, 6.C: 0.856284 | 9.300E−01 |
| 137.Polyethylene terephthalate, "mylar"<br>1.H: 0.041960, 6.C: 0.625016, 8.O: 0.333024 | 1.380E+00 |
| 138.Polymethyl methacrylate<br>1.H: 0.080541, 6.C: 0.599846, 8.O: 0.319613 | 1.190E+00 |
| 139.Polystyrene<br>1.H: 0.077421, 6.C: 0.922579 | 1.060E+00 |
| 140.Polytetrafluoroethylene, "teflon"<br>6.C: 0.240183, 9.F: 0.759818 | 2.250E+00 |
| 141.Polyvinyl chloride<br>1.H: 0.048382, 6.C: 0.384361, 17.Cl: 0.567257 | 1.406E+00 |
| 142.Radiochromic dye film (nylon base)<br>1.H: 0.101996, 6.C: 0.654396, 7.N: 0.098915, 8.O: 0.144693 | 1.080E+00 |
| 143.Testis (ICRU-44)<br>1.H: 0.106000, 6.C: 0.099000, 7.N: 0.020000, 8.O: 0.766000,<br>11.Na: 0.002000, 15.P: 0.001000, 16.S: 0.002000,<br>17.Cl: 0.002000, 19.K: 0.002000 | 1.040E+00 |
| 144.Tissue, soft (ICRU-44)<br>1.H: 0.102000, 6.C: 0.143000, 7.N: 0.034000, 8.O: 0.708000,<br>11.Na: 0.002000, 15.P: 0.003000, 16.S: 0.003000,<br>17.Cl: 0.002000, 19.K: 0.003000 | 1.060E+00 |
| 145.Tissue, soft (ICRU four-component)<br>1.H: 0.101174, 6.C: 0.111000, 7.N: 0.026000, 8.O: 0.761826 | 1.000E+00 |

| Material and the weight fractions of its components | Density, g/sm$^3$ |
|---|---|
| 146.Tissue-equivalent gas (methane based)<br>1.H: 0.101873, 6.C: 0.456177, 7.N: 0.035172, 8.O: 0.406778 | 1.064E−03 |
| 147.Tissue-equivalent gas (propane based)<br>1.H: 0.102676, 6.C: 0.568937, 7.N: 0.035022, 8.O: 0.293365 | 1.826E−03 |
| 148.Water, liquid<br>1.H: 0.111898, 8.O: 0.888102 | 1.000E+00 |

# Bibliography

Akilov, G. P., Makarov, B. M., and Khavin, V. P. (1969). *Elementary Introduction to the Theory of Integral.* Leningrad State University, Leningrad (in Russian).

Anikonov, D. S. (1994). Stefan-type problem for the transport equation. *Phys Dokl.* 39 (9), 599-602.

Anikonov, D. S. (1996). A formula for the gradient of the transport equation solution. *J. Inv. Ill-Posed Problems* 4 (2), 85–100.

Anikonov, D. S. (1997). Construction of the indicator of inhomogeneity for a medium under irradiation. *Dokl. Math.* 56 (3), 949–952.

Anikonov, D. S., Nazarov, V. G., and Prokhorov, I. V. (1997). Visible and invisible media in tomography. *Dokl. Math.* 56 (3), 955–958.

Anikonov, D. S. (1998). Comparison of two mathematical models in radiative transfer theory. *Dokl. Math.* 58 (1), 136–138.

Anikonov, D. S. (1999). Integro-differential heterogeneity indicator in tomography problem. *J. Inv. Ill-Posed Problems* 7 (1), 17–59.

Anikonov, D. S., Kovtanyuk, A. E., and Prokhorov, I. V. (1999). Tomography through the transport equation. In: *Proc. IMA Volumes in Mathematics and its Applications. Vol. 110. Computational Radiology and Imaging: Therapy and Diagnostics.* Springer-Verlag, New York, 33–44.

Anikonov, D. S. and Prokhorov, I. V. (1999). The importance of the radiation absorption coefficient in diagnosis of scattering and absorbing media. *Dokl. Math.* 60 (2), 264–266.

Anikonov, D. S. and Prokhorov, I. V. (2000). Some mathematical models of tomography for singular states of media. *Dokl. Math.* 61 (2), 293–297.

Anikonov, D. S. and Nazarov, V. G. (2001). Integro-differential indicator of inhomogeneity from incomplete data. *Dokl. Math.* 63 (1), 112–114.

Anikonov, D. S., Kovtanyuk, A. E., and Prokhorov, I. V. (2002). *Transport Equation and Tomography.* Inverse and Ill-Posed Problems Series. VSP, Utrecht.

Anikonov, D. S and Prokhorov, I. V. (2002). Necessary and sufficient conditions for the uniqueness of a solution to a tomography problem. *Comp. Math. and Math. Phys.* 42 (3), 353–362.

Case, K. M. and Zweifel, P. F. (1972). *Linear Transport Theory.* Addison-Wesley, London.

Ermakov, S. M. and Mikhailov, G. A. (1982). *Statistical Modelling.* Nauka, Moscow (in Russian).

Fano, U., Spencer, L. V., and Berger, M. J. (1963). *Transfer of Gamma-Radiation.* Gosatomizdat, Moscow (in Russian).

Fernandez, J. E., Hubbell, J. H., Hanson, A. L., and Spenser, L. V. (1993). Polarization effects on multiple scattering gamma transport. *Radiat. Phys. Chem.* 41 (4/5), 579–630.

Germogenova, T. A. (1986). *Local Properties of Solutions of the Transport Equation.* Nauka, Moscow (in Russian).

Henke, B. L., Gullikson, E. M., and Davis, J. C. (1993). X-ray interaction: photoabsorption, scattering, transmission, and reflection at $E = 50 \div 30000$ eV, $Z = 1 \div 92$. *Atomic Data and Nuclear Data Tables* 54 (2), 181–343.

Hubbell, J. H. and Seltzer, S. M. (1995). *Tables of X-Ray Mass Attenuation Coefficients and Mass Energy-Absorbtion Coefficients 1 keV to 20 MeV for Elements $Z = 1$ to 92 and 48 Additional Substances of Dosimetric Interest.* NISTIR-5632. Nat. Inst. Stand. and Technol., Gaithersburg.

Kolmogorov, A. N. and Fomin, S. V. *Elements of the Theory of Functions and Functional Analysis.* Dover Publ., New York, 1999.

Ladyzhenskaja, O. A. and Uralt'ceva, N. N. (1964). *Linear and Quasi-linear Equations of Elliptic Type.* Nauka, Moscow (in Russian).

Ladyzhenskaja, O. A. (1973). *Boundary Value Problems of Mathematical Physics.* Nauka, Moscow (in Russian).

Leypunskii, O. I., Novozhilov, B. V., and Sakharov, V. I. (1960). *Propagation of Gamma Quanta in Substance.* GIFML, Moscow (in Russian).

Prokhorov, I. V. (1996). Some properties of solutions of the transport equation. *Dal'nevost. Mat. Sb.* 2, 161–171 (in Russian).

Schwartz, L. (1981). *Cours d'Analysis.* Hermann, Paris.

Shilov, G. E. and Gurevich, B. L. (1964). *Integral, Measure and Derivative.* Nauka, Moscow (in Russian).

Tikhonov, A. N. and Samarskii, A. A. (1990). *Mathematical Physics.* Dover Publ., New York.

Vladimirov, V. S. (1961). Mathematical problems of one-velocity transport theory. *Trudy Mat. Inst. Steklov* 61, 3–158 (in Russian).

Zorich, V. A. (1981). *Mathematical Analysis. Pt 1.* Nauka, Moscow (in Russian).